Statistics for Industry and Technology

Series Editor

N. Balakrishnan
McMaster University
Department of Mathematics and Statistics
1280 Main Street West
Hamilton, Ontario L8S 4K1
Canada

Editorial Advisory Board

Max Engelhardt
EG&G Idaho, Inc.
Idaho Falls, ID 83415

Harry F. Martz
Group A-1 MS F600
Los Alamos National Laboratory
Los Alamos, NM 87545

Gary C. McDonald
NAO Research & Development Center
30500 Mound Road
Box 9055
Warren, MI 48090-9055

Kazuyuki Suzuki
Communication & Systems Engineering Department
University of Electro Communications
1-5-1 Chofugaoka
Chofu-shi
Tokyo 182
Japan

Statistical Models and Methods for Biomedical and Technical Systems

Filia Vonta
Mikhail Nikulin
Nikolaos Limnios
Catherine Huber-Carol
Editors

Birkhäuser
Boston • Basel • Berlin

Filia Vonta
Department of Mathematics and Statistics
University of Cyprus
CY-1678 Nicosia
Cyprus

Mikhail Nikulin
UFR Sciences et Modélisation
Université Victor Segalen Bordeaux 2
33076 Bordeaux Cedex
France

Nikolaos Limnios
Laboratoire de Mathématiques Appliquées
Université de Technologie de Compiègne
60205 Compiègne Cedex
France

Catherine Huber-Carol
Université Paris V
45 rue des Saints-Pères
75270 Paris Cedex 06
France

ISBN 978-0-8176-4464-2   e-ISBN 978-0-8176-4619-6

Library of Congress Control Number: 2007934439

Mathematics Subject Classification: 60K15, 62F03, 62G05, 62N01, 62P10, 60K20, 62F05, 62G10, 62N02, 62P30, 62F10, 62G20, 62N03, 62M02, 62F12, 62K05, 62N05, 62M05, 62F35

Printed on acid-free paper.

9 8 7 6 5 4 3 2 1

www.birkhauser.com

Contents

Preface   xix

Contributors   xxi

List of Tables   xxix

List of Figures   xxxiii

PART I: COX MODELS, ANALYSES, AND EXTENSIONS

**1 Extended Cox and Accelerated Models in Reliability,
with General Censoring and Truncation**   3
C. Huber-Carol and M. Nikulin

   1.1 Cox Model and Extensions   3

      1.1.1 The simple Cox model   3

      1.1.2 Nonhomogeneity in chronological time   4

      1.1.3 Effect not constant in time   5

      1.1.4 Omitted pertinent covariate: frailty models   5

   1.2 General Censoring and Truncations   6

      1.2.1 Definition   6

      1.2.2 Maximum likelihood estimation for frailty models   7

   1.3 Discrete Time: Logistic Regression Models for the
Retro-Hazard   8

   1.4 Accelerated Failure Time Models (AFT)   9

      1.4.1 Sedyakin principle   10

      1.4.2 Definition of AFT models   10

      1.4.3 Relationships between accelerated (AFT) and
proportional hazard (PH) models   11

      1.4.4 Relationships between Sedyakin and PH:
MPH models   12

      1.4.5 Generalized PH models (GPH) on $\mathcal{E}$ 12

      1.4.6 General models   13

      1.4.7 Modeling and homogeneity problem   13

   1.5 Correlated Survivals   15

      1.5.1 Introduction   15

1.5.2 Model in discrete time: Hierarchical dependencies   16
1.5.3 Definition of the models   16
1.5.4 Regression model   17
1.5.5 Estimation   17
References   18

**2 Corrected Score Estimation in the Cox Regression
Model with Misclassified Discrcte Covariates   23**
D. M. Zucker and D. Spiegelman

2.1 Introduction   24
2.2 Review of the Corrected Score Technique   25
2.3 Application to the Cox Survival Model   26
2.3.1 Setup   26
2.3.2 The method   27
2.4 Example   29
References   31

**3 A Varying-Coefficient Hazards Regression Model
for Multiple Cross-Effect   33**
H-D. I. Wu

3.1 Introduction   33
3.2 Illustration of the Piecewise-Constant Model   35
3.3 Estimation Under the Piecewise-Constant Setting   36
3.4 The Tests   37
3.4.1 Some spccific tests   37
3.5 Data Analysis   39
3.6 Discussion   41
References   42

**4 Closure Properties and Diagnostic Plots for the
Frailty Distribution in Proportional Hazards Models   43**
P. Economou and C. Caroni

4.1 Introduction   43
4.2 Closure Properties of the Individual Frailty Distribution   44
4.3 Diagnostic Plots   47
4.4 Application   48
4.5 Shared Frailty   49
References   53

5 Multivariate Survival Data with Censoring   55
S. Gross and C. Huber-Carol

5.1 Introduction   55

5.2 Definition of the Models   56
   5.2.1 Bivariate continuous model   56
   5.2.2 Generalization to p components   56
   5.2.3 Properties of the bivariate family   57
   5.2.4 General bivariate model   57
   5.2.5 The purely discrete model   58
   5.2.6 Simple examples of laws of type (5.1)   58
5.3 Some Usual Bivariate Models   59
   5.3.1 Clayton bivariate distribution   59
   5.3.2 Marshall-Olkin bivariate distribution   60
   5.3.3 Our quasi-Marshall-Olkin bivariate distribution   61
   5.3.4 Gumbel bivariate distribution   61
5.4 NPML Estimation   62
   5.4.1 Likelihood for the bivariate case   62
   5.4.2 NPML estimation   62
5.5 Concluding Remarks   64
References   64

PART II: RELIABILITY THEORY—DEGRADATION MODELS

6 Virtual (Biological) Age Versus Chronological Age   69
M. Finkelstein

6.1 Introduction   69
6.2 The Black Box Virtual Age   71
6.3 Information-Based Virtual Age   73
   6.3.1 Degradation curve   73
   6.3.2 Mean remaining lifetime   75
6.4 Virtual Age in a Series System   77
6.5 Concluding Remarks   80
References   80

7 A Competing Risks Model for Degradation and Traumatic Failure Times   83
V. Couallier

7.1 Introduction   83
7.2 The Degradation Failure—Estimation of F_A and F_{T_0} 84
7.3 A Joint Model with Both Degradation and Traumatic Failure Times   87
7.4 A Joint Model with Two Failure Modes   90
7.5 Conclusion   91
References   92

8 Generalized Birth and Death Processes as Degradation Models **95**

V. Rykov

8.1 Introduction and Motivation   95
8.2 Generalized B&D Process. Preliminary   96
8.3 Steady-State Distribution   98
8.4 Conditional Distribution Given Lifetime   99
8.5 An Example   103
8.6 Conclusion   106
References   106

9 Nonperiodic Inspections to Guarantee a Prescribed Level of Reliability **109**

C. T. Barker and M. J. Newby

9.1 Introduction   109
9.2 The Model   110
   9.2.1 The considered processes   110
   9.2.2 Maintenance actions and nonperiodic inspections   111
   9.2.3 Features of the model   114
9.3 Expected Total Cost   116
   9.3.1 Expression of the expected total cost   117
   9.3.2 Obtaining the solutions   118
9.4 Numerical Results and Comments   120
9.5 Conclusion   123
Appendix   124
References   125

10 Optimal Incomplete Maintenance for Weibull Failure Processes **127**

W. Kahle

10.1 Introduction   127
10.2 Kijima-Type Repairs   128
10.3 Parameter Estimation   129
10.4 Optimal Maintenance as Time Scale Transformation   131
10.5 Conclusion   135
References   135

11 Are Nonhomogeneous Poisson Process Models Preferable to General-Order Statistics Models for Software Reliability Estimation? **137**

S. Kundu, T. K. Nayak, and S. Bose

11.1 Introduction   137

11.2 Connections Between NHPP and GOS Models   140

11.3 Some Aspects of Inference   142

11.4 Simulation Results   143

11.5 Discussion   149

References   150

12 Multistate System Reliability Assessment by Using the Markov Reward Model   **153**

A. Lisnianski, I. Frenkel, L. Khvatskin, and Y. Ding

12.1 Introduction   153

12.2 Model Description   154

     12.2.1 Generalized MSS reliability measure   154

     12.2.2 Markov reward model: General description   155

     12.2.3 Rewards determination for MSS reliability computation   156

12.3 Numerical Example   157

12.4 Conclusions   166

References   167

PART III: INFERENTIAL ANALYSIS

13 Asymptotic Certainty Bands for Kernel Density Estimators Based upon a Bootstrap Resampling Scheme   **171**

P. Deheuvels and G. Derzko

13.1 Introduction and Results   171

13.2 An Example of Application   177

13.3 Proofs   182

     13.3.1 Proof of Theorem 13.1.1   182

References   185

14 Estimation of Rescaled Distribution   **187**

H. Läuter, M. Nikulin, and V. Solev

14.1 Introduction   187

14.2 Transportation Metric   188

14.3 Entropy, Duality of Metric Entropy   189

14.4 Expectation of $\kappa_{\mathfrak{C}}(P, P_n)$ 191

14.5 Minimum Distance Estimator   193

14.6 Empirical Process, Concentration Inequality   195

14.7 The Main Result   196

References   198

**15 Nested Plans for Sequential Change Point
     Detection—The Parametric Case**   **199**
P. Feigin, G. Gurevich, and Y. Lumelskii

15.1 Introduction and Notation   199
15.2 Definitions and Characteristics of Nested Plans   200
15.3 Multivariate Normal Distributions and Optimal
      Nested Plans   201
15.4 Nested Plans for One-Parameter Exponential
      Distributions   204
15.5 Numerical Examples and Comparisons   206
References   211

**16 Sampling in Survival Analysis and Estimation
     with Unknown Selection Bias and Censoring**   **213**
A. Guilloux

16.1 Introduction   213
16.2 Sampling in the Lexis Diagram   215
      16.2.1 Modeling the Lexis diagram   215
      16.2.2 Censored observations   217
16.3 Inference for the Distribution of the r.v. X 218
16.4 Inference for the Weight Function w 219
16.5 Simulation Study   220
References   223

17 Testing the Acceleration Function in Lifetime Models   **225**
H. Liero and M. Liero

17.1 Introduction   225
17.2 The Parametric ALT Model   226
17.3 The ALT Model with Nonparametric Baseline
      Distribution   229
17.4 The ALT Model with Parametric Baseline
      Distribution and Nonparametric Acceleration Function   231
17.5 The Nonparametric ALT Model   236
References   238

**18 Recent Achievements in Modified Chi-Squared
     Goodness-of-Fit Testing**   **241**
V. Voinov, R. Alloyarova, and N. Pya

18.1 Introduction   241
18.2 A Contemporary Status of the Theory of Modified
      Chi-Squared Tests   244

18.3 Some Recent Results 248

 18.3.1 Testing for normality 248

 18.3.2 Testing for the logistic probability distribution 249

 18.3.3 Testing for the three-parameter Weibull
   null hypothesis 250

 18.3.4 Testing for the power-generalized Weibull family 251

18.4 Conclusion 252

Appendix 253

References 255

19 Goodness-of-Fit Tests for Pareto Distribution 259
S. Gulati and S. Shapiro

19.1 Introduction 259

19.2 Type I Pareto Distribution 262

19.3 Test for the Type I Pareto Distribution 262

19.4 Power Study 264

19.5 Type II Pareto Distribution 265

19.6 Null Distribution of the Proposed Procedure and
   Power Study 268

19.7 Power of the Proposed Procedure 269

19.8 Examples 271

19.9 Conclusions 271

References 272

**20 Application of Inverse Problems in Epidemiology
and Biodemography 275**
A. Michalski

20.1 Introduction 275

20.2 Definition and Solution of Inverse Problem 277

20.3 Estimation on Incomplete Follow-Up 280

20.4 Estimation of HIV Infection Rate on the Dynamics
   of AIDS Cases 282

20.5 Estimation of Survival in the Wild 285

References 288

PART IV: ANALYSIS OF CENSORED DATA

**21 A Sampling-Based Chi-Squared Test for
Interval-Censored Data 295**
M. L. Calle and G. Gómez

21.1 Introduction 295

21.2 Johnson's Bayesian Chi-Squared Statistic 296

21.3 Sampling-Based Chi-Squared Test for
      Interval-Censored Data   298
      21.3.1 Iterative algorithm   299
      21.3.2 Asymptotic properties   299
      21.3.3 Decision criteria   302
21.4 Simulation Study   303
21.5 Discussion   304
References   305

**22 Semiparametric Regression Models for
    Interval-Censored Survival Data, With and
    Without Frailty Effects   307**
    P. Hougaard

22.1 Introduction   308
22.2 Parametric Models   309
22.3 Nonparametric Models   309
22.4 Proportional Hazards Models   311
22.5 Conditional Proportional Hazards (Frailty Model)   312
22.6 Extensions   313
22.7 Conclusion   316
References   316

**23 Exact Likelihood Inference for an Exponential Parameter
    Under Progressive Hybrid Censoring Schemes   319**
    A. Childs, B. Chandrasekar, and N. Balakrishnan

23.1 Introduction   319
23.2 Results for Type-I Progressive Hybrid Censoring   320
23.3 Results for Type-II Progressive Hybrid Censoring   326
23.4 Examples   328
References   330

PART V: QUALITY OF LIFE

**24 Sequential Analysis of Quality-of-Life Measurements
    Using Mixed Rasch Models   333**
    V. Sébille, J.-B. Hardouin, and M. Mesbah

24.1 Introduction   334
24.2 IRT Models   335
      24.2.1 The Rasch model   336
      24.2.2 Estimation of the parameters   336
24.3 Sequential Analysis   336
      24.3.1 Traditional sequential analysis   336
      24.3.2 Sequential analysis based on Rasch models   337
      24.3.3 The triangular test   339

24.4 Simulations   339
    24.4.1 Simulation design   339
    24.4.2 Results   340
24.5 Discussion—Conclusion   342
References   345

**25 Measuring Degradation of Quality-of-Life Related
to Pollution in the SEQAP Study**   **349**
S. Deguen, C. Segala, and M. Mesbah

25.1 Introduction   349
25.2 Material and Methods   350
    25.2.1 Finding questions, using previous knowledge,
        and focus groups   350
    25.2.2 Selecting questions, using a real sample,
        and psychometric methods   350
    25.2.3 From principal component analysis to
        Cronbach alpha curves   351
    25.2.4 Modern measurement models and graphical
        modeling   353
25.3 Results   354
    25.3.1 Rotated principal component analysis   355
    25.3.2 Backward Cronbach alpha curve   356
    25.3.3 Scoring procedure   356
    25.3.4 Correlation items to scores   356
    25.3.5 Rasch model   358
    25.3.6 External validation   359
25.4 Discussion   360
Appendix   361
References   367

26 A Bayesian Ponders "The Quality of Life"   **369**
M. Mesbah and N. D. Singpurwalla

26.1 Introduction and Overview   369
    26.1.1 Selective quotations on QoL   370
    26.1.2 Overview of this chapter   371
26.2 The Three-Party Architecture   372
26.3 The Rasch Model for $\mathcal{P}$s Input to QoL   374
    26.3.1 The case of a single dimension: $\mathcal{D}$'s
        assessment of θ_j 375
26.4 The Case of Multiple Dimensions: Fusing Information   376
    26.4.1 $\mathcal{D}$'s assessment of $\theta(\mathcal{D})$ 376
    26.4.2 Encoding the positive dependence between
        the θ_js   377

26.5 Defining the Quality of Life   378
26.6 Summary and Conclusions   379
References   380

PART VI: INFERENCE FOR PROCESSES

**27 On the Goodness-of-Fit Test for Some Continuous
Time Processes**   **385**
S. Dachian and Y. A. Kutoyants

27.1 Introduction   385
27.2 Diffusion Process with Small Noise   388
27.3 Ergodic Diffusion Processes   390
27.4 Poisson and Self-Exciting Processes   395
27.5 Simulation   400
References   402

**28 Nonparametric Estimation of Integral Functionals for
Semi-Markov Processes with Application in Reliability**   **405**
N. Limnios and B. Ouhbi

28.1 Introduction   405
28.2 The Semi-Markov Setting   406
28.3 Integral Functionals   409
28.4 Nonparametric Estimation of Moments   410
28.5 Confidence Intervals for the Moments   414
28.6 Numerical Application   415
References   416

29 Estimators for Partially Observed Markov Chains   **419**
U. U. Müller, A. Schick, and W. Wefelmeyer

29.1 Introduction   419
29.2 Nonparametric Estimators   420
       29.2.1 Full Observations   420
       29.2.2 Periodic Skipping   421
       29.2.3 Observing Two Out of Three   421
       29.2.4 Random Skipping   424
       29.2.5 Skipping at Random   424
29.3 Linear Autoregression   425
       29.3.1 Full Observations   425
       29.3.2 Observing One Out of Two   426
       29.3.3 Higher Lags   428
       29.3.4 Higher Order Autoregression   429
References   432

30 On Solving Statistical Problems for the Stochastic Processes by the Sufficient Empirical Averaging Method   **435**
A. Andronov, E. Chepurin, and A. Hajiyev

30.1 Introduction   435
30.2 Base Model   436
30.3 On a Class of Processes with the Complete Sufficient Statistics for the Plans of *A*-Type   437
30.4 On Complete Sufficient Statistics for a Class of Labeled Processes with the Plans of *B*-Type   439
30.5 On Procedures of Data Variant Generation   440
30.6 Numerical Examples   441
References   444

PART VII: DESIGNS

31 Adaptive Designs for Group Sequential Clinical Survival Experiments   **447**
E. V. Slud

31.1 Introduction   447
31.2 Decision-Theoretic Formulation   450
     31.2.1 Inference in a random-information environment   452
     31.2.2 Extended action affecting information growth   453
31.3 Two-Look Optimal Decision Rules   454
31.4 Modified Trial Designs with Accrual-Stopping   455
References   458

32 Optimal Two-Treatment Repeated Measurement Designs for Two Periods   **461**
S. Kounias and M. Chalikias

32.1 Introduction   461
32.2 Sequence Enumeration and the Model   462
     32.2.1 Enumeration of sequences   462
     32.2.2 The model   462
     32.2.3 Calculation of Q 463
32.3 Optimal Designs for Two Periods   465
     32.3.1 Optimal designs for direct effects   465
     32.3.2 Optimal designs for residual effects   466
     32.3.3 Optimal designs for direct and residual effects   467
     32.3.4 The model with interaction   468
References   469

PART VIII: MEASURES OF DIVERGENCE, MODEL SELECTION, AND SURVIVAL MODELS

33 Discrepancy-Based Model Selection Criteria Using Cross-Validation   **473**
J. E. Cavanaugh, S. L. Davies, and A. A. Neath

33.1 Introduction   474
33.2 Framework for Discrepancy-Based Selection Criteria   475
33.3 The Bias-Adjustment Approach to Developing a Criterion   476
33.4 The Cross-Validatory Approach to Developing a Criterion   477
33.5 Examples in the Linear Regression Setting   478
33.6 Linear Regression Simulations   480
Appendix   483
References   485

34 Focused Information Criteria for the Linear Hazard Regression Model   **487**
N. L. Hjort

34.1 Introduction: Which Covariates to Include?   487
34.2 Estimators in Submodels   489
34.3 Bias, Variance, and Mean Squared Error Calculations   491
34.4 Estimating the Risks   494
34.5 The FIC and the Weighted FIC   495
34.6 Exact Risk Calculations   497
34.7 Concluding Remarks   500
References   501

35 On Measures of Information and Divergence and Model Selection Criteria   **503**
A. Karagrigoriou and T. Papaioannou

35.1 Introduction   503
35.2 Classes of Measures   504
    35.2.1 Fisher-type measures   505
    35.2.2 Measures of divergence   506
    35.2.3 Entropy-type measures   507
35.3 Properties of Information Measures   508
35.4 Information Under Censoring and Truncation   510

35.5 Model Selection Criteria   513
    35.5.1 The expected overall discrepancy   513
    35.5.2 Estimation of the expected overall
        discrepancy   514
35.6 Discussion   515
References   516

36 Entropy and Divergence Measures for Mixed Variables   **519**
K. Zografos

36.1 Introduction   519
36.2 The Model   520
36.3 Entropy and Divergence in the Location Model   522
    36.3.1 φ-entropy in the location model   522
    36.3.2 ϕ-divergence in the location model   524
36.4 Sampling Properties   526
    36.4.1 Asymptotic distribution of $H_\varphi(f_{\widehat{\theta}})$ 526
    36.4.2 Asymptotic distribution of $D_\phi(f_{\widehat{\theta}_1}, f_{\widehat{\theta}_2})$ 529
36.5 Conclusions   532
References   532

PART IX: NEW STATISTICAL CHALLENGES

**37 Clinical Trials and the Genomic Evolution: Some
Statistical Perspectives**   **537**
P. K. Sen

37.1 Introduction   537
37.2 Biometry to Clinical Trial Methodology   538
37.3 Interim Analysis and Statistical Tests   540
37.4 Genomics Impact   545
References   549

Index   **553**

Preface

The material of this volume was inspired by papers presented at BIOSTAT2006, an international conference organized by the University of Cyprus and the European Seminar—"Mathematical Methods in Survival Analysis, Reliability and Quality of Life." The conference was a part of a series of conferences, workshops, and seminars organized or co-organized by the European Seminar over the years. BIOSTAT2006 took place in Limassol, Cyprus between May 29 to 31, 2006 with great success. It attracted over 100 participants from 30 countries. The aim of this event was to bring together scientists from all over the world that work in statistics in general and advance knowledge in fields related to biomedical and technical systems. The publication of this volume comes at a very special time because this year we are celebrating the tenth anniversary of the inauguration of the European Seminar.

The volume consists of selected papers presented at BIOSTAT2006 but it also includes other invited papers. The included papers nicely blend current concerns and research interests in survival analysis and reliability. There is a total of 37 papers which for the convenience of the readers are divided into the following nine parts.

- Cox Models, Analyses, and Extensions
- Reliability Theory - Degradation Models
- Inferential Analysis
- Analysis of Censored Data
- Quality of Life
- Inference for Processes
- Designs
- Measures of Divergence, Model Selection, and Survival Models
- New Statistical Challenges

The editors would like to thank all the authors for contributing their work to this book as well as all the anonymous referees for an excellent job in reviewing the papers and making their presentation the best possible. We would also like to thank Professor Alex Karagrigoriou whose help was invaluable during the organization of the conference as well as the preparation of this volume.

Thanks are also due to Professor N. Balakrishnan for his constant support and guidance, to Mr. Thomas Grasso for his assistance in the production of this volume and to Mrs. Debbie Iscoe for a highly professional job in typesetting this volume in a camera-ready form. Special thanks are due to the Department of Mathematics and Statistics of the University of Cyprus which financially supported the publication of this volume.

Nicosia, Cyprus   **F. Vonta**

Bordeaux, France   **M. Nikulin**

Compiègne, France   **N. Limnios**

Paris, France   **C. Huber-Carol**

Contributors

Alloyarova, R. Halyk Savings Bank of Kazakhstan, Almaty, Kazakhstan
RozaAl@halykbank.kz

Andronov, A. Faculty of Transport and Mechanical Engineering, Riga
Technical University, 1 Kalku Str., LV-1658, Riga, Latvia
lora@mailbox.riga.lv

Balakrishnan, N. Department of Mathematics and Statistics, McMaster
University, Hamilton, ON, Canada L8S 4K1
bala@mcmaster.ca

Barker, C. T. School of Engineering and Mathematical Sciences, The City
University, Northampton Square, London EC1V 0HB, England
c.t.barker@city.ac.uk

Bose, S. Department of Statistics, The George Washington University,
Washington, DC 20052, USA
sudip@gwu.edu

Calle, M. L. Systems Biology Department, Universitat de Vic, Sagrada
Familia, 7 08500 Vic, Spain
malu.calle@uvic.cat

Caroni, C. National Technical University of Athens, 9 Iroon Polytechniou,
Zografou, 157 80 Athens, Greece
ccar@math.ntua.gr

Cavanaugh, J. E. Department of Biostatistics C22-GH, College of Public
Health, The University of Iowa, Iowa City, IA 52242-1009, USA
joe-cavanaugh@uiowa.edu

Chalikias, M. Department of Mathematics, University of Athens, Greece
mchalikias@hotmail.com

Chandrasekar, B. Department of Statistics, Loyola College, Chennai 600 034, India
`bchandrasekar2003@yahoo.co.in`

Chepurin, E. Faculty of Mechanics and Mathematics, Moscow State University, Vorobyovi Gori, 119992, Moscow, Russia
`echepurin@rbcmail.ru`

Childs, A. Department of Mathematics and Statistics, McMaster University, Hamilton, ON, Canada L8S 4K1
`childsa@mcmaster.ca`

Couallier, V. Equipe Statistique Mathématique et ses Applications, UFR Sciences et Modélisation, Université Victor Segalen Bordeaux 2, 146 rue Leo Saignat, 31076 Bordeaux, France
`couallier@sm.u-bordeaux2.fr`

Dachian, S. Laboratoire de Mathématiques, Université Blaise Pascal, 63177 Aubière Cedex, France
`sdachian@math.univ-bpclermont.fr`

Davies, S. L. Pfizer Development Operations, Pfizer, Inc., La Jolla, CA, USA
`simon.davies2@pfizer.com`

Deguen, S. LAPSS, Ecole Nationale de Sante Publique, Rennes, France
`Severine.Deguen@ensp.fr`

Deheuvels, P. LSTA, Université Paris VI, 7 avenue du Château, F-92340 Bourg-la-Reine, France
`pd@ccr.jussieu.fr`

Derzko, G. Sanofi-Aventis Recherche, 371 rue du Professeur Joseph Blayac, F-34184, Montpellier Cedex 04, France
`Gerard.Derzko@sanofi-aventis.com`

Ding, Y. Center for Reliability and Risk Management, Sami Shamoon College of Engineering, Bialik/Basel Sts., Beer Sheva 84100 Israel
`PG02722465@ntu.edu.sg`

Economou, P. National Technical University of Athens, 9 Iroon Polytechniou, Zografou, 157 80 Athens, Greece
`polikon@math.ntua.gr`

Feigin, P. D. Faculty of Industrial Engineering and Management, Technion–Israel Institute of Technology, Haifa, Isreal 32000
`paulf@ie.technion.ac.il`

Finkelstein, M. Department of Mathematical Statistics, University of the Free State, Bloemfontein 9300, South Africa
FinkelM.SCI@mail.uovs.ac.za

Frenkel, I. B. Industrial Engineering and Management Department, Sami Shamoon College of Engineering, Bialik/Basel Sts., Beer Sheva 84100 Israel
iliaf@sce.ac.il

Gómez, G. Statistics and Operational Research Department, Universitat Politecnica de Catalunya, Despatx 210, Edifici C5, Campus Nord c/Jordi Girona 1-3, 08034 Barcelona, Spain
lupe.gomez@upc.edu

Gross, S. Director, Statistics, Consulting Laboratory, Department of Statistics and CIS, Baruch College of the City University of New York, New York, NY 10010, USA
Shulamith_Gross@baruch.cuny.edu

Guilloux, A. LSTA, Université Pierre et Marie Curie, 175 rue du Chevaleret, 75013 Paris, France
aguillou@ccr.jussieu.fr

Gulati, S. Department of Statistics, Florida International University, Miami, FL 33199, USA
gulati@fiu.edu

Gurevich, G. The Department of Industrial Engineering and Management, Sami Shamoon College of Engineering, Bialik/Basel Sts., Beer Sheva 84100, Israel
gregoryg@sce.ac.il

Hajiyev, A. Department of Probability and Statistics, Institute of Cybernetic, 9 F.Agayev Str., AZ1141, Baku, Azerbaijan
asaf@baku-az.net

Hardouin, J.-B. Laboratoire de Biostatistique, Faculté de Pharmacie, Université de Nantes, 1 rue Gaston Veil, 44035 Nantes Cedex 1, France
jean-benoit.hardouin@univ-nantes.fr

Hjort, N. L. Department of Mathematics, University of Oslo, P.B. 1053 Blindern N-0316 Oslo, Norway
nils@math.uio.no

Hougaard, P. Biostatistics Department, International Clinical Research, H. Lundbeck A/S, DK-250 Valby, Denmark
PHOU@lundbeck.com

Huber-Carol, C. Université René Descartes–Paris 5, 45 rue des
Saints-Péres, 75270 Paris, France
`catherine.huber@univ-paris5.fr`

Kahle, W. Institute of Mathematical Stochastics, Otto-von-Guericke
-University, Postfach 4120, D-39016 Magdeburg, Germany
`waltraud.kahle@mathematik.uni-magdeburg.de`

Karagrigoriou, A. Department of Mathematics and Statistics, University
of Cyprus, P.O. Box 20537, CY-1678 Nicosia, Cyprus
`alex@ucy.ac.cy`

Khvatskin, L. Center for Reliability and Risk Management, Sami Shamoon
College of Engineering, Bialik/Basel Sts., Beer Sheva 84100 Israel
`khvat@sce.ac.il`

Kounias, S. Department of Mathematics, University of Athens, Athens,
Greece
`skounias@math.uoa.gr`

Kundu, S. Department of Statistics, The George Washington University,
Washington, DC 20052, USA
`kundu@gwu.edu`

Kutoyants, Y. A. Laboratoire de Statistique et Processus, Université du
Maine, Av. Olivier Messiaen, 72085 Le Mans, Cedex 9, France
`kutoyants@univ-lemans.fr`

Läuter, H. Institute of Mathematics, University of Potsdam, D-14469
Potsdam, Germany
`laeuter@rz.uni-potsdam.de`

Liero, H. Institute of Mathematics, University of Potsdam, Potsdam,
Germany
`liero@rz.uni-potsdam.de`

Liero, M. Institute of Mathematics, Humboldt-University of Berlin,
Germany
`mliero@gmx.de`

Limnios, N. Université de Technologie de Compiègne, Laboratoire de
Mathématiques Appliquées, 60205 Compiègne Cedex, France
`Nikolaos.Limnios@utc.fr`

Lisnianski, A. The Israel Electric Corporation Ltd., P.O. Box 10, Bait
Amir, Haifa 3100, Israel
`anatoly-l@iec.co.il`

Lumelskii, Y. Faculty of Industrial Engineering and Management, Technion - Israel Institute of Technology, Haifa, ISRAEL 32000
lumelski@ie.technion.ac.il

Mesbah, M. Laboratoire de Statistique Théorique et Appliquée, Université Pierre et Marie Curie, Paris VI, 175 rue du Chevaleret, 75013 Paris, France
mesbah@ccr.jussieu.fr

Michalski, A. Institute of Control Sciences, Moscow, Russia
mpoctok@narod.ru

Müller U. U. Department of Statistics, Texas A& M University, College Station, TX 77843-3143, USA
uschi@stat.tamu.edu

Nayak, T. K. Department of Statistics, George Washington University, Washington, DC 20052, USA
tapan@gwu.edu

Neath, A. A. Department of Mathematics and Statistics, Southern Illinois University, Edwardsville, IL 62026, USA
aneath@siue.edu

Newby, M. J. School of Engineering and Mathematical Sciences, The City University, Northampton Square, London EC1V 0HB, UK
m.j.newby@city.ac.uk

Nikulin, M. UFR Sciences et Modelisation, Université Victor Segalen Bordeaux 2, 146 rue Leo Saignat, 33076 Bordeaux Cedex, France
nikou@sm.u-bordeaux2.fr

Ouhbi, B. Ecole Nationale Supérieure d'Arts et Métiers, Marjane II, Meknès Ismailia, B.P. 4024 Béni M'Hamed, Meknès, Maroc
ouhbib@yahoo.co.uk

Papaioannou, T. Department of Statistics and Insurance Science, University of Piraeus, 80 Karaoli and Demetriou, 18534 Piraeus, Greece
takpap@unipi.gr

Pya, N. Kazakhstan Institute of Management, Economics and Strategic Research, Almaty, Kazakhstan
pya@kimep.kz

Rykov, V. Institute for Information Transmission Problems RAS, Bol'shoy Karetny, 19, Moscow 127994, Russia
vladimir_rykov@mail.ru

Schick, A. Department of Mathematical Sciences, Binghamton University, Binghamton, NY 13902-6000, USA
anton@math.binghamton.edu

Sébille, V. Laboratoire de Biostatistique, Faculté de Pharmacie, Université de Nantes, 44035 Nantes Cedex 1, France
veronique.sebille@univ-nantes.fr

Segala, C. LSTA, Université Pierre et Marie Curie, Paris, France
sepia@sepia-sante.com

Sen, P. K. Department of Biostatistics, University of North Carolina at Chapel Hill, NC 27599-7420, USA
pksen@bios.unc.edu

Shapiro, S. Department of Statistics, Florida International University, Miami FL 33199, USA
shapiro@fiu.edu

Singpurwalla, N. D. Department of Statistics, The George Washington University, Washington, DC 20052, USA
nozer@gwu.edu

Slud, E. V. Mathematics Department, University of Maryland College Park, College Park, MD 20742, USA
evs@math.umd.edu

Solev, V. Steklov Institute of Mathematics at St. Petersburg, nab. Fontanki, 27 St. Petersburg 191023 Russia
solev@pdmi.ras.ru

Spiegelman, D. Departments of Epidemiology and Biostatistics, Harvard School of Public Health, Boston, MA 02115, USA
stdls@channing.harvard.edu

Voinov, V. Kazakhstan Institute of Management, Economics and Strategic Research, Almaty, Kazakhstan
voinovv@kimep.kz

Wefelmeyer, W. Mathematical Institute, University of Cologne, Weyertal 86-90, 50931 Cologne, Germany
wefelm@math.uni-koeln.de

Wu, H-D. I. Biostatistics Center and School of Public Health, China Medical University, Taichung 404, Taiwan
honda@mail.cmu.edu.tw

Zografos, K. Department of Mathematics, University of Ioannina, 451 10 Ioannina, Greece
kzograf@uoi.gr

Zucker, D. M. Department of Statistics, Hebrew University Mt. Scopus, Jerusalem, Israel
mszucker@mscc.huji.ac.il

List of Tables

Table 2.1   Estimated coefficients and standard errors for the Nurses   **30**
Health Study of the relationship between dietary calcium
intake and distal colon cancer incidence

Table 3.1   Analysis of first-ever stroke patients' two-year survivals   **41**

Table 9.1   Optimal values of the parameters a and b for the three   **123**
inspection scheduling functions

Table 11.1   Empirical performance of the MLE of model parameters   **145**
Table 11.2   Empirical performance of the MLEs of θ **146**
Table 11.3   Empirical performance of reliability estimators   **147**

Table 15.1   Out-of-control mean and standard deviation of the run   **207**
length of nested plans when the initial and the final distributions are multivariate normal with known different
means and the same covariance matrix

Table 15.2   Out-of-control ARL of the multivariate CUSUM para-   **208**
metric procedures (by simulation) and those of the pro-
posed nested plan for detecting a change in the mean of
the bivariate normal distribution

Table 15.3   Comparison of out-of-control ARLs for nested plans for   **209**
multivariate normal distribution for different values of parameters n and d: in-control ARL = 1000, $R = 1$

Table 15.4   Out-of-control expectation and standard deviation of the   **210**
run length of the CUSUM parametric procedures (by sim-
ulation) and those of the proposed nested plan (exact) for
detecting univariate normal shifts

Table 15.5   Out-of-control expectation and standard deviation of the   **210**
run length of the CUSUM parametric procedures (by simulation) and those of the proposed nested plan (exact) for
detecting a change in the parameter of the Pareto (θ, λ)
distribution

Table 16.1 $X \sim \Gamma(1, 0.5)$ **222**
Table 16.2 $X \sim \Gamma(1, 1.5)$ **222**

Table 18.1   Power of $Y2_n^2$, U_n^2, and $Y2_n^2 - U_n^2$ for two and four   **249**
Neyman–Pearson classes
Table 18.2   Power of HRM test for two Neyman–Pearson classes   **251**

Table 19.1   Power of the Pareto test for various alternate distributions, type I error $= 0.05$ **266**
Table 19.2   Power of the chi-square test for various alternate distributions, type I error $= 0.05$ **266**
Table 19.3   Power of the Pareto II test for the Weibull, type I error $= 0.05$ **269**
Table 19.4   Power of the Pareto II test for the gamma, type I error $= 0.05$ **270**
Table 19.5   Power of the Pareto II test for the half-normal and log-normal, type I error $= 0.05$ **270**

Table 20.1   Number of examined people, number of diagnosed malignant neoplasm cases, incidence estimates per 100,000   **282**
without and with adjustment for missing observations
Table 20.2   Simulated number of HIV-infected people by age (per   **285**
100,000) and its unstabilized and stabilized estimates

Table 21.1   Power to reject the null hypothesis $H_0 : X \sim \exp(\theta = 3)$ **304**

Table 23.1   Inference for θ **329**

Table 24.1   Type I error and power for the triangular test (TT) using   **340**
the method based on QoL scores or the Rasch model for
different values of the effect size and of the number of
items (nominal $\alpha = \beta = 0.05$, 1000 simulations)

Table 24.2   Sample size for the single-stage design (SSD) and aver-   **341**
age sample number (ASN) required to reach a conclusion
under H_0 and H_1 for the triangular test (TT) using the
method based on QoL scores or the Rasch model for different values of the effect size and of the number of items
(nominal $\alpha = \beta = 0.05$, 1000 simulations)

Table 24.3   Distribution of the standardized test statistics estimated   **343**
using the method based on QoL scores or the Rasch model
for different values of the number of items and for an
effect size equal to 0.5, assuming that the vector of item
parameter values β is either known or unknown (nominal
$\alpha = \beta = 0.05$, 1000 simulations)

Table 25.1   Rasch item parameter estimates for group 1   **358**

Table 25A.1   Original item list with French labels: 37 items   **361**
Table 25A.2   Rotated factors pattern   **363**
Table 25A.3   Pearson correlation coefficient between items and scores   **364**
Table 25A.4   External validation   **365**
Table 25A.5   New list of questions produced after the analysis: 32 items   **366**

Table 30.1   Estimates $\hat{\Psi}(u, 50)$ of ruin probability $\Psi(u, 50)$ **442**
Table 30.2   Estimates for probabilities $\{P_j(t)\}$ of the number of   **443**
customers in the system

Table 33.1   Selection results for AIC, AICc, PDC   **481**
Table 33.2   Selections results for C_p and PRESS   **482**

List of Figures

Figure 1.1   AIDS sample of right truncation.   **8**

Figure 1.2   Risk zone for right-censored and left-truncated discrete times.   **9**

Figure 3.1   Survival of 616 stroke patients in Taiwan.   **40**

Figure 4.1   Estimates of the survival function of the heart transplant data: Kaplan–Meier (broken line), Weibull with gamma frailty (bold line), and Weibull with inverse Gaussian frailty (lighter line).   **49**

Figure 4.2   Diagnostic plots for frailty distribution applied to the Stanford heart transplant data. The plotted points are $\eta(t)/\eta(0)$ against time; the envelopes are simulated 95 and 99 percentage points. Upper plot: Weibull–gamma mixture (=Burr distribution). Lower plot: Weibull–inverse Gaussian mixture.   **50**

Figure 7.1   Fatigue crack size propagation for alloy-A data.   **86**

Figure 7.2   (a) Predictors $(\hat{m}_i, \hat{c}_i)$ of (m_i, c_i) for alloy-A data and 95% confidence region for each estimation; (b) ecdf of predicted $\hat{m}_i$ and $\tilde{F}_m$.   **88**

Figure 7.3   Two estimations of F_{T_0} according to (7.4) and (7.5).   **88**

Figure 9.1   Surface representations of the expected total costs with different inspection scheduling functions, $k = 0.9$.   **121**

Figure 9.2   Surface representations of the expected total costs with different inspection scheduling functions, $k = 0.1$.   **122**

Figure 9.3   Optimal inspection scheduling functions.   **124**

Figure 10.1   The virtual age for Kijima-type repairs.   **129**

Figure 10.2   Mean number of failures under incomplete repair.   **130**

Figure 10.3   Operating time between failures: CDF and exponential   **131**
               Q–Q plot.
Figure 10.4   A discrete time transformation.   **133**
Figure 10.5   Weibull process without and with preventive maintenance **133**
               actions.

Figure 11.1   Comparison of $\hat{\gamma}_{1\{GO\}}(k)$ and $\hat{\gamma}_{1\{JM\}}(k)$ for (a) $\mu =$ **148**
               $20, \tau = 150$, $k = 20$, and (b) $\mu = 60, \tau = 200, k =$
               20. Horizontal broken line represents the true value of
               $\gamma_{1\{GO\}}(k)$.
Figure 11.2   Quartiles of $\hat{\mu}$ (solid line) and $\hat{\nu}$ (broken line) under the   **148**
               J–M model for (a) $\tau = 200$, and (b) $\tau = 300$.
Figure 11.3   Quartiles of $\hat{\gamma}_{1\{GO\}}(k)$ (solid curves) and $g(\nu, \theta)$ (broken   **149**
               curve) for (a) $\tau = 200$, $k = 20$, and (b) $\tau = 300$, $k = 40$.
               Horizontal broken line represents true $\gamma_{1\{GO\}}(k)$ for $\mu =$
               60 in plot (a) and for $\mu = 100$ in plot (b).

Figure 12.1   System with two online conditioners and one conditioner   **158**
               in cold reserve.
Figure 12.2   Calculation of the MSS average availability ($\mu = 100$ **160**
               year^{-1}).
Figure 12.3   MSS average availability dependent on mean time to re-   **161**
               pair.
Figure 12.4   Calculation of the mean total number of system failures   **162**
               ($\mu = 100$ year^{-1}).
Figure 12.5   Mean total number of system failures dependent on mean   **163**
               time to repair.
Figure 12.6   The state–space diagram for the transformed system with   **163**
               two online air conditioners and one in cold reserve with
               absorbing state.
Figure 12.7   Calculation of the mean time to system failure ($\mu = 100$ **165**
               year^{-1}).
Figure 12.8   Mean time to system failure dependent on mean time to   **165**
               repair.
Figure 12.9   Probability of MSS failure during one-year time interval   **167**
               depends on mean time to repair.

Figure 13.1   Certainty bands $\beta(2, 4)$, $n = 2000$, 1 bootstrap.   **173**
Figure 13.2   Certainty bands $\beta(2, 4)$, $n = 5000$, 1 bootstrap.   **174**
Figure 13.3   Repeated bootstrap bands $\beta(2, 4)$, $n = 5000$.   **174**

Figure 16.1   Age at inclusion.   **216**

Figure 16.2   Time-window study.   **220**

Figure 17.1   Histogram of the resampled betas.   **229**

Figure 17.2   Resampling under $\mathcal{H}$, $R = 1000$.   **235**

Figure 17.3   Resampled nonparametric regression estimates under the hypothesis and an alternative.   **236**

Figure 17.4   Histogram for simulations under the alternative. The histograms in the bottom show the results for "resampling cases."   **238**

Figure 18.1   Estimated powers as functions of the number of equiprobable cells r of $Y2_n^2$, U_n^2, and $Y2_n^2 - U_n^2$ tests versus the normal alternative. Sample size $n = 200$, type one error $\alpha = 0.05$.   **250**

Figure 18.2   Estimated powers as functions of the number of equiprobable cells r of $Y2_n^2$, U_n^2, and $Y2_n^2 - U_n^2$ tests versus exponentiated Weibull alternative $F(x) = \left[1 - \exp(-(x/\alpha)^\beta)\right]^\gamma$, $x, \alpha, \beta, \gamma > 0$, of Mudholkar *et al.* (1995). Sample size $n = 200$, type one error $\alpha = 0.05$.   **251**

Figure 20.1   Survival in the wild (open circuits), calculated and randomly disturbed survival among captured flies (crosses), estimate for survival in the wild corresponding to small value (dashed line) and selected value for regularization parameter (solid line).   **288**

Figure 21.1   Power of the proposed quantile chi-squared test for interval-censoring.   **305**

Figure 25.1   Graphical interpretation of the Rasch model.   **355**

Figure 25.2   Cronbach alpha curves for the three final groups.   **357**

Figure 25.3   Item characteristic curves for the group 1.   **359**

Figure 26.1 $\mathcal{D}$'s decision tree using QAL consideration (the unifying perspective of QAL).   **373**

Figure 26.2   Envelope showing the range of values for $p(\theta_j, \beta_{ij})$.   **375**

Figure 27.1   Threshold choice.   **401**

Figure 27.2   Limit power functions.   **402**

Figure 28.1   A three-state semi-Markov system.   **416**

Figure 28.2   Mean value of the integral functional estimation of the   **416**
three-state semi-Markov system and its 95% and 80%
nonparametric interval confidence.

Figure 31.1   Second look-time τ_2 in example of Section 31.3, for fixed   **455**
$\tau_1 = 0.42$, as a function of normalized statistic $U_1 = X(\tau_1)/\sqrt{\tau_1}$.

Figure 31.2   Rejection boundary at τ_2 as a function of $U_1 = X(\tau_1)/$ **456**
$\sqrt{\tau_1}$ in the optimized two-look procedure of Section 31.3.

Figure 31.3   Immediate rejection and acceptance boundaries, re-   **457**
spectively, $C_U/\sqrt{V_j}$ (plotted with filled dots) and
$C_{L,j}/\sqrt{V_j}$ (filled triangles) for normalized log-rank statistics $S_j/\sqrt{nV_j}$ in a particular case of the Koutsoukos *et
al.* (1998) boundaries described in Section 31.4

Figure 31.4   Accrual-stopping and final rejection boundaries, re-   **457**
spectively, $C_{A,j}/\sqrt{V_j}$ (plotted with filled squares) and
$C_{R,j}/\sqrt{V_j}$ (filled diamonds) for normalized log-rank
statistics $S_j/\sqrt{nV_j}$ in the same example of the Koutsoukos *et al.* (1998) boundaries as in Figure 31.3.

Figure 33.1   Expected discrepancies and criterion averages versus   **482**
number of regressors (set 3).

PART I
Cox Models, Analyses, and Extensions

1

Extended Cox and Accelerated Models in Reliability, with General Censoring and Truncation

Catherine Huber-Carol[1] **and Mikhail Nikulin**[2]

[1] *Université Paris 5 and Unité INSERM 870, Paris, France*
[2] *IMB, Université Victor Segalen, Bordeaux, France*

Abstract: We review recent developments in reliability or survival analysis. We consider various models for the time to failure or survival time, by a law on $\mathbb{R}^+$ that may depend on one or more factors. Inhomogeneity is taken into account by way of frailty models. The presence of censoring and truncation of a general type, more complex than the usual simple case of right censoring, induced the most recent developments on these topics. In the case of clusters of items or families of patients implying a possible dependence between multiple failure times, shared frailty models or hierarchical dependency models are considered.

Keywords and Phrases: Accelerated failure time models, censoring, clusters, correlated survival data, cross-effect, discrete time, extended Cox models, inhomogeneity problems, logistic model, survival data, truncation

1.1 Cox Model and Extensions

Let the failure time X have survival function $S(x) = P(X \geq x)$, density $f = -dS/dx$, hazard $\lambda(x) = f(x)/S(x)$, and cumulative hazard $\Lambda(x) = \int_0^x \lambda(u)du$.

1.1.1 The simple Cox model

The basic Cox model assumes that conditional on a p-dimensional covariate $Z = z$, the hazard rate verifies

$$\lambda(x|z) = \lambda_0(x)e^{(<\beta,z>)},$$

where β is an unknown p-dimensional parameter and λ_0 an unknown function of x. It is the most popular model because it leads to very easy interpretation of

3

the impact of each component of the covariate, over all when they are constant
in time. But it suffers some limitations. Let the covariates be constant in time at
the moment. First, the multiplicative dependence on the covariate z, assumed to
be exponential, could be replaced by a function $\varphi(z)$; the corresponding model
is called a proportional hazard (PH) model (see Definition 1.4.4). The second
limitation is that the model depends only on the time x elapsed between the
starting event (e.g., diagnosis) and the terminal event (e.g., death), and not on
the chronological time t; it is actually assumed to be homogeneous in chronological time. One could introduce a dependence on x and t. The third limitation is
that the effect of a given covariate is constant in time. This leads to the fact that
the survival functions $S(\cdot|z)$ and $S(\cdot|z')$ corresponding to two distinct values z
and z' of Z are always ordered, for example, $S(x|z) < S(x|z') \, \forall x$, without any
possibility of crossing. A fourth limitation is that if one pertinent covariate is
omitted, even if it is independent of the other covariates in the model, averaging
on the omitted covariate gives a new model that is no longer of Cox type, and if
it is treated as such, this leads to (possibly very) biased estimates [Bretagnolle
and Huber (1988)] of the regression coefficients β. Frailty models take care of
this case, introducing heterogeneity in the Cox model.

1.1.2   Nonhomogeneity in chronological time

In order to take into account the effect of the initial time t, there are several
possibilities: either add it, possibly categorized, as a $(p + 1)$th component of
covariate $Z = (Z_1, \ldots, Z_p)$ or have a baseline hazard which is both a function
of x and t, $\lambda_0 = \lambda_0(x; t)$. The second proposal is due to Pons (2000, 2002a) and
Pons and Visser (2000) who studied its asymptotic properties allowing for the
use of the following model,

$$\lambda(x|t, z) = \lambda_0(x; t)e^{<\beta, z(t+x)>}.$$

The usual Nelson–Aalen estimator for the cumulative hazard Λ is a kernel
estimate [Pons and Visser (2000)], with kernel K a continuous symmetric density, with support $[-1, +1]$ and $K_{h_n}(s) = (1/h_n)K(s/h_n)$, where $h_n \longrightarrow 0$ at a
convenient rate

$$\widehat{\Lambda_{n,X|S}}(x; s; \beta) = \sum_i \frac{K_{h_n}(s - S_i)\delta_i 1\{X_i \leq x\}}{nS^{(0)}},$$

where $S^{(0)}$ is defined as

$$S^{(0)} = (1/n)\sum_j K_{h_n}(s - S_j)Y_j(x)e^{<\beta, Z_j(S_j+x)>},$$

and $\widehat{\beta_n}$ maximizes the partial likelihood:

$$l_n(\beta) = \sum_i \delta_i[< \beta, Z_i(T_i^0) > - \ln\{nS^{(0)}(X_i; s; \beta)\}]\epsilon_n(S_i),$$

where $\epsilon_n(s) = 1\{s \in [h_n, \tau - h_n]\}$. Good asymptotic properties of those estimators were proved. Also a goodness-of-fit test was derived, as well as a test of H_0; the model is Cox, homogeneous in time; $\lambda_{X|S}(x;s) \equiv \lambda_X(x)$ against H_1; the model depends also on chronological time: $\lambda_{X|S}(x;s)$.

1.1.3 Effect not constant in time

The simplest way to involve effects not constant in time of some covariates is to consider that β is actually piecewise constant. This can be viewed as a breakpoint problem with the step function $\beta(x)$ having an unknown number k of steps (known to be bounded by a fixed constant k_0) as well as an unknown localization of the jumps, depending on the admissible complexity of the model. Another way is to consider that the constant ratio β may vary as a function of an observed covariate $Z_0 \in \mathbb{R}$: $\beta = \beta(Z_0)$, such that $Z_0 \sim f_0$ for some density f_0. The corresponding model [Pons (2000)] is

$$\lambda(t|Z_0, Z) = \lambda_0(t)e^{<\beta(Z_0), Z(t)>}.$$

Observations are $(T_i, \delta_i, Z_{i0}, Z_i)$, $T_i = T_i^0 \wedge C_i$, $\delta_i = 1\{T_i^0 \leq C_i\}, i = 1, \ldots, n$. The problem is to estimate $\beta(z_0)$ on a compact subset J_{Z_0} of the support of Z_0. $\hat{\beta}_n(z_0)$ maximizes the partial likelihood

$$l_{n,z_0}(\beta) = \sum_{i \leq n} \delta_i K_{h_n}(z_0 - Z_{i0})$$

$$\times \left[<\beta, Z_i(T_i)> - \ln\left\{ \sum_{j \leq n} K_{h_n}(z_0 - Z_{j0})Y_j(T_i)e^{<\beta, Z_j(T_i)>} \right\} \right],$$

and hence we get the following estimator of the cumulative hazard Λ_0

$$\widehat{\Lambda_n}(t) = \sum_{i:T_i \leq t} \frac{\delta_i}{S_n^{(0)}(T_i)},$$

where

$$S_n^{(0)}(s) = \sum_j Y_j(s)1\{Z_{j0} \in J_{Z_0}\}e^{<\hat{\beta}_n(Z_{j0}), Z_j(T_i)>}.$$

1.1.4 Omitted pertinent covariate: frailty models

Let the Cox model be true, but one component of the covariate Z is omitted or unobserved, say the $(p+1)$th component. $S(t|Z' = (z_1, \ldots, z_p))$ is equal to $S(t|Z = (z_1, \ldots, z_{p+1}))$ averaged on z_{p+1}. Denoting

$$\eta = e^{\beta_{p+1} z_{p+1}},$$

the corresponding model is a frailty model thus defined: η is a positive random variable, the survival of subject i, $i = 1, \ldots, n$, whose p-dimensional covariate z_i is observed and frailty η_i is not observed, but has known distribution function F_η on $I\!R^+$. The X_is are independent and their survival function S and hazard function h obey the following frailty model, where $\beta \in R^p$ is an unknown regression parameter, $\lambda(t)$ the unknown baseline hazard, and $\Lambda(t) = \int_0^\infty \lambda(u)du$ the baseline cumulative hazard.

$$h(t|z,\eta) = \eta e^{\beta^T z} \lambda(t) \tag{1.1}$$

$$S(t|z,\eta) = e^{-\eta e^{\beta^T z} \Lambda(t)}$$

$$S(t|z) = \int_0^\infty e^{-x e^{\beta^T z} \Lambda(t)} dF_\eta(x) = e^{-G(e^{\beta^T z} \Lambda(t))}, \tag{1.2}$$

where G is equal to $-\log$ of the Laplace transform of η:

$$G(y) = -\ln\left(\int_0^\infty e^{-uy} dF_\eta(u)\right). \tag{1.3}$$

The two most popular frailty distributions are the gamma [Clayton–Cuzick (1985) frailty model] with mean 1 and variance c, and the inverse Gaussian with mean 1 and variance $1/2b$; see, for example, Bagdonavicius and Nikulin (1998, 2002). The respective functions G defined in (1.3) are equal to:

$$G(x,c) = \frac{1}{c}\ln(1+cx), \qquad c > 0$$

$$G(x,b) = \sqrt{4b(b+x)} - 2b, \quad b > 0.$$

1.2   General Censoring and Truncation

1.2.1   Definition

Very often, the failure or survival time X is right-censored and classical statistical inference is obtained under this assumption. But it may also happen rather frequently that X is both-censored, in a more general way than on its right, and also truncated, so that the X_is are generally not observed. Instead, one observes two intervals (A_i, B_i), which are, respectively, the censoring interval, $A_i = [L_i; R_i]$, and the truncating interval $]\mathcal{L}_i; \mathcal{R}_i[$, such that $B_i \supset A_i$. This means that X_i is not observed but is known to lie inside A_i, and A_i itself is observed only conditionally on the fact that it is inside the truncating interval B_i. Otherwise, the corresponding subject is said to be "truncated;" that is, it does not appear in the sample. Finally, for the n subjects who are not truncated, the observations are (A_i, B_i, z_i), $i \in \{1, 2, \ldots, n\}$. When in model (1.2), there is no covariate and G is the identity, the nonparametric maximum likelihood estimate under general censoring and truncation is due to the early work of Turnbull (1976). It was then extended to the semiparametric Cox model by Alioum and Commenges (1996), and to the general frailty model (1.2) by Huber-Carol and Vonta (2004). The consistency of the NPML estimate of the density of X was proved [Huber-Carol *et al.* (2006)] under regularity conditions on the laws of X and of the censoring and truncation schemes.

1.2.2   Maximum likelihood estimation for frailty models

Under the above censoring and truncation scheme, the likelihood is proportional to

$$l(S) = \prod_{i=1}^{n} l_i(S_i) = \prod_{i=1}^{n} \frac{P_{S_i}(A_i)}{P_{S_i}(B_i)} = \prod_{i=1}^{n} \frac{\{S_i(L_i^-) - S_i(R_i^+)\}}{\{S_i(\mathcal{L}_i^+) - S_i(\mathcal{R}_i^-)\}}. \tag{1.4}$$

Following Turnbull (1976), we define the "beginning" set $\widetilde{L}$ and the "finishing" set $\widetilde{R}$, in order to take advantage of the fact that the likelihood is maximum when the values of $S_i(x)$ are the greatest possible for $x \in \widetilde{L}$ and the smallest possible for $x \subset \widetilde{R}$:

$$\widetilde{L} = \{L_i, 1 \le i \le n\} \cup \{\mathcal{R}_i, 1 \le i \le n\} \cup \{0\}$$

$$\widetilde{R} = \{R_i, 1 \le i \le n\} \cup \{\mathcal{L}_i, 1 \le i \le n\} \cup \{\infty\}.$$

Let

$$Q = \{[q_j' p_j'] : q_j' \in \widetilde{L} \ , \ p_j' \in \widetilde{R} \ , \ [q_j' p_j'] \cap \widetilde{L} = \varnothing \ , \ [q_j' p_j'] \cap \widetilde{R} = \varnothing\}$$

$$0 = q_1' \le p_1' < q_2' \le p_2' < \cdots < q_v' \le p_v' = \infty.$$

Then,

$$Q = \cup_{j=1}^{v} [q_j', p_j'] = C \cup W \cup D,$$

where

$$
\begin{aligned}
C &= \cup[q_j', p_j'] \quad \text{covered by at least one censoring set,} \\
W &= \cup[q_j', p_j'] \quad \text{covered by at least one truncating set,} \\
& \qquad\qquad\quad \text{but not covered by any censoring set,} \\
D &= \cup[q_j', p_j'] \quad \text{not covered by any truncating set.}
\end{aligned}
$$

The special case of $G \equiv Id$ and $\beta = 0$ was studied in detail in Turnbull (1976), followed by Frydman (1994) and Finkelstein et al. (1993). The above likelihood, for the general frailty model (1.2) as a function of the unknown β and Λ, is equal to

$$l(\Lambda, \beta | (A_i, B_i, z_i)_{i \in \{1,..,n\}}) = \prod_{i=1}^{n} \frac{\left\{ e^{-G(e^{\beta^T z_i} \Lambda(L_i^-))} - e^{-G(e^{\beta^T z_i} \Lambda(R_i^+))} \right\}}{\left\{ e^{-G(e^{\beta^T z_i} \Lambda(\mathcal{L}_i^+))} - e^{-G(e^{\beta^T z_i} \Lambda(\mathcal{R}_i^-))} \right\}}.$$

As in the special case where $G = Id$ and $\beta = 0$ in (1.2), the NPML estimator of Λ for the frailty model (1.1) is not increasing outside the set $C \cup D$ [Huber-Carol and Vonta (2004)]. Moreover, conditionally on the values of $\Lambda(q_j^-)$ and $\Lambda(p_j^+)$, $1 \le j \le m$, the likelihood does not depend on how the mass $\Lambda(p_j^+) - \Lambda(q_j^-)$ is distributed in the interval $[q_j, p_j]$. From this remark follows the estimation of Λ and β. The special case of $G = Id$ was studied by Alioum and Commenges (1996).

1.3   Discrete Time: Logistic Regression Models for the Retro-Hazard

A very classical example of censored and truncated survival data is the retrospective AIDS induction time for patients infected by blood transfusion [Kalbfleisch and Lawless (1989)]. See Figure 1.1. The starting date Y_1, infection time, is reached retrospectively from Y_2, the time of onset of AIDS. $0 < Y_1 + X \le b$ holds, which means that X is right-truncated by $b - Y_1$. When, moreover, one knows that Y_1 took place after the first transfusion, Y_0, X may be also left-censored by $Y_2 - Y_0$. We have there a censoring variable $C = Y_2 - Y_0$ and a truncating variable $T = b - Y_1$. We have there data that are left-censored and right-truncated. The treatment of this kind of data is the same as the treatment of right-censored left-truncated data, that is implied hereafter. Assuming now that, for those censored and truncated data, time is discrete, with values $\{1, 2, \ldots, k\}$. X is the survival, C the right-censoring and T the left-truncating

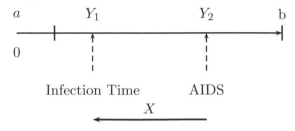

$X = Y_2 - Y_1$: AIDS induction time.

Figure 1.1. AIDS example of right-truncation.

variable, they are independent, and the model for X is the logistic model for the retro-hazard $h^*(t)dt = [f(t)dt]/[1 - S(t)]$:

$$\log \frac{h^*(t|Z(t) = z)}{1 - h^*(t|Z(t) = z)} = \langle \beta, z \rangle, \ \ t \in \{1, 2, \ldots, T\}.$$

Gross and Huber (1992) obtain nonparametric estimators and tests for the saturated model when all covariates are categorical, for the three laws of X, the survival, C the censoring, and T the truncation, using a special partial likelihood. In Figure 1.2, observations take place in the hatched triangle, due to left-truncation, and the risk set at time i is the hatched rectangle.

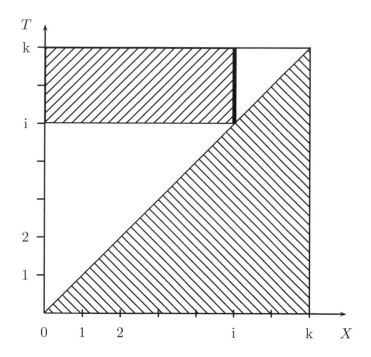

Figure 1.2. Risk zone for right-censored and left-truncated discrete times.

1.4 Accelerated Failure Time Models (AFT)

Enforced controlled stresses are meant to reduce the time on test. It is used in particular for tires, brakes, and more generally for planes and train equipment, hence the need for a transfer functional [Bagdonavicius and Nikulin (1997, 1998)] allowing an interpolation from the time to failure under enforced stress to the time to failure under regular stress, the Sedyakin principle.

1.4.1 Sedyakin principle

Let $\mathcal{E}_1$ be the set of constant stresses and $\mathcal{E}_2$ the step stresses, thus defined:

$$\mathcal{E}_2 = \{Z(\cdot) : Z(t) = Z_1 \; \mathbb{1}\{0 \le t \le t_0\} + Z_2 \; \mathbb{1}\{t > t_0\}; Z_1, Z_2 \in \mathcal{E}_1\}.$$

The Sedyakin principle may then be formulated as follows for step stresses.

Definition 1.4.1 (Sedyakin principle (A_S) on $\mathcal{E}_2$) Let $Z_1(\cdot)$ and $Z_2(\cdot)$ be two stresses. We say that $t_1 \sim t_2$ if $S(t_1|Z_1(\cdot)) = S(t_2|Z_2(\cdot))$. If $Z_1(\cdot) = Z_1$ constant, $Z_2(\cdot) = Z_2$ constant, and $Z(t) = Z_1 \; \mathbb{1}\{0 \le t \le t_1\} + Z_2 \; \mathbb{1}\{t > t_1\}$, then the Sedyakin principle (A_S) on $\mathcal{E}_2$ holds if

$$\lambda(t_1 + s|Z(\cdot)) = \lambda(t_2 + s|Z_2).$$

Let $\mathcal{E}$ be the set of the general stresses that are p-dimensional left-continuous processes having right limits. Then, the Sedyakin principle for general stress is the following.

Definition 1.4.2 (Generalized Sedyakin principle (A_{GS}) on $\mathcal{E}$). A model obeys the generalized Sedyakin assumption (A_{GS}) if there exists a function g such that

$$\lambda(t|Z(s) \; 0 \le s \le t) = g(Z(t), S(t|Z(s); 0 \le s \le t)).$$

It means that the hazard rate $\lambda(t|Z(\cdot))$ is independent of the past conditionally on $\Lambda(t|Z(s), 0 \le s < t)$:

$$(\lambda(t|Z(\cdot)))^{\stackrel{\Lambda(t|Z(\cdot))}{\perp}} \mathcal{F}_{t^-}$$

or equivalently on $S(t|Z(s), 0 \le s < t)$ sometimes called the *resource*.

1.4.2 Definition of AFT models

Loosely speaking, an accelerated model is a model based on a given survival function G and a transformation $\alpha(t)$ of time t, where α is a nondecreasing function: $S(t) = G(\alpha(t))$. This acceleration $(\alpha > Id)$ or deceleration $(\alpha < Id)$ takes place through a positive function r of the stress $Z(s)$; $0 < s \le t$.

Definition 1.4.3 (AFT model on $\mathcal{E}$) A model is AFT on $\mathcal{E}$ if there exists a survival function G and a positive function r such that:

$$S(t|Z(s), 0 \le s \le t) = G\left(\int_0^t r(Z(s))ds\right) \; \forall Z \in \mathcal{E}.$$

In the simple case of a constant stress $Z \in \mathcal{E}_1 : Z = z_0$:

$$S(t|Z) = G(r(z_0)t) \; \forall Z \in \mathcal{E}_1. \qquad (*)$$

There is a relationship between the Sedyakin (A_{GS}) and AFT models [Meeker and Escobar (1998), Bagdonavicius and Nikulin (2000b)]: A_{GS} and $(*)$ hold $\iff \exists q > 0, r > 0$ such that

$$\lambda(t|Z(\cdot)) = r(Z(t)) * q(S(t|Z(\cdot))).$$

An AFT model on $\mathcal{E}_2$ is such that if Z_1 and Z_2 are constant stresses, and $Z(t) = Z_1 \ \mathbb{1}\{0 \leq t \leq t_1\} + Z_2 \ \mathbb{1}\{t > t_1\}$, then

$$t_2 \quad = \quad \frac{r(Z_1)}{r(Z_2)} \sim t_1$$

$$S(t|Z(\cdot)) \quad = \quad \begin{cases} S(t|Z_1), & 0 \leq t < t_1 \\ S(t - t_1 + t_2|Z_2), & t \geq t_1 \end{cases}.$$

1.4.3 Relationships between accelerated (AFT) and proportional hazard (PH) models

The Cox model is a particular case of the more general proportional hazard (PH) models:

Definition 1.4.4 (PH model) A PH model on $\mathcal{E}$ is such that, for two positive functions r and λ_0, the hazard rate verifies:

$$\lambda(t|Z(\cdot)) = r(Z(t)) \, \lambda_0(t) \ \forall Z(\cdot) \in \mathcal{E}.$$

Then $\Lambda(t|Z(\cdot)) = \int_0^t r(Z(s)) d\Lambda_0(s)$ and $S(t|Z(\cdot)) = e^{-\int_0^t r(Z(s)) d\Lambda_0(s)}$, where $\Lambda_0(t) = \int_0^t \lambda_0(s) ds$, and $S_0(t) = e^{-\Lambda_0(t)}$. The simple case of a PH model on $\mathcal{E}_1$ gives $\lambda(t|Z) = r(Z)\lambda_0(t) \quad \forall Z \in \mathcal{E}_1$. The corresponding survival is then $S(t|Z) = S_0^{r(Z)}(t) = e^{-r(Z)\Lambda_0(t)}$. Let $\rho(Z_1, Z_2) = r(Z_2)/r(Z_1)$. Then $S(t|Z_2) = S(t|Z_1)^{\rho(Z_1, Z_2)}$. If PH holds on $\mathcal{E}_2$, then $\forall Z(\cdot) \in \mathcal{E}_2$ such that for two constant stresses Z_1 and Z_2, $Z(t) = Z_1 \ \mathbb{1}\{0 \leq t \leq t_1\} + Z_2 \ \mathbb{1}\{t > t_1\}$,

$$\lambda(t|Z(\cdot)) = \begin{cases} \lambda(t|Z_1) = r(Z_1)\lambda_0(t), \ 0 \leq t \leq t_1 \\ \lambda(t|Z_2) = r(Z_2)\lambda_0(t), \ t > t_1 \end{cases}$$

and

$$S(t|Z(\cdot)) = \begin{cases} S(t|Z_1), & 0 \leq t \leq t_1 \\ S(t|Z_2)\frac{S(t_1|Z_1)}{S(t_1|Z_2)}, & t > t_1 \end{cases}.$$

1.4.4 Relationships between Sedyakin and PH: MPH models

Bagdonavicius and Nikulin (2002) define a proportional hazard model that obeys the Sedyakin principle.

Definition 1.4.5 (Modified PH model: MPH) A model is Sedyakin (A_{GS}) on $\mathcal{E}$ and PH on $\mathcal{E}_1$ and called MPH if and only if, for two functions r and λ_0,

$$\lambda(t|Z(\cdot)) = r(Z(t))\lambda_0 \left(\Lambda_0^{-1} \left(\frac{\Lambda(t|Z(\cdot))}{r(Z(t))} \right) \right).$$

If MPH holds on $\mathcal{E}_2$, then $\forall Z(\cdot) \in \mathcal{E}_2$ such that for two constant stresses Z_1 and Z_2:

$$
\begin{aligned}
Z(t) &= Z_1 \, \mathbb{1}\{0 \le t \le t_1\} + Z_2 \, \mathbb{1}\{t > t_1\} \\
t_2 &= S^{-1}((S(t_1, Z_1))^{\rho(Z_2, Z_1)})
\end{aligned}
$$

then

$$
S(t|Z(\cdot)) = \left\{
\begin{array}{ll}
S(t|Z_1), & 0 \le t < t_1 \\
S(t - t_1 + t_2|Z_2), & t \ge t_1
\end{array}
\right. .
$$

1.4.5 Generalized PH models (GPH) on $\mathcal{E}$

Bagdonavicius and Nikulin (1998, 2002) define two distinct generalized PH models, GPH1 and GPH2.

Definition 1.4.6 (GPH1) A model is GPH1 if and only if, for two positive functions r and λ_0, the hazard λ verifies

$$\lambda(t|Z(\cdot)) = r(Z(t)) * q\{\Lambda(t, Z(\cdot))\} * \lambda_0(t).$$

When $q \equiv 1$ this is simply a PH model, whereas $\lambda_0(t) \equiv \lambda_0$ constant gives the AFT model.

Definition 1.4.7 (GPH2) A model is GPH2 if and only if, for two positive functions u and λ_0,

$$\lambda(t|Z(\cdot)) = u(Z(t), \Lambda(t|Z(\cdot))) * \lambda_0(t).$$

$\lambda_0(t) \equiv \lambda_0$ constant gives a GS model on $\mathcal{E}$, and $u(Z, s) = r(Z)q(s)$ gives a GPH1 model. Model GPH1 holds on $\mathcal{E}$ if and only if there exist two survival functions G and S_0 such that

$$S(t|Z(\cdot)) = G\left\{ \int_0^t r(Z(s))dH(S_0(s)) \right\},$$

where $H = G^{-1}$. Function f_G defined as

$$f_G(t|Z(\cdot)) = H(S(t|Z(\cdot)))$$

is called the *transfer functional*. It is the G-resource used until time t under stress Z. It is actually a transfer of quantiles. More about these models and other time transformation models can be found in Wu *et al.* (2002), Scheike (2006), Nikulin and Wu (2006), Dabrowska and Doksum (1998), and Wu (2006), among others.

1.4.6 General models

There are many relationships between those models. One can construct a general model that contains most of the models defined above.

1. Accelerated model (AFT)

$$\lambda(t|Z) = r(Z)q\{S(t|Z)\}.$$

2. Generalized proportional models of type 1 (GPH1)

$$\lambda(t|Z) = r(Z)q\{\Lambda(t)\}$$

   include the following submodels:

$$
\begin{aligned}
q(v) &= 1 && (PH)\\
q(v) &= (1+v)^{\gamma+1}\\
q(v) &= e^{\gamma v}\\
q(v) &= \frac{1}{(1+\gamma v)}.
\end{aligned}
$$

3. Generalized proportional models of type 2 (GPH2)

$$\lambda(t|Z) = u\{Z, \Lambda(t|Z)\}\lambda_0(t)$$

whose submodels correspond to various choices of function u.

1.4.7 Modeling and homogeneity problem

General models, considered here, are very useful not only for construction of goodness-of-fit tests for the PH model but they also give the possibility of constructing goodness-of-fit tests for a data homogeneity hypothesis. Following Bagdonavicius and Nikulin (2005) we give three models here, each including the PH model.

Generalized proportional hazards (GPH) model on $\mathcal{E}_1$:

$$\lambda(t,|Z) = e^{\beta^T Z}(1 + \gamma e^{\beta^T Z}\Lambda_0(t))^{\frac{1}{\gamma}-1} * \lambda_0(t).$$

This model has the following properties on $\mathcal{E}_1$: the ratios of the hazard rates increase, decrease, or are constant; and the hazard rates and the survival function do not intersect in the interval $(0, \infty)$.

Simple cross-effects (SCE) model $\mathcal{E}_1$:

$$\lambda(t, |Z) = e^{\beta^T Z}\{1 + e^{(\beta+\gamma)^T}\Lambda_0(t)\}^{e^{-\gamma^T Z}-1} * \lambda_0(t).$$

The SCE model has the following properties on $\mathcal{E}_1$: the ratios of the hazard rates increase, decrease, or are constant; and the hazard rates and the survival function do not intersect or intersect once in the interval $(0, \infty)$.

Multiple cross-effects (MCE) model $\mathcal{E}_1$:

$$\lambda(t, |Z) = e^{\beta^T Z}\left(1 + \gamma^T Z \Lambda_0(t) + \delta^T Z \Lambda_0^2(t)\right)\lambda_0(t).$$

The MCE model has the next properties on $\mathcal{E}_1$: the ratios of the hazard rates increase, decrease, or are constant, the hazard rates and the survival function do not intersect, intersect once or twice in the interval $(0, \infty)$.

The parameter γ is one-dimensional for the GPH model and m-dimensional for the SCE model; the parameter δ is m-dimensional. The PH model is a particular case with $\gamma = 1$ (GPH), $\gamma = 0$ (SCE), and $\delta = \gamma = 0$ (MCE). The homogeneity (no lifetime regression) takes place if $\gamma = 1$, $\beta = 0$ (GPH), $\gamma = 0$, $\beta = 0$ (SCE), $\beta = \delta = \gamma = 0$ (MCE). At the end let us consider the so-called Hsieh model (2001), which is also a SCE model. According to the idea of Hsieh, one possible way to obtain a cross-effect of hazard rates is to take a power function of Λ_0:

$$\Lambda_x(t) = r(x_1)\Lambda_0^{\rho(x_2)}(t), \quad \lambda_x(t) = r(x_1)\rho(x_2)\Lambda_0^{\rho(x_2)-1}(t)\lambda_0(t),$$

where $x = (x_1, x_2), x_1, x_2 \in E_1$, $r(\cdot), \rho(\cdot) : E \to R_+^1$. Using natural parameterization $r(x_1) = e^{\beta^T x_1}$ and $\rho(x_2) = e^{\gamma^T x_2}$ we have the model

$$\Lambda_x(t) = e^{\beta^T x_1}\Lambda_0^{e^{\gamma^T x_2}}(t).$$

In the particular case $x_1 = x_2 = x$ the obtained model is

$$\lambda_x(t) = e^{(\beta+\gamma)^T x}\Lambda_0^{e^{\gamma^T x}-1}(t)\lambda_0(t).$$

For any two covariates x, y the ratio $\lambda_x(t)/\lambda_y(t)$ is increasing from 0 to ∞ or decreasing from ∞ to 0. So we have a cross-effect of the hazard rates. About estimation, testing, and computational methods for all models considered here, see, for example, Tsiatis (1981), Cheng *et al.* (1995), Dabrowska (2005, 2006), Hsieh (2001), Wu (2004, 2006, 2007), Martinussen and Scheike (2006), Slud and Vonta (2004), Huber-Carol *et al.* (2006), and Zeng and Lin (2007), among others.

1.5 Correlated Survivals

1.5.1 Introduction

We first present several examples of data having the structure of correlated survival data. In diabetic retinopathy, the cluster is constituted by each diabetic patient. The survival time is the time to blindness onset for each eye separately. Two types of covariates may have an impact on the time to onset: the treatment, called a structural covariate, cluster covariates such as sex and age, and individual covariates such as past history of each eye. The time to onset is censored by death prior to blindness. In animal experiments on litters of rats, each litter is a cluster, and the treatment is a supposed carcinogenic product injected regularly into each rat. The survival time is the time to onset of a tumor. Again the structural covariate is the treatment, the individual covariates are sex, age, and weight. The censoring takes place when death occurs before the onset of a tumor. In genetic epidemiology, the cluster is a pair of twins or a family. The survival time is the age at onset of a specific chronic disease. The structural covariates are the position inside the family (father, mother, male sibling, etc.) and individual covariates are sex, and so on. Time is again censored by death or lost to followup. The following picture illustrates the data structure.

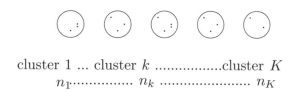

cluster 1 ... cluster k ....cluster K

n_1................ n_k .... n_K

Classical proposals to take into account the correlation induced by the clusters are frailty or copula models. There are two kinds of frailty well distinguished by Parner (1998). First, is *shared frailty*, which is more appropriate for taking into account inhomogeneity than dependence, as it gives the possibility of estimating the frailty distribution parameter when only one of two twins is observed. Second is *shared and correlated frailty*. Gross and Huber (2002) proposed a logisticlike family model in discrete time, related to hierarchical log-linear models which is detailed in the next section.

1.5.2 Model in discrete time: Hierarchical dependencies

X_{ki} is the survival time of subject i in cluster k, and C_{ki} is the associated right-censoring time. Actually, what is observed is:

$$T_{ki} = X_{ki} \wedge C_{ki} \qquad \text{observed duration.}$$
$$D_{ki} = I\{X_{ki} \le C_{ki}\} \text{ death indicator.}$$

Globally data are summarized by the pair of variables (T, D) or else the two-dimensional process (R, Y), where R is the couple of the "at risk" and event processes:

$$T = \{T_{ki}; 1 \le k \le K ; 1 \le i \le n_k\}$$
$$D = \{D_{ki}; 1 \le k \le K ; 1 \le i \le n_k\}$$

$$R_{ki}(t) = \begin{cases} 1 & \text{if } T_{ki} \ge t \\ 0 & \text{otherwise} \end{cases}$$

$$Y_{ki}(t) = \begin{cases} 1 & \text{if } D_{ki}T_{ki} = t \\ 0 & \text{otherwise.} \end{cases}$$

In the case of discrete time, if N is the maximum size of the clusters, data are summarized through two arrays of 0 and 1, of dimension $T \times N \times K$: $R_{T \times N \times K}$, the at-risk array, and the event array $Y_{T \times N \times K}$.

1.5.3 Definition of the models

The model parameters are $p_{r,y}(t)$ such that

$$P(Y = y | R = r; t) = \frac{1}{c(r,t)} \exp\left\{ \sum_{\substack{0 < r' \le r \\ 0 \le y' \le r' \wedge y}} p_{r',y'}(t) \right\}$$

and the normalization constant is c(r,t):

$$c(r,t) = 1 + \sum_{s' \le r} \exp\left\{ \sum_{\substack{0 < r' \le r \\ 0 < y'' \le r' \wedge y'}} p_{r',y''}(t) \right\}.$$

Each model is characterized by the set $\mathcal{R}$ of those parameters $p_{r,y}$ that are equal to 0 and is thus denoted $\mathcal{H}(\mathcal{R})$; the saturated model is the one for which this set is the empty set $\emptyset$. Especially interesting are the so-called hierarchical models defined below.

Definition 1.5.1 (Hierarchical models $\mathcal{H}(\mathcal{R})$) A model is said to be hierarchical if all $p_{r,y}$ such that $r \notin \mathcal{R}$ are equal to 0, where $\mathcal{R}$ is a family of subsets of $\{1, 2, \ldots, N\}$, such that for any R in $\mathcal{R}$ and $R' \subset R$, $R' \in \mathcal{R}$.

Definition 1.5.2 (Model of order k, $\mathcal{H}_k$) If all $p_{r,y}$ such that $\sum_i r_i > k$ are equal to 0, the corresponding model is called a model of order k and called $\mathcal{H}_k$, as all interactions up to order k are included, whereas interactions of order greater than k are excluded.

Models $\mathcal{H}_k$ are a special case of hierarchical models. More generally, a model may be defined by the pair $(\mathcal{R}, \mathcal{Y})$ such that $p_{r,y} = 0$ except if $r \in \mathcal{R}$ and $y \in \mathcal{Y}$, $y \subset \mathcal{Y}$.

1.5.4 Regression model

Let us now include covariates in the models: The $p_{r,y}$ are modeled linearly in terms of time t and individual profiles, and the partial likelihood is a function of the following counts of clusters at time t,

$$N(r, y, t) = \text{count of clusters s.t.} \begin{cases} \text{risk set} & = r \\ \text{jump set} & = y \end{cases}$$

$$N(r, t) = \text{count of clusters s.t. risk set} = r.$$

1.5.5 Estimation

Theorem 1.5.1 (Sufficient statistics) *Under the general model of dependence $(\mathcal{R}, \mathcal{Y})$ and with some regularity conditions fulfilled, the sufficient statistics for the parameters of the model are the counts $N(r, t)$ and $N(r, y, t)$ for $t \in \{1, 2, \ldots, T\}$ and $(r, y) \in \mathcal{R} \otimes \mathcal{Y}$.*

Under right censoring, the same counts are the only statistics involved in the partial likelihood. One can prove consistency and asymptotic normality: p^* = true set of p parameters $(\mathcal{R}^*, \mathcal{Y}^*) \subset (\mathcal{R}, \mathcal{Y}) \equiv (r^*, y^*)$ combinations, for which $P^*(R = r^*)$ and $P^*(Y = y^*|R = r^*, t)$ are strictly positive. Σ = matrix of the second derivatives of the log-likelihood with respect to the parameters p_{r^*,y^*}, whose general entry, for $p_{r_0^*, y_0^*}(t), p_{r_1^*, y_1^*}(t)$, is, dropping the asterisk,

$$\Sigma_{p_{r_0, y_0}(t), p_{r_1, y_1}(t)}$$
$$= \sum_{\{r: \, r \geq r_0 \vee r_1\}} N(r, t)\{P\{Y(t) \geq (y_0 \vee y_1)|R(i) = r\}$$
$$- P\{Y(t) \geq y_0|R(t) = r\}P\{Y(t) \geq y_1|R(t) = r\}\}.$$

As the number of clusters K tends to infinity,

$$\frac{N(r, t)}{K} \xrightarrow{a.s.} P^*(r, t),$$

the true probability that $R(t) = r$. Similarly,

$$\frac{N(r, y, t)}{K} \xrightarrow{a.s.} P^*(r, y, t),$$

the true joint probability that $R(t) = r$ and $Y(t) = y$, for $t \in \{1, 2, \ldots, T\}$. Consequently,

$$\frac{\Sigma}{K} \xrightarrow{a.s.} \Sigma^*,$$

with typical entry:

$$\Sigma^*_{p_{r_0,y_0}(t), p_{r_1,y_1}(t)}$$

$$= \frac{1}{K} \sum_{\{r:\, r \geq r_0 \vee r_1\}} P^*(r, t)\{P^*\{Y(i) \geq (y_0 \vee y_1)|R(t) = r\}$$

$$- P^*\{Y(t) \geq y_0|R(t) = r\}P^*\{Y(t) \geq y_1|R(t) = r\}\} \, .$$

Theorem 1.5.2 (Consistency and as. normality) *If*

1. *For all (r', y') included in the model there exists a pair (r, y), also included in the model and such that $r \supseteq r'$ and $s \supseteq s'$, and $P^*(R = r)$ and $P^*(Y = y|R = r, t)$ are strictly positive,*

2. *Σ is nonsingular in a neighborhood of the true value p^* of the parameters, as K tends to infinity; the partial likelihood estimate $\widehat{p_K}$ of the parameters p is consistent and asymptotically normal:*

$$\sqrt{K}(\widehat{p_K} - p_0) \xrightarrow{\mathcal{L}} N(0, \Sigma^{*-1}).$$

References

1. Alioum, A. and Commenges, D. (1996). A proportional hazards model for arbitrarily censored and truncated data, *Biometrics*, **52**, 512–524.

2. Bagdonavicius, V. and Nikulin, M. (1997). Transfer functionals and semiparametric regression models, *Biometrika*, **84**, 365–378.

3. Bagdonavicius, V. and Nikulin, M. (1998). *Additive and multiplicative semiparametric models in accelerated life testing and survival analysis*, Queen's papers in Pure and Applied Mathematics, Queen's University, Kingston, Ontario, Canada.

4. Bagdonavicius, V. and Nikulin, M. (1999). Generalized proportional hazards model based on modified partial likelihood, *LIDA*, **5**, 323–344.

5. Bagdonavicius, V. and Nikulin, M. (2000a). On goodness of fit for the linear transformation and frailty models, *Statistics and Probability Letters*, **47**, 177–188.

6. Bagdonavicius, V. and Nikulin, M. (2000b). On nonparametric estimation in accelerated experiments with step stresses, *Statistics*, **33**, 349–365.

7. Bagdonavicius, V. and Nikulin, M. (2002). *Accelerated Life Models. Modeling and Statistical Analysis*, Chapman and Hall, Boca Raton, FL.

8. Bagdonavicius, V. and Nikulin, M. (2005). Statistical analysis of survival and reliability data with multiple crossings of survival functions, *Comptes Rendus de l'Academie des Sciences de Paris, Series I*, **340**, 377–382.

9. Bretagnolle, J. and Huber, C. (1988). Effects of omitting covariates in Cox's model for survival data, *Scandinavian Journal of Statistics*, **15**, 125–138.

10. Cheng, S. C., Wei, L. J., and Ying Z. (1995). Analysis of transformation models with censored data, *Biometrika*, **82**, 835–846.

11. Clayton, D. G. and Cuzick, J. (1985). Multivariate generalization of the proportional hazards model (with discussion), *Journal of the Royal Statistical Society, Series A*, **148**, 82–117.

12. Dabrowska, D. (2005). Quantile regression in transformation models, *Sankhya*, **67**, 153–187.

13. Dabrowska, D. (2006). Information bounds and efficient estimation in a class of censored transformation models, Web page: arXiv:math.ST/0608088 v1 3 Aug 2006.

14. Dabrowska, D. (2006). Estimation in a class of semi-parametric transformation models, In *Second Eric L. Lehmann Symposium – Optimality* (Ed., J. Rojo), Institute of Mathematical Statistics, Lecture Notes and Monograph Series, **49**, 166–216.

15. Dabrowska, D. M. and Doksum, K. A. (1988). Partial likelihood in transformation model with censored data, *Scandinavian Journal of Statistics*, **15**, 1–23.

16. Finkelstein, D. M., Moore, D. F., and Shoenfeld, D. A. (1993). A proportional hazards model for truncated AIDS data, *Biometrics*, **49**, 731–740.

17. Frydman, H. (1994). A note on nonparametric estimation of the distribution function from interval-censored and truncated observations, *Journal of the Royal Statistical Society, Series B*, **56**, 71–74.

18. Gross, S. and Huber, C. (1992). Regression models for truncated survival data, *Scandinavian Journal of Statistics*, **19**, 193–213.

19. Gross, S. and Huber, C. (2002). A new family of multivariate distributions for survival data, In *Goodness of Fit Tests and Model Validity*, pp. 255–266, Birkhaüser, Boston.

20. Hsieh, F. (2001). On heteroscedastic hazards regression models: Theory and application, *Journal of the Royal Statistical Society, Series B*, **63**, 63–79.

21. Huber-Carol, C. and Vonta, F. (2004). Frailty models for arbitrarily censored and truncated data, *Lifetime Data Analysis*, **10**, 369–388.

22. Huber-Carol, C., Solev, V., and Vonta, F. (2006). Estimation of density for arbitrarily censored and truncated data, In *Probability, Statistics and Modelling in Public Health* (Eds., M. Nikulin, D. Commenges, C. Huber), pp. 246–265, Springer-Verlag, New York.

23. Kalbfleisch, J.D. and Lawless, J.F. (1989). Inference on retrospective ascertainment: An analysis of the data on transfusion-related AIDS, *Journal of the American Statistical Association*, **84**, 360–372.

24. Martinussen, T., Scheike, T. (2006). *Dynamic Regression Models for Survival Analysis*, Springer-Verlag, New York.

25. Meeker, W. Q. and Escobar L. (1998), *Statistical Methods for Reliability Data*, John Wiley & Sons, New York.

26. Nikulin, M. and Wu, H-D.I. (2006). Flexible regression models for carcinogenesis studies, In *Probability and Statistics, 10* (Eds., I. Ibragimov and V. Sudakov), pp. 78–101, Academy of Sciences of Russia, St. Petersburg.

27. Parner, E. (1998). Asymptotic theory for the correlated gamma-frailty model, *Annals of Statistics*, **26**, 183–214.

28. Pons, O. and Visser, M. (2000). A non-stationary Cox model, *Scandinanvia Journal of Statistics*, **24**, 619–639.

29. Pons, O. (2000). Nonparametric estimation in a varying-coefficient Cox model, *Mathematical Methods in Statistics*, **9**, 376–398.

30. Pons, O. (2002a). Inference in extensions of the Cox model for heterogeneous populations, In *Goodness-of-fit Tests and Validity of Models* (Eds., C. Huber-Carol, N. Balakrishnan, M. S. Nikulin, and M. Mesbah), pp. 211–225, Birkhaüser, Boston.

31. Pons, O. (2002b). Estimation in a Cox regression model with a change-point at an unknown time, *Statistics*, **36**, 101–124.

32. Scheike, T. (2006). A flexible semiparametric transformation model for survival data, *Lifetime Data Analysis*, **12**, 461–480.

33. Slud, E. V. and Vonta, F. (2004). Consistency of the NPML estimator in the right-censored transformation model, *Scandinavian Journal of Statistics*, **31**, 21–41.

34. Tsiatis, A. A. (1981). A large sample study of Cox's regression model, *Annals of Statistics*, **9**, 93–108.

35. Turnbull, B. W. (1976). The empirical distribution function with arbitrarily grouped, censored and truncated data, *Journal of the Royal Statistical Society*, **38**, 290–295.

36. Wu, H-D. I. (2004). Effect of ignoring heterogeneity in hazards regression, In *Parametric and Semiparametric Models with Applicatiions to Reliability, Survival Analysis, and Quality of Life*, pp. 239–252, Birkhaüser, Boston.

37. Wu, H-D. I. (2006). Statistical inference for two-sample and regression models with heterogeneity effects: A collected-sample perspective, In *Probability, Statistics and Modelling in Public Health* (Eds., M. Nikulin, D. Commenges, and C. Huber), pp. 452–465, Springer-Verlag, New York.

38. Wu, H-D. I. (2007). A partial score test for difference among heterogeneous populations, *Journal of Statistical Planning and Inference*, **137**, 527–537.

39. Wu, H-D. I., Hsieh, F., and Chen C.-H. (2002). Validation of a heteroscedastic hazards regression model, *Lifetime Data Analysis*, **8**, 21–34.

40. Zeng, D. and Lin, D. (2007). Maximum likelihood estimation in semiparametric regression models with censored data, *Journal of the Royal Statistical Society*, **69**, 1–30.

2

Corrected Score Estimation in the Cox Regression Model with Misclassified Discrete Covariates

David M. Zucker[1] **and Donna Spiegelman**[2]

[1]*Department of Statistics, Hebrew University, Jerusalem, Israel*
[2]*Departments of Epidemiology and Biostatistics, Harvard School of Public Health, Boston, MA, USA*

Summary: We consider Cox proportional hazards regression when the covariate vector includes error-prone discrete covariates along with error-free covariates that may be discrete or continuous. The misclassification in the discrete error-prone covariates is allowed to be of arbitrary form. Building on work of Nakamura and his colleagues, we develop a corrected score method for this setting. The method can handle all three major study designs (internal validation design, external validation design, and replicate measures design), both functional and structural error models, and time-dependent covariates satisfying a certain "localized error" condition. This chapter presents the method, briefly describes its asymptotic properties, and illustrates it on data from a study of the relationship between dietary calcium intake and distal colon cancer. Zucker and Spiegelman (2007, 2008) present further details on the asymptotic theory and a simulation study under Weibull survival with a single binary covariate having known misclassification rates. In these simulations, the method presented here performed similarly to related methods we have examined in previous work. Specifically, our new estimator performed as well as or, in a few cases, better than the full Weibull maximum likelihood estimator. In further simulations for the case where the misclassification probabilities are estimated from an external replicate measures study our method generally performed well. The new estimator has a broader range of applicability than many other estimators proposed in the literature, including those described in our own earlier work, in that it can handle time-dependent covariates with an arbitrary misclassification structure.

Keywords and Phrases: Errors in variables, nonlinear models, proportional hazards

2.1   Introduction

Many regression analyses involve explanatory variables that are measured with error. It is well known that failing to account for covariate error can lead to biased estimates of the regression coefficients. For linear models, theory for handling covariate error has been developed over the past 50 or more years; Fuller (1987) provides an authoritative exposition. For nonlinear models, theory has been developing over the past 25 or so years. Carroll *et al.* (2006) provide a comprehensive summary of the development to date; currently, the covariate error problem for nonlinear models remains an active research area. In particular, beginning with Prentice (1982), a growing literature has developed on the Cox (1972) proportional hazards survival regression model when some covariates are measured with error. In this chapter, we focus on discrete covariates subject to misclassification, which are of interest in many epidemiological studies.

Three basic design setups are of interest. In all three designs, we have a main survival cohort for which surrogate covariate measurements and survival time data are available on all individuals. The designs are as follows: (1) the internal validation design, where the true covariate values are available on a subset of the main survival cohort; (2) the external validation design, where the measurement error distribution is estimated from data outside the main survival study; and (3) the replicate measurements design, where replicate surrogate covariate measurements are available, either on a subset of the survival study cohort or on individuals outside the main survival study. Also, two types of models for the measurement error are of interest [see Fuller (1987, p. 2) and Carroll *et al.* (2006, Section 1.2)]: structural models, where the true covariates are random variables, and functional models, where the true covariates are fixed values. Structural model methods generally involve estimation of some aspect of the distribution of the true covariate values; in functional model methods, this process is avoided.

The Cox model with covariate error has been examined in various settings. Zucker and Spiegelman (2007, 2008) give a detailed review of the existing work. Much of this work focuses on the independent additive error model, under which the observed covariate value is equal to the true value plus a random error whose distribution is independent of the true value. For discrete covariates subject to misclassification, this model practically never holds, and so the methods built upon it do not apply. Other methods exist, but are subject to various limitations. There is a need for a convenient method for all three study designs that can handle general measurement error structures, both functional and structural models, and time-dependent covariates. The aim of our work is to provide such a method for the case where the error-prone covariates are discrete, with misclassification of arbitrary form. Our method builds on a corrected score approach developed by Akazawa *et al.* (1998) for generalized linear models. We begin by reviewing their work, and we then present our extension to the Cox model.

2.2 Review of the Corrected Score Technique

We work with a sample of n independent individuals. Associated with each individual i is a response variable T_i and a p-vector of covariates $\mathbf{X}_i$. The conditional density or mass function of T_i given $\mathbf{X}_i$ is denoted by $f(t|\mathbf{X}_i, \boldsymbol{\theta})$, where $\boldsymbol{\theta}$ is a q-vector of unknown parameters, which includes regression coefficients and auxiliary parameters such as error variances. We have in mind mainly generalized linear models such as linear, logistic, and Poisson regression, but we present the theory in a general way. We denote the true value of $\boldsymbol{\theta}$ by $\boldsymbol{\theta}_0$. Extending Akazawa *et al.* (1998), we partition the vector $\mathbf{X}_i$ into $\mathbf{W}_i$ and $\mathbf{Z}_i$, where $\mathbf{W}_i$ is a p_1-vector of error-prone covariates and $\mathbf{Z}_i$ is a p_2-vector of error-free covariates. We denote the observed value of $\mathbf{W}_i$ by $\tilde{\mathbf{W}}_i$. The vector $\mathbf{W}_i$ is assumed to be discrete, with its possible values (each one a p_1-vector) denoted by $\mathbf{w}_1, \ldots, \mathbf{w}_K$. The range of values of $\tilde{\mathbf{W}}_i$ is assumed to be the same as that for $\mathbf{W}_i$. We denote by $k(i)$ the value of k such that $\tilde{\mathbf{W}}_i = \mathbf{w}_k$. The vector $\mathbf{Z}_i$ of error-free covariates is allowed to be either discrete or continuous. We denote $A_{kl}^{(i)} = \Pr(\tilde{\mathbf{W}}_i = \mathbf{w}_l | \mathbf{W}_i = \mathbf{w}_k, \mathbf{Z}_i, T_i)$, which defines a square matrix $\mathbf{A}^{(i)}$ of classification probabilities. As the notation indicates, we allow the classification probabilities to depend on $\mathbf{Z}_i$ and T_i (e.g., through a suitable model). This feature can be useful in certain applications; in others, it is sensible to assume that the same classification probabilities apply to all individuals. We assume for now that $\mathbf{A}^{(i)}$ is known. We denote by $\mathbf{B}^{(i)}$ the matrix inverse of $\mathbf{A}^{(i)}$. We assume this inverse exists, which will be the case if the misclassification is not too extreme [cf. Zucker and Spiegelman, (2004, Appendix A.1)]. When individual i is a member of an internal validation sample, for the estimation of $\boldsymbol{\theta}$ we set $\tilde{\mathbf{W}}_i = \mathbf{W}_i$ and replace $\mathbf{A}^{(i)}$ by the identity matrix.

Define $\mathbf{u}(t, \mathbf{w}, \mathbf{z}, \boldsymbol{\theta}) = [\partial/\partial\boldsymbol{\theta}] \log f(t|\mathbf{w}, \mathbf{z}, \boldsymbol{\theta})$ and $\mathbf{u}_i(\boldsymbol{\theta}) = \mathbf{u}(T_i, \mathbf{W}_i, \mathbf{Z}_i, \boldsymbol{\theta})$. The classical normalized likelihood score function when there is no covariate error is then given by $\mathbf{U}(\boldsymbol{\theta}) = n^{-1} \sum_i \mathbf{u}_i(\boldsymbol{\theta})$, and the maximum likelihood estimate (MLE) is obtained by solving the equation $\mathbf{U}(\boldsymbol{\theta}) = \mathbf{0}$. Under classical conditions, $E_{\boldsymbol{\theta}_0}[\mathbf{U}(\boldsymbol{\theta}_0)] = \mathbf{0}$ and the MLE is consistent and asymptotically normal. The idea of the corrected score approach is to find a function $\mathbf{u}^*(t, \tilde{\mathbf{w}}, \mathbf{z}, \boldsymbol{\theta})$ such that

$$E[\mathbf{u}^*(T_i, \tilde{\mathbf{W}}_i, \mathbf{Z}_i, \boldsymbol{\theta})|\mathbf{W}_i, \mathbf{Z}_i, T_i] = \mathbf{u}(T_i, \mathbf{W}_i, \mathbf{Z}_i, \boldsymbol{\theta}). \tag{2.1}$$

Then, with $\mathbf{u}_i^*(\boldsymbol{\theta}) = \mathbf{u}^*(T_i, \tilde{\mathbf{W}}_i, \mathbf{Z}_i, \boldsymbol{\theta})$, we use the modified likelihood score function $\mathbf{U}^*(\boldsymbol{\theta}) = n^{-1} \sum_i \mathbf{u}_i^*(\boldsymbol{\theta})$ in place of $\mathbf{U}(\boldsymbol{\theta})$ as the basis for estimation.

The estimation equation thus becomes $\mathbf{U}^*(\boldsymbol{\theta}) = \mathbf{0}$. In the case of discrete error-prone covariates, as shown by Akazawa *et al.* (1998), a function $\mathbf{u}^*$ satisfying (2.1) is given by a simple formula:

$$\mathbf{u}_i^*(\boldsymbol{\theta}) = \sum_{l=1}^{K} B_{k(i)l}^{(i)} \mathbf{u}(T_i, \mathbf{w}_l, \mathbf{Z}_i, \boldsymbol{\theta}). \tag{2.2}$$

Let $\mathbf{J}_i(\boldsymbol{\theta})$ be the matrix with elements $J_{i,rs}(\boldsymbol{\theta}) = (\partial/\partial\theta_s)u_{i,r}(\boldsymbol{\theta})$ and let $\mathbf{J}_i^*(\boldsymbol{\theta})$ be defined correspondingly with $\mathbf{u}_i^*$ in place of $\mathbf{u}_i$.

Under the typical conditions assumed in generalized estimation equations (GEE) theory, the estimator $\hat{\boldsymbol{\theta}}$ will be consistent and asymptotically normal. The limiting covariance matrix $\mathbf{V}$ of $\sqrt{n}(\hat{\boldsymbol{\theta}} - \boldsymbol{\theta}_0)$ can be estimated using the sandwich estimator $\hat{\mathbf{V}} = \mathbf{D}(\hat{\boldsymbol{\theta}})^{-1}\mathbf{H}(\hat{\boldsymbol{\theta}})\mathbf{D}(\hat{\boldsymbol{\theta}})^{-1}$, where $\mathbf{H}(\boldsymbol{\theta}) = n^{-1}\sum_i \mathbf{u}_i^*(\boldsymbol{\theta})$ $\mathbf{u}_i^*(\boldsymbol{\theta})^T$ and $\mathbf{D}(\boldsymbol{\theta}) = -n^{-1}\sum_i \mathbf{J}_i^*(\boldsymbol{\theta})$.

The case where there are replicate measurements $\tilde{\mathbf{W}}_{ij}$ of $\tilde{\mathbf{W}}$ on the individuals in the main study can be handled in various ways. A simple approach is to redefine the quantity $\mathbf{u}_i^*(\boldsymbol{\theta})$ given in (2.2) by replacing $B_{k(i)l}^{(i)}$ with the mean of $B_{k(i,j)l}^{(i)}$ over the replicates for individual i, with $k(i,j)$ defined as the value of k such that $\tilde{\mathbf{W}}_{ij} = \mathbf{w}_k$. The development then proceeds as before.

2.3   Application to the Cox Survival Model

2.3.1   Setup

We now show how to apply the foregoing corrected score approach to the Cox model. Denote the survival time by T_i° and the censoring time by C_i. The observed survival data then consist of the observed follow-up time $T_i = \min(T_i^\circ, C_i)$ and the event indicator $\delta_i = I(T_i^\circ \leq C_i)$. We let $Y_i(t) = I(T_i \geq t)$ denote the at-risk indicator. We assume the failure process and the censoring process are conditionally independent given the covariate process in the sense described by Kalbfleisch and Prentice (2002, Sections 6.2 and 6.3).

The covariate structure is as described in the preceding section, except that the covariates are allowed to be time-dependent, so that we write $k(i,t)$ and $\mathbf{Z}_i(t)$. We assume that the measurement error process is "localized" in the sense that it depends only on the current true covariate value. More precisely, the assumption is that, conditional on the value of $\mathbf{X}_i(t)$, the value of $\tilde{\mathbf{W}}_i(t)$ is independent of the survival and censoring processes and of the values of $\mathbf{X}_i(s)$ for $s \neq t$. This assumption is plausible in many settings, for example, when the main source of error is technical or laboratory error, or reading/coding error, as with diagnostic X-rays and dietary intake assessments. With no change in the theory, the classification probabilities $A_{kl}^{(i)}$ can be allowed to depend upon t. This extension permits accounting for improvements in measurement techniques over time. In addition, if internal validation data are available, this extension allows us to dispense with the localized error assumption.

In the proportional hazards model, the hazard function is taken to be of the form $\lambda(t|\mathbf{X}(t)) = \lambda_0(t)\psi(\mathbf{X}(t); \boldsymbol{\beta})$, with $\lambda_0(t)$ being a baseline hazard function of unspecified form. The function $\psi(\mathbf{x}; \boldsymbol{\beta})$, which involves a p-vector $\boldsymbol{\beta}$ of unknown regression parameters which are to be estimated, represents the relative risk for an individual with covariate vector $\mathbf{x}$. The classical Cox model assumes $\psi(\mathbf{x}; \boldsymbol{\beta}) = e^{\boldsymbol{\beta}^T \mathbf{x}}$. In line with Thomas (1981) and Breslow and Day (1993, Section 5.1(c)), we allow a general relative risk function $\psi(\mathbf{x}; \boldsymbol{\beta})$ which is assumed to be positive in a neighborhood of the true $\boldsymbol{\beta}$ for all $\mathbf{x}$ and to be twice differentiable with respect to the components of $\boldsymbol{\beta}$. We assume further that $\psi(\mathbf{x}; \mathbf{0}) = 1$, which simply means that $\boldsymbol{\beta} = \mathbf{0}$ corresponds to no covariate effect. In many applications, it will be desirable to take $\psi(\mathbf{x}; \boldsymbol{\beta})$ to be a function that is monotone in each component of $\mathbf{x}$ for all $\boldsymbol{\beta}$. We let $\boldsymbol{\beta}_0$ denote the true value of $\boldsymbol{\beta}$.

2.3.2   The method

We now describe the method. Let $\psi_r'(\mathbf{x}; \boldsymbol{\beta})$ denote the partial derivative of $\psi(\mathbf{x}; \boldsymbol{\beta})$ with respect to β_r and define $\xi_r(\mathbf{x}; \boldsymbol{\beta}) = \psi_r'(\mathbf{x}; \boldsymbol{\beta})/\psi(\mathbf{x}; \boldsymbol{\beta})$. Then the classical Cox partial likelihood score function in the case with no measurement error is given by

$$U_r(\boldsymbol{\beta}) = \frac{1}{n}\sum_{i=1}^{n} \delta_i \left(\xi_r(\mathbf{X}_i(T_i); \boldsymbol{\beta}) - \frac{e_{1r}(T_i)}{e_0(T_i)} \right), \qquad (2.3)$$

where

$$e_0(t) = \frac{1}{n}\sum_{j=1}^{n} Y_j(t)\psi(\mathbf{X}_j(t); \boldsymbol{\beta}), \;\; e_{1r}(t) = \frac{1}{n}\sum_{j=1}^{n} Y_j(t)\psi_r'(\mathbf{X}_j(t); \boldsymbol{\beta}).$$

Now define

$$\psi_i^*(t, \boldsymbol{\beta}) = \sum_{l=1}^{K} B_{k(i,t)l}^{(i)}\psi(\mathbf{w}_l, \mathbf{Z}_i(t); \boldsymbol{\beta}), \;\; \eta_{ir}(t, \boldsymbol{\beta}) = \sum_{l=1}^{K} B_{k(i,t)l}^{(i)}\psi_r'(\mathbf{w}_l, \mathbf{Z}_i(t); \boldsymbol{\beta}),$$

$$\xi_{ir}^*(t, \boldsymbol{\beta}) = \sum_{l=1}^{K} B_{k(i,t)l}^{(i)}\xi_r(\mathbf{w}_l, \mathbf{Z}_i(t); \boldsymbol{\beta}), \;\; e_0^*(t) = \frac{1}{n}\sum_{j=1}^{n} Y_j(t)\psi_j^*(t, \boldsymbol{\beta}),$$

$$e_{1r}^*(t) = \frac{1}{n}\sum_{j=1}^{n} Y_j(t)\eta_{jr}(t, \boldsymbol{\beta}).$$

Then our proposed corrected score function is the following obvious analogue of (2.3):

$$U_r^*(\boldsymbol{\beta}) = \frac{1}{n} \sum_{i=1}^{n} \delta_i \left(\xi_{ir}^*(T_i, \boldsymbol{\beta}) - \frac{e_{1r}^*(T_i)}{e_0^*(T_i)} \right). \tag{2.4}$$

As before, the proposed corrected score estimator is the solution to $\mathbf{U}^*(\boldsymbol{\beta}) = \mathbf{0}$, where $\mathbf{U}^*$ denotes the vector whose components are U_r^*.

Using an iterated expectation argument, under the localized error assumption, we can show that

$$E[Y_i(t)\psi_i^*(t, \boldsymbol{\beta})|\mathbf{X}_i(t)] = E[Y_i(t)\psi(\mathbf{X}_i(t); \boldsymbol{\beta})|\mathbf{X}_i(t)], \tag{2.5}$$

$$E[Y_i(t)\eta_{ir}^*(t, \boldsymbol{\beta})|\mathbf{X}_i(t)] = E[Y_i(t)\psi_r'(\mathbf{X}_i(t), \boldsymbol{\beta})|\mathbf{X}_i(t)], \tag{2.6}$$

$$E[Y_i(t)\xi_{ir}^*(t, \boldsymbol{\beta})|\mathbf{X}_i(t)] = E[Y_i(t)\xi_r(\mathbf{X}_i(t), \boldsymbol{\beta})|\mathbf{X}_i(t)]. \tag{2.7}$$

Thus, referring to the quantity in parentheses in (2.4), the first term and the numerator and denominator of the second term all have the correct expectation. It follows that $\mathbf{U}^*(\boldsymbol{\beta})$ is an asymptotically unbiased score function.

Accordingly, under standard conditions such as those of Andersen and Gill (1982) and of Prentice and Self (1983), our corrected score estimator will be consistent and asymptotically normal. The asymptotic covariance matrix of $\sqrt{n}(\hat{\boldsymbol{\beta}} - \boldsymbol{\beta}_0)$ may be estimated by the sandwich formula $\hat{\mathbf{V}} = \mathbf{D}(\hat{\boldsymbol{\beta}})^{-1}\mathbf{H}(\hat{\boldsymbol{\beta}})\mathbf{D}(\hat{\boldsymbol{\beta}})^{-1}$. Here $\mathbf{D}(\boldsymbol{\beta})$ is -1 times the matrix of derivatives of $\mathbf{U}^*(\boldsymbol{\beta})$ with respect to the components of $\boldsymbol{\beta}$ and $\mathbf{H}(\boldsymbol{\beta})$ is an empirical estimate of the covariance matrix of $\sqrt{n}\,\mathbf{U}^*(\boldsymbol{\beta})$.

We note again that, for the internal validation design, the available true $\mathbf{W}$ values can be used in the estimation of $\boldsymbol{\beta}$ by replacing $\tilde{\mathbf{W}}_i$ with $\mathbf{W}_i$ and $\mathbf{A}^{(i)}$ by the identity matrix when individual i is in the internal validation sample. Alternatively, the hybrid scheme of Zucker and Spiegelman (2004, Section 5) can be used. Also, the case where there are replicate measurements $\tilde{\mathbf{W}}_{ij}$ of $\tilde{\mathbf{W}}$ on the individuals in the main study can be handled as described at the end of the preceding section.

In Zucker and Spiegelman (2007, 2008) we give an outline of the asymptotic argument, explicit expressions for the matrices $\mathbf{H}$ and $\mathbf{D}$, an estimator of the cumulative hazard function, and an extension of the theory to the case where the classification matrix $\mathbf{A}^{(i)}$ is estimated. We also give results of a finite-sample simulation study under Weibull survival with a single binary covariate having known misclassification rates. The performance of the method described here was similar to that of related methods we have examined in previous work [Zucker and Spielgelman (2004) and Zucker (2005)]. Specifically, our new estimator performed as well as or, in a few cases, better than the full Weibull maximum likelihood estimator. We also present simulation results for our method for the case where the misclassification probabilities are estimated from an external replicate measures study. Our method generally performed well in these simulations.

2.4 Example

We illustrate our method on data from the Nurses Health Study concerning the relationship between dietary calcium (Ca) intake and incidence of distal colon cancer [Wu *et al.* (2002, Table 4)]. The data consist of observations on female nurses whose calcium intake was assessed through a food frequency questionnaire (FFQ) in 1984 and were followed up to May 31, 1996 for distal colon cancer occurrence. Our analysis includes data on 60,575 nurses who reported in 1984 that they had never taken calcium supplements, and focuses on the effect of baseline calcium intake after adjustment for baseline body mass index (BMI) and baseline aspirin use. In line with Wu *et al.*'s analysis, we use the classical Cox relative risk function $\psi(\boldsymbol{\beta}; \mathbf{x}) = e^{\boldsymbol{\beta}^T \mathbf{x}}$, and, as in Wu *et al.*'s Table 4, we work with a binary "high Ca" risk factor defined as 1 if the calcium intake was greater than 700 mg/day and 0 otherwise. Note that one glass of milk contains approximately 300 mg of calcium. BMI is expressed in terms of the following categories: <22 kg/m^2, 22 to <25 kg/m^2, 25 to <30 kg/m^2, and 30 kg/m^2 or greater. Aspirin use is coded as yes (1) or no (0). Thus, our model has five explanatory variables, one for the binary risk factor (W), three dummy variables for BMI (Z_1, Z_2, Z_3), and one for aspirin use (Z_4). BMI and aspirin use status are assumed to be measured without error.

It is well known that the FFQ measures dietary intake with some degree of error and more reliable information can be obtained from a diet record (DR) [Willett (1998, Chapter 6)]. We thus take W to be the Ca risk factor indicator based on the DR and $\tilde{W}$ to be the Ca risk factor indicator based on the FFQ. The classification probabilities are estimated using data from the Nurse's Health Study validation study [Willett (1998, pp. 122–126)]. The estimates obtained were $\Pr(\tilde{W} = 0 | W = 0) = 0.78$ and $\Pr(\tilde{W} = 1 | W = 1) = 0.72$, with corresponding estimated standard errors of 0.042 and 0.046.

Table 2.1 presents the results of the following analyses: (1) a naive classical Cox regression analysis ignoring measurement error, corresponding to an assumption that there is no measurement error; (2) our method with $\mathbf{A}$ assumed known and set according to the foregoing estimated classification probabilities, ignoring the estimation error in these probabilities; and (3) our method with $\mathbf{A}$ estimated as above with the estimation error in the probabilities taken into account (main study/external validation study design).

The results followed the expected pattern. Adjusting for the misclassification in calcium intake had a marked effect on the estimated relative risk for high calcium intake. Accounting for the error in estimating the classification probabilities increased (modestly) the standard error of the log relative risk estimate. The relative risk estimates for high calcium intake and corresponding 95% confidence intervals obtained in the three analyses were as follows.

Table 2.1. Estimated coefficients and standard errors for the Nurses Health Study of the relationship between dietary calcium intake and distal colon cancer incidence

Method	High Calcium		BMI of 22 to <25		BMI of 25 to <30		BMI of 30+		Aspirin Use	
	Estimate	Std Err	Estimate	Std Err	Estimate	Std Err	Estimate	Std Err	Estimate	Std Err
Cox	−0.3448	0.1694	0.6837	0.2240	0.5352	0.2395	0.5729	0.2876	−0.4941	0.1954
CS0	−0.7121	0.3690	0.7124	0.2247	0.5776	0.2419	0.6157	0.2892	−0.4994	0.1955
CS1	−0.7121	0.3832	0.7124	0.2249	0.5776	0.2423	0.6157	0.2896	−0.4994	0.1955

Cox = Classical Cox regression analysis.

CS0 = Corrected score method, observed classification matrix taken as known.

CS1 = Corrected score method, accounting for uncertainty in the classification matrix.

Method	Estimate	95% CI
Naive Cox	0.71	[0.51,0.99]
A known	0.49	[0.24,1.01]
A estimated	0.49	[0.23,1.04]

The misclassification adjustment had a small effect on the estimated regression coefficients for the BMI dummy variables and essentially no effect on the estimated regression coefficient for aspirin use.

References

1. Akazawa, K., Kinukawa, N., and Nakamura, T. (1998). A note on the corrected score function corrected for misclassification, *Journal of the Japan Statistical Society*, **28**, 115–123.

2. Andersen, P. K. and Gill, R. D. (1982). Cox's regression model for counting processes: A large sample study, *The Annals of Statistics*, **10**, 1100–1120.

3. Breslow, N. and Day, N. E. (1993). *Statistical Methods in Cancer Research*, Volume 2: *The Design and Analysis of Cohort Studies*, Oxford University Press, Oxford.

4. Carroll, R. J., Ruppert, D., Stefanski, L. A., and Crainiceanu, C. M. (2006). *Measurement Error in Nonlinear Models: A Modern Perspective*, 2nd ed. Chapman and Hall/CRC, Boca Raton.

5. Cox, D. R. (1972). Regression models and life-tables (with discussion), *Journal of the Royal Statistical Society, Series B*, **34**, 187–220.

6. Fuller, W. A. (1987). *Measurement Error Models*, John Wiley & Sons, New York.

7. Kalbfleisch, J. D. and Prentice, R. L. (2002). *The Statistical Analysis of Failure Time Data*, 2nd ed. John Wiley & Sons, New York.

8. Prentice, R. (1982). Covariate measurement errors and parameter estimation in a failure time regression model, *Biometrika*, **69**, 331–342.

9. Prentice, R. L. and Self, S. G. (1983). Asymptotic distribution theory for Cox-type regression models with general relative risk form, *The Annals of Statistics*, **11**, 804–812.

10. Thomas, D. C. (1981). General relative-risk models for survival time and matched case-control analysis, *Biometrics*, **37**, 673–686.

11. Willett, W. C. (1998). *Nutritional Epidemiology*, 2nd ed., Oxford University Press, New York.

12. Wu, K., Willett, W. C., Fuchs, C. S., Colditz, G. A., and Giovannucci, E. L. (2002). Calcium intake and risk of colon cancer in women and men, *Journal of the National Cancer Institute*, **94**, 437–446.

13. Zucker, D. M. (2005). A pseudo partial likelihood method for semiparametric survival regression with covariate errors, *Journal of the American Statistical Association*, **100**, 1264–1277.

14. Zucker, D. M. and Spiegelman, D. (2004). Inference for the proportional hazards model with misclassified discrete-valued covariates, *Biometrics,* **60**, 324–334.

15. Zucker, D. M. and Spiegelman, D. (2007). Corrected score estimation in the proportional hazards model with misclassified discrete covariates. Technical Report, Hebrew University. Available online at http://pluto.mscc.huji.ac.il/~mszucker.

16. Zucker, D. M. and Spiegelman, D. (2008). Corrected score estimation in the proportional hazards model with misclassified discrete covariates, *Statistics in Medicine*, in press.

3

A Varying-Coefficient Hazards Regression Model for Multiple Cross-Effect

Hong-Dar Isaac Wu

School of Public Health and Biostatistics Center, China Medical University, Taiwan

Abstract: We consider a piecewise-constant varying-coefficient model to account for survival data with multiple crossings. Estimating procedures are provided, and a class of tests is constructed in order to impose varying coefficients for some specific covariates, or for some other purposes. Analysis of the survival of Taiwan's stroke patients is reported to illustrate the applications.

Keywords and Phrases: Time-varying effect, heteroscedasticity, multiple crossings, proportional hazards, nonproportional hazards

3.1 Introduction

In event-history data analysis where the effect of a specific variable is the main interest, the problem of dealing with time-varying effects has become more important in recent years. In contrast with the proportional hazards (PH) model [Cox (1972)], many authors have devoted themselves to the study of the varying-coefficient PH (PH^{VC}) model. For example, see Murphy and Sen (1991), Murphy (1993), Martinussen and Scheike (2006), and Tian et al. (2005) among others. Without regard to the space of time, the PH^{VC} model basically still estimates the homogeneity effect over the space of covariate(s). By *homogeneity* we mean that there is a common effect between two covariate-specific subpopulations represented by different values of the covariate, say Z, or of the configurations of several covariates. On the contrary, *heterogeneity* states that the effect is different and diverse over the covariate space of Z. The variable Z can either be observed or unobserved. Examples of modeling observed and unobserved heterogeneity include the heteroscedastic hazards regression (HHR) model [Hsieh (2001)] and the frailty model [Vaupel (1979) and Hougaard (1986)], respectively. This study focuses on the former case. In addition to capturing the heterogeneity effect, the HHR model also has the merit of modeling time-varying effects by the hazard function:

$$\lambda(t; \mathbf{z}, \mathbf{x}) = \lambda_0(t) e^{\gamma^T \mathbf{x}(t)} \{\Lambda_0(t)\}^{e^{\gamma^T \mathbf{x}(t)} - 1} e^{\beta^T \mathbf{z}(t)}, \qquad (3.1)$$

where $\mathbf{z}(t)$ and $\mathbf{x}(t)$ are two sets of predictable time-dependent covariates, and $\Lambda_0(t) = \int_0^t \lambda_0(u) du$ is the baseline cumulative hazard. In view of the intrinsic time-varying property of the hazard ratio implied by (3.1), it is possible to extend the HHR model to incorporate varying-coefficient settings. Hereafter we denote the varying-coefficient HHR model as an HHR^{VC} model with its functional form stated in Section 3.2. Contrasting with the PH model, the most significant goals are certainly to make feasible the incorporation of parameter γ, and to convince us about the use of time-varying $\beta(t)$ and $\gamma(t)$ [see (3.2) below]. Motivation of this extension can be interpreted as follows. First, the inter-relation among groups in terms of survivor or cumulative hazard functions may be diverse in time. An apparent phenomenon is the multiple cross-effect (MCE) studied by Bagdonavičius and Nikulin (2005). Second, cure-fraction (CF) appeared in many clinical and oncological studies in which the survival of cancer patients receiving surgery followed by (or prior to) chemo- and/or radiotherapies are of concern. However, the definition of "cure" still needs to be clarified. The probability of cure needs to be handled. Finally, if the data cannot be suitably described by a simpler model (such as the PH or PH^{VC} model) and can be well described by the extended model (such as the HHR^{VC}), it is also sensible to consider the extended class from the viewpoint of model fitting.

The HHR^{VC} model can deal with survival data with time-diversity (e.g., MCE) and cure-fraction simultaneously, within a reasonable range of observational period. The purpose of this chapter is to study the applicability and model validity problems of HHR^{VC}. For the latter, we assume HHR^{VC} as the alternative hypothesis and test whether the varying-coefficient setting can be further simplified. Section 3.2 introduces the piecewise-constant setting of the HHR^{VC} model. Estimation and model validity procedures are provided in Sections 3.3 and 3.4. In Section 3.5 we report actual data analysis concerning the mortality of stroke patients with comorbidities. Finally, implications of the varying-coefficient model and some practical issues of data analysis are discussed.

3.2 Illustration of the Piecewise-Constant Model

Piecewise-constant setting

Model (3.1) can be extended to allow for varying coefficients:

$$\lambda_{\mathbf{z},\mathbf{x}}(t) = \lambda_0(t)\{\Lambda_0(t)\}^{e^{\gamma(t)\mathbf{z}}-1}e^{\beta(t)\mathbf{z}+\gamma(t)\mathbf{x}}, \tag{3.2}$$

where $e^{\beta(t)\mathbf{z}}$ is referred to as the *risk function*, and $e^{\gamma(t)\mathbf{x}}$ as the *heteroscedasticity component*. For an easy exposition, we adopt notations only with the univariate case and, in the sequel, $\mathbf{z} = \mathbf{x}$. Due to the fact that the partial likelihood does not eliminate the baseline hazard, there are three time-dependent parameters, ($\Lambda_0(t)$ (or $\lambda_0(t)$), $\beta(t)$, and $\gamma(t)$) to be estimated simultaneously. We use the *piecewise-constant approximation* method [Murphy and Sen (1991), Murphy (1993), and Marzec and Marzec (1997)] to make it compatible with the approach of Hsieh (2001). Let $[0, \tau]$ be the observational period, and $0 = \tau_0 < \tau_1 < \cdots < \tau_m = \tau$ be a set of cutoff points. The following piecewise-constant approximations are adopted.

$$
\begin{aligned}
\overline{\Lambda}_0(t) &= \int_0^t \sum_1^m \alpha_j \mathbf{1}_{(\tau_{j-1}<u\leq\tau_j)} du, \\
\overline{\beta}(t) &= \sum_1^m \beta_j \mathbf{1}_{(\tau_{j-1}<t\leq\tau_j)}, \\
\overline{\gamma}(t) &= \sum_1^m \gamma_j \mathbf{1}_{(\tau_{j-1}<t\leq\tau_j)}.
\end{aligned}
\tag{3.3}
$$

Thus the HHR^{VC} model considered in this chapter has the following "pieces" of hazard and cumulative hazard.

$$
\begin{aligned}
\overline{\lambda}(t;\mathbf{z}) &= \alpha_j\{\overline{\Lambda}_0(t)\}^{\sigma_j-1}\sigma_j\mu_j, \quad \tau_{j-1} < t \leq \tau_j, \\
\overline{\Lambda}(t;\mathbf{z}) &= \overline{\Lambda}(\tau_{j-1};\mathbf{z}) + [\{\overline{\Lambda}_0(t)\}^{\sigma_j} - \{\overline{\Lambda}_0(\tau_{j-1})\}^{\sigma_j}]\mu_j, \quad \tau_{j-1} < t \leq \tau_j,
\end{aligned}
\tag{3.4}
$$

where $\overline{\lambda}(\cdot)$ denotes the approximation of $\lambda(\cdot)$, $\sigma_j = e^{\gamma_j^T\mathbf{z}}$, $\mu_j = e^{\beta_j^T\mathbf{z}}$, and $\overline{\Lambda}(\tau_0;\mathbf{z}) = \overline{\Lambda}_0(\tau_0) = 0$. Formula (3.4) is very useful in understanding the HHR^{VC} model and the accompanying random number generation in simulation studies [because we can simply use the relation $S(\cdot) = \exp\{-\Lambda(\cdot)\}$, and equate it to a Uniform(0,1)-random number].

The reasons why we consider (3.2) [or (3.4)] for modeling multiple-crossings are: (i) the HHR model without varying coefficient gives only a *one-time crossing*; and (ii) although the PH model with varying-coefficient risk function produces multiple crossings, the intersubpopulation effect is still homogeneous *at any fixed time point.* An example of data analysis in Section 3.5 illustrates the feasibility, where the probability of "cure" is actually a heterogeneity effect. By model (3.2), suitably modulating the baseline hazard also contributes to model "multiple cross-effects plus cure-fraction," albeit a *monotonic* $\gamma(t)$ is inevitably demanded.

3.3 Estimation Under the Piecewise-Constant Setting

Suppose there are n randomly right-censored observations $T_1 < T_2 < \cdots < T_n$, which can be survival or censoring times. Let $\lambda_i(t; \mathbf{z}(t), \mathbf{x}(t))$, $N_i(t)$ and $Y_i(t))$ be the intensity process, counting process, and the associated at-risk indicator for the ith individual at time t, and denote

$$S_{\mathbf{J}}(t) = (1/n) \sum_{i=1}^{n} Y_i(t) \mathbf{J}(t) e^{\overline{\beta}(t)\mathbf{z}_i + \overline{\gamma}(t)\mathbf{x}_i} \{\overline{\Lambda}_0(t)\}^{e^{\overline{\gamma}(t)\mathbf{x}_i} - 1}, \qquad (3.5)$$

with possibly time-dependent covariates $\mathbf{J}(t) = 1, \mathbf{z}_i(t), \mathbf{x}_i(t)$, or $\mathbf{v}_i(t) \equiv \mathbf{x}_i(t)$ $\{1 + e^{\overline{\gamma}(t)\mathbf{x}_i} \log \overline{\Lambda}_0(t)\}$. It is straightforward to use the following Breslow-type equation (3.6) for the baseline cumulative hazard and estimating equations (3.7) and (3.8) for β_js and γ_js.

$$\overline{\Lambda}_0(t) = \sum_{i=1}^{n} \int_0^t \frac{dN_i(u)}{nS_1(u)}, \qquad (3.6)$$

$$M_{2j} \equiv \frac{1}{\sqrt{n_j}} \sum_{i=1}^{n} \int_{\tau_{j-1}}^{\tau_j} \left\{ \mathbf{z}_i - \frac{S_{\mathbf{z}}}{S_1} \right\} dN_i(u) = 0, \quad j = 1, 2, \ldots, m, \qquad (3.7)$$

and

$$M_{3j} \equiv \frac{1}{\sqrt{n_j}} \sum_{i=1}^{n} \int_{\tau_{j-1}}^{\tau_j} \left\{ \mathbf{v}_i - \frac{S_{\mathbf{v}}}{S_1} \right\} dN_i(u) = 0, \quad j = 1, 2, \ldots, m. \qquad (3.8)$$

In addition, $\mathbf{M}_j = (M_{2j}, M_{3j})^T$, and $\mathcal{A}_j$ with elements

$$A_{j,ll'} = (1/n) \sum \int \mathrm{E}\{dM_{lj}(u) dM_{l'j}(u)\} du, \quad (l, l' = 2, 3)$$

is the covariation matrix between M_{2j} and M_{3j}. By imposing several technical conditions, large-sample properties of $\{(\widehat{\beta}_j, \widehat{\gamma}_j)\}_{j=1}^{m}$ and $\widehat{\Lambda}_0(t)$ can be established.

3.4 The Tests

In this section we study the HHR^{VC} model, starting from the consideration of the following statistic [Hsieh (2001) and Wu *et al.* (2002)]:

$$\mathcal{T}_{\textbf{degen}} = \sum_{j=1}^{m}\{\mathbf{M}_j^T \mathcal{A}_j^{-1}\mathbf{M}_j\}_{(\widehat{\beta}_j,\widehat{\gamma}_j,\widehat{\Lambda}_0)}$$

with the parameters of interest being evaluated piecewise at $(\beta_j,\gamma_j) = (\widehat{\beta}_j,\widehat{\gamma}_j)$, $\forall j$, where $\widehat{\beta}_j$ and $\widehat{\gamma}_j$ are the piecewise estimates solved from (3.7) and (3.8). The statistic $\mathcal{T}_{\textbf{degen}}$ has a degenerate value of 0; named *"degenerate"* because all degrees of freedom were *consumed* at each segment. However, it offers an important clue to constructing tests for model validity. For example, the test studied in Wu *et al.* (2002) can be viewed as a special case when the HHR model is treated as a submodel of HHR^{VC}. By this perspective, $\mathcal{T}_{\textbf{degen}}$ can be amended to augment the degrees of freedom to $2m-2$ for the purpose of testing the validity of the HHR model, simply by replacing all β_js and γ_js with the overall estimates $\widehat{\beta}$ and $\widehat{\gamma}$, respectively, and by using $\widetilde{\mathcal{A}}_j^{\circ}$ (defined below) instead of $\mathcal{A}_j$.

3.4.1 Some specific tests

The test considered in this section is constructed by assuming that the HHR^{VC} model is true, and then testing for a subset of the parameters at a given value. Now we define some notations used in the following context. For example, if $\theta = (\theta_1,\ldots,\theta_p)$ and $\theta_{\mathbf{k}} = (\theta_1,\theta_2)$ are a subset of θ, then $\theta_{(\mathbf{k})} \equiv \theta\backslash\theta_{\mathbf{k}} = (\theta_3,\theta_4,\ldots,\theta_p)$, and $\theta = \theta_{\mathbf{k}} \cup \theta_{(\mathbf{k})} = \theta_{(\mathbf{k})} \cup \theta_{\mathbf{k}}$. In this case, $\omega_{\mathbf{k}} = \{1,2\}$, and $\omega_{(\mathbf{k})} = \{3,4,\ldots,p\}$. Moreover $\underline{\mathbf{M}} = (M_{21},\ldots,M_{2m},M_{31},\ldots,M_{3m})$, and, if $\theta_{\mathbf{k}^*} = (\theta_1,\theta_3)$, then $\theta_{\mathbf{k}}\backslash\theta_{\mathbf{k}^*} = \theta_2$ and $\theta_{\mathbf{k}}\cap\theta_{\mathbf{k}^*} = \theta_1$. We say in this example that $\theta_{\mathbf{k}}$ is the **k**-component of θ. Hereafter let us define $\theta = (\beta_1,\ldots,\beta_m,\gamma_1,\ldots,\gamma_m)$. In order to test the hypothesis $H_0 : \theta_{\mathbf{k}} = \theta_{\mathbf{k}0}$ versus $H_a : \theta_{\mathbf{k}} \neq \theta_{\mathbf{k}0}$ at some $\theta_{\mathbf{k}0}$, the proposed statistic is:

$$\mathcal{T}_{\mathbf{k}} = \sum_{j=1}^{m}\{\widetilde{\mathbf{M}}_j^T \widetilde{\mathcal{A}}_j^{\circ^{-1}}\widetilde{\mathbf{M}}_j\}_{\widehat{\theta}_{(\mathbf{k})}\cup\theta_{\mathbf{k}0}},$$

for which $\widetilde{\mathbf{M}}_j^T = (M_{2j},M_{3j}) \cap \{M_l \in \underline{\mathbf{M}} : l \in \omega_{\mathbf{k}}\}$ and $\widetilde{\mathcal{A}}_j^{\circ^{-1}} = \{\widetilde{\mathbf{A}}_{j,kk} - \widetilde{\mathbf{A}}_{j,k(k)}\widetilde{\mathbf{A}}_{j,(k)(k)}^{-1}\widetilde{\mathbf{A}}_{j,(k)k}\}^{-1}$ with $\widetilde{\mathcal{A}}_j^{\circ}$ being the covariation submatrix of $\widetilde{\mathbf{M}}_j$ associated with the **k**-component. Here a submatrix $\mathbf{B}_{k(k^*)}$ of $\mathbf{B}$ is defined as only keeping the **k**-component of $\mathbf{B}$ *in row* and with "deleting the **k***-component of $\mathbf{B}$" *in column*, and so on. Note that $\mathcal{T}_{\mathbf{k}}$ is basically a score-type test. Another useful test to be compared with the above $\mathcal{T}_{\mathbf{k}}$-test is the (full-) likelihood ratio test, which is not discussed in the present study.

Test for varying effect of a specific covariate

If the HHR^{VC} is the underlying model and piecewise-constant approximation is utilized, then the $T_{\{\cdot\}}$-statistic can be amended to test for varying effect *with respect to a specific covariate*. For example, if we want to test for constant heteroscedasticity [i.e., $\gamma(t) = \gamma_0, \forall t$, for some constant γ_0], the test statistic can be constructed as

$$\mathcal{T} = \sum_{j=1}^{m} \{\widetilde{\mathbf{M}}_j^T \widetilde{\mathcal{A}}_j^{\circ^{-1}} \widetilde{\mathbf{M}}_j\}_{(\widehat{\beta}_j, \gamma_0, \widehat{\Lambda}_0)}.$$

In practice γ_0 is substituted by an overall estimate $\widehat{\gamma}$. That is, assuming the HHR^{VC} model, our hypotheses are $H_0 : \gamma_1 = \cdots = \gamma_m = \gamma_0$ versus $H_a : \gamma_j$s are not all equal. If we set $\gamma_0 = \widehat{\gamma}$, the statistic $T_{\{\cdot\}}$ will be a χ^2_{m-1}-variate approximately.

Test for the varying-coefficient PH model

There are tests and diagnostic plots proposed to check for varying effects under the PH^{VC}-based framework [Murphy (1993), Valsecchi *et al.* (1996), Marzec and Marzec (1997), and Martinussen and Scheike (2006)]. Here we propose a test $\mathcal{T}_{\mathbf{phvc}}$ for the PH^{VC} model by assuming HHR^{VC} as the alternative hypothesis. This $\mathcal{T}_{\mathbf{phvc}}$-test can be compared with the performance of several tests proposed in Marzec and Marzec (1997) (which are omnibus). To this purpose, $\mathcal{T}_{\mathbf{phvc}}$ has the same form with $\mathcal{T}_{\mathbf{k}}$, except for being evaluated at $(\widehat{\beta}_j, 0, \widehat{\Lambda}_0)$ at the jth segment. Under the hypotheses $H_0: \gamma_j = 0, \forall j$ versus $H_a:$ at least one of the γ_js is not equal to 0; $\mathcal{T}_{\mathbf{phvc}}$ is distributed as χ^2_m for large n.

Test for equality

A commonly used test for equality is the log-rank test in the K-sample problem. The current $\mathcal{T}_{\{\cdot\}}$ can now be modified to test for equality among groups represented by different covariate values. Consider the hypotheses: $H_0: \beta_j = \gamma_j = 0, \forall j$; and $H_a:$ at least one of β_js and γ_js is not equal to 0. The statistic $(\mathcal{T}_{\mathbf{equal}})$ evaluated at H_0 is distributed as χ^2_{2m} asymptotically. Note that the proposed test for equality can be applied under a cure model. When the cure probabilities are large for distinct groups, a genuine difference among groups could be masked (or ignored) by these large probabilities of cure. However, the proposed test may have good power in testing the difference. In this case, it is also appealing to compare the performance of the present $\mathcal{T}$ with the modified score test studied by Bagdonavičius and Nikulin (2005) under their multiple cross-effect (MCE) model.

3.5   Data Analysis

The methods discussed above are implemented on stroke patients' survival data collected *retrospectively* from six regional teaching hospitals (bed number larger than 200) of central Taiwan during January 2002 to December 2003. These data comprise 616 individuals who experienced acute stroke with subtypes of cerebral hemorrhage, cerebral infarct, or transient ischemic attack. The zero-time point is defined as the time of an inpatient's hospitalization; and potential variables for explaining mortality rate include age, sex, disease subtype, length of hospital stay (LOS), comorbidity status of diabetes mellitus (DM) and/or hypertension, and so on. Some of the patients also have the Glasgow coma scale (GCS) and Barthel index data ascertained from hospital records. For a simple exposition, we only investigate the impact of comorbidity on the hazards. The Kaplan–Meier (KM) survival estimates exhibit multiple crossings and a high cure (or nonsusceptible to death) probability. For the other variables, sex and LOS are not significant, age has a nonhomogeneous effect, and the hazards among different stroke subtypes satisfy proportionality. Furthermore, the GCS and Barthel functional index are not recorded in a unified manner and are missing by a large proportion. So the subsequent analysis based on HHR^{VC} is basically *univariate*. The only variable used for interpreting the mortality is "comorbid disease status"; it is dichotomized into two groups: those *with* and *without* the coexistence of either DM or hypertension. The impact of comorbidity on the death rate of acute strokes is still inconclusive. Our analysis in this section attempts to disclose the time-varying property of relative hazards between the two groups of patients. However, the influential part of this kind of data is: there is a very high proportion of patients who still survive at the endtime of the study period.

The KM estimates are displayed in Figure 3.1, accompanied by a pair of survival curves obtained from the HHR^{VC} estimates. In order to give a clear comparison, the KM and HHR^{VC} survival estimates are plotted only within the range of $t \leq 697$ with $0.85 \leq S(t) \leq 1$, because a large proportion of patients survive beyond 697 days. The estimate proposed in the current study fits well to the nonparametric KM survivals. If we denote the failure or censoring time as T, the sample is divided into four segments ($m = 4$): those with $T < 10$, $10 \leq T < 35$, $35 \leq T < 244$, and $244 \leq T \leq 697$. The selected four segments contain 25, 13, 16, and 22 noncensored failure times in 25, 13, 16, and 562 observations. That means that the first three have no right-censoring cases, and

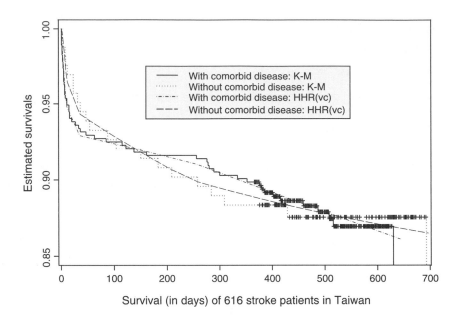

Figure 3.1. Survival of 616 stroke patients in Taiwan.

the last one has 540 censored observations. As a whole, the data have 76 failures, and censoring proportion is $540/616 = 87.7\%$. Here we do not put an artificial adjustment to get a better fit. These four segments are selected to control balanced sample sizes between segments as well as between the two groups, so that each segment contains *no less than* four noncensored failures for both groups. For group 1 (without comorbidity) [versus group 2 (with comorbidity)], there are 4[21], 4[9], 8[8], and 5[17] failures. Table 3.1 reports the *point estimates* of parameters $(\alpha_j, \beta_j, \gamma_j)$ for $j = 1, 2, 3, 4$ under the HHR^{VC} model. According to this result, the rate ratio [$\widehat{\text{RR}}(t)$, for $\tau_{J-1} < t \le \tau_J$] can be calculated from (3.3) and (3.4) as

$$e^{\beta_J + \gamma_J} \{ \alpha_J(t - \tau_{J-1}) + \sum_{j=1}^{J-1} \alpha_j(\tau_j - \tau_{j-1}) \}^{e^{\gamma_J} - 1}.$$

The $\mathcal{T}_{\mathbf{hetvc}}$-test for varying heteroscedasticity has a realized value of $\chi_3^2 = 44.83$ (p-value < 0.001); and the $\mathcal{T}_{\mathbf{equal}}$-statistic is $\chi_8^2 = 11.72$ (p-value $= 0.164$), indicating that the acute stroke patients' survival within two years is irrespective of the comorbid diseases discussed in this study and that, using HHR^{VC}, time-varying heteroscedasticity should be included.

Table 3.1. Analysis of first-ever stroke patients' two-year survivals

Segment($j =$)	1	2	3	4	Test
α_j	3.673	0.592	0.062	0.104	$\mathcal{T}_{\mathbf{hetvc}} = 44.83 (p = 0.000)$
β_j	2.143	0.150	3.202	4.065	$\mathcal{T}_{\mathbf{equal}} = 11.72 (p = 0.164)$
γ_j	0.628	0.010	-4.751	-6.654	

3.6 Discussion

The results of Table 3.1 have some important implications. First, the baseline parameter estimates $\hat{\alpha}$s are decreasing, revealing overall declination in the risk of death of stroke patients. This phenomenon confounds with the time-varying property of β and γ. In particular, the decreasing baseline hazard and the decreasing heteroscedasticity (to a large negative value) together result in the large proportions of cured patients for each group. Second, the baseline-hazard parameters modulate the overall trend of incidence of events, $\beta(t)$ reflects the relative location or strength, and $\gamma(t)$ captures the shape or heterogeneity that interacted with time. The global validity of HHR^{VC} is only diagnosed by visualized fitness in Figure 3.1. How to construct an omnibus (or global) test for the goodness-of-fit of the HHR^{VC}-model remains an issue.

For a regression set-up with multiple regressors, not all variables have varying effect, and not all the varying coefficients have the same crossing point(s). This involves the strategy of data analysis. Here we propose plotting Kaplan–Meier estimates for each specific covariate after an adequate grouping. The covariates without crossings in KM estimates are suggested not to be put in the heteroscedasticity component. For those with cross-effect, practitioners need to decide the cut-off points $\{\tau_j\}$. In practice, the selected cut-off intervals $(\tau_{j-1}, \tau_j]$ should not contain more than one crossing point. Finally, for the parametric approach, we also suggest the application of a Weibull-type regression model equipped with time-varying parameters to deal with multiple cross-effect problems possibly combined with a cure probability.

Acknowledgments

This study was partly supported by Grant NSC94-2118-M-039-001, National Science Council of Taiwan.

References

1. Bagdonavičius, V. B. and Nikulin, M. S. (2005). Statistical analysis of survival and reliability data with multiple crossings of survival functions, *Comptes Rendus Academie de Sciences du Paris, Series I*, **340**, 377–382.

2. Cox, D. R. (1972). Regression models and life-tables (with discussion), *Journal of the Royal Statistical Society, Series B*, **34**, 187–220.

3. Hougaard, P. (1986). Survival models for heterogeneous populations derived from stable distributions, *Biometrika*, **73**, 387–396.

4. Hsieh, F. (2001). On heteroscedastic hazards regression models: Theory and application, *Journal of the Royal Statistical Society, Series B*, **63**, 63–79.

5. Martinussen, T. and Scheike, T. H. (2006). *Dynamic Regression Models for Survival Data*, Springer-Verlag, New York.

6. Marzec, L. and Marzec, P. (1997). On fitting Cox's regression model with time-dependent coefficients, *Biometrika*, **84**, 901–908.

7. Murphy, S. A. (1993). Testing for a time dependent coefficient in Cox's regression model. *Scandinavian Journal of Statistics*, **20**, 35–50.

8. Murphy, S. A. and Sen, P. K. (1991). Time-dependent coefficients in a Cox-type regression model, *Stochastic Processes and Their Applications*, **39**, 153–180.

9. Tian, L., Zucker, D., and Wei, L. J. (2005). On the Cox model with time-varying regression coefficients, *Journal of the American Statistical Association*, **100**, 172–183.

10. Valsecchi, M. G., Silvestri, D., and Sasieni, P. (1996). Evaluation of long-term survival: Use of diagnostics and robust estimators with Cox's proportional hazards model, *Statistics in Medicine*, **15**, 2763–2780.

11. Vaupel, J. W. (1979). The impact of heterogeneity in individual frailty on the dynamics of mortality, *Demography*, **16**, 439–454.

12. Wu, H.-D. I., Hsieh, F., and Chen, C.-H. (2002). Validation of a heteroscedastic hazards regression model, *Lifetime Data Analysis*, **8**, 21–34.

4

Closure Properties and Diagnostic Plots for the Frailty Distribution in Proportional Hazards Models

P. Economou and C. Caroni

Department of Mathematics, National Technical University of Athens, Athens, Greece

Abstract: Starting from the distribution of frailty amongst individuals with lifetimes between t_1 and t_2, we construct a graphical diagnostic for the correct choice of frailty distribution in a proportional hazards model. This is based on a closure property of certain frailty distributions in the case $t_2 \to \infty$ (i.e., among survivors at time t_1), namely that the conditional frailty distribution has the same form as the unconditional, with some parameters remaining the same. We illustrate the plot on the Stanford heart transplant data. We investigate the application of the same principle to the case of shared frailty, where the members of a cluster share a common value of frailty. A similar plot can be used when the cluster lifetime is defined as the shortest lifetime of the cluster's members. Other definitions of cluster lifetime are less useful for this purpose because the closure property does not apply.

Keywords and Phrases: Lifetime data, frailty, shared frailty, proportional hazards, graphical diagnostics

4.1 Introduction

Frailty models are widely used in the analysis of lifetime data because they provide a simple and convenient way of introducing heterogeneity between individuals or between groups. The frailty Z is an unobserved random effect which affects the lifetime distribution in a similar way to any observed covariates. In the proportional hazards framework, it has a multiplicative effect on some baseline hazard function h_b, so that the hazard function for an individual with frailty $Z = z$ is given by

$$h\left(t|z;\mathbf{x}\right) = ze^{\beta'\mathbf{x}}h_b(t), \tag{4.1}$$

where $\mathbf{x}$ is a vector of possibly time-dependent covariates. An important extension is to the shared frailty model. This applies to data structures where individuals are grouped naturally into clusters (e.g., members of a family, patients treated in the same unit, samples of material cut from the same piece) and correlation is expected between the failure times within a cluster. The model induces this correlation by assuming that the members of a cluster share the same value of frailty. Individual failure times are conditionally independent given the frailty. Assuming proportional hazards again, the hazard function h_{mj} of individual $j = 1, \ldots, q_m$ in cluster $m = 1, \ldots, k$ which has frailty z_m becomes (without covariates)

$$h_{mj}\left(t|z_m\right) = z_m h_b(t). \tag{4.2}$$

The conditional joint survivor function of the q_m members of the mth cluster is

$$S\left(t_1, t_2, \ldots, t_{q_m}|z_m\right) = e^{-z_m \sum_{j=1}^{q_m} H_b(t_{mj})}, \tag{4.3}$$

where H_b is the cumulative hazard function. If there are measured covariates common to all members of the cluster, represented by the possibly time-dependent vector $\mathbf{x}$, then H_b is usually replaced by $H_b^{\mathbf{x}}(t) = \int_0^t e^{\beta'\mathbf{x}}h_b(u)du$.

In order to apply the proportional hazards model for individual or shared frailty, a specific frailty distribution has to be assumed. Diagnostic tools should be available to enable the modeller to test the assumption. Our purpose in this chapter is to discuss diagnostic plots for the frailty distribution in proportional hazards models, both for individual frailty and shared frailty. Our method is based on closure properties of the frailty distribution, which we extend in the following section. We consider only fully parametric models for both the frailty and the baseline hazard function.

4.2   Closure Properties of the Individual Frailty Distribution

We assume that the frailty distribution in a proportional hazards individual frailty model is given by the p.d.f.

$$g(z; \eta_1(\alpha), \ \eta_2(\alpha)) = \frac{e^{-[z, \ \psi(z)][\eta_1(\alpha), \ \eta_2(\alpha)]'}}{\Phi(\alpha)} \ \xi(z), \ \ z > 0. \tag{4.4}$$

This is an exponential family distribution with z as one of its canonical statistics. In general, η_2 and α are vectors. We prove the following new result on a conditional distribution of frailty among the subset of individuals whose lifetime falls in the interval (t_1, t_2).

Theorem 4.2.1 *If the p.d.f. of the frailty distribution* $G(\eta_1(\alpha), \eta_2(\alpha))$ *in the population is given by (4.4), then the distribution of frailty among individuals who die in the interval* (t_1, t_2) *is the negative mixture:*

$$
\begin{aligned}
g(z|t_1 < T < t_2) &= pg(z; \eta_1(\alpha) + H_b^{\times}(t_1), \eta_2(\alpha)) \\
&\quad - (1-p)g(z; \eta_1(\alpha) + H_b^{\times}(t_2), \eta_2(\alpha)),
\end{aligned}
\tag{4.5}
$$

where $p = \frac{S_T(t_1)}{S_T(t_1) - S_T(t_2)}$ *and* $S_T(t)$ *is the unconditional survivor function.*

PROOF. The p.d.f. of frailty Z conditional on $T \in (t_1, t_2)$ is given by

$$
\begin{aligned}
g(z|t_1 < T < t_2) &= \frac{\int_{t_1}^{t_2} f(u, z)du}{\int_0^{\infty} \int_{t_1}^{t_2} f(u, z)dudz} \\
&= \frac{\int_{t_1}^{t_2} f(u|z)g(z)du}{\int_0^{\infty} \int_{t_1}^{t_2} f(u|z)g(z)dudz},
\end{aligned}
\tag{4.6}
$$

where $f(t, z)$ is the joint p.d.f. of T and Z and $f(t|z)$ is the p.d.f. of t conditional on z. Noticing that

$$
\int_{t_1}^{t_2} f(u, z)du = e^{-zH_b^{\times}(t_1)} - e^{-zH_b^{\times}(t_2)}
\tag{4.7}
$$

we have

$$
g(z|t_1 < T < t_2) = \frac{g(z)e^{-zH_b^{\times}(t_1)} - e^{-zH_b^{\times}(t_2)}}{\int_0^{\infty} e^{-zH_b^{\times}(t_1)} - e^{-zH_b^{\times}(t_2)}dz}
\tag{4.8}
$$

which after some algebra leads to the relation

$$
\begin{aligned}
g(z|t_1 < T < t_2) &= \frac{\Phi_1^*(\alpha)}{\Phi(\alpha)(S_T(t_1) - S_T(t_2))} g(z; \eta_1(\alpha) + H_b^{\times}(t_1), \eta_2(\alpha)) \\
&\quad - \frac{\Phi_1^*(\alpha)}{\Phi(\alpha)(S_T(t_1) - S_T(t_2))} g(z; \eta_1(\alpha) + H_b^{\times}(t_2), \eta_2(\alpha))
\end{aligned}
\tag{4.9}
$$

but $\Phi_i^*(\alpha)$ is given by

$$
\Phi_i^*(\alpha) = \int_0^{\infty} e^{-[z, \, \psi(z)][\eta_1(\alpha) + H_b^{\times}(t_i), \, \eta_2(\alpha)]'} = \Phi(\alpha)S_T(t_i)
\tag{4.10}
$$

and hence the required result. ∎

Corollary 4.2.1 *The frailty distribution among survivors at time t has p.d.f.*

$$f(z|T > t) = \frac{e^{-[z, \, \psi(z)][\eta_1^*(\alpha), \, \eta_2(\alpha)]'}}{\Phi^*(\alpha)} \, \xi(z), \quad z > 0, \tag{4.11}$$

where $\eta_1^*(\alpha) = \eta_1(\alpha) + H_b^{\times}(t)$ and $\Phi^*(\alpha) = \Phi(\alpha)S_T(t)$. It thus belongs to the same family as the original frailty distribution, but with a different value for η_1, the element of the parameter vector corresponding to z.

PROOF. Let $t_2 \to \infty$ in Theorem 4.2.1. Then $S_T(t_2) \to 0$, $p \to 1$ and the above result follows. ∎

Corollary 4.2.2 *The p.d.f. of the frailty distribution among individuals dying before time t is*

$$g(z|T < t_2) = \frac{1}{1 - S_T(t_2)} f_Z(z) - \frac{S_T(t_2)}{1 - S_T(t_2)} \, g(z; \eta_1(\mathbf{a}) + H_b^{\times}(t_2), \eta_2(\mathbf{a})). \tag{4.12}$$

PROOF. Let $t_1 = 0$ in Theorem 4.2.1. ∎

A third interesting special case could be obtained by letting $t_2 \to t_1$, which leads to the distribution of frailty among individuals dying at time t_1. This has a closure property similar to Corollary 4.2.1. However, this result is most conveniently proved directly, as follows.

Theorem 4.2.2 *If the frailty distribution G belongs to an exponential family similar to (4.4) but with $\log z$ among its canonical statistics in addition to z, then the distribution of frailty among those dying at time t is in the same family, but with different values of the parameters.*

PROOF. The proportional hazards model implies that the lifetime distribution conditional on $Z = z$ is

$$f(t|z) = zh_b(t)\exp\{-zH_b^{\times}(t)\}. \tag{4.13}$$

Hence write down the joint distribution of frailty and lifetime $f(t, z) = f(t|z)g(z)$, then integrate z out to obtain the unconditional $f(z)$ and hence obtain $g(z|t)$ as $f(t, z)/f(t)$. ∎

Applied to the special case of gamma frailty with shape parameter θ and scale parameter λ, this result shows that the distribution of frailty among individuals dying at time t is also gamma, with shape parameter $\theta + 1$ and scale parameter $\lambda + H_b^{\times}(t)$. Other popular frailty distributions can be fit into this framework by adding $\log z$ as a canonical statistic but with parameter initially equal to zero; the frailty distribution among those dying at time t then has a nonzero value of this parameter. For example, the inverse Gaussian distribution can be regarded as a special case of the generalized inverse Gaussian distribution, to which the closure property applies.

The distributions of frailty among survivors at time t and among those dying at time t were first given by Vaupel *et al.* (1979), assuming a gamma distribution. The extension to exponential families was made by Hougaard (1984).

4.3   Diagnostic Plots

Corollary 4.2.1 states that the parameter $\eta_2(\alpha|t)$ of the frailty distribution among survivors at time t, which for simplicity we now write as $\eta_2(t)$, is the same for all t. For gamma frailty, this is the shape parameter. A diagnostic plot based on this property was developed by Economou and Caroni (2005). For an earlier application of the idea of employing various degrees of truncation in order to check a model, see Hougaard *et al.* (1992). The method of Economou and Caroni (2005) is to fit the assumed model, such as gamma frailty with Weibull lifetimes, firstly to the original full dataset and subsequently to survivors at times $t_1, t_2, \ldots$ (these could be the observed lifetimes or just an arbitrary set of time points). In these subsequent fits the lifetime distribution's parameters are taken as equal to the values estimated from the full data, instead of re-estimating them each time. If the assumed frailty distribution is correct, and assuming also that the Weibull lifetime distribution is correctly specified, then the plot of each element of $\eta_2(t)$ against time should be a horizontal line starting from $\eta_2(0)$, which is the estimate obtained upon fitting the model to the full set of data. Note that in general η_2 is a vector. For example, for the generalized inverse Gaussian distribution with parameters $(\lambda, \delta, \gamma)$ with p.d.f.

$$g(z) = \frac{(\gamma/\delta)^\lambda}{2K_\lambda(\delta\gamma)} z^{\lambda-1} e^{-\frac{1}{2}\left(\delta^2 z^{-1} + \gamma^2 z\right)}, \tag{4.14}$$

where $K_\lambda(.)$ is the modified Bessel function of the third kind with index λ, the two components of η_2 are $\lambda^2 - 1$ and δ^2. A separate plot should be constructed for each component of η_2. As an alternative to plotting $\eta_2(t)$, we may plot $\eta_2(t)/\eta_2(0)$ against time: the points on this plot should be scattered around a horizontal line starting from one. The advantage of this alternative plot is that it is conceptually easy (although quite time-consuming computationally) to add a simulated envelope to aid the assessment of whether the line is horizontal [Economou and Caroni (2005)].

The other consequence of the closure property in Theorem 4.2.1 is that the parameter η_1 corresponding to the canonical statistic z changes to $\eta_1 + H_b(t)$

when the data are restricted to survivors at time t. If the baseline lifetime distribution is Weibull with parameters β and α, then $H_b(t) = (t/\alpha)^\beta$. It seems that it could be possible to base another diagnostic plot on this property, checking that the estimate $\eta_1(t)$ based on survivors at time t does follow the correct form when plotted against $\eta_1(0) + H_b(t)$. This would be checking simultaneously the frailty distribution and the lifetime distribution. It is probably not very fruitful to pursue this second plot because the plot already suggested does the job of checking the frailty distribution assuming the lifetime distribution, and other methods can be used to check the lifetime distribution. Furthermore, it is often necessary to place a constraint on the parameters for identifiability. For example, in the case of the gamma–Weibull mixture, the two scale parameters are not separately identifiable. Hence the gamma scale parameter might be set equal to one, so in practice it would not be possible to construct this second plot.

The other closure property, Theorem 4.2.2, does not seem to be practically useful either. Any failure time will occur only once in a sample of continuous data, or a small number of times because of rounding. Therefore, it is either impossible to fit the distribution of frailty among those dying at a specified time, or it has to be fit to such a small amount of data that random variation is too large to allow the expected pattern in the parameter estimates to be seen. Grouping nearby failure times to increase the sample size does not solve the problem, because the correct result to apply in that case is given by Theorem 4.2.1, which does not have the simplicity of the closure result.

4.4   Application

In order to illustrate the use of the diagnostic plots and show their effectiveness, we use the well-known Stanford heart transplant data on the survival times of 103 patients (28 right-censored). The data were obtained from Kalbfleisch and Prentice (2002). We used only the survival or censoring time and ignored the covariates that are available for some of the patients.

Figure 4.1 shows the Kaplan–Meier estimate of the survival function, together with the fitted curves obtained from the two parametric models, that is, Weibull lifetimes mixed with either gamma frailty (this gives the Burr distribution of lifetimes) or inverse Gaussian frailty. In both models, the mean of the frailty distribution was set equal to one. The Burr distribution seems to be the better fit. Figure 4.2 shows two diagnostic plots. The upper one refers to the mixture of Weibull lifetimes with gamma frailty. At each observed survival time t we re-estimate the gamma shape parameter $\eta(t)$ using the data from the survivors beyond t. The quantity $\eta(t)/\eta(0)$ [where $\eta(0)$ is the value obtained

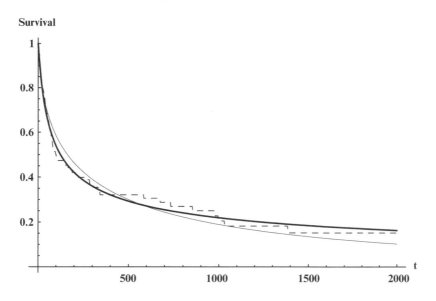

Figure 4.1. Estimates of the survival function of the heart transplant data: Kaplan–Meier (broken line), Weibull with gamma frailty (bold line), and Weibull with inverse Gaussian frailty (lighter line).

using all the data, i.e., at time zero] is plotted against time. The envelopes plotted on the graph are the smoothed 95% and 99% limits obtained by applying the same computational procedure to 200 sets of data of the same size, simulated from the Burr distribution with parameters equal to the estimates at time zero in the actual data [Economou and Caroni (2005)]. The plotted points are visually very close to a horizontal line and after the first few values, which fall on the lower confidence bound, are well inside the confidence limits. This indicates that the gamma frailty distribution is an acceptable model (assuming that the Weibull is the correct baseline survival distribution). The lower part of Figure 4.2 shows the results of applying exactly the same procedure when the inverse Gaussian distribution was used for frailty instead of the gamma. After about $t = 40$, the plotted points follow a clear trend away from the value one and fall consistently outside the simulated confidence limits. This indicates that the inverse Gaussian frailty distribution is not acceptable for these data (again assuming Weibull survival as the baseline).

4.5 Shared Frailty

In the case of shared frailty, the distribution of the random variable Z is over the clusters, not the individuals. Therefore in order to extend the above ideas to

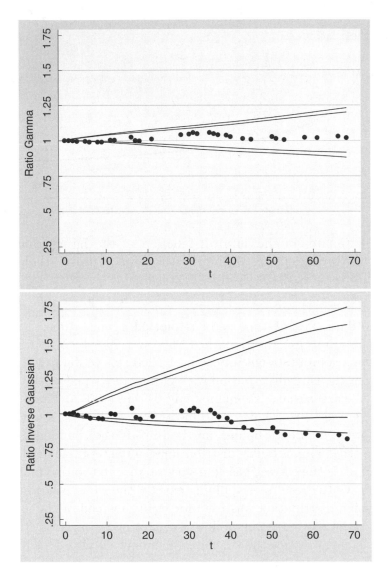

Figure 4.2. Diagnostic plots for frailty distribution applied to the Stanford heart transplant data. The plotted points are $\eta(t)/\eta(0)$ against time; the envelopes are simulated 95 and 99 percentage points. Upper plot: Weibull–gamma mixture (=Burr distribution). Lower plot: Weibull–inverse Gaussian mixture.

shared frailty, we need to define what is meant by saying that a cluster survives at time t. Two possibilities are as follows.

Minimum definition

The "death" of a cluster occurs when any of its members dies. If the first event in a cluster is a right-censoring, then the cluster has to be treated as right-censored at that point in time, as if all its members were censored together [this is homogeneous censoring; Hougaard (2000)]. Hence the lifetime distribution of a cluster of size m is given by the random variable $T_{(1)} = \min_{i=1,...,m} T_i$. The survivor function of the cluster given frailty z and assuming that all the members of a cluster share common values of the covariates, is

$$S_{(1)}(t|z) = (S(t|z))^m, \qquad (4.15)$$

hence properties at the cluster level are basically the same as those found already for individual frailty. In particular, the closure property of Corollary 4.2.1 to Theorem 4.2.1 applies. It is easy to see that the parameter denoted earlier as η_1 becomes $\eta_1 + mH_b^{\times}(t)$ and η_2 remains unchanged.

Maximum definition

Another possible definition of the death of a cluster is that the cluster "dies" when all its members have died. Any censoring therefore means that the cluster's lifetime is censored too. The lifetime distribution of a cluster of size m is given by the random variable $T_{(m)} = \max_{i=1,...,m} T_i$. In this case the closure property does not extend neatly. The statements in Theorem 4.2.1 concerning η_1 and η_2 still hold, but the term $\xi(z)$ also changes, to

$$\xi^*(z) = \xi(z) \left\{ 1 - \left(1 - e^{-zH_b^{\times}(t)}\right)^m \right\}. \qquad (4.16)$$

Both of these definitions can be written as special cases of defining a cluster as "surviving" if at least r of its members are alive. The maximum definition corresponds to $r = 1$ and the minimum definition to $r = m$. The simple closure property applies only to the minimum definition and for this reason we consider only this definition from here onwards.

Whatever the definition of a cluster's lifetime, the analysis for shared frailty can be carried out in two ways, corresponding to two kinds of likelihood function. In the first, the cluster is the unit of analysis, and a surviving cluster at time t enters the likelihood as one observation (the cluster's lifetime). This is called the cluster-level approach. In the second likelihood, we use the individual lifetimes of the surviving clusters' surviving members. This is the individual-level approach. In both approaches, we consider only uninformative right-censoring.

We assume that the dataset is ordered by $t_i < t_u$ for $i < u$, where $t_m = \min_{1 \le j \le q_m} t_{mj}$ is the lifetime of the mth cluster under the minimum definition. The likelihood for estimation among surviving clusters at time t_{m_0} in the cluster-level approach is given by

$$L_{t_{m_0}}\left(\eta_1(\alpha), \eta_2(\alpha)\right) = \prod_{m=m_0+1}^{k} h_m(t_m)^{\delta_m} S_m(t_m), \qquad (4.17)$$

where the censoring indicator δ_m is equal to one or zero for uncensored or censored cluster lifetimes, respectively, $S_m(t)$ is the survivor function of the mth cluster conditional on its lifetime being greater than t_{m_0} (but not conditional on z), and $h_m(t)$ is the corresponding hazard function for this cluster given by $h_m(t) = -\partial/\partial t \log S_m(t)$, where $S_m(t) = S_T(t, t, \ldots, t)/S_T(t_{m_0}, t_{m_0}, \ldots, t_{m_0})$. In the individual level approach, the likelihood at t_{m_0} is

$$\prod_{m=m_0+1}^{k} \left[\prod_{j \in R_m} \left(-\frac{\partial}{\partial t_{mj}} \right) S_{T|T_{(1)}>t_{m_0}}(t_{m1}, t_{m2}, \ldots, t_{mq_m}) \right], \qquad (4.18)$$

where R_m is the subset of uncensored observations in the mth cluster; that is, $R_m = \{j : j \in \{1, 2, \ldots, q_m\}$, and $\delta_{mj} = 1\}$, $S_{T|T_{(1)}>t_{m_0}}(t_{m1}, t_{m2}, \ldots, t_{mq_m})$ is the joint survivor function of the mth cluster's members given that their minimum is bigger than t_{m_0}. This is

$$S_{T|T_{(1)}>t_{m_0}}(t_{m1}, t_{m2}, \ldots, t_{mq_m}) = \frac{S_T(t_{m1}, t_{m2}, \ldots, t_{mq_m})}{S_T(t_{m_0}, t_{m_0}, \ldots, t_{m_0})}. \qquad (4.19)$$

Given particular survival functions and frailty distributions, direct maximisation of the likelihoods can be carried out straightforwardly, in MATHEMATICA, for example.

Because we already know from the application of the idea to individual frailty that these diagnostic plots work, the only question arising in the case of shared frailty is which of the two likelihood functions should be used. The first has the advantage of simplicity; the second uses more information and should be substantially more powerful. The answer obviously depends on the size of the sample, the degree of heterogeneity, and the amount of censoring. It also depends on the frailty distribution (our experience so far is that it is easier to reject gamma frailty than inverse Gaussian). Because the individual-level approach is time-consuming to carry out, we recommend using it in large samples only as a further check on a distribution which seems acceptable under the cluster-level approach. For small samples, the individual-level approach is recommended.

Acknowledgements

P. Economou's graduate studies are supported by a grant from the Papakyri-
akopoulos Foundation.

References

1. Economou, P. and Caroni, C. (2005). Graphical tests for the assumption of
   gamma and inverse Gaussian frailty distributions, *Lifetime Data Analysis*,
   11, 565–582.

2. Hougaard, P. (1984). Life table methods for heterogeneous populations: Distributions describing the heterogeneity, *Biometrika*, **71**, 75–83.

3. Hougaard, P. (2000). *Analysis of Multivariate Survival Data*, Springer-Verlag,
   New York.

4. Hougaard, P., Harvald, B., and Holm, N. V. (1992). Measuring the similarities between the lifetimes of adult Danish twins born between 1881–1930.
   Journal of the American Statistical Association, **87**, 17–24.

5. Kalbfleisch, J. D. and Prentice, R. L. (2002). *The Statistical Analysis of
   Failure Time Data* (2nd ed.), John Wiley & Sons, New York.

6. Vaupel, J. A., Manton, K. G., and Stallard, E. (1979). The impact of heterogeneity in individual frailty on the dynamics of mortality, *Demography*,
   16, 439–454.

5

Multivariate Survival Data With Censoring

Shulamith Gross[1] **and Catherine Huber-Carol**[2]

[1] *Baruch College of the City University of New York, Department of Statistics and CIS, NY, USA*
[2] *Université Paris V, René Descartes, Paris, France and INSERM U 780*

Abstract: We define a new class of models for multivariate survival data, in continuous time, based on a number of cumulative hazard functions, along the lines of our family of models for correlated survival data in discrete time [Gross and Huber-Carol (2000, 2002)]. This family is an alternative to frailty and copula models. We establish some properties of our family and compare it to Clayton's and Marshall–Olkin's and derive nonparametric partial likelihood estimates of the hazards involved in its definition.

Keywords and Phrases: Survival data, cluster data, right-censoring, continuous time, hazard rates

5.1   Introduction

Much attention has been paid to multivariate survival models and inference since the early work of Hougaard, and his recent book (2004) on the subject. Studies on twins led to the development of papers on bivariate distributions and, more generally, the analysis of family data or clusters data led to more general models for correlated survival data. One way of dealing with this problem is to use copula or frailty models [see, e.g., Bagdonavicius and Nikulin (2002) for a review of those models]. Among the most usual bivariate models, one finds Clayton's, Marshall–Olkin's, and Gumbel's models. We present here a model for continuous multivariate data based on the same idea as the one we used in the discrete case [Gross and Huber-Carol (2002)], and which is closely related to a multistate process. We define our class of models in detail for the special case of bivariate data, and generalize this class to any dimension. We then obtain properties of these models and compare them to the usual ones cited above. We then derive NPML estimators for the functions involved and derive their asymptotic properties.

5.2   Definition of the Models

5.2.1   Bivariate continuous model

Let $\mathcal{L}$ be the class of continuous univariate cumulative hazard functions on $I\!\!R^+$:

$$\mathcal{L} = \{\Lambda : I\!\!R^+ \to I\!\!R^+, \text{ continuous, nondecreasing}, \Lambda(0) = 0, \Lambda(t) \xrightarrow[t\to\infty]{} \infty\}.$$

Definition 5.2.1 (Bivariate continuous model) Given any five members $\Lambda_{11}^{01}, \Lambda_{11}^{10}, \Lambda_{11}^{00}, \Lambda_{01}^{00}, \Lambda_{10}^{00}$ of $\mathcal{L}$, we define a joint bivariate survival function S on $I\!\!R^+ \times I\!\!R^+$ by

$$
\begin{aligned}
\text{for } x < y, \ dS(x,y) &= \exp\{-\Lambda_{11}^{01}(x) - \Lambda_{11}^{10}(x) - \Lambda_{11}^{00}(x)\}d\Lambda_{11}^{01}(x) \\
&\quad \times \exp\{-(\Lambda_{01}^{00}(y) - \Lambda_{01}^{00}(x))\}d\Lambda_{01}^{00}(y) \\
\text{for } y < x, \ dS(x,y) &= \exp\{-\Lambda_{11}^{01}(y) - \Lambda_{11}^{10}(y) - \Lambda_{11}^{00}(y)\}d\Lambda_{11}^{10}(y) \\
&\quad \times \exp\{-(\Lambda_{10}^{00}(x) - \Lambda_{10}^{00}(y))\}d\Lambda_{10}^{00}(x) \\
\text{for } y = x, \ dS(x,y) &= \exp\{-\Lambda_{11}^{01}(x) - \Lambda_{11}^{10}(x) - \Lambda_{11}^{00}(x)\}d\Lambda_{11}^{00}(x). \quad (5.1)
\end{aligned}
$$

We propose the family (5.1) of bivariate distributions as an alternative to the bivariate probabilies defined by frailties or copulas. It is easy to verify that S thus defined is actually a bivariate survival function, and that a necessary and sufficient condition for the corresponding probability to be absolutely continuous (AC) with respect to λ^2, the Lebesgue measure on $I\!\!R^2$, is that $\Lambda_{11}^{00} \equiv 0$. Otherwise, part of the mass is on the diagonal of $I\!\!R^2$.

5.2.2   Generalization to p components

When more than two components are involved, say p, then our hierarchical class of models is defined in a similar way, involving now a number of cumulative hazards $K(p)$ equal to

$$K(p) = \sum_{k=0}^{p-1} C_p^{p-k} C_{p-k}^1 \qquad (5.2)$$

when the multivariate law is absolutely continuous with respect to λ^p, the Lebesgue measure on $I\!\!R^p$, and

$$K(p) = \sum_{k=0}^{p-1} C_p^{p-k} (2^{p-k} - 1) \qquad (5.3)$$

when simultaneous jumps are allowed.

5.2.3 Properties of the bivariate family

Theorem 5.2.1 *For all bivariate survival functions defined above and such that $\Lambda_{11}^{00} \equiv 0$, we have the following conditional hazard rates $\forall s < t \in \mathbb{R}^+$.*

$$
\begin{aligned}
P(X = dt, Y > t | X \geq t, Y \geq t) &= d\Lambda_{11}^{01}(t) \\
P(X > t, Y = dt | X \geq t, Y \geq t) &= d\Lambda_{11}^{10}(t) \\
P(X = dt | X \geq t, Y < t) &= d\Lambda_{10}^{00}(t) = P(X = dt | X \geq t, Y = ds) \\
P(Y = dt | Y \geq t, X < t) &= d\Lambda_{01}^{00}(t) = P(Y = dt | Y \geq t, X = ds).
\end{aligned}
$$

Conversely, if there exist $\Lambda_{11}^{10}, \Lambda_{11}^{01}, \Lambda_{10}^{00}, \Lambda_{01}^{00}$, cumulative hazard functions in $\mathcal{L}$ such that the joint law satisfies the above equations, then the joint survival function of (X, Y) satisfies (5.1).

Theorem 5.2.2 *If (X, Y) has survival function S given by (5.1), then X and Y are independent and S is absolutely continuous with respect to λ^2 if and only if*

$$
\Lambda_{11}^{00} \equiv 0; \quad \Lambda_{11}^{01} \equiv \Lambda_{10}^{00}; \quad \Lambda_{11}^{10} \equiv \Lambda_{01}^{00}.
$$

5.2.4 General bivariate model

A version of our model (5.1), in discrete time, was introduced in Gross and Huber-Carol (2000). The two models are embedded in the following general model. Let $\mathcal{L}^*$ be the set of cumulative hazards with possible jumps on an at most denumerable set of points $\mathcal{D} \in \mathbb{R}^+$:

$$
\mathcal{L}^* = \{\Lambda : \mathbb{R}^+ \to \mathbb{R}^+, \Lambda \text{ nondecreasing}, \Lambda(0) = 0, \Lambda(t) \xrightarrow[t \to \infty]{} \infty\}.
$$

Definition 5.2.2 (General bivariate model) Given any five members Λ_{11}^{01}, $\Lambda_{11}^{10}, \Lambda_{11}^{00}, \Lambda_{01}^{00}, \Lambda_{10}^{00}$ of $\mathcal{L}^*$ and $\mathcal{D} = \{x_1, \ldots, x_m, \ldots\}$ the ordered set of discontinuity points of the Λs we define a joint bivariate survival function S on $\mathbb{R}^+ \times \mathbb{R}^+$ by

For $x < y$

$$dS(x,y) \;=\; \prod_{t<x}(1 - \Lambda_{11}^{01}(dt) - \Lambda_{11}^{10}(dt) - \Lambda_{11}^{00}(dt)) \; \Lambda_{11}^{01}(dx)$$

$$\times \prod_{x \le t < y} (1 - \Lambda_{01}^{00}(dt))\Lambda_{01}^{00}(dy)$$

and for $x > y$

$$dS(x,y) \;=\; \prod_{t<y}(1 - \Lambda_{11}^{01}(dt) - \Lambda_{11}^{10}(dt) - \Lambda_{11}^{00}(dt)) \; \Lambda_{11}^{10}(dy)$$

$$\times \prod_{y \le t < x} (1 - \Lambda_{10}^{00}(dt))\Lambda_{10}^{00}(dx). \tag{5.4}$$

Finally for $y = x$

$$dS(x,x) \;=\; \prod_{t<x}(1 - \Lambda_{11}^{01}(dt) - \Lambda_{11}^{10}(dt) - \Lambda_{11}^{00}(dt)) \; \Delta\Lambda_{11}^{00}(x).$$

If $\mathcal{D} = \emptyset$, then (5.4) simplifies to (5.1).

5.2.5   The purely discrete model

Definition 5.2.3 (Purely discrete model) Let $\lambda(u) = \Lambda(u^+) - \Lambda(u^-)$, for all five Λs involved in (5.4), assumed to be purely discontinuous, with jumps in $\mathcal{D} = \{x_k, k \in I\!N\}$. Then define

For $x_i < x_j$,

$$P(X = x_i, Y = x_j) \;=\; \prod_{k<i}(1 - \lambda_{11}^{01}(x_k) - \lambda_{11}^{10}(x_k) - \lambda_{11}^{00}(x_k))\lambda_{11}^{01}(x_i)$$

$$\times \prod_{i<k<j}(1 - \lambda_{01}^{00}(x_k))\lambda_{01}^{00}(x_j).$$

For $x_i > x_j$,

$$P(X = x_i, Y = x_j) \;=\; \prod_{k<j}(1 - \lambda_{11}^{01}(x_k) - \lambda_{11}^{10}(x_k) - \lambda_{11}^{00}(x_k))\lambda_{11}^{10}(x_j)$$

$$\times \prod_{j<k<i}(1 - \lambda_{10}^{00}(x_k))\lambda_{10}^{00}(x_i).$$

For $x_i = x_j$,

$$P(X = x_i, Y = x_i) \;=\; \prod_{k<i}(1 - \lambda_{11}^{01}(x_k) - \lambda_{11}^{10}(x_k) - \lambda_{11}^{00}(x_k))\lambda_{11}^{00}(x_i).$$

5.2.6   Simple examples of laws of type (5.1)

Let a, b, c, d be four strictly positive constants and $d\Lambda_{11}^{01}(t) = a$, $d\Lambda_{11}^{10}(t) = b$, $d\Lambda_{10}^{00}(t) = c$, $d\Lambda_{01}^{00}(t) = d$. Then, denoting S the bivariate survival, we have:

$$\begin{aligned}
\frac{d^2 S(x,y)}{dxdy} &= e^{-(a+b)x}ae^{-d(y-x)}d \quad \text{if} \quad x < y \\
&= e^{-(a+b)y}be^{-c(x-y)}c \quad \text{if} \quad x > y.
\end{aligned}$$

Although all four hazard rates are constant, the marginals of these distributions are not exponential. Other simple examples arise from replacing the above exponential hazards by other families, such as Weibull or Pareto.

5.3 Some Usual Bivariate Models

Among the most usual bivariate models, one finds Clayton's, Marshall–Olkin's, and Gumbel's models.

5.3.1 Clayton bivariate distribution

The Clayton survival function (1978), parametrized by Oakes (1989) is given by

$$S(x,y) = P(X_1 > x, X_2 > y) = [S_1(x)^{-(\theta-1)} + S_2(y)^{-(\theta-1)} - 1]^{\frac{-1}{\theta-1}}, \quad (5.5)$$

where $\theta \in]1, +\infty[$ and $S_1(x)$ and $S_2(y)$ are the marginal survival functions for X_1 and X_2. The limiting distribution, when $\theta \to 0$ has independent components. We change parameter, letting

$$a = \frac{1}{\theta - 1} \quad \theta > 1; \ a > 0.$$

Genest *et al.* (1995) propose a pseudo-likelihood (PL) estimate for a. Their PL is based on a copula defining the joint distribution function $F(x,y) = c_\alpha(F_1(x), F_2(y))$. It is the product, for all observations (x_i, y_i), of the second partial derivative of $c_\alpha(u,v)$ with respect to u and v. u and v are further respectively replaced by $\widehat{F_1(x)}$ and $\widehat{F_2(y)}$. With our copula acting on the survival rather than on the d.f., the corresponding PL is derived below. If

$$S_a(u,v) \quad = \quad [u^{-1/a} + v^{-1/a} - 1]^{-a},$$

the pseudo-likelihood is equal to

$$\prod_{i=1}^{n} \left[\frac{\partial^2 S_a(u,v)}{\partial u \partial v} \right]_{u=\widehat{S_1}(x_i), v=\widehat{S_2}(y_i)}.$$

As

$$\frac{\partial^2 S_a(u,v)}{\partial u \partial v} = \left(1 + \frac{1}{a}\right) \frac{1}{uv} e^{-\frac{1}{a}\log(uv)} [u^{-\frac{1}{a}} + v^{-\frac{1}{a}} - 1]^{-a-2}$$

one can compute easily the PL substituting the Kaplan–Meier estimates $\widehat{S_1}$ and $\widehat{S_2}$ for S_1 and S_2.

5.3.2   Marshall–Olkin bivariate distribution

Let λ_1, λ_2 and λ_{12} be three positive constants and S the bivariate survival function

$$S(x_1, x_2) = P(X_1 \geq x_1, X_2 \geq x_2) = e^{-\lambda_1 x_1 - \lambda_2 x_2 - \lambda_{12}(x_1 \vee x_2)}. \qquad (5.6)$$

It is clear that the bivariate Marshall–Olkin is not absolutely continuous with respect to λ^2 as

$$P(X_1 > X_2) + P(X_2 > X_1) = \frac{\lambda_1 + \lambda_2}{\lambda_1 + \lambda_2 + \lambda_{12}}. \qquad (5.7)$$

Moreover, denoting $min = 1\{x_1 < x_2\} + 2 * 1\{x_2 < x_1\}$ and $max = 1\{x_1 > x_2\} + 2 * 1\{x_2 > x_1\}$, the density at point (x_1, x_2); $x_1 \neq x_2$ may be written as

$$f(x_1, x_2) = \lambda_{\min}(\lambda_{\max} + \lambda_{12})e^{-(\lambda_1 x_1 + \lambda_2 x_2 + \lambda_{12} x_{\max})}. \qquad (5.8)$$

The deficit to one is due to the fact that there is a probability mass equal to

$$\frac{\lambda_{12}}{\lambda_1 + \lambda_2 + \lambda_{12}}$$

on the diagonal. The linear density on the diagonal is equal to

$$f_0(x) = \lambda_{12} e^{-(\lambda_1 x + \lambda_2 x + \lambda_{12} x)} \qquad (5.9)$$

as can be derived from looking at the following limit

$$\lim_{dt \to 0} \frac{1}{dt}(S(t,t) - S(t, t+dt) - S(t+dt, t) + S(t+dt, t+dt)).$$

The corresponding hazards in our scheme would be

$$\lambda_{11}^{01}(t) = \frac{P(X_1=t, X_2>t)}{P(X_1 \geq t, X_2 \geq t)} = \lambda_1; \; \lambda_{10}^{00}(t) = \frac{P(X_1=t, X_2 \leq t)}{P(X_1 \geq t, X_2 \leq t)} = \lambda_1 + \lambda_{12}$$

$$\lambda_{11}^{10}(t) = \frac{P(X_1>t, X_2=t)}{P(X_1 \geq t, X_2 \geq t)} = \lambda_2; \; \lambda_{01}^{00}(t) = \frac{P(X_2=t, X_1 \leq t)}{P(X_1 \leq t, X_2 \geq t)} = \lambda_2 + \lambda_{12}$$

$$\lambda_{11}^{00}(t) = \lambda_{12}.$$

This can be seen from the following example of our class of distributions defined below.

5.3.3 Our quasi-Marshall–Olkin bivariate distribution

Let a bivariate distribution be defined as in (5.1), the hazards being equal to

$$(11) \xrightarrow{\lambda_{11}^{01} \equiv \lambda_1 \equiv \alpha} (01) \xrightarrow{\lambda_{01}^{00} \equiv \lambda_2 + \lambda_{12} \equiv \beta + \gamma} (00)$$

$$(11) \xrightarrow{\lambda_{11}^{10} \equiv \lambda_2 \equiv \beta} (10) \xrightarrow{\lambda_{01}^{00} \equiv \lambda_1 + \lambda_{12} \equiv \alpha + \gamma} (00)$$

and λ_{11}^{00} being identically null. Let us denote

$$\begin{aligned} Y &= \min(X_1, X_2) \\ Z &= \max(X_1, X_2). \end{aligned}$$

Following the log-likelihood L derived earlier, we obtain

$$\begin{aligned} L(x_1, x_2) \\ &= 1\{x_1 < x_2\} * [-(\alpha + \beta)y + \log(\alpha) - (\beta + \gamma)(z - y) + \log(\beta + \gamma)] \\ &\quad + 1\{x_2 < x_1\} * [-(\alpha + \beta)y + \log(\beta) - (\alpha + \gamma)(z - y) + \log(\alpha + \gamma)] \\ &= -(\alpha + \beta)y - \gamma(z - y) + 1\{x_1 < x_2\} * [\log(\alpha(\beta + \gamma)) - \beta(z - y)] \\ &\quad + 1\{x_2 < x_1\} * [\log(\beta(\alpha + \gamma)) - \alpha(z - y)]. \end{aligned}$$

In order to compare our distribution with that of Marshall–Olkin's, let $g(x_1, x_2)$ be the density

$$g(x_1, x_2) = \lambda_{\min}(\lambda_{\max} + \lambda_{12})e^{-(\lambda_1 x_1 + \lambda_2 x_2 + \lambda_{12}(x_{\max} - x_{\min}))}. \tag{5.10}$$

One can see that only $x_{\max}$ is replaced by $x_{\max} - x_{\min}$. As a result,

$$\int_0^\infty g(x_1, x_2)dx_1 dx_2 = 1.$$

It is an A.C. distribution. If we add the λ_{11}^{00} as in the preceding paragraph, we get the Marshall–Olkin distribution.

5.3.4 Gumbel bivariate distribution

The Gumbel bivariate exponential distribution is part of the general Morgenstern proposal for bivariate distributions

$$F(x, y) = F_1(x)F_2(y)[1 + \alpha(1 - F_1(x))(1 - F_2(y))], \quad (-1 \le \alpha \le 1), \tag{5.11}$$

where F_1 and F_2 are the respective marginal distribution functions for X and Y. Gumbel bivariate exponential is thus equal to

$$F(x, y) = (1 - e^{-x})(1 - e^{-y})[1 + \alpha e^{-x}e^{-y}] \quad (x \ge 0, y \ge 0, -1 \le \alpha \le 1). \tag{5.12}$$

In order to simulate this law, one may notice that the conditional distribution of Y with respect to X is given by

$$P(Y \leq y | X = x) = (1 - \alpha(2e^{-x} - 1))(1 - e^{-y}) + \alpha(2e^{-x} - 1)(1 - e^{-2y}). \quad (5.13)$$

5.4 NPML Estimation

5.4.1 Likelihood for the bivariate case

Let $X = (X_{i1}, X_{i2})$ be the bivariate survival time of cluster i, $i \in \{1, 2, \ldots, n\}$. The clusters are assumed to be independent. X_{i1} and X_{i2} may possibly be right-censored by a bivariate censoring time $C = (C_{i1}, C_{i2})$, independent of X, so that the observed bivariate time is $T = (X_{i1} \wedge C_{i1}, X_{i2} \wedge C_{i2}) \equiv (T_{i1}, T_{i2})$. The indicator of noncensoring is denoted $\delta = (\delta_{i1}, \delta_{i2}) \equiv (1\{T_{i1} = X_{i1}\}, 1\{T_{i2} = X_{i2}\})$. Let then $R(t) = (R_{i1}(t), R_{i2}(t))$ and $N(t) = (N_{i1}(t), N_{i2}(t))$ be, respectively, the associated at-risk and counting processes defined for $i \in \{1, 2, \ldots, n\}$ and $j \in \{1, 2\}$ as

$$\begin{aligned} R_{ij}(t) &= 1\{t < T_{ij}\} \\ N_{ij}(t) &= \delta_{ij} 1\{t \geq T_{ij}\}. \end{aligned}$$

The likelihood will be expressed in terms of the following hazards defined for $X = (X_1, X_2)$.

$$\begin{aligned} \lambda_{11}^{01}(t)dt &= P(t \leq X_1 \leq t + dt | X_1 \geq t, X_2 > t) \\ \lambda_{11}^{10}(t)dt &= P(t \leq X_2 \leq t + dt | X_1 > t, X_2 \geq t) \\ \lambda_{10}^{00}(t)dt &= P(t \leq X_1 \leq t + dt | X_1 \geq t, X_2 < t) \\ \lambda_{01}^{00}(t)dt &= P(t \leq X_2 \leq t + dt | X_1 < t, X_2 \geq t). \end{aligned}$$

The likelihood for the n clusters is the product $V = \prod_{i=1}^{n} V_i$ where each V_i may be written as

$$\begin{aligned} V_i &= \prod_t (1 - \lambda_{11}^{10}(t)dt - \lambda_{11}^{01}(t)dt)^{R_1(t)R_2(t)} (\lambda_{11}^{10}(t))^{R_1(t^-)R_2(t^-)dN_1(t)} \\ &\times (\lambda_{11}^{01}(t))^{R_1(t^-)R_2(t^-)dN_2(t)} \prod_t (1 - \lambda_{10}^{10}(t)dt)^{R_1(t)(1-R_2(t))\delta_2} \\ &\times \prod_t (1 - \lambda_{01}^{01}(t)dt)^{R_2(t)(1-R_1(t))\delta_1} (\lambda_{10}^{10}(t)dt)^{R_1(t)(1-R_2(t))\delta_2 dN_1(t)} \\ &\times (\lambda_{01}^{01}(t)dt)^{R_2(t)(1-R_1(t))\delta_1 dN_2(t)}. \end{aligned}$$

5.4.2 NPML estimation

Maximization of the log-likelihood (NPML) implies jumps of the Λs at (ordered) times T_k, $k = 1, 2, \ldots, K$ when an event occurred $[\delta_{ij} = 1$ for some $(i, j)]$. Let us introduce the quantities

$$
\begin{aligned}
\tau_1(i) &= 1\{T_{i1} < T_{i2}\}; & \tau_2(i) &= 1\{T_{i2} < T_{i1}\} \\
\tau(i) &= 1\{T_{i1} = T_{i2}\} \\
a_k &= \Lambda_{11}^{01}(T_k^+) - \Lambda_{11}^{01}(T_k^-); & b_k &= \Lambda_{11}^{10}(T_k^+) - \Lambda_{11}^{10}(T_k^-) \\
c_k &= \Lambda_{10}^{00}(T_k^+) - \Lambda_{10}^{00}(T_k^-); & d_k &= \Lambda_{01}^{00}(T_k^+) - \Lambda_{01}^{00}(T_k^-);
\end{aligned}
$$

and the counts

$$
\begin{aligned}
s_1(i) &= \sum_{i'} 1\{T_{i1} \le T_{i'1} \wedge T_{i'2}\}; & s_3(i) &= \sum_{i'} \tau_2(i')1\{T_{i'2} \le T_{i1} \le T_{i'1}\}\} \\
s_2(i) &= \sum_{i'} 1\{T_{i2} \le T_{i'1} \wedge T_{i'2}\}; & s_4(i) &= \sum_{i'} \tau_1[i']1\{T_{i'1} \le T_{i2} \le T_{i'2}\}\}.
\end{aligned}
$$

Then the log-likelihood is equal to

$$
\begin{aligned}
L = {}& -\sum_i a_i\delta_{i1}\tau_1(i)s_1(i) - \sum_i b_i\delta_{i2}\tau_2(i)s_2(i) + \sum_i \delta_{i1}\tau_1(i)\log(a_i) \\
& \sum_i \delta_{i2}\tau_2(i)\log(b_i) - \sum_i c_i\delta_{i1}\tau_2(i)b_is_3(i) - \sum_i d_i\delta_{i2}\tau_1(i)b_is_4(i) \\
& \sum_i \delta_{i1}\tau_2(i)\log(c_i) + \sum_i \delta_{i2}\tau_1(i)\log(d_i).
\end{aligned}
$$

By the derivation of L with respect to the jumps a_i, b_i, c_i, d_i, we obtain the following NPML estimates,

$$
\widehat{a}_i = \frac{\delta_{i1}\tau_1(i)}{s_1(i)}; \quad \widehat{b}_i = \frac{\delta_{i2}\tau_2(i)}{s_2(i)}; \quad \widehat{c}_i = \frac{\delta_{i1}\tau_2(i)}{s_3(i)}; \quad \widehat{d}_i = \frac{\delta_{i2}\tau_1(i)}{s_4(i)}.
$$

In order to derive the asymptotic properties of the NPML estimates, one rewrites them in terms of the associated counting processes and martingales, an example of which is given below. Let

$$
\mathcal{F}(t) = \sigma(N_{i1}(s), N_{i2}(s), R_{i1}(s), R_{i2}(s), s < t) \tag{5.14}
$$

be a filtration. We define four point processes N with associated presence at risk processes Y, for each case: jump of individual 1 (respectively, 2) in the presence (respectively, absence) of the other element of the pair. For the jumps of X_1 in the presence of X_2, this gives rise to

$$
\begin{aligned}
N_{i,11:01}(t) &= 1\{X_{i1} \le t, X_{i1} < X_{i2} \wedge C_{i1} \wedge C_{i2}\} \\
&= \int_0^t R_{i1}(s)R_{i2}(s)dN_{i1}(s) \\
Y_{i,11}(t) &= 1\{X_{i1} \wedge X_{i2} \wedge C_{i1} \wedge C_{i2} \ge t\} \\
&= R_{i1}(t)R_{i2}(t) \\
M_{i,11:01}(t) &= N_{i,11:01}(t) - \int_0^t Y_{i,11}(u)d\Lambda_{11}^{01}(u).
\end{aligned}
$$

The corresponding results will appear in a further paper still in progress together with simulations of our models and Clayton and Cuzick's.

5.5   Concluding Remarks

The proposed model could be considered as a multistate model, where the successive states are the actual composition of the subset of the cluster that is *still at risk* after some members have experienced the expected event. In a future work, we shall introduce covariates such as clusters and individual covariates as well as the time elapsed between two successive states of the cluster. Let us finally remark that the parallel with semi-Markov models for multistate models is not straightforward. This is due to the fact that, for example, in the bivariate case, when the pair is in state $(0, 1)$ the cumulative hazard Λ_{01}^{00} starts from 0 and not from the time s at which the first member of the pair experienced the event. Making the parallel perfect would lead to a new family of models having all properties of semi-Markov multistate models, to which could be applied all results already obtained, for example, by Huber-Carol et al. (2006).

References

1. Bagdonavicius, V. and Nikulin, M. (2002). *Accelerated Life Models*, Chapman & Hall/CRC, Boca Raton, FL.

2. Clayton, D. G. (1978). A model for association in bivariate life tables and its application in epidemiological studies of familial tendency in chronic disease incidence, *Biometrika*, **65**, 543–552.

3. Clayton, D. G. and Cuzick, J. (1985). Multivariate generalizations of the proportional hazards model (with discussion), *Journal of the Royal Statistical Society, Series A*, **148**, 82–117.

4. Genest, C., Ghoudi, K., and Rivest, L.-P. (1995). A semi-parametric estimation procedure of dependence parameter in multivariate families of distributions, *Biometrika,* **82**, 543–552.

5. Gross, S. and Huber-Carol, C. (2000). Hierarchical dependency models for multivariate survival data with censoring, *Lifetime Data Analysis,* **6**, 299–320.

6. Gross, S. and Huber-Carol, C. (2002). A new family of multivariate distributions for survival data, In *Goodness of Fit Tests and Model Validity* (Eds., C. Huber-Carol, N. Balakrishnan, M. S. Nikulin, and M. Mesbah), pp. 255–266, Birkhäuser, Boston.

7. Hougaard, P. (2004). *Analysis of Multivariate Survival Data*, Springer-Verlag, New York.

8. Huber-Carol, C., Pons, O., and Heutte, N. (2006). Inference for a general semi-Markov model and a sub-model for independent competing risks, In *Probability, Statistics and Modelling in Public Health* (Eds., M. Nikulin, D. Commenges, and C. Huber), pp. 231–244, Springer-Verlag, New York.

9. Lee, J. C., Wei, L. J., and Ying, Z. (1993). Linear regression analysis for highly stratified failure time data, *Biometrics*, **58**, 643-649.

10. Marschall, A. W. and Olkin, I. (1967). A multivariate exponential distribution, *Journal of the American Statistical Association*, **62**, 30–44.

11. Oakes, D. (1989). Bivariate survival models induced by frailties, *Journal of the American Statistical Association*, **84**, 487–493.

12. Ross, E. A. and Moore, D. (1999). Modeling clustered, discrete, or grouped time survival data with covariates, *Biometrics*, **55**, 813–819.

PART II
RELIABILITY THEORY—DEGRADATION MODELS

6

Virtual (Biological) Age Versus Chronological Age

Maxim Finkelstein

Department of Mathematical Statistics, University of the Free State, Bloemfontein, South Africa and Max Planck Institute for Demographic Research, Rostock, Germany

Abstract: The age of a deteriorating object is described by the corresponding process of degradation and is compared with the chronological age. A "black box" approach is considered, when deterioration depends on the environment and can be modeled by the accelerated life model. In, for example, the more severe environment, deterioration is more intensive, which means that objects are aging faster and, therefore, the corresponding virtual age is larger than the chronological age in a baseline environment. The second approach is based on considering an observed level of individual degradation and on its comparison with some average, "population degradation." The virtual age of the series system is also defined via the corresponding weighting of individual virtual ages.

Keywords and Phrases: Virtual age, degradation, aging distributions, failure rate, mean remaining lifetime

6.1 Introduction

According to numerous theories [see, e.g., Yashin *et al.* (2000) for references] the nature of biological aging is in some "wearing" (damage accumulation). For instance, damage accumulation can be due to nonideal repair mechanisms or (and) accumulation of deleterious mutations. These processes are stochastic and therefore it is natural to apply to organisms some concepts and approaches used in stochastic modeling of degrading (aging) engineering systems. The analogies should not be, however, interpreted too literally, which means that the implications of the corresponding stochastic modeling should be considered rather carefully.

Stochastic deterioration is usually described by the increasing failure (mortality) rate (IFR) lifetime distributions. For instance, adult mortality of humans (and of some other species as well) follows the Gompertz distribution with exponentially increasing mortality rate. We implicitly assume in this chapter the IFR-aging property of underlying lifetime distributions.

Virtual (biological) age of a degrading system can be probably considered as some elusive concept, but it certainly makes sense, if reasonably defined, and the goal of this chapter is to consider and to discuss different approaches to defining this notion.

It should be noted that chronological age of a system or of an organism is informative as some overall trivial marker of aging only for degrading objects. This age is the same for all individuals in a cohort and the cohort setting is especially important in Section 6.2, where different environments (regimes) are considered, although some generalizations on the period setting can be also performed in this case [Finkelstein (2006)].

Degradation in a more severe environment is usually more intensive, which means that objects are aging faster in some appropriate statistical sense. Therefore, in Section 6.2 we define and discuss a *statistical (black box) virtual age* and compare it with the chronological age in some baseline environment. Environment is understood rather generally: it can be, for example, electrical stress or temperature for engineering systems and, for example, climate, nutrition, lifestyle, and so on for organisms.

Degradation, however, is a stochastic process and therefore individuals age differently. Assume for simplicity that deterioration of an object can be modeled by a single, predictable, increasing stochastic process. Observing its state at a specific time can give under certain assumptions an indication of a "true" age defined by the level of the observed deterioration. We call this characteristic an *information-based virtual (biological) age* of a system or of an organism. If, for instance, someone 50 years old looks like and has the vital characteristics (blood pressure, level of cholesterol, etc.) of an "ordinary" 35 year-old one, we can say that this observation indicates that his virtual (biological) age can be estimated as 35. This is, of course, a rather vague statement, which can be made more precise for some simple, specific model settings and under certain assumptions. In Sections 6.2 and 6.3 we consider and discuss several possible approaches to defining virtual (biological) age of objects.

Another really challenging problem is to define a virtual age of a system with components in series having different virtual ages. An intuitive setting of this problem in a biological aging context is given by Vaupel *et al.* (2004): "Biological age may be better captured by the average age of individual, i.e., by some appropriate measure of the average age of the organs, body parts or cells of an individual-than by his chronological age." Based on results of previous sections, possible ways of solving this problem by specific weighting of virtual ages of components are considered in Section 6.4.

It should be noted that there exist several dependent biomarkers of aging in the organism (e.g., cell proliferation, metabolism, the rate of information processes), which can result in different estimates of the virtual age. A proper weighting of these individual virtual ages presents an interesting problem for future biological research and the corresponding stochastic modeling as well.

In this chapter we discuss some simple possibilities for a formal probabilistic definition of "objective aging." Evidently, other approaches can be also suggested and discussed. Although numerous authors have mentioned a notion of biological age, as far as we know, there are no papers with formal, stochastically based definitions. From now on we mostly use for definiteness the term "virtual age" omitting the term "biological."

6.2   The Black Box Virtual Age

Consider a degrading object (or a cohort) in a fixed *baseline environment* with a lifetime distribution $F_b(t)$. Let another statistically identical individual (or a cohort) be subject to, for example, a more *severe environment* (regime). Denote the corresponding lifetime distribution by $F_s(t)$. It is clear that degradation under the second regime is more intensive, therefore, the biological age of an individual, which survived under this regime in $[0, t)$ will be larger than t. We call this age the *black box virtual age* in the second regime.

To formalize the approach, assume that the lifetimes for two regimes comply with a general accelerated life model (ALM) [Cox and Oakes (1984) and Finkelstein (1999)] of the following form.

$$F_s(t) = F_b(W(t)), \qquad W(0) = 0, W(t) > t, \qquad t \in (0, \infty), \qquad (6.1)$$

where $W(t)$ is an increasing to infinity function and an evident condition $W(t) > t$ is due to the fact that the second regime is more severe than the baseline one. In fact, $W(t)$ is a scale transformation function. Note that only the linear case of this model was thoroughly investigated in the literature. Equation (6.1) explicitly suggests that the black box virtual age of an object, which has been operating for time t in a more severe environment, is $W(t)$, compared with the baseline chronological age t.

Definition 6.2.1 Assume that an impact of a more severe environment on a lifetime random variable can be described by the ALM (6.1), which is a widely used assumption for deteriorating objects [Bagdonavicius and Nikulin (2002)].

Then the function $W(t)$ defines the black box virtual age of an object in this environment, whereas the age in the baseline environment is the chronological one t.

Given the corresponding mortality rates $\mu_b(t)$ and $\mu_s(t)$, the function $W(t)$ can be obtained from Equation (6.1):

$$\exp\left\{-\int_0^t \mu_s(u)du\right\} = \exp\left\{-\int_0^{W(t)} \mu_b(u)du\right\},$$

therefore,

$$\int_0^t \mu_s(u)du = \int_0^{W(t)} \mu_b(u)du. \tag{6.2}$$

Remark 6.2.1 Under certain assumptions the function $W(t)$ can be estimated from the failure data [Bagdonavicius and Nikulin (2002)]. It should also be noted that (6.1) follows immediately from the assumption that one environment is more severe than the other: $F_s(t) > F_b(t)$, $t > 0$; therefore (6.1) is not stringent at all. The only restriction can come from the additional assumption that $W(t)$ should be an increasing function.

Remark 6.2.2 It is worth noting that the well-known time-dependent proportional hazards model

$$\mu_s(t) = w(t)\mu_b(t), \qquad w(t) > 1, \tag{6.3}$$

which is also often used for modeling the impact of environment, is not usually suitable for modeling deterioration [Bagdonavicius and Nikulin (2002)] due to its memoryless property, whereas the future behavior of degrading objects usually should, at least, depend on the accumulated damage. One can explicitly see the difference between the two models by differentiating Equation (6.2) and comparing the obtained mortality rate with (6.3):

$$\mu_s(t) = w(t)\mu_b(W(t)), \tag{6.4}$$

where $w(t) = W'(t)$.

Example 6.2.1 (a) Let mortality rates in both regimes be increasing power functions (Weibull law):

$$\mu_b(t) = \alpha t^\beta, \qquad \mu_s(t) = \mu t^\nu, \qquad \alpha, \beta, \mu, \nu > 0.$$

Assume that $\nu > \beta$; $\mu > \alpha$. This will be sufficient for $\mu_s(t) > \mu_b(t)$, $t > 1$, which describes in terms of mortality rates that the second regime is more severe than the baseline one (the case $0 < t \le 1$ can be considered in a similar way). Then the corresponding statistical virtual age is defined by Equation (6.2) as an increasing function:

$$W(t) = \left(\frac{\mu(\beta+1)}{\alpha(\nu+1)}\right)^{1/(\beta+1)} t^{\frac{\nu+1}{\beta+1}}.$$

In order for inequality $W(t) > t$ for $t > 1$ to hold, the following additional restriction on parameters is sufficient: $\mu(\beta + 1)/\alpha(\nu + 1) > 1$.

Let mortality rates in both regimes be ordered exponential functions (Gompertz law):

$$\mu_b(t) = a_b e^{b_b t}, \qquad \mu_s(t) = a_s e^{b_s t}, \qquad a_s > a_b > 0, \qquad b_s > b_b > 0;$$
$$\mu_s(t) > \mu_b(t), \qquad t > 0.$$

Then, similar to the previous example:

$$W(t) = \frac{\log[(a_b b_s - a_s b_b) + a_s b_b e^{b_s t}] - \log(a_b b_s)}{b_b}.$$

Thus, $W(t)$ is an increasing function and $W(0) = 0$. Condition $W(t) > t$ can be met by some additional assumptions on the constants involved.

When $a_s = k a_b$, $b_s = k b_b$, where $k > 1$, we arrive at a linear ALM with $W(t) = kt$, which is a simplified example that speaks for itself.

6.3 Information-Based Virtual Age

In the previous section no additional information on a system's deterioration was available. However, deterioration is a stochastic process and individuals age differently. Observation of a state of a system at time t under certain assumptions can give an indication of its virtual (but, in fact, real) age defined by the level of deterioration. Two possible ways of defining the information-based virtual age are considered in this section.

6.3.1 Degradation curve

We start with a meaningful example, which helps us to understand the issue of the information-based virtual age.

Example 6.3.1 Consider a system of $n+1$ components (one initial component and n cold standby identical ones) with constant mortality rates μ. The failure occurs when the last component fails. The possible biological interpretation is the limited number of repairs [Vaupel and Yashin (1987)] or cell replications. When a cell divides, one of the daughter cells will have a maintained telomere length; the other will have a shorter length [Olofsson (2000)]. When this length is shorter than some critical value, the cell stops dividing. It is clear that this process can be modeled in the suggested way, whereas the assumption of constant mortality rates on each stage can be relaxed (see later). Alternatively, one can think about a redundant biological organ or a part. In this case the model can be easily modified from cold standby (switched off) to hot standby (functioning) redundant components.

The mortality rate of the described system is an increasing function of the following form [Hoyland and Rausand (1993)]:

$$\mu_{n+1}(t) = \frac{\mu e^{-\mu t}(\mu t)^n / n!}{e^{-\mu t} \sum_0^n \frac{(\mu t)^i}{i!}}. \tag{6.5}$$

The number of failed components observed at time t is a natural measure of accumulated degradation in $[0, t]$ for this setting. Denote by T_{n+1} the time to failure of the described system. Consider the following conditional expectation (in fact, this is a conditional compensator for the corresponding counting process).

$$D(t) \equiv E[N(t), |N(t) \le n] = E[N(t) | T_{n+1} > t]$$
$$= \frac{e^{-\lambda t} \sum_0^n i \frac{(\lambda t)^i}{i!}}{e^{-\lambda t} \sum_0^n \frac{(\lambda t)^i}{i!}}, \tag{6.6}$$

where $N(t)$ is a number of events in the interval $[0, t]$ for the Poisson process with rate μ. As we observe an operable system, relation (6.6) defines the expected value of the number of its failures (measure of degradation) on condition of survival in $[0, t]$. The function $D(t)$ is monotonically increasing, $D(0) = 0$, and $\lim_{t \to \infty} D(t) = n$. This function defines an average degradation curve for the defined system. If our observation is $0 \le k \le n$ (the number of failed components at time t lies on this curve), then the information-based virtual age is just equal to the chronological age t.

Denote the corresponding information-based virtual age by $V(t)$. Our definition for this specific model is:

$$V(t) = D^{-1}(k), \tag{6.7}$$

where $D^{-1}(t)$ is an inverse function of $D(t)$. If $k = D(t)$, then $V(t) = D^{-1}(D(t)) = t$, which means that if the observation lies on the degradation curve, then the corresponding virtual age is equal to the chronological one. Similarly,

$$k < D(t) \Rightarrow V(t) < t, \qquad k > D(t) \Rightarrow V(t) > t.$$

Thus, in this example, the information-based virtual age is obtained via the average degradation curve $D(t)$.

We can simplify the model even further, assuming that n is sufficiently large. Then $D(t) = \mu t$ (in fact, this equality is approximate) and in accordance with (6.7):

$$V(t) = \frac{k}{\mu}.$$

Let, for instance, $\mu = 0.001(hr)^{-1}$ and the observation at time t (chronological age) is $k = 2$. This means that the virtual age is $200\,hr$ and it obviously does not depend on t.

Remark 6.3.1 As operation of convolution preserves the IFR property, the approach of this example can be generalized to the case of IFR components. Due to this fact, the mortality rates $\mu_n(t), n = 1, 2, \ldots$ are also increasing in this case and therefore the corresponding function $D(t)$ as well.

The general case of degrading objects can be considered in the same line. Let D_t be an increasing stochastic process of degradation with a mean $D(t)$. Assume for simplicity that this is a *process with independent increments,* and therefore it possesses the Markov property. Similar to (6.7), observation d_t at time t defines the information-based virtual age. Formally:

Definition 6.3.1 Let D_t be an increasing, with independent increments, stochastic process of degradation with a mean $D(t)$, and let d_t be an observation at time t.

Then the information-based virtual age is defined as

$$V(t) = D^{-1}(d_t).$$

Remark 6.3.2 It is clear that it is reasonable to apply the suggested approach to smoothly varying (predictable) stochastic processes of deterioration. Most of the aging processes in organisms are of this kind. However, Example 6.3.1 shows that formally the approach can also be used for the jump processes as well. The natural assumption in this case is that the jumps should be relatively small in comparison with the values of $D(t)$.

6.3.2 Mean remaining lifetime

The alternative way of defining $V(t)$ is via the information-based remaining lifetime [Finkelstein (2001)]. The mean remaining lifetime (MRL) at t of an object with a lifetime distribution $F(x)$ (in demographic and biological literature this notion is called the *life expectancy at t*) is defined in a standard way [Barlow and Proschan (1975)] as

$$M(t) = \int_0^\infty F(x|t)dx \equiv \int_0^\infty \frac{\bar{F}(t+x)}{\bar{F}(t)}dx. \tag{6.8}$$

We must compare $M(t)$ with the mean information-based remaining lifetime, denoted by $M_I(t)$. Let, as previously, d_t denote the observed level of degradation at time t. We now consider this value as a new initial value for a degradation process and denote by $M_I(t)$ the mean time to failure in this case.

For instance, in Example 6.3.1: $d_t = k$, the number of the failed components, which means that $M_I(t) = (n+1-k)/\mu$, as the mean lifetime of one component is $1/\mu$.

Definition 6.3.2 The information-based virtual age of a degrading system is given by the following equation,

$$V(t) = t + (M(t) - M_I(t)). \tag{6.9}$$

Thus, the information-based virtual age is the chronological one plus the difference between the "ordinary" and the information-based mean remaining lifetimes. If, for example, $M(t) = t_1 < t_2 = M_I(t)$, then $V(t) = t - (t_2 - t_1) < t$ and we have an additional expected $t_2 - t_1$ years of life for an object, compared with the "no information" version. It can be shown that under natural assumptions $M_I(t) - M(t) < t$ [Finkelstein and Vaupel (2006)], which ensures that $V(t)$ is positive.

Example 6.3.2 Consider a system of two independent, statistically identical components in parallel (hot redundancy) with exponential lifetime distributions. The time-to-failure survival function is $\bar{F}(t) = \exp\{-2\mu t\} - 2\exp\{-\mu t\}$ and

$$M(t) = \int_0^\infty \frac{2\exp\{-\mu t\} - \exp\{-2\mu t\}\exp\{-\mu x\}}{2 - \exp\{-\mu x\}} dx. \tag{6.10}$$

Assume that our observation at time t is two operable components. Then

$$M_I(t) = M(0) = \int_0^\infty \bar{F}(x)dx = \frac{1.5}{\mu}.$$

It is clear that $M(t)$ is monotonically decreasing from $1.5/\mu$ to $1/\mu$ as $t \to \infty$. Therefore it follows from Definition (6.9) that $0 < V(t) < t$, which means that the information-based virtual age in this case is smaller than the calendar age t. If observation is one operable component, then the virtual age is larger than t: $V(t) > t$. For given values of μ the exact values of $M(t)$ [and therefore of $V(t)$] can be easily numerically calculated using Equation (6.10).

Remark 6.3.3 An obvious question arises: what measure of virtual age to use? In accordance with our reasoning, the suggested possibility in the absence of information on the state of the object is the black box virtual age, which is defined for different regimes. When this information is available, the choice depends on the description of the aging process. If the degradation curve can be modeled by an observed, increasing stochastic process and the criterion of failure (death) is not well defined, then the first choice is the approach based on Equation (6.7). On the other hand, when the failure time distribution based on the corresponding stochastic process with different initial values (and therefore the corresponding mean remaining lifetime) can be defined, then Equation (6.9) should be preferably used.

6.4 Virtual Age in a Series System

As already mentioned in the introduction, defining the age of an organism, which consists of differently aging parts is a challenging unsolved problem [Vaupel et al. (2004)]. For instance, assume that there are two components in series and the first one has a much higher relative level of degradation than the second one, meaning that the corresponding virtual ages are also different. How do we define the virtual age of a system as a whole? It is clear that some averaging should be performed on the basis of the corresponding survival probabilities. We approach this problem using different definitions of virtual age.

We start with considering the statistical virtual age discussed in Section 6.2. In accordance with Equation (6.1), the survival functions of a series system of n statistically independent components under the baseline and a more severe environment are

$$\bar{F}_b(t) = \prod_1^n \bar{F}_{bi}(t); \qquad \bar{F}_s(t) = \prod_1^n \bar{F}_{bi}(W_i(t)), \qquad (6.11)$$

respectively, where $W_i(t)$ is the virtual age of the ith component and we assume that the model (6.1) holds for every component. The virtual age of the system $W(t)$ is obtained from the following equation,

$$\bar{F}_b(W(t)) = \prod_1^n \bar{F}_{bi}(W_i(t)) \qquad (6.12)$$

or, equivalently,

$$\int_0^{W(t)} \sum_1^n \mu_{bi}(u)du = \sum_1^n \int_0^{W_i(t)} \mu_{bi}(u)du. \qquad (6.13)$$

Therefore, this is a rather formal solution of the problem based on Equation (6.2).

Example 6.4.1 Let $n = 2$. Assume that $W_1(t) = t$, $W_2(t) = 2t$, which means that the first component is somehow protected from the stress (environment). Equation (6.13) turns into

$$\int_0^{W(t)} (\mu_{b1}(u) + \lambda_{b2}(u))du = \int_0^t \mu_{b1}(u)du + \int_0^{2t} \mu_{b2}(u)du.$$

Assume that the mortality rates are linear: $\mu_{b1}(t) = \mu_1 t$, $\mu_{b2}(t) = \mu_2 t$. Then

$$W(t) = t\sqrt{\frac{\mu_1 + 4\mu_2}{\mu_1 + \mu_2}}. \qquad (6.14)$$

The result is similar for mortality rates increasing as arbitrary power functions. If the components are statistically identical in the baseline environment ($\mu_1 = \mu_2$), then $W(t) = \sqrt{5/2}t \approx 1.6t$, which means that the statistical virtual age of a system with chronological age t is approximately $1.6t$. It is clear that the weight of components is eventually defined by the relationship between μ_1 and μ_2. When, for example, the ratio of μ_1 and μ_2 tends to 0, the virtual age of a system tends to $2t$; the virtual age of the second component.

A similar example can be easily considered, when all mortality rates are exponential functions with different parameters, but in this case there is no analytical solution and $W(t)$ should be obtained numerically.

As in the previous section, two approaches for defining the information-based virtual age of a system are considered. First, we weight ages in the series system of n degrading components in accordance with the importance (sensitivity) of the components with respect to the failure of a system. The most critical component is the one in which probability of failure is the highest. Let $V_i(t)$ denote the information-based virtual age of the ith component with mortality rate $\mu_i(t)$ in a series system of n statistically independent components. Then the virtual age of a system at time t can be defined as an expected value of the virtual age of a failed in $[t, t+dt)$ component:

$$V(t) = \sum_1^n \frac{\mu_i(t)}{\mu_s(t)} V_i(t), \tag{6.15}$$

where $\mu_s(t) = \sum_1^n \mu_i(t)$ is the mortality rate of the series system. This definition means, specifically, that the virtual age of a less reliable component should be weighted with the highest probability. If all virtual ages are equal $V_i(t) = \tilde{V}(t)$, $i = 1, 2, \ldots, n$, then $V(t) = \tilde{V}(t)$, which shows the "consistency" of Definition (6.15).

Example 6.4.2 Let

$$V_1(t) = \nu_1 t, \qquad V_2(t) = \nu_2 t, \qquad \mu_1(t) = \mu_1 e^{bt}, \qquad \mu_2(t) = \mu_2 e^{bt},$$

where $\nu_1, \nu_2, \mu_1, \mu_2, b > 0$. Then

$$V(t) = \frac{\mu_1 \nu_1 + \mu_2 \nu_2}{\mu_1 + \mu_2} t.$$

The second approach is based on the notion of the MRL function (life expectancy). A positive feature of this approach is that unlike (6.15), there is no direct link between the virtual age at the chronological time t and the probability of failure in $[t, t+dt)$. The survival function of a series system n of components and the survival function for a remaining lifetime are

$$\bar{F}(x) = \prod_1^n \bar{F}_i(x), \qquad \bar{F}(x|t) = \frac{\bar{F}(x+t)}{\bar{F}(x)} = \prod_1^n \bar{F}_i(x|t),$$

respectively. The corresponding MRL can be obtained, using this definition and Equation (6.8). Denote now by $F_{I,i}(x,t)$ the information-based distribution function of the remaining lifetime for the ith component. Then the corresponding MRL and the information-based MRL for the series system are defined as

$$M(t) = \int_0^\infty \prod_1^n \bar{F}_i(x|t), \qquad M_I(t) = \int_0^\infty \prod_1^n \bar{F}_{I,i}(x,t), \qquad (6.16)$$

respectively, where $\bar{F}_{I,i}(x,t)$ denotes the survival function for the information-based remaining lifetime with observation at time t. Finally, Equation (6.9) should be used for obtaining the information-based virtual age of a series system in this case.

Example 6.4.3 The functions $M(t)$ and $M_I(t)$ can usually be easily obtained numerically. But in certain cases some reasonable qualitative conclusions can be made. Consider two systems of the type described in Example 6.3.1, connected in series. The first system has parameters μ and n (as in Example 6.3.1), and the second η and m, respectively. It is clear that

$$\frac{1}{\mu + \eta} < M(t) < M(0),$$

where $M(t)$ for $t \in [0, \infty)$ can be obtained numerically using (6.16). Assume, that for some time t, our observation is no standby components are left in both systems, which means that the mean remaining lifetime is $1/(\mu + \eta)$. In accordance with Equation (6.9), the information-based virtual age of our series system in this case is

$$V(t) = t + \left(M(t) = \frac{1}{\mu + \eta} \right) > t,$$

which obviously illustrates the fact that this observation indicates a higher level of deterioration than the one that corresponds to the chronological age t.

Remark 6.4.1 The case of several biomarkers of aging, as mentioned in the introduction, can be considered as a special important problem for future research. It is clear that it should not necessarily be modeled by the corresponding series system; therefore the weighting should be performed in some different way. In addition, the dependence between the biomarkers is crucial for this "multivariate" case.

6.5 Concluding Remarks

Virtual (biological) age can be considered as some elusive concept, but it certainly makes sense, if properly defined. This chapter is probably the first step in *formalizing* this important notion. It should be noted, however, that the developed approaches are considered under some simplifying assumptions, but it is hoped that our reasoning can also be used for more general settings.

We described simple univariate models of deterioration just to illustrate this reasoning. Several other well-known models of aging [see, e.g., the review by Yashin *et al.* (2000)], described by stochastic processes, can also be used. It is essential, especially for the developed information-based approach, that the first passage time probabilities for the corresponding processes be well defined for different initial conditions.

Further studies should be conducted both in the direction of a more adequate stochastic modeling and, of course, in applying the developed reasoning to organisms and their parts.

References

1. Bagdonavicius, V. and Nikulin, M. (2002). *Accelerated Life Models. Modeling and Statistical Analysis*, Chapman & Hall, London.

2. Barlow, R. and Proschan, F. (1975). Statistical theory of reliability and life testing, In *Probability Models*, Holt, Rinehart, & Winston, New York.

3. Cox D. R. and Oakes D. (1984). *Analysis of Survival Data*, Chapman & Hall, London.

4. Finkelstein, M. S. (1999). Wearing-out components in variable environment, *Reliability Engineering and System Safety*, **66**, 235–242.

5. Finkelstein, M. S. (2001). How does our *n*-component system perform? *IEEE Transactions on Reliability*, **50**, 414–418.

6. Finkelstein, M. S. (2006). Mortality in varying environment, In *Probability, Statistics and Modelling in Public Health*, (Eds., M. Nikulin, D. Commenges, and C. Huber), pp. 145–157, Springer-Verlag, New York.

7. Finkelstein, M. S. and Vaupel J. W. (2006). The relative tail of longevity and the mean remaining lifetime, *Demographic Research*, **14**, 111–138.

8. Hoyland, A. and Rausand, M. (1993). *System Reliability Theory. Models and Statistical Methods*, John Wiley & Sons, New York.

9. Natvig, B. (1990). On information-based minimal repair and reduction in remaining system lifetime due to a failure of a specific module, *Journal of Applied Probability*, **27**, 365–375.

10. Olofsson, K. (2000). Branching process model of telomere shortening, *Communications in Statistics—Stochastic Models*, **16**, 167–177.

11. Ross, S. M. (1996). *Stochastic Processes*, John Wiley & Sons, New York.

12. Vaupel, J., Baudisch, A., Dolling, M., Roach, D., and Gampe, J. (2004). The case for negative senescence, *Theoretical Population Biology*, **65**, 339–351.

13. Vaupel, J. W. and Yashin, A. I. (1987). Repeated resuscitation: How life saving alters life tables, *Demography*, **4**, 123–135.

14. Yashin, A., Iachin, I., and Begun, A. S. (2000). Mortality modeling: A review, *Mathematical Population Studies*, **8**, 305–332.

7

A Competing Risks Model for Degradation and Traumatic Failure Times

Vincent Couallier

Equipe Statistique Mathématique et ses Applications, Université Victor Segalen Bordeaux 2, France

Abstract: We are interested here in some failure times due to wear or aging. The main aim is to jointly model the degradation process and one (or more) associated failure time(s). Two main joint models exist. The first one considers a failure time which is directly defined by the degradation process (degradation failure) as a hitting time of growth curve with random coefficients; the second one considers that the degradation influences the hazard rate of a failure time by a conditional definition of its survival function (traumatic failure). When both modes of failure exist, only the first one is observed. Very often, longitudinal observations of degradation values (measured with error) are available for each item until the first failure. We are mainly interested here in the nonparametric estimation of the cumulative intensity function of the traumatic failure time and related reliability characteristics.

Keywords and Phrases: Degradation failure time, traumatic failure time, nonlinear mixed regression, Nelson–Aalen estimator

7.1 Introduction

Degradation data modeling presents an attractive alternative in the assessment and improvement of reliability of components from which the overall system reliability can be deduced. If a component is monitored during its operation time, periodical tests can provide either the simple information that the component performs well (and thus is at risk for a failure) or quantitative information giving the level of degradation in a specified scale at every time measurement. Thus the degradation process can sometimes be observed and monitored through some quantitative characteristics. Examples of such degradation characteristics for monitoring degradation processes include the wear of tires [de Oliveira and Colosimo (2004)], gain of transistors [Whitmore (1995)], or degradation of fluorescent lamps [Tseng *et al.* (1995)] or catalytic converters for automobiles [Barone *et al.* (2001)], among others.

The usual traumatic failure time then has to be related to the evolution of the degradation process. Two main joint models exist. The first one considers a failure time which is directly defined by the degradation process; the second one considers that the degradation process influences the distribution of the failure time through a conditional definition of its hazard rate.

Let us assume that the degradation of an item is given by the sample path of a nondecreasing real-valued right-continuous and left-hand limited stochastic process $Z(t)$, $t \in I$. Lawless and Crowder (2004) and Couallier (2004) consider gamma processes, Kahle and Wendt (2004) and Lehmann (2004) consider marked point processes, and Whitmore and Schenkelberg (1997) consider Wiener diffusion processes. In the following, we make the assumption that

$$Z(t) = \mathcal{D}(t, A), \qquad t > 0, \tag{7.1}$$

where $\mathcal{D}$ is a differentiable and nondecreasing parametric function of the time and A is a random variable in $\mathbb{R}^p$ which takes account of the variability of the degradation evolution. The model reduces here to a nonlinear growth curve model with random coefficients where, for each individual $i = 1, \ldots, n$ the unknown real degradation is $Z^i(t) = \mathcal{D}(t, A_i)$ where A_i is the realization of A for the ith item and the observed degradation values are

$$Z_j^{i|obs} = \mathcal{D}(t_{ij}, A_i) + \epsilon_j^i, \tag{7.2}$$

measured at times t_{ij}, $j = 1, \ldots, n_i$ where the ϵ_j^i are error measurements of the degradation values.

7.2   The Degradation Failure—Estimation of F_A and F_{T_0}

We consider the lifetime T_0 which is the first time of crossing a fixed ultimate threshold z_0 for $Z(t)$,

$$T_0 = \inf\{t \in I, Z(t) \geq z_0\}.$$

The failure time T_0 is sometimes called soft failure (or failure directly due to wear) because in most industrial applications, z_0 is fixed and the experiment voluntarily ceases at the time the degradation process reaches the level z_0 or just after this time. Known results about parametric models of degradation failure time T_0 give the distribution function of T_0 with respect to the distribution function of $Z(t)$ or A.

For instance, Padgett and Tomlinson (2004) use the fact that if Z is a Gaussian process with positive drift then T_0 follows an inverse Gaussian distribution; de Oliveira and Colosimo (2004) assume the path model $Z(t) = a + bt$ where a is fixed (unknown) and b is Weibull(α, β). Then T_0 follows an inverse Weibull whose parameters depend on z_0, a, α, and β. Yu (2003) assumes the decreasing path model $Z(t) = -\beta t^\alpha$ where α is fixed and $\beta \sim LN(\mu, \sigma^2)$; then $T_0 \sim LN((\ln(-z_0) - \mu)/\alpha, \sigma^2/\alpha^2)$.

As an example, we analyze the following 21 degradation curves describing the fatigue crack propagation in aluminium alloy materials where at time $t = 0$; the initial crack size is 0.9 inches for all items [Meeker and Escobar (1998)]. The crack-lengths are measured every 10,000 cycles until the degradation level exceeds 1.6 inches. Figure 7.1 is a plot of the crack-length measurements versus time (in million cycles) joined by straight lines. Denoting by $g(., m, C)$ the solution of a simple version of the deterministic Paris-rule model [Dowling (1993)]

$$\frac{dg}{dt}(t, m, C) = C\sqrt{\pi g(t, m, C)}^m,$$

it is found that

$$g(t, m, C) = \left(0.9^{\frac{(2-m)}{2}} + \frac{2-m}{2}C\sqrt{\pi}^m t\right)^{\frac{2}{(2-m)}}.$$

Each curve is well fit by a Paris curve with unit-to-unit coefficients $A^i = (m_i, C_i)$ fit on each item. The failure due to degradation is defined as the time where the curve reaches the threshold $z_0 = 1.6$ inches. The aim is thus to estimate the distribution functions $F_{(m,C)}$ and F_{T_0} with the noisy measurements of degradation for each item without assuming that $F_{(m,C)}$ lies in a parametric family of distribution functions. For purely parametric estimation of degradation curves with maximum likelihood estimation of the d.f. of the failure time T_0 only due to wear, we refer to Meeker and Escobar (1998) and references therein.

Each individual path leads to a prediction $(\hat{A}_i)$ of unknown (A_i) by the nonlinear least squares method. For all i, a predictor $\hat{A}^i$ is computed with the nonlinear least squares method with observed degradation values Z_{ij}^{obs}, $j = 1, \ldots, n_i$:

$$\hat{A}_i = \text{argmin}_{a \in \mathbb{R}^p}(Z_{ij}^{obs} - \mathcal{D}(t_{ij}, a))' \Sigma_i^{-1}(Z_{ij}^{obs} - \mathcal{D}(t_{ij}, a)),$$

where Σ_i^{-1} is the variance matrix of $\epsilon_1^i, \ldots, \epsilon_{n_i}^i$. The simplest case of independent and identically distributed random variables ϵ_j^i with common variance σ^2 leads

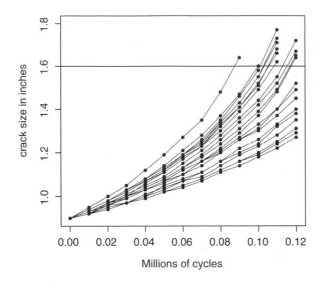

Figure 7.1. Fatigue crack size propagation for alloy-A data.

to the $n_i \times n_i$ diagonal matrix $\Sigma_i = \sigma^2 Id$. Several temporal correlation structures can be included in the variance matrix [see Couallier (2006)].

Bagdonavicius and Nikulin (2004) have shown under technical assumptions that the pseudo-empirical cumulative distribution function

$$\hat{\hat{F}}_A(a) = 1/n \sum_{i=1}^{n} \mathbf{1}_{\{\hat{A}^i \leq a\}},$$

is a uniformly consistent estimator of F_A. Instead of plugging the $\hat{A}^i$'s in the unknown empirical measure $P(E) = 1/n \sum_{i=1}^{n} 1(A^i \in E)$, we propose here to use the approximate distribution function of $\hat{A}^i$ around A^i which is asymptotically Gaussian with mean zero. Asymptotic results hold when n_i tends to infinity. The error terms can be assumed to be normally distributed but this is not necessary to get the asymptotic normality of $\hat{A}_i$ [see Seber and Wild (2005) for technical details]. Let us denote by $\hat{\Sigma}_i$ the estimated variance matrix given by the numerical least square method. If, for all i, $\hat{A}^i - A^i \sim \mathcal{N}(0, \hat{\Sigma}_i)$ then a estimator of the cumulative distribution function F_A is

$$\widetilde{F}_A(a) = \frac{1}{n} \sum_{i=1}^{n} \int_{\mathbb{R}^p} 1_{(u<a)} f_{\mathcal{N}(\hat{A}^i, \hat{\Sigma}_i)}(u) du, \qquad (7.3)$$

and its estimated density function is a mixing of normal densities

$$\tilde{f}_A(a) = \frac{1}{n} \sum_{i=1}^{n} f_{\mathcal{N}(\hat{A}^i, \hat{\Sigma}_i)}(a).$$

Marginal distributions are easily deduced. For each coordinate A_k of A, the estimated cumulative distribution function is

$$\widetilde{F}_{A_k}(a) = \frac{1}{n} \sum_{i=1}^{n} \Phi\left(\frac{a - \hat{A}_k^i}{\hat{\sigma}_k^i}\right),$$

where $\hat{\sigma}_k^{2i}$ is the estimated variance of $\hat{A}_k^i$ and Φ is the cumulative distribution function of the standard normal law.

The distribution function of T_0 is estimated either by calculating the pseudo-failure times $\hat{T}_0^i = h(z_0, \hat{A}_i)$ and plugging it in the unknown empirical cumulative distribution function of T_{0i}, $i = 1 \cdots n$:

$$\hat{F}_{T_0}(t) = \frac{1}{n} \sum_{i=1}^{n} 1_{\{h(z_0, \hat{A}^i) \leq t\}}, \tag{7.4}$$

or by using $P(T_0 \leq t) = P(\mathcal{D}(t, A) \geq z_0)$ to obtain

$$\widetilde{F}_{T_0}(t) = \int 1_{\{\mathcal{D}(t,a) \geq z_0\}} d\widetilde{F}_A(a). \tag{7.5}$$

The last formula requires numerical computation. We give a Monte Carlo procedure to calculate it. Because $\widetilde{F}_A$ is a Gaussian mixture, $\widetilde{F}_{T_0}$ is obtained by:

1. For large B, $(B = 10{,}000)$, simulate B realizations $(A_k)_{\{k=1,\ldots,B\}}$ of A, with d.f. $\widetilde{F}_A$; that is, B times do,

   (a) Draw at random i in $\{1, \ldots, n\}$.

   (b) Simulate a random vector A with d.f. $N(\hat{A}_i, \hat{\Sigma}_i)$.

2. Compute the pseudo lifetimes $T_{0k} = h(z_0, A_k)$, $k = 1, \ldots, B$.

3. Compute $\hat{F}_{T_0}(t) \approx \frac{Card\{k | T_{0k} \leq t\}}{B}$.

7.3   A Joint Model with Both Degradation and Traumatic Failure Times

As in Bagdonavicius and Nikulin (2004) and Couallier (2004), we define the traumatic failure time T with the conditional survival function given the past degradation process as

$$P(T > t | Z(s), 0 \leq s \leq t) = \exp\left(-\int_0^t \lambda_T(Z(s)) ds\right). \tag{7.6}$$

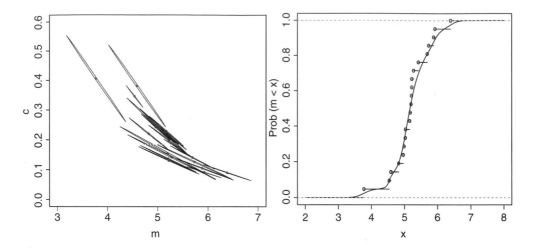

Figure 7.2. (a) Predictors $(\hat{m}_i, \hat{c}_i)$ of (m_i, c_i) for alloy-A data and 95% confidence region for each estimation; (b) ecdf of predicted $\hat{m}_i$ and $\widetilde{F}_m$.

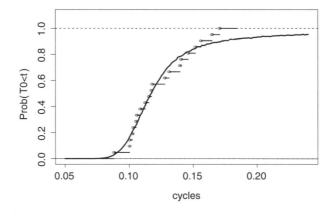

Figure 7.3. Two estimations of F_{T_0} according to (7.4) and (7.5).

λ_T is a nondecreasing function living in the degradation domain. The aim is to estimate this failure rate which depends on the chronological time only through the degradation process. The higher the degradation is, the higher the instantaneous probability of failure for an at-risk item will be. Also, the conditional survival function depends on the whole past degradation process. In this model, contrarily to T_0, the traumatic failure time T can occur even if the degradation level is low. Of course its survival function depends on the degradation function. In fact, the hazard function for the traumatic failure time T is determined by the value of the degradation process at time t because (7.6) involves

$$P(t < T \le t + \Delta | T > t, Z(t) = z) = \lambda_T(z)\Delta + o(\Delta), \quad \text{as } \Delta \longrightarrow 0.$$

Thus $\lambda_T(z)$ is proportional to the conditional probability of a traumatic failure in the small interval $(t, t + \delta)$ given that the unit survives at time t and that the degradation has reached the value z at time t.

We assume that T and T_0 are two competing failure times whose distribution functions are related to the degradation process $Z(t) = \mathcal{D}(t, A), t \geq 0$ defined in (7.1). Thus each failure time can be considered as a censoring time for the other because we only observe the minimum of T and T_0. T and T_0 are also assumed to be conditionally independent given $A = a$ where A is the random parameter vector of the degradation curve. The observed failure time is $U = \min\{T, T_0\}$. For instance, if $U = T_0$, we do not observe the traumatic failure time T. The function

$$\Lambda_T(z) = \int_0^z \lambda_T(s)ds,$$

is the cumulative intensity function of T in the degradation space. The definition (7.6) reduces here to

$$R_T(t|A = a) = P(T > t|A = a) = \exp\left(-\int_0^t \lambda_T(\mathcal{D}(s, a))ds\right).$$

For each item $i = 1, \ldots, n$, by denoting $T_0^i = \inf\{j \in \{1, \ldots, n_i\}|Z_j^i \geq z_0\}$, we observe $U^i = \min(T^i, T_0^i, t_{n_i}^i)$ and $\delta^i = 1(U^i = T^i)$ where $t_{n_i}^i$ is the last time of observation. The random coefficients $(A_i)_{(i=1,\ldots,n)}$ are deduced from degradation measurements before the failure time. In fact, if observed degradation data follow (7.2), nonlinear regression methods will provide predictors $\hat{A}^i$s which will be assumed to be closed to the unknown $\hat{A}^i$s. In the following, in a first step, we just assume that the A_is are known. In a second step, the A_is are replaced with their predictors $\hat{A}^i$.

In order to get nonparametric estimates of the cumulative intensity function Λ, the conditional survival function $R_T(t|A = a)$ and the survival function $R_T(t) = E_A(R(t|A))$, we use the fact that, denoting $h(., a)$ the inverse function of $\mathcal{D}(., a)$ we have

$$
\begin{aligned}
R_T(t|Z(s), 0 \leq s \leq t) &= P(T > t|A = a) \\
&= \exp\left[-\int_{\mathcal{D}(0,a)}^{\mathcal{D}(t,a)} h'(z, a)d\Lambda_T(z)\right]. \quad (7.7)
\end{aligned}
$$

Let us denote by Z_i the last observed degradation value (reached at time U_i), $Z_i = \mathcal{D}(U_i, A_i)$; then a Doob–Meyer decomposition of some counting process in the degradation space leads to a nonparametric estimator of Λ_T [Bagdonavicius and Nikulin (2004)]

$$\hat{\Lambda}_T(z) = \sum_{\delta_i=1, Z_i \leq z} \left(\frac{1}{\sum_{j, Z_j \geq Z_i} h'(Z_i, A^j)}\right). \quad (7.8)$$

Formulae (7.7) and (7.8) lead to the following estimate for the conditional survival function $\hat{R}_T(t|A = a)$

$$
\begin{aligned}
\hat{R}_T(t|A = a) &= \exp\left[-\int_{\mathcal{D}(0,a)}^{\mathcal{D}(t,a)} h'(z,a)d\hat{\Lambda}(z)\right] \\
&= \exp\left(-\sum_{i:\delta_i=1,Z_i\leq\mathcal{D}(t,a)} h'(Z_i,a)\frac{1}{\sum_{j:Z_j\geq Z_i} h'(Z_i,A_j)}\right).
\end{aligned}
$$

The estimation of the survival function R_T requires integration with respect to F_A because $R_T(t) = P(T > t) = \int R_T(t|A = a)dF_A(a)$. By using the empirical cumulative distribution function $\hat{F}_A$ as an estimate of F_A we get

$$
\begin{aligned}
\hat{R}_T(t) &= \int \exp\left[-\int_{\mathcal{D}(0,a)}^{\mathcal{D}(t,a)} h'(z,a)d\hat{\Lambda}_T(z)\right]d\widetilde{F}_A(a) \\
&= \frac{1}{n}\sum_{k=1}^{n} \exp\left(-\sum_{i:\delta_i=1,Z_i\leq\mathcal{D}(t,A_k)} h'(Z_i,A_k)\frac{1}{\sum_{j:Z_j\geq Z_i} h'(Z_i,A_j)}\right).
\end{aligned}
$$

Note that because the degradation curves are measured with errors, the A_is are not observed. In that case A_i has to be replaced by $\hat{A}_i$ and $\hat{F}_A$ by $\hat{\tilde{F}}_A$ or $\widetilde{F}_A$ in the formulae; see Section 7.2.

The overall survival function R_U of the failure time $U = min(T_0,T)$ is estimated by

$$
\begin{aligned}
\hat{R}_U(t) &= \int\left[\exp-\int_0^{\mathcal{D}(t,a)} h'(z,a)d\hat{\Lambda}_T(z)\right]1_{t<h(z_0,a)}d\hat{F}_\Lambda(a) \\
&= \frac{1}{n}\sum_{k=1}^{n} \exp\left[-\int_0^{\mathcal{D}(t,A_k)} h'(z,A_k)d\hat{\Lambda}_T(z)\right]1_{t<h(z_0,A_k)} \\
&= \frac{1}{n}\sum_{k=1}^{n} 1_{t<h(z_0,A_k)} \\
&\quad \times \exp\left(-\sum_{i:\delta_i=1,Z_i\leq\mathcal{D}(t,A_k)} h'(Z_i,A_k)\frac{1}{\sum_{j:Z_j\geq Z_i} h'(Z_i,A_j)}\right).
\end{aligned}
$$

7.4   A Joint Model with Two Failure Modes

Consider that degradation data are not observable until the failure time U which is the minimum of the degradation failure T_0 and the traumatic failure T. In that case we observe for $i = 1\ldots n$ the failure times $U^i = \min(T^i,T_0^i)$, the censoring indicators $\delta^i = 1_{(U^i = T^i)}$, and Z_i the degradation values at time U_i. If we assume that items are new at time zero, it is natural to consider linear degradation curves $Z^i(t) = A_i.t$ where A_i is a real-valued random variable that can be obtained from the failure time U_i and the degradation value Z_i by $A_i = Z_i/U_i$ (of course, some situations might be better described by another relationship than a linear trend; the only hypothesis here is that the random coefficient A_i can be recovered with one degradation measurement). The results of the last section hold and give

$$\hat{\Lambda}_T(z) = \sum_{i:\delta_i=1, Z_i \leq z} \frac{1}{\sum_{j:Z_j \geq Z_i} U_j/Z_j},$$

$$\hat{R}(t|A = a) = \exp\left(-\frac{1}{a} \sum_{i:\delta_i=1, Z_i \leq at} \frac{1}{\sum_{j:Z_j \geq Z_i} U_j/Z_j}\right),$$

$$\hat{R}_T(t) = P(T > t) = \frac{1}{n} \sum_{k=1}^{n} \exp\left(-\frac{U_k}{Z_k} \sum_{i:\delta_i=1, Z_i \leq Z_k t/U_k} \frac{1}{\sum_{j:Z_j \geq Z_i} U_j/Z_j}\right),$$

$$\hat{R}_U(t) = P(U > t) = \frac{1}{n} \sum_{k=1}^{n} 1_{(t < z_0 U_k/Z_k)}$$

$$\times \exp\left(-\frac{U_k}{Z_k} \sum_{i:\delta_i=1, Z_i \leq Z_k t/U_k} \frac{1}{\sum_{j:Z_j \geq Z_i} U_j/Z_j}\right).$$

7.5 Conclusion

Some statistical approaches to model and estimate the relationship between degradation and failure data were considered here. When the aging process due to cumulated wear and tiredness is observed, longitudinal degradation data are often a rich source of reliability information and offer many advantages over failure time data: degradation data are observed before the failure; some information about degradation status is available even for censored failure times. The joint model includes either a traumatic failure time whose hazard function is determined by the value of the degradation process [the essential point is that given the value of $Z(t)$, the hazard does not depend on t itself] or a degradation failure time defined as a first hitting time of the degradation process. Both failure time can obviously be considered in a competing risk model with degradation data.

Acknowledgements

The author wants to thank an anonymous referee for his careful reading and insightful comments and suggestions.

References

1. Bagdonavicius, V. and Nikulin, M. (2000). Estimation in degradation models with explanatory variables, *Lifetime Data Analysis*, **7**, 85–103.

2. Bagdonavicius, V. and Nikulin, M. (2004). Semiparametric analysis of degradation and failure time data with covariates, In *Parametric and Semiparametric Models with Applications to Reliability, Survival Analysis, and Quality of Life*, Birkhäuser, Boston.

3. Barone, S., Guida, M., and Pulcini, G. (2001). A stochastic degradation model of catalytic converters performances, In *MECA'01 International Workshop on Modeling and Control in Automotive engines*, technical paper.

4. Couallier, V. (2004). Comparison of parametric and semiparametric estimates in a degradation model with covariates and traumatic censoring, In *Parametric and Semiparametric Models with Applications to Reliability, Survival Analysis, and Quality of Life*, Birkhäuser, Boston.

5. Couallier, V. (2006). Some recent results on joint degradation and failure time modeling, In *Probability, Statistics and Modelling in Public Health* (Eds., M. Nikulin, D. Commenges, and C. Huber), Springer-Verlag, New York.

6. Dowling, N. E. (1993). *Mechanical Behavior of Materials*, Prentice Hall, Englewood Cliffs, NJ.

7. Kahle, W. and Wendt, H. (2004). On a cumulative damage process and resulting first passages times, *Applied Stochastic Models in Business and Industry*, **20**, 17–26.

8. Lawless, J. and Crowder, M. (2004). Covariates and random effects in a gamma process model with application to degradation and failure, *Lifetime Data Analysis*, **10**, 213–227.

9. Lehmann, A. (2004). On a degradation-failure model for repairable items, In *Semiparametric Models and Applications to Reliability, Survival Analysis and Quality of Life* (Eds., M. Nikulin, M. Mesbah, N. Balakrishnan, and N. Limnios), Birkhäuser, Boston.

10. Meeker, W. Q. and Escobar, L. (1998). *Statistical Analysis for Reliability Data*, John Wiley & Sons, New York.

11. de Oliveira, V. R. B. and Colosimo, E. A. (2004). Comparison of methods to estimate the time-to-failure distribution in degradation *Tests. Qual. Reliab. Eng. Int.*, **20**, 363–373.

12. Padgett, W. J. and Tomlinson, M. A. (2004). Inference from accelerated degradation and failure data based on Gaussian process models, *Lifetime Data Analysis*, **10**, 191–206.

13. Seber, G. A. F. and Wild, C. J. (2005), *Nonlinear Regression*, John Wiley & Sons, New York.

14. Tseng, S. T., Hamada, M., and Chiao, C. H. (1995). Using degradation data from a factorial experiment do improve fluorescent lamp reliability, *Journal of Quality Technology*, **27**, 363–369.

15. Whitmore, G. A. (1995). Estimating degradation by a Wiener diffusion process subject to measurement error, *Lifetime Data Analysis*, **1**, 307–319.

16. Whitmore, G. A. and Schenkelberg, F. (1997). Modelling accelerated degradation data using Wiener diffusion with a time scale transformation, *Lifetime Data Analysis*, **3**, 27–45.

17. Yu, H. F. (2003). Designing an accelerated degradation experiment by optimizing the estimation of the percentile, *Quality and Reliability Engineering International*, **19**, 197–214.

8

Generalized Birth and Death Processes as Degradation Models

Vladimir Rykov

Institute for Information Transmission Problems RAS, Bol'shoy Karetny, Moscow, Russia

Abstract: To model degradation processes in technical and biological objects generalized birth and death processes are introduced and studied.

Keywords and Phrases: Degradation models, generalized birth and death processes, quasi-stationary state probabilities

8.1 Introduction and Motivation

Traditional studies of technical systems' reliability mainly deal with their survival function (s.f.) and steady-state probabilities (s.s.p.) for renewable systems. For biological objects the hazard rate function (h.r.f.) is a more informative characteristic. Because there are no infinitely long living objects and any repair is possible only from the state of partial failure, the modelling of the degradation process during the lifetime of an object is the most interesting topic. From the mathematical point of view the degradation during the object's lifetime can be described by the birth and death (B&D) type process with absorbing state. For this process the conditional state probability distribution given the object's lifetime is the most interesting characteristic. The closed form solution for this characteristic is not a simple problem even for a usual B&D process. But it is possible to calculate the limiting values at infinity (so-called quasi-stationary distributions). The problem of existence of quasi-stationary distributions for B&D processes has a long history [see, e.g., van Doorn (1991), Kijima *et al.* (1997) and the bibliography therein], where this problem was considered for a B&D process with absorbtion at the state $\{-1\}$ with the help of the spectral representation technique, proposed in Karlin and McGregor (1957). Recently intensive attention to the aging and degradation models for technical and biological objects has been paid. The aging and degradation models suppose the

95

study of systems with gradual failures for which multistate reliability models were elaborated [for the history and bibliography see, e.g., Lisniansky and Levitin (2003)]. In some of our previous papers [see Dimitrov *et al.* (2002), Rykov and Dimitrov (2002), Dimitrov *et al.* (2004)] the model of a complex hierarchical system was proposed and the methods for its steady-state and time-dependent characteristics investigation was done. Controllable fault-tolerance reliability systems were considered in Rykov and Efrosinin (2004) and Rykov and Buldaeva (2004).

In the present chapter a generalized B&D process as a model for degradation and aging processes of technical and biological objects is proposed. Conditional state probabilities given the object's lifetime and their limiting values when $t \rightarrow \infty$ are calculated. The variation of the model parameters allows us to consider various problems of aging and degradation control.

8.2   Generalized B&D Process. Preliminary

Most up-to-date complex technical systems as well as biological objects with sufficiently high organization during their lifetime pass over different states of evolution and existence. In the simplest case it can be modelled by the B&D type process. Suppose that the states of an object are completely ordered, its transitions only into neighboring states are possible, and their intensities depend on the time spent in the present state. Consider firstly the general case of the process with denumerable set of states $E = \{1, 2, \ldots\}$. To describe the object behavior by a Markov process let us introduce an enlarged state space $\mathcal{E} = E \times [0, \infty)$ and consider the two-dimensional process $Z(t) = \{S(t), X(t)\}$, where the first component $S(t) \in E$ shows the object's state, and the second one $X(t) \in [0, \infty)$ denotes the time spent in the state since the last entrance into it. Denote by $\alpha_i(x)$ and $\beta_i(x)$ $(i \in E)$ the transition intensities from the state i to the states $i + 1$ and $i - 1$, respectively under the condition that the time spent at the state i equals to x.

Remark 8.2.1 If the staying time at state i is considered as a minimum of two independent random variables (r.v): times A_i and B_i until the transition into the states $i + 1$ and $i - 1$, respectively, with cumulative distribution functions (c.d.f.) $A_i(x)$, $B_i(x)$, probability density functions (p.d.f.) $a_i(x)$, $b_i(x)$, and mean values $a_i = \int [1 - A_i(x)] \, dx$, $b_i = \int [1 - B_i(x)] \, dx$, then the introduced process can be considered as a special case of a semi-Markov process (SMP) [see Korolyuk and Turbin (1976)], with conditional transition p.d.f.s $\alpha_i(x)$ and $\beta_i(x)$. Nevertheless, the above formalization opens new possibilities for their investigations and, moreover, in the degradation models we are studying the conditional probability state distribution given the lifetime, that was not investigated previously.

Denote by $\pi_i(t, x)$ the p.d.f. of the process $Z(t)$ at time t,

$$\pi_i(t, x)dx = \mathbf{P}\{S(t) = i, \ x \le X(t) < x + dx\} \qquad (i \in E).$$

These functions satisfy Kolmogorov's system of differential equations

$$\frac{\partial \pi_i(t, x)}{\partial t} + \frac{\partial \pi_i(t, x)}{\partial x} = -(\alpha_i(x) + \beta_i(x))\pi_i(t, x), \qquad 0 \le x \le t < \infty, \quad (8.1)$$

with the initial and boundary conditions

$$\left.\begin{array}{rcl} \pi_1(t, 0) &=& \delta(t) + \int\limits_0^t \pi_2(t, x)\beta_2(x)dx \\[2mm] \pi_i(t, 0) &=& \int\limits_0^t \pi_{i-1}(t, x)\alpha_{i-1}(x)dx + \int\limits_0^t \pi_{i+1}(t, x)\beta_{i+1}(x)dx \end{array}\right\}. \qquad (8.2)$$

In the following we suppose the process to be nonreducible and nondegenerated. The conditions for this in terms of SMP might be found, for example, in Jacod (1971) and McDonald (1978). For the nonreducible, nondegenerated generalized B&D process Equation (8.1) with initial and boundary conditions (8.2) has a unique solution over all time axes.

It is possible to show by the method of characteristics [Petrovsky (1952)], that its solution has the form

$$\pi_i(t, x) = g_i(t - x)(1 - A_i(x))(1 - B_i(x)), \qquad 0 \le x \le t < \infty, \qquad i \in E, \ (8.3)$$

where functions $g_i(t)$ according to the initial and boundary conditions (8.2) satisfy the system of equations

$$\left.\begin{array}{rcl} g_1(t) &=& \delta(t) + \int\limits_0^t g_2(t - x)(1 - A_2(x)b_2(x))dx, \\[2mm] g_i(t) &=& \int\limits_0^t g_{i-1}(t - x)a_{i-1}(x)(1 - B_{i-1}(x))dx \\[2mm] && + \int\limits_0^t g_{i+1}(t - x)(1 - A_{i+1}(x)b_{i+1}(x))dx \end{array}\right\}. \qquad (8.4)$$

The form of these equations shows that their solution should be found in terms of Laplace transforms (LTs). Therefore by passing to the LTs with respect to both variables into relations (8.3) one can get

$$\tilde{\tilde{\pi}}_i(s, v) \equiv \int\limits_0^\infty e^{-st} \int\limits_0^t e^{-vx} \pi(t, x)\, dx\, dt = \tilde{g}_i(s)\tilde{\gamma}_i(s + v), \qquad (8.5)$$

where $\tilde{g}_i(s)$ are the LTs of the functions $g_i(t)$, and the functions $\tilde{\gamma}_i(s)$ are

$$\tilde{\gamma}_i(s) = \int\limits_0^\infty e^{-st}(1 - A_i(t))(1 - B_i(t))dt \qquad (i \in E).$$

From the other side by passing to the LTs in the system (8.4) one gets

$$\left.\begin{aligned}
\tilde{g}_1(s) - \tilde{g}_2(s)\tilde{\psi}_2(s) &= 1 \\
-\tilde{g}_{i-1}(s)\tilde{\phi}_{i-1}(s) + \tilde{g}_i(s) - \tilde{g}_{i+1}(s)\tilde{\psi}_{i+1}(s) &= 0
\end{aligned}\right\}, \qquad (8.6)$$

where the functions $\tilde{\phi}_i(s)$ and $\tilde{\psi}_i(s)$ for all $i \in E$ are given by the relations

$$\tilde{\phi}_i(s) = \int\limits_0^\infty e^{-sx}a_i(x)(1 - B_i(x))dx, \qquad \tilde{\psi}_i(s) = \int\limits_0^\infty e^{-sx}(1 - A_i(x))b_i(x)dx.$$

The closed-form solution of this system in the general case even in the simplest case of the usual B&D process is not possible. Nevertheless, it provides calculation of different characteristics of the process. Consider some of them.

8.3   Steady-State Distribution

For calculation of the process $Z(t)$ stationary macrostate probabilities (m.s.p.)

$$\pi_i(t) = \int\limits_0^t \pi_i(t, x)dx = \int\limits_0^t g_i(t - x)(1 - A_i(x))(1 - B_i(x))dx, \qquad (8.7)$$

we use the connection between asymptotic behavior of functions at infinity and their LTs at zero. Letting $\tilde{\gamma}_i(0) = \gamma_i$ and taking into account that according to (8.5) $\tilde{\pi}_i(s) = \tilde{\tilde{\pi}}_i(s, 0)$, we find

$$\pi_i = \lim_{t\to\infty} \pi_i(t) = \lim_{s\to 0} s\tilde{\pi}_i(s) = \gamma_i \lim_{s\to 0} s\tilde{g}_i(s) = \gamma_i g_i, \qquad (8.8)$$

where $g_i = \lim_{s\to 0} s\tilde{g}_i(s)$, which should be calculated for the problem solution. For this we use Equations (8.6). Denote $\phi_i = \tilde{\phi}_i(0)$, $\psi_i = \tilde{\psi}_i(0)$, and note that $\phi_i + \psi_i = 1$, and $\phi_1 = 1$. The following theorem holds.

Theorem 8.3.1 *For the generalized B&D process stationary regime existence the convergence of the following series is necessary.*

$$g_1^{-1} = \sum_{1 \le i < \infty} \gamma_i \prod_{1 \le j \le i} \frac{\phi_{j-1}}{\psi_j} < \infty. \qquad (8.9)$$

In this case the stationary m.s.p. are given by the formulas

$$\pi_1 = g_1\gamma_1, \qquad \pi_i = g_1\gamma_i \prod_{1 \le j \le i} \frac{\phi_{j-1}}{\psi_j}, \qquad i = 2, 3, \ldots. \tag{8.10}$$

PROOF. Suppose that the limits (8.8) exist. Multiplying Equations (8.6) by s, passing to the limit when $s \to 0$, and taking into account the above notations and relations from these equations one gets the recursive relations

$$g_i\phi_i - g_{i+1}\psi_{i+1} = g_{i-1}\phi_{i-1} - g_i\psi_i, \qquad i = 2, 3 \ldots. \tag{8.11}$$

Because of $\phi_1 = 1$, from the first of Equations (8.6) it follows that $g_1\phi_1 - g_2\psi_2 = 0$. With the help of the last recursive relation it is possible to calculate coefficients g_i and find the stationary m.s.p. in form (8.10), for which the converges of the series (8.9) is necessary. ∎

Moreover, from the form of the stationary m.s.p. the next important corollary follows.

Corollary 8.3.1 *The stationary m.s.p. of generalized B&D process are insensitive to the shape of distributions $A_i(x)$, $B_i(x)$ and depend only on jump probabilities up and down an embedded random walk, and mean time of the process staying in the given states,*

$$\phi_i = \mathbf{P}\{A_i \le B_i\}, \qquad \psi_i = \mathbf{P}\{A_i > B_i\}, \qquad \gamma_i = \mathbf{E}[\min A_i, B_i].$$

PROOF. Follows from the formulas (8.9) and (8.10). ∎

In the case of exponential distributions $A_i(x) = 1 - e^{-\alpha_i x}$ and $B_i(x) = 1 - e^{-\beta_i x}$ the formulas (8.10) are reduced to the s.s.p. of the usual B&D process.

8.4 Conditional Distribution Given Lifetime

For many phenomena, especially for degradation processes, the absorbing process model is more appropriate. For the generalized B&D process with absorbing state $n + 1$ in Equations (8.1) one should put $\alpha_{n+1}(x) = \beta_{n+1}(x) \equiv 0$. In this case the equation for the p.d.f. $\pi_{n+1}(t)$ takes the form

$$\frac{\partial \pi_{n+1}(t, x)}{\partial t} + \frac{\partial \pi_{n+1}(t, x)}{\partial x} = 0, \tag{8.12}$$

with the initial and boundary condition

$$\pi_{n+1}(t, 0) = \int_0^t \pi_n(t, x)\alpha_n(x)dx. \tag{8.13}$$

Thus, all p.d.f.s $\pi_i(t, x)$ $(i = \overline{1, n})$ have the same form (8.3) as before. But the p.d.f. $\pi_{n+1}(t, x)$, being a constant over characteristics, is

$$\pi_{n+1}(t, x) = g_{n+1}(t - x), \tag{8.14}$$

where due to the boundary conditions (8.13) it follows that

$$g_{n+1}(t) = \int_0^t g_n(t - x) a_n(x)(1 - B_n(x)) dx. \tag{8.15}$$

From the systems of Equations (8.1), (8.2), (8.12), and (8.13) it follows that the m.s.p.s $\pi_i(t)$ $(i = \overline{1, n})$ represent the probabilities of the object to be in some state jointly with its lifetime T,

$$\pi_i(t) = \mathbf{P}\{S(t) = i, \ t < T\}, \qquad (i = \overline{1, n}),$$

whereas the m.s.p. $\pi_{n+1}(t)$ represents the distribution of this period,

$$\pi_{n+1}(t) = \mathbf{P}\{T \leq t\}.$$

For the degradation problem investigation, more useful and adequate characteristics are the conditional state probabilities given the object lifetime for which the following representations are true.

$$\bar{\pi}_i(t) \equiv \mathbf{P}\{S(t) = i \ |t < T\} = \frac{\pi_i(t)}{R(t)}, \qquad (i = \overline{1, n}),$$

where the s.f. of the object is

$$R(t) = 1 - \pi_{n+1}(t) = \mathbf{P}\{T > t\}. \tag{8.16}$$

We are interested in asymptotic behavior of these conditional probabilities at infinity. To find their limits at infinity, it is necessary to show that the asymptotic behavior of the s.f. $R(t)$ coincide with the asymptotic behavior of the m.s.p.s $\pi_i(t)$. We do that with the help of their LTs. The LTs $\tilde{\pi}_i(s)$ of the m.s.p.s $\pi_i(t)$ have the same form (8.5) as before, and for m.s.p. $\tilde{\pi}_{n+1}(s)$ according to (8.14) and (8.15) it holds

$$\tilde{\pi}_{n+1}(s) = \int_0^\infty e^{-st} \int_0^t g_{n+1}(t - x) \, dx dt = \frac{1}{s} \tilde{g}_{n+1}(s) = \frac{1}{s} \tilde{\phi}_n(s) g_n(s). \tag{8.17}$$

For the functions $\tilde{g}_i(s)$ $(i = \overline{1, n})$ the first n of Equations (8.6) take place, the matrix form of which is

$$\Psi(s) \underrightarrow{\tilde{g}(s)} = e_1, \tag{8.18}$$

where $\Psi(s)$ is the matrix of coefficients of the n first equations of the system (8.6). Denote also by $\Psi_i(s)$ the matrix, obtained from this one by changing its ith column with the vector of the right-hand side of the system (vector $\vec{e}_1$), and by $\Delta(s)$ and $\Delta_i(s)$ the determinants of these matrices. Then taking into account the expressions (8.5) and (8.17), and the solution of the system (8.18) in terms of Kramer's rule, one can get

$$
\left.
\begin{array}{rl}
\tilde{\pi}_i(s) &= \tilde{\gamma}_i(s)\tilde{g}_i(s) = \tilde{\gamma}_i(s)\frac{\Delta_i(s)}{\Delta(s)} \qquad (i = \overline{1,n}) \\[2mm]
\tilde{\pi}_{n+1}(s) &= \frac{\tilde{\phi}_n(s)}{s}\tilde{g}_n(s) = \frac{\tilde{\phi}_n(s)}{s}\frac{\Delta_n(s)}{\Delta(s)}
\end{array}
\right\}.
\tag{8.19}
$$

Due to the definition all functions $\tilde{\pi}_i(s)$ $(i = \overline{1,n})$ and $\tilde{R}(s)$ are analytical in right the half-plane, $Re\, s \geq 0$. Suppose that all these functions at the left half-plane have only a finite number of singular points. [This is true, e.g., if all functions $\tilde{\phi}_i(s)$, $\tilde{\psi}_i(s)$ are meromorphic.] Therefore, according to the inverse LT formulae the behavior of their originals is determined with their singularities in the left half-plane [Lavrent'ev and Shabat (1958)].

$$
\pi_i(t) = \sum \mathrm{res}\{\tilde{\pi}_i(s_k)e^{s_k t}\}, \qquad R(t) = \sum \mathrm{res}\{\tilde{R}(s_k)e^{s_k t}\},
$$

where the summations go over all singularities of appropriate functions.

Suppose that for all these functions the singular point s_1 with a minimal module is defined with the root of the characteristic equation

$$
\Delta(s) = 0,
\tag{8.20}
$$

and suppose that in its neighborhood the function $\Delta(s)$ has a pole of the first order.

Theorem 8.4.1 *If the singular point s_1 for all functions $\tilde{\pi}_i(s)$ $(i = \overline{1,n})$ and $\tilde{R}(s)$ with a minimal module is determined by the root of the characteristic equation (8.20), then the asymptotic behavior of the m.s.p.s $\pi_i(t)$ and the s.f. $R(t)$ when $t \to \infty$ coincides. This provides the existence of the limits*

$$
\bar{\pi}_i = \lim_{t \to \infty} \bar{\pi}_i(t) = \frac{\tilde{\pi}_i(s_1)}{\tilde{R}(s_1)} = \gamma_i(s_1)\frac{\Delta_i(s_1)}{\Delta_R(s_1)}.
$$

PROOF. From the last of relations (8.19) it follows that the function $\tilde{\pi}_{n+1}(s)$ can be represented in the form

$$
\tilde{\pi}_{n+1}(s) = \frac{\tilde{\phi}_n(s)}{s}\frac{\Delta_n(s)}{\Delta(s)} = \frac{B}{s} + \frac{\Delta_R(s)}{\Delta(s)},
$$

with some coefficient B and some function $\Delta_R(s)$. Let us show that the coefficient B equals one, $B = 1$. Really, from the definition it follows that

$$
B = \lim_{s \to 0} s\tilde{\pi}_{n+1}(s) = \lim_{s \to 0} \tilde{\phi}_n(s)g_n(s) = \phi_n g_n(0) = \phi_n\frac{\Delta_n(0)}{\Delta(0)}.
$$

Denote $\Psi = \Psi(0)$, $\Psi_n = \Psi_n(0)$ and consider the matrix $\Psi - \phi_n\Psi_n$. Because $\phi_1 = 1$ and $\phi_i + \psi_i = 1$ for all $i = \overline{1, n}$, the sum of elements of rows of the matrix Ψ except the last elements are equal to the zero row. Because the matrix Ψ_n differs from Ψ only with the last column, thus the sum elements of all rows of the matrix $\Psi - \phi_n\Psi_n$ except elements of its last column are also zero row. Consider now the elements of the last column. At the first place in it is an element $-\phi_n$, at the before-last one is an element $-\psi_n$, and at the last one is an element $1 = \phi_n + \psi_n$. Thus, the rows of the matrix $\Psi - \phi_n\Psi_n$ are linearly dependent, and, therefore, its determinant equals zero. From this fact it follows that $\phi_n\Delta_n(0) = \Delta(0)$ and consequently $B = (\phi_n\Delta_n(0))/\Delta(0) = 1$. At least from this it follows that the function $\tilde{R}(s)$ can be presented as

$$\tilde{R}(s) = \frac{\Delta_R(s)}{\Delta(s)}.$$

Thus, the asymptotic behavior of the s.f. $R(t)$ when $t \to \infty$ also as all m.s.p.s $\pi_i(t)$ is determined by the maximal root s_1 of the characteristic equation $\Delta(s) = 0$.

To evaluate the precise value of the limit it is necessary to note that the values of the limit are determined by the residuals of the functions $\tilde{\pi}_i(s)$ and $\tilde{R}(s)$ at this point,

$$A_{i1} = \lim_{s \to s_1} (s - s_1)\tilde{\pi}_i(s) = \lim_{s \to s_1} (s - s_1)\frac{\Delta_i(s)}{\Delta(s)} = \frac{\Delta_i(s_1)}{\dot{\Delta}(s_1)};$$

$$A_{R1} = \lim_{s \to s_1} (s - s_1)\tilde{R}(s) = \lim_{s \to s_1} (s - s_1)\frac{\Delta_R(s)}{\Delta(s)} = \frac{\Delta_R(s_1)}{\dot{\Delta}(s_1)}.$$

Therefore, when $t \to \infty$ the limiting value is

$$\bar{\pi}_i = \lim_{t \to \infty} \frac{\pi_i(t)}{R(t)} = \frac{\tilde{\pi}_i(s_1)}{\tilde{R}(s_1)} = \gamma(s_1)\frac{\Delta_i(s_1)}{\Delta_R(s_1)}.$$

■

To investigate the h.r.f. behavior at infinity it is necessary to remark that the p.d.f. of an object's lifetime due to (8.14)–(8.16) equals

$$f(t) = -\dot{R}(t) = \dot{\pi}_{n+1}(t) = g_{n+1}(t) = \int_0^t g_n(t - x)a_n(x)(1 - B_n(x))dx.$$

Thus,

$$\tilde{f}(s) = \tilde{\phi}_n(s)\tilde{g}_n(s) = \tilde{\phi}_n(s)\frac{\Delta_n(s)}{\Delta(s)}.$$

Therefore, because in the conditions of the previous theorem the behavior of p.d.f. $f(t)$ and the s.f. $R(t)$ at infinity coincide, the limit of h.r.f. $h(t)$ at infinity also exists. This consideration could be formulated as a theorem.

Theorem 8.4.2 *Under the conditions of Theorem 8.4.1 there exists the limit*

$$h = \lim_{t\to\infty} h(t) = \phi_n(s_1)\frac{\Delta_n(s_1)}{\Delta_R(s_1)}.$$

PROOF. Follows from the above considerations.   ■

To illustrate the above results let us consider an object with only three states: normal functioning N, degradation D, and failure F.

8.5   An Example

Suppose for simplicity that the times-to-failure in the normal N and the degeneration D states are exponentially distributed with parameters λ and ν, respectively, but the repair times are generally distributed with c.d.f. $B(x)$ and the conditional p.d.f. $\beta(x)$. Moreover suppose that the direct transition from the normal state into the failure state are also possible with intensity γ. The transition graph is presented in the figure below.

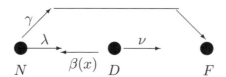

The marked transition graph of the process, for example.

In accordance with the given transition structure, Kolmogorov's system of differential equations for system state probabilities has the form

$$\left.\begin{array}{rcl}
\frac{d\pi_N(t)}{dt} &=& -(\lambda+\gamma)\pi_N(t) + \int_0^t \beta(x)\pi_D(t,x)dx \\[2mm]
\frac{\partial\pi_D(t,x)}{\partial t} + \frac{\partial\pi_D(t,x)}{\partial x} &=& -(\nu+\beta(x))\pi_D(t,x) \\[2mm]
\frac{d\pi_F(t)}{dt} &=& \gamma\pi_N(t) + \nu\int_0^t \pi_D(t,x)\,dx
\end{array}\right\} \qquad (8.21)$$

with the initial and the boundary conditions

$$\left.\begin{array}{rcl}
\pi_D(t,0) &=& \lambda\pi_N(t), \\
\pi_N(0) &=& 1, \quad \pi_D(0,0) = \pi_F(0) = 0.
\end{array}\right\}. \qquad (8.22)$$

The s.f. of the system is

$$R(t) = 1 - \pi_F(t) = 1 - \int_0^t [\gamma \pi_N(u) + \nu \pi_D(u)] \, du, \qquad (8.23)$$

where

$$\pi_D(t) = \int_0^t \pi_D(t, x) \, dx. \qquad (8.24)$$

The solution of the second equation from the system (8.21) according to (8.3) can be given in the form

$$\pi_D(t, x) = g_D(t - x)e^{-\nu x}(1 - B(x)),$$

and using the boundary condition (8.22) gives

$$\pi_D(t, x) = \lambda \pi_N(t - x)e^{-\nu x}(1 - B(x)). \qquad (8.25)$$

The following equation

$$\frac{d\pi_N(t)}{dt} = -(\lambda + \gamma)\pi_N(t) + \lambda \int_0^t \beta(x)\pi_N(t - x)e^{-\nu x}(1 - B(x))dx \qquad (8.26)$$

is the result of the substitution of this solution into the first equation of the system (8.21). In terms of LT with the initial condition (8.22) the last equation is

$$s\tilde{\pi}_N(s) - 1 = -(\lambda + \gamma)\tilde{\pi}_N(s) + \lambda \tilde{b}(s + \nu)\tilde{\pi}_N(s),$$

where $\tilde{b}(s) = b(x)dx$ is a LT of the p.d.f. $b(x)$. Therefore

$$\tilde{\pi}_N(s) = \left[s + \gamma + \lambda(1 - \tilde{b}(s + \nu)) \right]^{-1}. \qquad (8.27)$$

The calculation of the LT $\tilde{\pi}_D(s)$ of the function $\pi_D(t)$, using the formulae (8.24), (8.25), and (8.27) gives

$$\tilde{\pi}_D(s) = \int_0^\infty e^{-st} \int_0^t \pi_D(t, x) \, dx = \frac{\lambda(1 - \tilde{b}(s + \nu))}{(s + \nu)(s + \gamma + \lambda(1 - \tilde{b}(s + \nu)))}. \qquad (8.28)$$

At least for the LT $\tilde{\pi}_F(s)$ of the function $\pi_F(t)$ from the last of equations (8.21) one can find

$$s\tilde{\pi}_F(s) = \gamma \tilde{\pi}_N(s) + \nu \tilde{\pi}_D(s) = \frac{\gamma(s + \nu) + \lambda\nu(1 - \tilde{b}(s + \nu))}{(s + \nu)(s + \gamma + \lambda(1 - \tilde{b}(s + \nu)))}. \qquad (8.29)$$

Therefore, the LT of the s.f. (8.23) is

$$\tilde{R}(s) = \frac{1}{s} - \tilde{\pi}_F(s) = \frac{s + \nu + \lambda(1 - \tilde{b}(s + \nu))}{(s + \nu)(s + \gamma + \lambda(1 - \tilde{b}(s + \nu)))}. \qquad (8.30)$$

From the last expression one can find the mean lifetime of the object

$$m_F = \tilde{R}(0) = \frac{\nu + \lambda(1 - \tilde{b}(\nu))}{\nu(\gamma + \lambda(1 - \tilde{b}(\nu)))}. \tag{8.31}$$

For calculation of the limiting values of the conditional state probabilities given the lifetime we use the above procedure. In the considered case the characteristic equation (8.20) has a form

$$\Delta(s) = (s + \nu)(s + \gamma + \lambda(1 - \tilde{b}(s + \nu))) = 0. \tag{8.32}$$

One of its roots is $s = -\nu$. The second root is determined by the equation $(s + \gamma + \lambda(1 - \tilde{b}(s + \nu))) = 0$ or

$$\tilde{b}(s + \nu) = 1 + \frac{s + \gamma}{\lambda}. \tag{8.33}$$

Because the function $\tilde{b}(s+\nu)$ is a completely monotone one [Feller (1966)], that is, monotonically decreases, concave upward, takes the value 1 at the point $s = -\nu$ and $\tilde{b}(\nu) < 1 + \gamma/\lambda$, then Equation (8.33) has a unique negative root, and its value depends on the sign of the difference $\gamma - \nu$. If $\gamma \geq \nu$ the root of this equation, which we denote by s_1, is less than $-\nu$, $s_1 \leq -\nu$. On the other hand if $\gamma < \nu$ the root of this equation s_1 is greater than $-\nu$, $s_1 > -\nu$. Thus, when $\gamma \geq \nu$ the maximal root of the equation (8.33) is $-\nu$, and therefore,

$$\left.\begin{aligned}
\bar{\pi}_N &= \lim_{t \to \infty} \bar{\pi}_N(t) = \lim_{t \to \infty} \frac{\pi_N(t)}{R(t)} = \lim_{s \to -\nu} \frac{\tilde{\pi}_N(s)}{\tilde{R}(s)} = \frac{1}{1 + \lambda m_B} \\
\bar{\pi}_D &= \lim_{t \to \infty} \bar{\pi}_D(t) = \lim_{t \to \infty} \frac{\pi_D(t)}{R(t)} = \lim_{s \to -\nu} \frac{\tilde{\pi}_D(s)}{\tilde{R}(s)} = \frac{\lambda m_B}{1 + \lambda m_B}
\end{aligned}\right\}; \tag{8.34}$$

that is, if the death intensity from the normal state is greater than the death intensity resulting from degradation, then the limiting distribution of the conditional state probabilities is determined by the parameter $\rho = \lambda m_B$.

From another side, under condition $\gamma < \nu$ the greatest root of the characteristic equation (8.32) is the root of Equation (8.33), and consequently

$$\left.\begin{aligned}
\bar{\pi}_N &= \lim_{t \to \infty} \bar{\pi}_N(t) = \lim_{s \to s_1} \frac{\tilde{\pi}_N(s)}{\tilde{R}(s)} = \frac{s_1 + \nu}{s_1 + \nu + \lambda(1 - \tilde{b}(s_1 + \nu))} \\
\bar{\pi}_D &= \lim_{t \to \infty} \bar{\pi}_D(t) = \lim_{s \to s_1} \frac{\tilde{\pi}_D(s)}{\tilde{R}(s)} = \frac{\lambda(1 - \tilde{b}(s_1 + \nu))}{s_1 + \nu + \lambda(1 - \tilde{b}(s_1 + \nu))}
\end{aligned}\right\}. \tag{8.35}$$

Therefore, if the death intensity from the normal state is less than the same as a degradation result, then the limiting distribution of the conditional probabilities strongly depends on the value s_1 of the Equation (8.33) root. Note that in the case where direct transitions from the normal state to the failure state are impossible (i.e., when $\gamma = 0$) the second case takes place.

8.6   Conclusion

Generalized birth and death processes, which are a special class of semi-Markov processes are introduced for modelling the degradation processes. The special parametrization of the processes allows us to give a more convenient presentation of the results. Special attention is focused on the conditional state probabilities given the lifetime, which are the most interesting for the degradation processes.

In conclusion the author thanks the referee for his or her remarks, which allowed us to improve the chapter's presentation.

Acknowledgements

The chapter was partially supported by the RFFI Grants No. 04-07-90115 and No 06-07-90929.

References

1. Dimitrov, B., Green Jr., D., Rykov, V., and Stanchev P. (2004). Reliability model for biological objects, In *Longevity, Aging and Degradation Models. Transactions of the First Russian-French Conference (LAD-2004)* (Eds., V. Antonov, C. Huber, M. Nikulin, and V. Polischook), Vol. 2, pp. 230–240, Saint Petersburg State Politechnical University, Saint Petersburg, Russia.

2. Dimitrov, B., Rykov, V., and Stanchev, P. (2002). On multi-state reliability systems, In *Proceedings MMR-2002*, Trondheim, Norway.

3. van Doorn, E. A. (1991). Quasi-stationary distributions and convergence to quasi-stationarity of birth-death processes, *Advances in Applied Probability*, **26**, 683–700.

4. Feller, W. (1966). *An Introduction to Probability Theory and its Applications Vol. II*, John Wiley & Sons, New York.

5. Jacod, J. (1971). Theorems de renouvellement et classification pour les chaines semi-Markoviennes, *Annals of the Institute of Henri Poincaré, Section B*, **7**, 83–129.

6. Karlin, S. and McGregor, J. L. (1957). The differential equations of birth-and-death processes, and the Stieltjes moment problem, *Transactions of the American Mathematical Society*, **85**, 489–546.

7. Kijima, M., Nair, M. G., Pollet, P. K., and van Doorn, E. A. (1997). Limiting conditional distributions for birth-death processes, *Advances in Applied Probability*, **29**, 185–204.

8. Korolyuk, V. S. and Turbin, A. F. (1976). *Semi-Markov Processes and Their Applications*, Kiev: "Naukova dumka," (In Russian)

9. Lavrent'ev, M. A. and Shabat, B. V. (1958). *Methods of the Theory of Complex Variable Functions*, Fismatgis, Moscow.

10. Lisniansky, A. and Levitin, G. (2003). *Multi-State System Reliability. Assessment, Optimization and Application*, World Scientific, Singapore.

11. McDonald, D. (1978). On semi-Markov and semi-regenerative processes. I, II. *Zeitschrift fur Wahrscheinlichkeitstheorie und Verwandte Gebiete*, **42**, 261–377; *Annals of Probability*, **6**, 995–1014.

12. Petrovsky, I. G. (1952). *Lectures on the Theory of Usual Differential Equations*, M.-L.: GITTL. (In Russian)

13. Rykov, V. and Dimitrov, B. (2002). On multi-state reliability systems, In *Applied Stochastic Models and Information Processes*, pp. 128–135, Proceedings of the International Seminar, Petrozavodsk. See also http://www.jip.ru/2002-2-2-2002.htm.

14. Rykov, V. and Efrosinin, D. (2004). Reliability control of biological systems with failures, In *Longevity, Aging and Degradation Models. Transactions of the First Russian-French Conference (LAD-2004)* (Eds., V. Antonov, C. Huber, M. Nikulin, and V. Polischook), Vol. 2, pp. 241–255, Saint Petersburg State Politechnical University, Saint Petersburg, Russia.

15. Rykov, V. and Buldaeva E. (2004). On reliability control of fault tolerance units: Regenerative approach, In *Transactions of XXIV International Siminar on Stability Problems for Stochastic Modes*, Jurmala, Latvia, Transport and Telecommunication Institute, Riga, Latvia.

9

Nonperiodic Inspections to Guarantee a Prescribed Level of Reliability

C. T. Barker and M. J. Newby

*The City University School of Engineering and Mathematical Sciences,
Northampton Square, London, England*

Abstract: A cost-optimal nonperiodic inspection policy is derived for complex
multicomponent systems. The model takes into consideration the degradation
of all the components in the system with the use of a Bessel process with drift.
The inspection times are determined by a deterministic function and depend on
the system's performance measure. The nonperiodic policy is developed by evaluating the expected lifetime costs and the optimal policy by an optimal choice
of inspection function. The model thus gives a guaranteed level of reliability
throughout the life of the project.

Keywords and Phrases: Wiener process, Bessel process, regenerative process

9.1   Introduction

The aim of the chapter is to derive a cost-optimal inspection and maintenance
policy for a multicomponent system whose state of deterioration is modelled
with the use of a Markov stochastic process. Each component in the system undergoes a deterioration described by a Wiener process. The proposed
model takes into account the different deterioration processes by considering a
multivariate state description $\mathbf{W}_t$. The performance measure R_t of the system
is a functional on the underlying process and is not monotone. Decisions are
made by setting a critical level for the process. Because it is nonmonotone the
performance measure can cross the critical level in both directions but will eventually grow without limit. Our decisions are thus based on the probability that
the performance measure never returns below the critical level. By choosing the
critical level appropriately we thus guarantee a minimum level of reliability.

9.2   The Model

9.2.1   The considered processes

A system S consisting of N components (or subsystems) is considered. It is assumed that each component experiences its own way of deteriorating through time and that the N deteriorations are independent; that is, the deterioration of any component has no influence on the deterioration of the $N-1$ remaining components. The proposed model takes into account the different N deterioration processes as follows. Each component undergoes a deterioration described by a Wiener process. The components are labelled C_i, $i \in \{1, \ldots, N\}$ and the corresponding Wiener processes are $W_t^{(i)}$, $i \in \{1, \ldots, N\}$, where

$$W_t^{(i)} = \mu_i t + \sigma B_t^{(i)}, \qquad \forall i \in \{1, \ldots, N\}. \tag{9.1}$$

The above Wiener processes have different drift terms (the μ_is) but for simplicity the volatility terms (σ) are assumed identical and each component is assumed to be new at time $t = 0$: $W_0^{(i)} = 0$. The independence is modelled by considering N independent Brownian motions $B_t^{(i)}$s. The next step consists in considering the following N-dimensional Wiener process:

$$\mathbf{W}_t = \left(W_t^{(1)}, W_t^{(2)}, \ldots, W_t^{(N)} \right)$$
$$= \underline{\mu} t + \sigma \mathbf{B}_t \tag{9.2}$$
$$\mathbf{W}_0 = \underline{0}$$

with

$$\underline{\mu} = \begin{pmatrix} \mu_1 \\ \vdots \\ \mu_N \end{pmatrix}, \qquad \mathbf{B}_t = \begin{pmatrix} B_t^{(1)} \\ \vdots \\ B_t^{(N)} \end{pmatrix}. \tag{9.3}$$

Decisions are based on a summary measure of performance which corresponds to a functional on the underlying process $A(W_t)$, as in Newby and Barker (2006). In this study the functional used to describe the system's performance measure is the Euclidean norm R_t,

$$R_t = \|\mathbf{W}_t\|_2$$
$$= \sqrt{\sum_{i=1}^{N} (W_t^{(i)})^2} \ . \tag{9.4}$$

R_t is the radial part of a drifting Brownian motion starting at the origin; it therefore corresponds to a Bessel process with drift $Bes_0(\nu, \mu)$ starting at the origin with index ν and drift μ [Rogers and Pitman (1980)], where:

$$\nu = \frac{1}{2}N - 1 \quad \text{and} \quad \mu = \sqrt{\sum_{i=1}^{N} \mu_i^2}. \tag{9.5}$$

Remark 9.2.1 The radial part of a Brownian motion with drift starting from any other point $R_0 \neq 0$ does not correspond to a Bessel process with drift $Bes_X(\nu, \mu)$ [Rogers and Pitman (1980)].

9.2.2   Maintenance actions and nonperiodic inspections

The model proposed in this chapter aims at giving an optimal maintenance and inspection policy. The efficiency of the policy entirely depends on the inspection times and the type of maintenance on the system.

Maintenance actions are determined by comparing the observed system state R_t with a critical level ξ. However, rather than considering the first hitting time at this threshold, decisions are based on the last exit time from this critical level. For a general process X_t the last exit time is

$$H_\xi^x = \sup_{t \in \mathbb{R}^+} \{X_t \leq \xi | X_0 = x\}.$$

In a monotone process both the first hitting time and last exit times are stopping times and the distributions of these times are relatively straightforward to obtain. The Bessel process R_t describing the performance measure is nonmonotone so that the last exit time is not a stopping time but the probability $\mathbb{P}[H_\xi^0 \leq t]$ is known.

Decision rules for maintenance are made with the help of a maintenance function. In our particular case, the process chosen is the Euclidean norm of an n-dimensional Wiener process which corresponds to a Bessel process only when the process starts from the initial state 0. Hence it is a necessity to always consider the process starting from state 0. This rules out the usual repair model, that describes the effect of maintenance on the system by determining a new starting point for the process. The problem is tackled by considering changes in the value of the critical threshold ξ, rather than a new starting point for the process, and hence affects the time taken to traverse the distance to the critical threshold. After a repair the system is described by the same process starting from zero but with the critical threshold reduced to the distance between the repaired state and the original threshold. We introduce a repair function which models the amount by which the threshold is lowered after undertaking a repair on the system. The function introduced is denoted by d and if $\{\tau_1, \tau_2, \ldots\}$ refer to the inspection times, d may be defined as

$$d : \mathbb{R}^+ \to \mathbb{R}^+ \qquad R_{\tau_i} \mapsto d(R_{\tau_i}). \tag{9.6}$$

It is a function of the performance measure of the system at inspection times. The choice for d is made among the set of bijective functions. The bijective property for d is required when the derived cost functions are numerically evaluated with an appropriate choice of quadrature points. The idea is that rather than considering R_t starting from a new initial state after the maintenance action with the same threshold value ξ, we reset the value R_{τ_i} to 0 and consider a lower threshold $\xi' = \xi - d(R_{\tau_i})$. This may also be regarded as a shift of the x-axis of amount $d(R_{\tau_i})$ upwards. As far as the decision problem is concerned, the Markov property of the process is exploited and allows a copy of the original process to be considered:

$$\mathbb{P}[R_t < \xi \mid R_0 = x] = \mathbb{P}[R'_t < \xi - x \mid R'_0 = 0] \tag{9.7}$$

with

$$\begin{aligned} R_t &= \|\mathbf{W}_t\|_2 \\ R'_t &= \|\mathbf{W}_{\tau_i^+ + t} - \mathbf{W}_{\tau_i^+}\|_2 \end{aligned} \tag{9.8}$$

Recall that $\mathbf{W}_t$ is the n-dimensional process describing the state of the system. The process observed to be in state $\mathbf{W}_{\tau_i}$ is repaired instantaneously and restarts in state $\mathbf{W}_{\tau_i^+}$ where $\|\mathbf{W}_{\tau_i^+}\|_2 = x$: the repair undertaken on the system can therefore be interpreted as a componentwise repair. R'_t is an equivalent process with the same probability structure and starting at the origin. In the more usual notation

$$\mathbb{P}^x[R_t < \xi] = \mathbb{P}^0[R'_t < \xi - x] \tag{9.9}$$

with the superscript indicating the starting point.

The proposed model considers a nonperiodic inspection policy, the reason for this being that it is a more general approach and often results in policies with lower costs, particularly in cases where high costs of lost production are taken into consideration. Rather than considering a dynamic programming problem as did Newby and Dagg (2004), the optimization problem is simplified by using an inspection scheduling function m as introduced in Grall *et al.* (2002). The scheduling function is a decreasing function of $d(R_{\tau_i})$, the amount by which the threshold is decreased, and determines the amount of time until the next inspection time

$$m : \quad \begin{aligned} \mathbb{R}^+ &\to [m_{\min}, m_{\max}] \\ d(R_{\tau_i}) &\mapsto m[d(R_{\tau_i})]. \end{aligned} \tag{9.10}$$

With τ_i ($i \in \mathbb{N}$) denoting the times at which the system is inspected and R_{τ_i} its performance, the next inspection time τ_{i+1} is deduced using the relation

$$\tau_{i+1} = \tau_i + m[d(R_{\tau_i})]. \tag{9.11}$$

Consequently, it is the state of the performance measure that determines the next inspection time. The choice for m is made among the set of decreasing functions

$$\forall i, j \in \mathbb{N} : d\left(R_{\tau_i}\right) \leq d\left(R_{\tau_j}\right) \Leftrightarrow m\left[d\left(R_{\tau_i}\right)\right] \geq m\left[d\left(R_{\tau_j}\right)\right]. \tag{9.12}$$

This allows us to model the fact that the worse the performance of the system is (and hence the lower the value for the new critical threshold after repair is) the more frequently it needs to be inspected. We note that the great advantage with this approach is that it preserves continuity within the model. The approach here is to optimize the total expected cost with respect to the inspection scheduling function. The inspection functions form a two-parameter family and these two parameters, a and b, are allowed to vary to locate the optimum values. The function can be thus written $m\left[.\,|\,a,\,b\right]$ leading to a total expected cost function $v_\xi\left(a, b\right)$ which is optimized with respect to a and b. The two parameters are defined in the following way,

$$
\begin{aligned}
m\left[0\,|\,a,\,b\right] &= a, \\
m\left[R_t\,|\,a,\,b\right] &= \alpha, \qquad \text{if } R_t \geq b,
\end{aligned}
\tag{9.13}
$$

for some fixed chosen value $\alpha \in [0, a]$. From the above, we may deduce that $m_{min} = \alpha$ and $m_{max} = a$. These parameters have physical interpretations:

(i) Parameter a corresponds to the amount of time elapsed before the first inspection (i.e., when the system is new)

(ii) Parameter b controls changes in frequency of inspections.

As the choice of inspection scheduling functions is made among the set of decreasing functions, one may deduce

$$\forall i \in \mathbb{N}, \qquad \tau_{i+1} - \tau_i \leq a.$$

(That is, the amount of time between any two consecutive inspections will not exceed a.) Moreover, the parameter b sets a lower bound for the process R_t below which the system's performance is assumed to be insufficient; this therefore justifies a periodic inspection of the system of period α.

To ensure tractability of the optimization and of the effects of the chosen function on the optimal cost, choices for m are confined within the set of polynomials of order less than or equal to 2. We note, however, that the proposed models are not restricted to this choice of inspection scheduling functions and can be extended to any other type of function. Particular attention is paid to the convexity or concavity property of m; this allows different rates of inspections as time passes to be considered. The following three expressions for m are investigated,

$$m_1\left[x\,|\,a,\,b\right] = \max\left\{1, a - \frac{a-1}{b}x\right\} \tag{9.14}$$

$$m_2\left[x\,|\,a,\,b\right] = \begin{cases} \dfrac{(x-b)^2}{b^2}(a-1) + 1, & 0 \leqslant x \leqslant b \\ 1, & x > b \end{cases} \tag{9.15}$$

$$m_3\left[x\,|\,a,\,b\right] = \begin{cases} -\left(\dfrac{\sqrt{a-1}}{b}x\right)^2 + a, & 0 \leqslant x \leqslant b \\ 1, & x > b \end{cases} \tag{9.16}$$

with $a > 1$ in all cases. Note that if $a = 1$ the policy becomes a periodic inspection policy with period $\tau = a = 1$ and in the case where $a < 1$ the policy inspects less frequently for a more deteriorated system.

Remark 9.2.2 In the rest of the chapter, the notations $m(x)$ and $v_{\xi-x}$ are used rather than $m(x|a,b)$ and $v_{\xi-x}(a,b)$, for clarity.

The function m_1 resembles the inspection scheduling function considered in the numerical example section of Grall *et al.* (2002) and constitutes a reference for our numerical results. Note that whereas the time until the next inspection decreases rather quickly when dealing with m_2, m_3 allows greater time between the inspections when the state of the system is still small. The function m_2 might be thought appropriate for a system experiencing early failures (infant mortality), whereas m_3 is more appropriate for a system that is unlikely to fail in its early age.

9.2.3   Features of the model

Model assumptions

1. Without loss of generality, it is assumed that the system's initial performance is maximum (i.e., $R_0 = 0$) with initial critical threshold ξ.

2. Inspections are nonperiodic, perfect (in the sense that they reveal the true state of the system), and they are instantaneous.

3. Maintenance actions are instantaneous.

4. The system's performance is only known at inspection times, however, the moment at which the performance does not meet the prescribed criteria is immediately known (self-announcing): the system is then instantaneously replaced by a new one with cost C_f.

5. Each inspection incurs a fixed cost C_i.

6. Each maintenance action on the system incurs a cost determined by a function C_r. It is a function of the performance of the system at inspection time.

Settings for the model

1. The state space in which the process R_t evolves is partitioned by the critical threshold ξ as follows.

$$\mathbb{R}^+ = [0, \xi) \cup [\xi, +\infty). \qquad (9.17)$$

Because the process R_t is nonmonotone, the first time at which the process hits the threshold ξ is not considered as the time at which the system fails. Instead, we use the transience and positivity properties of the process to define the system as unsafe when it has escaped from the interval $[0, \xi)$. This time is the last exit time $H^0_\xi = \sup_{t \in \mathbb{R}^+} \{R_t \leq \xi | R_0 = 0\}$.

2. The system is inspected at inspection times $\{\tau_1, \tau_2, \ldots\}$. The time between inspections τ_{i-1} and τ_i is T_i, $i \in \mathbb{N}$ and is determined by using an inspection scheduling function m, described in Section 9.2.2. The sequence of inspection times $(\tau_i)_{i \in Z^+}$ is strictly increasing and satisfies:

$$\tau_0 = 0$$

$$\tau_i = \sum_{k=1}^{i} T_k \qquad (9.18)$$

$$T_i = \tau_i - \tau_{i-1}, \qquad i \geq 1.$$

At inspection time τ_i, the corresponding system's state is R_{τ_i} and appropriate maintenance action (repair or do nothing) is undertaken. Let τ_i^* denote the times at which the system is replaced: at such times the process $(R_t)_{t \geq 0}$ is reset to zero. These times are regeneration times and allow us to derive an expression for the total expected cost of inspection and maintenance.

3. At inspection time $t = \tau$ (prior to any maintenance action), the system's performance is R_τ.

4. Given that the system's initial performance is maximum (i.e., $R_0 = 0$), decisions on the level of maintenance (replacement or imperfect maintenance) are made on the basis of the indicator function $\mathbf{1}_{\{H^0_\xi > \tau\}}$. By this it is meant that decisions on whether to replace the system are taken on the basis of the process having definitively escaped from the interval $[0, \xi)$.

5. Deterministic maintenance at inspection time is modelled with the use of the following maintenance function,

$$d(x) = \begin{cases} x, & x < \frac{\xi}{K} \\ kx, & x \geq \frac{\xi}{K} \end{cases} \tag{9.19}$$

with corresponding cost function

$$C_r(x) = \begin{cases} 0, & x < \frac{\xi}{K} \\ 100, & x \geq \frac{\xi}{K} \end{cases} \tag{9.20}$$

with constants $k \in (0,1]$ and $K \in (1,+\infty)$. The constant k determines the amount of repair undertaken on the system; K is arbitrarily chosen and sets the region of repairs for the system.

9.3   Expected Total Cost

In this section we propose an expression for the expected total cost of inspections and maintenance. The Markov property of the Bessel process allows the total cost to be expressed via a recursive approach: a conditioning argument on the threshold value is considered. The notation $V_{\xi-x}$ is used to denote the total cost of maintenance, where $\xi - x$ refers to the threshold value. The maintenance decisions are made using the exit time from the region of acceptable performance. The time $H^0_{\xi-x}$ can never be known by observation because observing any up-crossing of the threshold reveals a potential exit time but there remains the possibility of a further down-crossing and up-crossing in the future. This is the meaning of the fact that $H^0_{\xi-x}$ is not a stopping time. In a nonprobabilistic context, the process $H^0_{\xi-x}$ is described by a noncausal model. The difficulty is readily resolved because the probability that the last exit time occurs before the next inspection is known. In the light of these observations the decision rules are formulated as follows.

- $\mathbf{1}_{\{H^0_{\xi-x}>m(x)\}} = 1$: performance of the system (evaluated with respect to the last time the process hits the critical threshold) meets the prescribed criteria until the next scheduled inspection. Upon inspection, the system's performance is $R_{m(x)}$. The system is inspected, and a cost of inspection C_i is considered. The maintenance brings the system state of degradation back to a lower level $d\left(R_{m(x)}\right)$ with cost $C_r\left(R_{m(x)}\right)$. Future costs enter by looking at the process starting from the origin and with the new critical threshold set up equal to $\xi - d\left(R_{m(x)}\right)$. The system is then next inspected after $m\left[d\left(R_{m(x)}\right)\right]$ units of time.

- $\mathbf{1}_{\{H^0_{\xi-x}>m(x)\}} = 0$: the performance fails to meet the prescribed criteria between two inspections. The system is replaced with cost C_f and the process restarts from the origin. Future costs are then taken into consideration by looking at the process starting from the origin and with the new critical threshold set up equal to ξ.

9.3.1 Expression of the expected total cost

We first give the expression for the total cost and then take the expectation. This is done by considering the above different scenarios

$$
\begin{aligned}
V_{\xi-x} &= \left(C_i + V_{\xi-d(R_{m(x)})} + C_r\left(R_{m(x)}\right)\right)\mathbf{1}_{\{performance\ acceptable\}} \\
&\quad + (C_f + V_\xi)\,\mathbf{1}_{\{performance\ not\ acceptable\}} \\
&= \left(C_i + V_{\xi-d(R_{m(x)})} + C_r\left(R_{m(x)}\right)\right)\mathbf{1}_{\{H^0_{\xi-x}>m(x)\}} \\
&\quad + (C_f + V_\xi)\,\mathbf{1}_{\{H^0_{\xi-x}\leq(x)\}}.
\end{aligned}
\tag{9.21}
$$

Taking the expectation leads to:

$$
\begin{aligned}
v_{\xi-x} &= \mathbb{E}[V_{\xi-x}] \\
&= \mathbb{E}\left[(C_f+V_\xi)\,\mathbf{1}_{\{H^0_{\xi-x}\leq m(x)\}}\right] \\
&\quad + \mathbb{E}\left[\left(C_i + V_{\xi-d(R_{m(x)})} + C_r\left(R_{m(x)}\right)\right)\mathbf{1}_{\{H^0_{\xi-x}>m(x)\}}\right] \\
&= (C_f+v_\xi)\,\mathbb{E}\left[\mathbf{1}_{\{H^0_{\xi-x}\leq m(x)\}}\right] \\
&\quad + \mathbb{E}\left[\left(C_i + V_{\xi-d(R_{m(x)})} + C_r\left(R_{m(x)}\right)\right)\mathbf{1}_{\{H^0_{\xi-x}>m(x)\}}\right] \\
&= (C_f+v_\xi)\,\mathbb{P}\left[H^0_{\xi-x}\leq m(x)\right] \\
&\quad + \int_0^{+\infty}\left(C_i + C_r(y) + v_{\xi-d(y)}\right)\mathbb{P}\left[H^0_{\xi-x}>m(x)\right]f^0_{m(x)}(y)\,dy \\
&= (C_f+v_\xi)\,\mathbb{P}\left[H^0_{\xi-x}\leq m(x)\right] \\
&\quad + \int_0^{+\infty}\left(C_i + C_r(y) + v_{\xi-d(y)}\right)\mathbb{P}\left[H^0_{\xi-x}>m(x)\right]f^0_{m(x)}(y)\,dy.
\end{aligned}
\tag{9.22}
$$

Using the density of the last hitting time h^0_ξ and the transition density f^0_t of the process R_t

$$
\begin{aligned}
v_{\xi-x} &= (C_f+v_\xi)\int_0^{m(x)} h^0_{\xi-x}(t)\,dt \\
&\quad + \int_0^{+\infty}\left(C_i + C_r(y) + v_{\xi-d(y)}\right)\left(1 - \int_0^{m(x)} h^0_{\xi-x}(t)\,dt\right)f^0_{m(x)}(y)\,dy
\end{aligned}
$$

$$
\begin{aligned}
= \; & C_i \left(1 - \int_0^{m(x)} h_{\xi-x}^0 (t)\, dt \right) + (C_f + v_\xi) \int_0^{m(x)} h_{\xi-x}^0 (t)\, dt \\
& + \left(1 - \int_0^{m(x)} h_{\xi-x}^0 (t)\, dt \right) \int_0^{+\infty} C_r (y)\, f_{m(x)}^0 (y)\, dy \\
& + \int_0^{+\infty} v_{\xi-d(y)} \left(1 - \int_0^{m(x)} h_{\xi-x}^0 (t)\, dt \right) f_{m(x)}^0 (y)\, dy. \qquad (9.23)
\end{aligned}
$$

In (9.22) the expected value $\mathbb{E}\left[V_{\xi-d(R_{m(x)})} \mathbf{1}_{\{H_{\xi-x}^0 > m(x)\}} \right]$ is required. The expected value is derived by using the conditional independence of $H_{\xi-x}^0$ and R_τ. The independence allows the factorization of the integrals as shown in the appendix.

Rearranging (9.23) above gives

$$
v_{\xi-x} = Q(x) + \lambda(x)\, v_\xi + \int_0^{d^{-1}(\xi)} v_{\xi-d(y)} K\{x, y\}\, dy, \qquad (9.24)
$$

where

$$
\lambda(x) = \int_0^{m(x)} h_{\xi-x}^0 (t)\, dt
$$

$$
Q(x) = (1 - \lambda(x)) \left(C_i + \int_0^{+\infty} C_r (y)\, f_{m(x)}^0 (y)\, dy \right) + C_f \lambda(x) \qquad (9.25)
$$

$$
K\{x, y\} = \left(1 - \int_0^{m(x)} h_{\xi-x}^0 (t)\, dt \right) f_{m(x)}^0 (y).
$$

Note that now the limit in the integral in (9.24) is finite. The justification for this change of limit is that the expected cost $v_{\xi-x}$ is assumed to be zero when the critical threshold is negative. Indeed, a negative threshold in the model would either mean that the system never reaches a critical state or that it is always in a failed state; hence no maintenance action needs to be considered, setting the expected cost of maintenance to zero.

9.3.2   Obtaining the solutions

The equation (9.24) is solved numerically: an approximation to the continuous problem is constructed by discretizing the integrals giving a set of linear matrix equations. The discrete problem is solved using the methods described in Press *et al.* (1992). First, note that at $t = 0$ the system is new. Under this condition, we rewrite Equation (9.24) as follows.

$$
v_{\xi-x} = Q(x) + \lambda(x)\, v_{\xi-x} + \int_0^{d^{-1}(\xi)} v_{\xi-d(y)} K\{x, y\}\, dy. \qquad (9.26)
$$

Yielding to the following Fredholm equation,

$$\{1 - \lambda(x)\}v_{\xi-x} = Q(x) + \int_0^{d^{-1}(\xi)} v_{\xi-d(y)} K\{x, y\} \, dy. \tag{9.27}$$

Rewriting (9.24) as (9.27) does not affect the solution to the equation and will allow the required solution to be obtained by a homotopy argument based on ξ. Indeed both Equations (9.24) and (9.27) are identical when $x = 0$; we therefore solve Equation (9.27) and get the solution for $x = 0$. The Nystrom routine with the N-point Gauss–Legendre rule at the points y_j, $j \in \{1, \ldots, N\}$ is applied to (9.27); we get

$$\{1 - \lambda(x)\}v_{\xi-x} = Q(x) + \sum_{j=1}^{N} v_{\xi-d(y_j)} K\{x, y_j\} w_j. \tag{9.28}$$

We then evaluate the above at the following appropriate points $x_i = d(y_i)$ and obtain:

$$\{1 - \lambda(x_i)\}v_{\xi-x_i} = Q(x_i) + \sum_{j=1}^{N} v_{\xi-d(y_j)} K\{x_i, y_j\} w_j, \tag{9.29}$$

which, because $v_{\xi-x_i}$ and $v_{\xi-d(y_i)}$ are evaluated at the same points, can be rewritten in the following matrix form,

$$(\mathbf{D} - \mathbf{K})\mathbf{v} = \mathbf{Q}, \tag{9.30}$$

where:

$$\begin{aligned}
\mathbf{v}_i &= v_{\xi-x_i} \\
\mathbf{D}_{i,j} &= (1 - \lambda(x_i)) \, \mathbf{1}_{\{i=j\}} \\
\mathbf{K}_{i,j} &= K\{x_i, y_j\} w_j \\
\mathbf{Q}_i &= Q(x_i).
\end{aligned} \tag{9.31}$$

Having obtained the solution at the quadrature points by solving inversion of the matrix $\mathbf{D} - \mathbf{K}$, we get the solution at any other quadrature point x by simply using Equation (9.28) as an interpolatory formula.

Remark 9.3.1 $K\{x, y\}$ in (9.25) is the product of a density function by a survival function hence it is bounded by the maximum of the density which, by the Fredholm alternative, ensures that the equation in (9.30) has a solution (i.e., $\mathbf{D} - \mathbf{K}$ is invertible).

Because we are interested in a system which is new at time $t = 0$, we just choose the quadrature point $x_i = 0$, which justifies that rewriting (9.24) as (9.27) does not affect the solution to the equation.

9.4   Numerical Results and Comments

This section presents results from numerical experiments. The values of the parameters for the process used to model the degradation of the system and the different costs used were chosen arbitrarily to show some important features of the inspection policy. The initial value for the critical threshold is $\xi = 5$, the Bessel process considered is $Bes_0\,(0.5, 1)$, and the values for the cost of inspection and the cost of failure are $C_i = 50$ and $C_f = 200$.

The corresponding costs of repair are chosen to be dependent on the state of the system found at inspection as follows.

$$C_r\,(y) = \begin{cases} 0, & y < \frac{\xi}{2} \\ \\ 100, & y \geq \frac{\xi}{2}. \end{cases} \tag{9.32}$$

The purpose of the present model is to find an optimal inspection policy for the expected total cost of inspection and maintenance of the system. Three different types of inspection policies are considered with the use of the three inspection scheduling functions m_1, m_2, and m_3 defined in Section 9.2.2. The expected total costs are minimized with respect to the two parameters a and b.

The numerical results for the case of small maintenance on the system ($k = 0.9$) are shown in Figure 9.1. In the case of a large amount of maintenance ($k = 0.1$), the numerical results are shown in Figure 9.2. The optimal values a_i^*, b_i^*, and v_i^* ($i = \{1, 2, 3\}$) for a, b, and v_ξ, respectively, in the different scenarios, are summarized in Table 9.1.

We first note that the surfaces obtained clearly show the presence of an optimal policy for each inspection function considered. In the case $k = 0.1$ with inspection function m_2, the optimal inspection policy seems to strongly depend on parameter a only, which is the first time of inspection of the system. The choice for b does not seem to be of much importance.

Even if the optimal inspection policy gives a value b^* which is less than ξ, we note that the choice $b > 5\,(\equiv \xi)$ is not meaningless: indeed the value R_{τ_i} of the process at inspection time τ_i may be greater then ξ: it is the last hitting time of ξ by the process that defines the process as unsafe.

From Table 9.1, we note that the optimal costs are smaller for $k = 0.1$ than for $k = 0.9$. This makes sense, because in both cases the same values for the costs were considered: the case $k = 0.1$ corresponding to more repair, the system will tend to deteriorate slower and therefore will require less maintenance resulting in a smaller total cost. In both cases $k = 0.9$ and $k = 0.1$, we note that the value for v^* increases with the convexity of the inspection function: $v_3^* < v_1^* < v_2^*$.

Plots of the optimal inspection functions in Figure 9.3 show that the smallest value for a is a_3, corresponding to the first inspection time for a new system

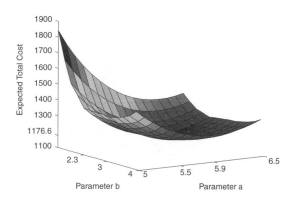

(a) Inspection function: m_1

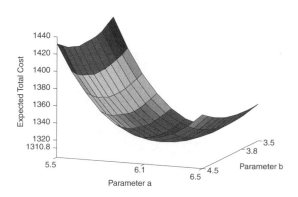

(b) Inspection function: m_2

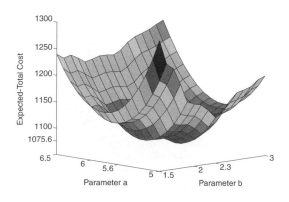

(c) Inspection function: m_3

Figure 9.1. Surface representations of the expected total costs with different inspection scheduling functions, $k = 0.9$.

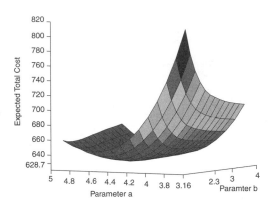

(a) Inspection function: m_1

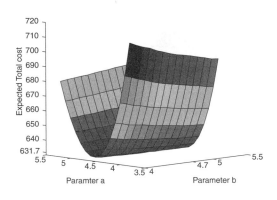

(b) Inspection function: m_2

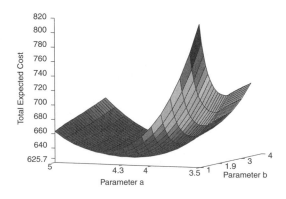

(c) Inspection function: m_3

Figure 9.2. Surface representations of the expected total costs with different inspection scheduling functions, $k = 0.1$.

Table 9.1. Optimal values of the parameters a and b for the three inspection scheduling functions

Inspection Policies		$k = 0.9$	$k = 0.1$
	a_1^*	5.9	4.5
m_1	b_1^*	2.3	2.3
	v_1^*	1176.6	628.73
	a_2^*	6.1	4.5
m_2	b_2^*	3.8	4.7
	v_2^*	1310.8	631.71
	a_3^*	5.6	4.3
m_3	b_3^*	2.3	1.9
	v_3^*	1089.3	625.67

when inspection function m_3 is used. However, when the value of the process reaches some value (rather close to 0), the function m_3 crosses m_1 and m_2 to lie above them. It then crosses m_2 a second time to return below it. We may deduce that for this process an optimal policy is first to allow a long time between the inspections, then to change strategy drastically to a small interval or an almost periodic inspection policy of period 1. This change of inspection decision within the same policy m_3 happens earlier when $k = 0.1$.

9.5 Conclusion

The proposed model provides optimal nonperiodic inspection policies for a complex multicomponent system whose state is described by a multivariate Wiener process. Decisions are made on the basis of the state of a performance measure defined by the Euclidean norm of the multivariate process and the last exit time from an interval rather than the first hitting time. The models are optimized in the sense that they result in a minimum expected maintenance cost, whose expression uses a conditioning argument on the critical threshold's value. The nonperiodicity of the inspection times is modelled with the use of an inspection scheduling function, introduced in Grall *et al.* (2002), which determines the next time to inspect the system based on the value of the performance measure at inspection time. The numerical results obtained show the presence of a cost-optimal inspection policy in each of the six cases, where different inspection functions and different amounts of repair are considered. Attention is paid to

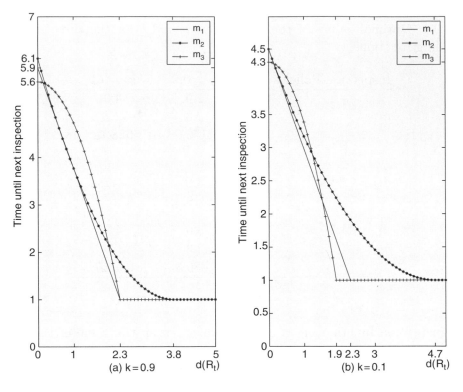

Figure 9.3. Optimal inspection scheduling functions.

the influence of the convexity of the inspection function on the optimal expected total cost: the value for the optimal cost v^* increases with the convexity of the inspection function.

Appendix

Let $f_{R_{m(x)}, H^0_{\xi-x}}$ be the joint probability density function of the process at time $m(x)$ and the last exit time from the interval $[0, \xi - x)$. We may deduce:

$$
E\left[V_{\xi-d(R_{m(x)})} \times \mathbf{1}_{\{H^0_{\xi-x} > m(x)\}} \right]
$$

$$
= \int_0^{+\infty} \int_0^{+\infty} v_{\xi-d(y)} \times \mathbf{1}_{\{t > m(x)\}} f_{R_{m(x)}, H^0_{\xi-x}}(y, t)\, dy\, dt
$$

$$
= \int_0^{+\infty} \int_0^{+\infty} v_{\xi-d(y)} \times \mathbf{1}_{\{t > m(x)\}} f_{R_{m(x)} | H^0_{\xi-x} = t}(y)\, h^0_{\xi-x}(t)\, dy\, dt
$$

$$
= \int_{m(x)}^{+\infty} \int_0^{+\infty} v_{\xi-d(y)} f_{R_{m(x)} | H^0_{\xi-x} > m(x)}(y)\, h^0_{\xi-x}(t)\, dy\, dt
$$

$$= \int_{m(x)}^{+\infty} h_{\xi-x}^0 (t) \int_0^{+\infty} v_{\xi-d(y)} f_{R_{m(x)}|H_{\xi-x}^0 > m(x)} (y) \, dy \, dt$$

$$= \int_{m(x)}^{+\infty} h_{\xi-x}^0 (t) \, dt \int_0^{+\infty} v_{\xi-d(y)} f_{R_{m(x)}} (y) \, dy$$

$$= \left(1 - \int_0^{m(x)} h_{\xi-x}^0 (t) \, dt \right) \int_0^{+\infty} v_{\xi-d(y)} f_{R_{m(x)}} (y) \, dy$$

$$= \left(1 - \int_0^{m(x)} h_{\xi-x}^0 (t) \, dt \right) \int_0^{+\infty} v_{\xi-d(y)} f_{m(x)}^0 (y) \, dy.$$

The conditional independence allows the replacement of $f_{R_{m(x)}|H_{\xi-x}^0 > m(x)}$ by $f_{R_{m(x)}}$: as $H_{\xi-x}^0 > m(x)$, the process may still be in the region $[0, \xi - x)$ and hence the region of integration remains $[0, +\infty)$.

References

1. Barker, C. T. and Newby, M. J. (2006). Inspection and maintenance planning for complex multi-component systems, In *Proceedings of ALT'2006, ISTIA*, Angers, France.

2. Grall, A., Dieulle, L., Berenger, C., and Roussignol, M. (2002). Continuous-time predictive-maintenance scheduling for a deteriorating system, *IEEE Transaction on Reliability*, **51**, 141–150.

3. Newby, M. J. and Barker, C. T. (2006). A bivariate process model for maintenance and inspection planning, *Pressure Vessels and Piping*, **83**, 270–275.

4. Newby, M. J. and Dagg, R. (2004). Optimal inspection and perfect repair, *IMA Journal of Management Mathematics*, **15**(2), 175–192.

5. Pitman, J. W. and Yor, M. (1981). Bessel Process and Infinitely Divisible Laws, Stochastic Integrals, *Lecture Notes in Mathematics*, Springer Berlin.

6. Press, W. H., Teukolsky, S. A., Vetterling, W. T., and Flannery, B. P. (1992). *Numerical Recipes in C, 2nd Edition*, Cambridge Univerity Press, New York.

7. Revuz, D. and Yor, M. (1991). *Continuous Martingale and Brownian Motion*, Springer-Verlag, New York.

8. Rogers, L. C. G. and Pitman, J. W. (1980). Markov functions, *Annals of Probability*, **9**, 573–582.

10

Optimal Incomplete Maintenance for Weibull Failure Processes

Waltraud Kahle

Otto-von-Guericke-University, Institute of Mathematical Stochastics, Magdeburg, Germany

Abstract: We consider an incomplete repair model; that is, the impact of repair is not minimal as in the homogeneous Poisson process and not "as good as new" as in renewal processes but lies between these boundary cases. The repairs are assumed to affect the failure intensity following a virtual age process affect of the general form proposed by Kijima. In previous works field data from an industrial setting were used to fit several models. In most cases the estimated rate of occurrence of failures was that of an underlying exponential distribution of the time between failures. In this chapter it is shown that there exist maintenance schedules under which the failure behavior of the failure–repair process becomes a homogeneous Poisson process.

Keywords and Phrases: Incomplete repair, Poisson process, renewal process, virtual age, hazard rate, optimal maintenance

10.1 Introduction

In this research, we are concerned with the statistical modeling of repairable systems. Our particular interest is the operation of electrical generating systems. As in repairable systems, we assume the failure intensity at a point in time depends on the history of repairs. In the environment under investigation, it was observed that maintenance decisions were regularly carried out. We assume that such actions affected the failure intensity. Specifically, we assume that maintenance actions served to adjust the virtual age of the system in a Kijima-type manner [Kijima *et al.* (1988) and Kijima (1989)]. Kijima proposed that the state of the machine just after repair can be described by its so-called virtual age which is smaller (younger) than the real age. In his framework, the rate of occurrence of failures (ROCOF) depends on the virtual age of the system.

Our immediate interest was to obtain an operating/repair effects model consistent with data obtained from a selected hydroelectric turbine unit within the British Columbia Hydro-Electric Power Generation System. The data collected over the period January 1977 to December 1999 contains 496 sojourns with 160 failures. Two types of repairs are recorded by maintenance personnel: major repairs and minor repairs. The classification of repairs into these two categories is made at the time of the repair. Within this period, 50 major repairs and 96 minor repairs were conducted. All 50 major repairs occurred from a censor decision (i.e., a decision to shut the system down). Furthermore, of the 96 minor repairs, 1 of them was undertaken immediately following a failure. The remaining 95 were censored minor repairs. In addition to sojourn and censor times of these stoppages, the data also included the times to repair the system. These times ranged from a smallest of 1 minute to a largest of 66,624 minutes (or approximately 46 days).

In this chapter, we assume that the baseline failure intensity of the system follows a Weibull distribution

$$\lambda(x) = \frac{\beta}{\alpha}\left(\frac{x}{\alpha}\right)^{\beta-1}, \qquad \beta > 0, \qquad \alpha > 0.$$

10.2   Kijima-Type Repairs

Consider the impact of repairs. A system (machine) starts working with an initial prescribed failure rate $\lambda_1(t) = \lambda(t)$. Let t_1 denote the random time of the first sojourn. At this time t_1 the item will be repaired with the degree ξ_1. When the system is minimally repaired then the degree is equal to one, and if the repair makes the system as good as new then this degree is zero. The virtual age of the system at the time t_1, following the repair, is $v_1 = \xi_1 t_1$, implying the age of the system is reduced by maintenance actions. The distribution of the time until the next sojourn then has failure intensity $\lambda_2(t) = \lambda(t - t_1 + v_1)$. Assume now that t_k is the time of the kth ($k \geq 1$) sojourn and that ξ_k is the degree of repair at that time. We assume that $0 \leq \xi_k \leq 1$, for $k \geq 1$.

After repair the failure intensity during the $(k+1)$th sojourn is determined by

$$\lambda_{k+1}(t) = \lambda(t - t_k + v_k), \qquad t_k \leq t < t_{k+1}, k \geq 0,$$

where the virtual age v_k is for Kijima's Type II imperfect repair model

$$v_k = \xi_k(v_{k-1} + (t_k - t_{k-1}));$$

that is, the repair resets the intensity of failure proportional to the virtual age.

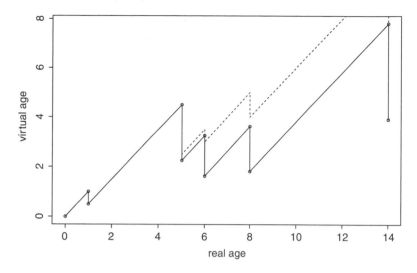

Figure 10.1. The virtual age for Kijima-type repairs.

Kijima's Type I imperfect repair model suggests that upon failure, the repair undertaken could serve to reset the intensity only as far back as the virtual age at the start of working after the last failure. That is:

$$v_k = t_{k-1} + \xi_k(t_k - t_{k-1}).$$

The process defined by $v(t, \xi_k, k = 1, 2, \ldots) = t - t_k + v_k$, $t_k \leq t < t_{k+1}$, $k \geq 0$ is called the *virtual age process* [Last and Szekli (1998)].

In Figure 10.1 the virtual age is shown for both types of repair. Figure 10.2 shows the mean number of failures over time for a minimal repair process (the Weibull process) where the degree of repair is 1, for the Weibull renewal process, where the degree of repair is 0, and, further, for some degrees of repair between 0 and 1 under Kijima Type II. In the two extreme cases, the expected number of failures is the cumulative hazard function $(t/\alpha)^\beta$ for the Weibull process and the solution of the renewal equation for the Weibull renewal process. In the general case an explicit calculation of the expected number of failures is possible only for some very special cases. In the plot 100 failure processes with 50 failures were simulated with parameters $\alpha = 1$, $\beta = 1.5$. Each line shows the mean number of failures from these 100 simulations for the degrees of repair 1, 0.5, 0.3, 0.05, and 0.

10.3 Parameter Estimation

In Gasmi et al. (2003) a generalized Kijima-type model was considered, where a major repair gives an additional impact. It was shown that the likelihood function can be developed from the general likelihood function for observation of

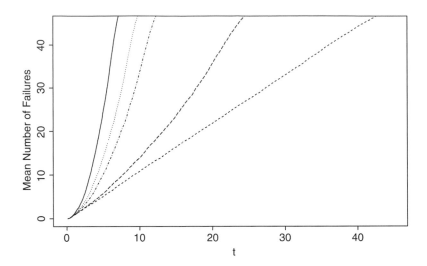

Figure 10.2. Mean number of failures under incomplete repair.

point processes [Liptser and Shiryayev (1978)]. Furthermore, the likelihood ratio statistic can be used to find confidence estimates for the unknown parameters.

The numerical results for this data file are surprising. Under different assumptions about the repair actions (renewals, Kijima Type I or II, mixture of Kijima-type repairs and renewals in dependence on the time required for repair) a value for β was estimated approximately to be 1; see Gasmi et al. (2003). That is, the failure intensity is more or less constant. But in this case the failure behavior does not depend on maintenance actions.

One of the reasons for this could be that for real systems, maintenance actions depend on the state of the system. In Kahle and Love (2003) it was assumed that each maintenance action has its own degree of repair which is assumed to be

$$\xi_k = 1 - \Phi(\log(r_k) - 2.4),$$

where ξ_k is the degree of repair after the kth failure or shut down, r_k is the repair time after the kth sojourn, and Φ is the distribution function of the standard normal distribution. The constant 2.4 is the estimated mean value of the log repair times. The estimated variance of the log repair times is about 1. It is easy to see that we get a degree of repair ξ_k of nearly 1.0 for very small repair times (which means that the age of the system after repair is the same as before the failure or shutdown) and a ξ_k of approximately 0.0 for long repair times (the system is perfectly repaired).

For this model we get the following estimates for the parameters of the baseline Weibull intensity:

$$\hat{\beta} = 2.305 \qquad \hat{\alpha} = 134{,}645 \text{ min};$$

that is, the assumption that each maintenance action has its own degree of repair leads to an estimate of the shape parameter of $\hat{\beta} = 2.305$. This really increasing failure rate is in agreement with the experiences of maintenence engineers.

10.4 Optimal Maintenance as Time Scale Transformation

The results, mentioned in the previous sections, suggest that in practice the engineers make a good maintenance policy; that is, they make repairs in connection with the state of the system. The idea is that such a policy makes the apparent failure behavior of a system to be that of an exponential distribution. This is consistent with our data. In Figure 10.3 we see the cumulative distribution function of the operating time between failures together with the fitted CDF of an exponential distribution and the Q–Q plot (observed quantiles against the quantiles of the exponential model). These plots suggest reasonable agreement with the exponential model if we consider only the failure process and ignore all maintenance events.

Definition 10.4.1 A maintenance policy is called **failure rate optimal**, if the state-dependent preventive maintenance actions lead to a constant ROCOF of the failure process.

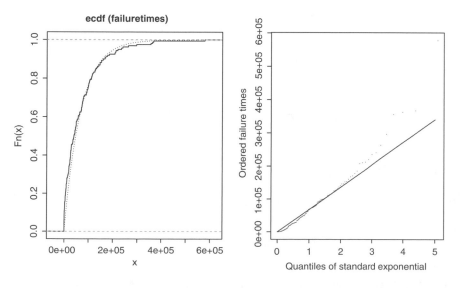

Figure 10.3. Operating time between failures: CDF and exponential Q–Q plot.

Following an idea in Finkelstein (2000) we assume that by repair actions, the time scale is transformed by a function $W(t)$. Let $\Lambda_0(t)$ be the baseline cumulative hazard function and let $\Lambda_1(t) = \Lambda_0(W(t))$ be the resulting hazard after a transformation of the time scale. For the Weibull hazard

$$\Lambda_0(t) = (t/\alpha)^\beta$$

and $W(t) = t^{1/\beta}$ we get

$$\Lambda_1(t) = \Lambda_0(t^{1/\beta}) = \frac{t}{\alpha^\beta},$$

that is, the hazard function of an exponential distribution with parameter $\lambda_1 = 1/\alpha^\beta$.

In practice we have repair actions at discrete time points, which lead to the question of the degrees of repair at these points. Let us consider two examples. In both examples we assume that after a failure the system is repaired minimally. In addition, maintenance decisions were regularly carried out. We assume that maintenance actions served to adjust the virtual age of the system in a Kijima-type manner.

Example 10.4.1 Assume that the distances between maintenance actions are constant and all repair actions follow the Kijima Type I repair process. Let $t_1, t_2, \ldots$ be the time points of maintenance actions and $\Delta = t_k - t_{k-1}$, $k = 1, 2, \ldots$, where $t_0 = 0$, be the constant distance between maintenances. Then it is possible to find a discrete time transformation which consists of different degrees of repair. Let the sequence of degrees be

$$\xi_k = \frac{k^{1/\beta} - (k-1)^{1/\beta}}{\Delta^{1-1/\beta}}.$$

Then the virtual age v_n of the system at time $t_n = n \cdot \Delta$ can be found to be

$$v_n = \Delta \sum_{k=1}^{n} \xi_k = \Delta \sum_{k=1}^{n} \frac{k^{1/\beta} - (k-1)^{1/\beta}}{\Delta^{1-1/\beta}} = (n \cdot \Delta)^{1/\beta}.$$

Example 10.4.2 Again we assume that the distances between maintenance actions are constant, but now we consider the Kijima Type II repair process. In this case the appropriate sequence of degrees of repair is

$$\xi_k = \frac{k^{1/\beta}}{(k-1)^{1/\beta} + \Delta^{1-1/\beta}}.$$

In both cases the sequence is decreasing; that is, with increasing time the repairs must become better.

It should be noted that in the case of time scale transformation it is not necessary to make a difference between Kijima Type I and II. In both examples the virtual age at maintenance points was re-set to those of the continuous time transformation as shown in Figure 10.4.

In Figure 10.5 are shown the cumulative hazard functions for a Weibull process without maintenance (solid line) and for maintenance actions every $\Delta = .1$ time units (broken line). For this, a Weibull process with parameters

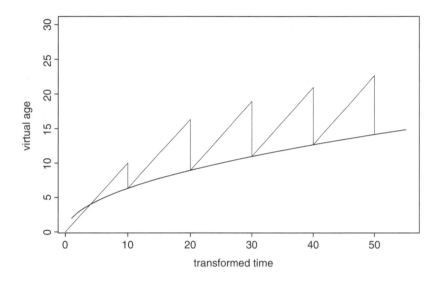

Figure 10.4. A discrete time transformation.

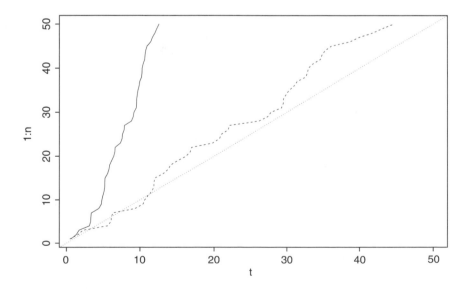

Figure 10.5. Weibull process without and with preventive maintenance actions.

$\alpha = 1$ and $\beta = 2.5$ and 30 failures was simulated. The difference $\Delta = .1$ between maintenance actions is relatively small, and the empirical cumulative hazard function of the process with preventive maintenance is close to that of a Poisson process. The dotted line shows the theoretical cumulative hazard function of an homogeneous Poisson process.

There are many other possibilities for finding failure-rate optimal mainte-nance policies. One other very simple policy is to consider constant degrees of repair. It is easy to see that in this case the repair actions must take place more often with increasing time.

By preventive maintenance it is always possible to get a ROCOF which lies under that of the corresponding homogeneous Poisson process:

Theorem 10.4.1 *Let be given a Weibull failure process with cumulative hazard $H_0(t) = (t/\alpha)^\beta$. We assume that after a failure the system is minimally repaired. In addition, at times $t_k = \Delta \cdot k$ preventive maintenance actions are undertaken. If the distance between maintenance actions $\Delta < \alpha$ and the virtual age v after a maintenance is the solution of*

$$(v + \Delta)^\beta - v^\beta = \Delta, \tag{10.1}$$

then for the resulting ROCOF $H^*(t)$ holds

$$H^*(t) \leq \frac{t}{\alpha^\beta}.$$

PROOF. First, let us note that Equation (10.1) has a unique solution, because the derivative of $(v + \Delta)^\beta - v^\beta - \Delta$ with respect to v is positive and its value is less than 0 for $v = 0$ and greater than 0 for large v. The proposition of the theorem then follows very simply from the following figure.

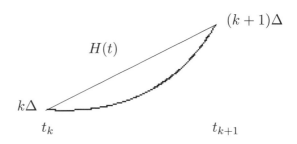

10.5 Conclusion

We have considered failure-rate optimal maintenance under the assumption, that the maintenance action has an impact between the two extreme cases of minimal repair and renewal. For finding cost-optimal maintenance it is necessary to define a cost function which describes the costs of repair actions according to the degree of repair. Furthermore, additional assumptions about times of maintenance actions must be made, because there is the possibility of frequently making small repairs or rarely large repairs that cause the same costs.

References

1. Finkelstein, M. S. (2000). Modeling a process of nonideal repair, In *Recent Advances in Reliability Theory* (Eds., N. Limnios and M. Nikulin), pp. 41–53, Birkhäuser, New York.

2. Gasmi, S., Love, C. E., and Kahle, W. (2003). A general repair/proportional hazard framework to model complex repairable systems, *IEEE Transactions on Reliability*, **52**, 26–32.

3. Kahle, W. and Love C. E. (2003). Modeling the influence of maintenance actions, In *Mathematical and Statistical Methods in Reliability* (Eds., B. H. Lindquist and K. A. Doksum), pp. 387–400, World Scientific, Singapore.

4. Kijima, M. (1989). Some results for repairable systems with general repair, *Journal of Applied Probability*, **26**, 89–102.

5. Kijima, M., Morimura, H., and Suzuki, Y. (1988). Periodical replacement problem without assuming minimal repair, *European Journal of Operational Research*, **37**, 194–203.

6. Last, G. and Szekli, R. (1998). Stochastic comparison of repairable systems by coupling, *Journal of Applied Probability*, **35**, 348–370.

7. Liptser, R. S. and Shiryayev, A. N. (1978). *Statistics of Random Processes, Vol. II*, Springer-Verlag, New York.

11

Are Nonhomogeneous Poisson Process Models Preferable to General-Order Statistics Models for Software Reliability Estimation?

Subrata Kundu, Tapan K. Nayak, and Sudip Bose

Department of Statistics, George Washington University, Washington, DC, USA

Abstract: As alternatives to general order statistics (GOS) models, several nonhomogeneous Poisson process (NHPP) models have been proposed in the literature for software reliability estimation. It has been known that an NHPP model in which the expected number of events (μ) over $(0, \infty)$ is finite (called an NHPP-I process) is a Poisson mixture of GOS processes. We find that the underlying GOS model better fits the data in the sense that it has a larger likelihood than the NHPP-I model. Also, among unbiased estimators for an NHPP-I model, if an estimator is optimal for estimating a related feature of the underlying GOS model, then it is also optimal for the NHPP-I estimation problem. We conducted a simulation study to compare maximum likelihood estimators for one NHPP-I model and for its corresponding GOS model. The results show for small μ and small debugging time the estimators for NHPP-I model are unreliable. For longer debugging time the estimators for the two models behave similarly. These results and certain logical issues suggest that compared to an NHPP-I model, its underlying GOS model may better serve for analyzing software failure data.

Keywords and Phrases: Failure rate, maximum likelihood, Poisson mixture, software debugging, software error

11.1   Introduction

Software is a critical part of the operational technology of all major organizations. Software has grown rapidly in size and complexity in recent years. This greater size and complexity has been accompanied by an increase in the rate

137

of software failures. Software errors (bugs) have caused various system failures with severe consequences and economic losses; see Pham (2000, Section 1.1) for some significant examples. In principle, software can be error-free, but in reality, no method is available for creating perfect software, although existing tools and guidelines are helpful in achieving high quality. Before a new piece of software (a program) is put into operation, it is tested with diverse inputs to detect the bugs hidden in the program. Whenever the program fails or gives a wrong output, attempts are made to identify the error that caused the failure and fix it. However, removal of all errors cannot be assured through testing. Also, greater testing effort generally yields higher quality but costs more time and money. One therefore wants to assess the reliability of software to help decide when to release it. Statistical analysis of software failure data can help in this assessment of reliability.

There are some fundamental differences between software and hardware reliability. Software failure is due to imperfect code, whereas material deterioration is a major cause of hardware failures. Hence technological advances can improve the reliability of hardware, but not of software. On the other hand, software does not deteriorate over time and, in fact, continued usage, resulting in bugs being discovered and fixed, should improve the reliability of software. Furthermore, hardware can be replicated to introduce redundancy, and thus improve reliability, but this does not help with software as each copy of a program contains exactly the same bugs. Thus, many of the methods of reliability theory that work for modeling reliability of physical systems are not well suited for modeling software reliability. For further discussion see the following books: Musa *et al.* (1987), Xie (1991), Singpurwalla and Wilson (1999), and Pham (2000).

We focus on modeling of usual software failure data which are generated by testing the software for a fixed amount of time τ with varied inputs and recording the failure times. We also assume that upon each failure during the testing period, efforts are made to detect and remove the error that caused the failure, and time is measured in processor running time, excluding debugging and idle time. Specifically, the random observables that constitute the data are: the number of failures during testing (R) and the successive failure times $0 \leq T_{(1)} \leq \cdots \leq T_{(R)} \leq \tau$. We do not consider other variations of testing such as error seeding [Duran and Wiorkowski (1981)] or recapture debugging [Nayak (1988, 1991)].

One of the earliest and most discussed software reliability models, introduced by Jelinski and Moranda (1972), assumes perfect debugging and that the detection times of the errors are independently and identically distributed exponential random variables. These assumptions have been modified and generalized to produce many other models. One important class of models, called the general order statistics (GOS) models [see, e.g., Miller (1986) and Raftery (1987)], is based on the following two assumptions.

Assumption 1. Whenever the software fails, the error causing the failure is detected and corrected completely without inserting any new errors; that is, the debugging process is perfect.

Assumption 2. The software initially contains an unknown number of errors ν, and the detection times of those errors are independently and identically distributed (iid) with a common density $f_\theta(x)$, where θ is an unknown parameter, possibly vector-valued.

In the Jelinski and Moranda (J–M) model, $f_\theta(x)$ is an exponential density function. The assumptions of perfect debugging and independent and identical distribution of detection times of the errors have been criticized as unrealistic [see, e.g., Musa *et al.* (1987)].

Another class of software reliability models that has received considerable attention in recent years postulates that the failure counts follow a nonhomogeneous Poisson process (NHPP). Let $M(t)$ denote the number of failures observed in the time interval $(0, t]$ and let $m(t) = E[M(t)]$, which is a nondecreasing function of t. An NHPP model specifies the functional form of the intensity function $\lambda(t) = d/dt\, m(t)$, letting it depend on some unknown parameters. The Goel and Okumoto (1979) model (G–O) is one of the earliest NHPP models for software reliability, in which the intensity function $\lambda(t)$ is assumed to be

$$\lambda(t) = \mu\theta\exp(-\theta t), \qquad \mu > 0, \qquad \theta > 0.$$

The expected number of failures $m(t)$ in time $(0, t]$, which is also the cumulative intensity rate $\Lambda(t) = \int_0^t \lambda(u)du$ is given by $\Lambda(t) = m(t) = \mu(1 - \exp(-\theta t))$.

The NHPP models in which $m(\infty) < \infty$ (i.e., the expected number of failures in infinite testing is finite), are called NHPP-I models [Kuo and Yang (1996)], and those with $m(\infty) = \infty$ are called NHPP-II models. As we discuss in the next section, all NHPP-I models can be expressed as mixtures of GOS models. This suggests that inferences based on an NHPP-I model would be closely related to those based on the underlying GOS model. In this chapter we further explore the logical implications of the mixture representation and compare the maximum likelihood estimators (MLE) for an NHPP-I model and the MLEs for its underlying GOS model. In Section 11.2, we discuss the mixture representation and argue that for software reliability estimation, it may be more appropriate to use the underlying GOS model than the NHPP-I model. In Section 11.3, we consider model selection via maximized likelihood and unbiased estimation of parametric functions. We show that based on likelihood comparison, the underlying GOS model better fits the data than the NHPP-I model. We also find that unbiased estimation of a parametric function under an NHPP-I model is closely connected to unbiased estimation of a related quantity in the underlying GOS model. In Section 11.4, we present results from a simulation study evaluating certain maximum likelihood estimators for the G–O model and for the J–M model. We considered these two models because they are the most commonly discussed NHPP-I and GOS models and they are closely connected. The results show that choice of the model has little effect when the sample information is large, otherwise the J–M estimators have smaller variation. We make some concluding remarks in Section 11.5.

11.2 Connections Between NHPP and GOS Models

Some connections between NHPP-I and GOS models have already been discussed in the literature [Langberg and Singpurwalla (1985), Musa *et al.* (1987), and Kuo and Yang (1996)]. Firstly, a Poisson (μ) mixture (on the initial number of errors ν) of a GOS model yields an NHPP-I model. The rate function of the resulting NHPP-I model is $\lambda_\theta(t) = \mu f_\theta(t)$ where $f_\theta(t)$ is the probability density function (pdf) of the detection time of each error in the GOS model. It is also true that any given NHPP-I process with rate function $\lambda(t)$ and mean function $m(t)$ can be expressed as a Poisson mixture of GOS processes with $\mu = \lim_{t\to\infty} m(t)$ and $f(t) = \lambda(t)/\mu$. In particular, the Goel–Okumoto NHPP model can be expressed as a mixture of the Jelinski–Moranda model, by allowing the parameter ν to have a Poisson distribution with parameter μ. Other examples of NHPP-I models include the models proposed by Goel (1985) where $\lambda(t) = \mu\theta\alpha t^{\alpha-1}\exp(-\theta t^\alpha)$, and Littlewood (1984) where $\lambda(t) = \mu[1 - (\theta/(\theta + t))]^\alpha$ among others.

The likelihood function for an NHPP-I model with $\lambda_\theta(t) = \mu f_\theta(t)$ is

$$f_{NHPP-I}(r, t_{(1)}, \ldots, t_{(r)}|\mu, \theta) = \mu^r e^{-\mu F_\theta(\tau)} \prod_{i=1}^{r} f_\theta(t_{(i)}),$$

and it is a Poisson mixture of the GOS likelihood:

$$f_{NHPP-I}(r, t_{(1)}, \ldots, t_{(r)}|\mu, \theta) = \sum_{\nu=0}^{\infty} f_{GOS}(r, t_{(1)}, \ldots, t_{(r)}|\nu, \theta)\frac{e^{-\mu}\mu^\nu}{\nu!}, \quad (11.1)$$

where

$$
\begin{aligned}
f_{GOS}(r, t_{(1)}, \ldots, t_{(r)}|\nu, \theta) &= f_{\nu,\theta}(r) f_\theta(t_{(1)}, \ldots, t_{(r)}|r) \\
&= \left[\binom{\nu}{r} \{F_\theta(\tau)\}^r \{1 - F_\theta(\tau)\}^{\nu-r} \right] \times \left[r! \prod_{i=1}^{r} \frac{f_\theta(t_{(i)})}{F_\theta(\tau)} \right] \\
&= \frac{\nu!}{(\nu - r)!} \left[\prod_{i=1}^{r} f_\theta(t_{(i)}) \right] [1 - F_\theta(\tau)]^{\nu-r}
\end{aligned}
$$

is the likelihood function for a GOS model.

We just discussed that an NHPP-I model can be obtained as a Poisson mixture of models. Conversely, a GOS process can be obtained from an NHPP process by conditioning on $M(\infty)$ [see, e.g., Kuo and Yang (1996)]. Specifically, let $M(t)$ be an NHPP-I process with rate function $\lambda_\theta(t) = \mu f_\theta(t)$, where $f_\theta(t)$ is a pdf. Then, conditional on $M(\infty) = \nu$, $M(t)$ is a GOS process with initial number of errors ν and the pdf of detection time of each error $f_\theta(t)$.

We now explore some logical implications of the above connections on the choice between the two models for estimating software reliability. Among several metrics for measuring software reliability we focus on $\gamma_1(k)$ = the probability of failure-free operation of the debugged program between time τ and $\tau + k$. The length of the future time interval (k) depends on the usage of the software; it is short for a specific mission and is much longer in commercial applications. The theoretical expressions for $\gamma_1(k)$ under a GOS model and under an NHPP-I model with rate function $\lambda(t)$, respectively, are

$$\gamma_{1-GOS}(k) = \left(\frac{1 - F_\theta(\tau + k)}{1 - F_\theta(\tau)}\right)^{(\nu - R)} \tag{11.2}$$

$$\gamma_{1-NHPP}(k) = \exp[\Lambda(\tau) - \Lambda(\tau + k)], \tag{11.3}$$

where $\Lambda(t) = \int_0^t \lambda(u)du$.

From the mixture representation, failures under an NHPP-I model may be regarded as generated by a two-step process. First a quantity ν is generated from a Poisson distribution with parameter μ. Once ν is chosen (generated), failure times are generated from a GOS process with initial number of errors ν and detection time pdf $f_\theta(x)$. The parameter μ has no further role in failure occurrences over the entire time horizon $(0, \infty)$. From this viewpoint, the observed data as well as all future failures occur according to a GOS process with an unknown ν (generated from the Poisson (μ) distribution), and hence it would be more reasonable to use the underlying GOS process for data analysis and reliability estimation.

Another point to note is that for an NHPP-I model, the expression for $\gamma_1(k)$ in (11.3) does not depend on the data. Logically, the reliability should depend on how many errors are detected and removed during the testing period. In contrast, Equation (11.2) shows that the reliability under a GOS model depends on the data through R. From the connections between NHPP-I and GOS models discussed earlier, it follows that $\gamma_{1-NHPP}(k)$ is the average, with respect to the distribution of ν given the data, of $\gamma_{1-GOS}(k)$. Because the average, that is, $\gamma_{1-NHPP}(k)$ is independent of the data, it may be more meaningful to use the GOS model and estimate $\gamma_{1-GOS}(k)$. In the next section we provide a decision-theoretic rationale for estimating parametric functions for the underlying GOS model.

11.3   Some Aspects of Inference

For choosing between two models, one may fit them to the observed data and then select the better-fitting model. Between an NHPP-I model and its underlying GOS model, we find that the underlying GOS model gives a better fit in the sense of having a larger likelihood. This follows from the mixture representation (11.1) of NHPP-I models. Let us write L_{NHPP} and L_{GOS} for the two likelihoods. Then, from (11.1), we get

$$L_{NHPP}(\mu, \theta) = \sum_{\nu=0}^{\infty} L_{GOS}(\nu, \theta) \frac{e^{-\mu} \mu^{\nu}}{\nu!} \leq \sup_{\nu, \theta} L_{GOS}(\nu, \theta). \qquad (11.4)$$

From (11.4), it follows that $\sup_{\mu, \theta} L_{NHPP}(\mu, \theta) \leq \sup_{\nu, \theta} L_{GOS}(\nu, \theta)$; that is, the maximized likelihood for the underlying GOS model is at least as large as that for the NHPP-I model. Thus, based on likelihood comparison, the underlying GOS model is preferable to the NHPP-I model.

Let us now consider unbiased estimation of a function $h(\mu, \theta)$ for an NHPP-I model. In this section we use X to denote the data. Let $\delta(X)$ be an unbiased estimator (UE) of $h(\mu, \theta)$ and let $g_\delta(\nu, \theta) = E_{X|\nu, \theta}[\delta(X)]$, where $E_{X|\nu, \theta}$ denotes expectation under the corresponding GOS model. Now, unbiasedness of δ implies that

$$E_{\nu|\mu}[g_\delta(\nu, \theta)] = h(\mu, \theta) \qquad \text{for all } \mu, \theta, \qquad (11.5)$$

where $E_{\nu|\mu}$ denotes expectation with respect to the Poisson (μ) distribution of ν. Because a Poisson (μ) random variable has a complete family of distributions [for $\mu \in (0, \infty)$ or in general μ taking all values in a set that contains a nonempty open interval], there exists at most one function $g_\delta(\nu, \theta)$ satisfying (11.5) and hence $g_\delta(\nu, \theta)$ does not depend on δ. In other words, if $h(\mu, \theta)$ is unbiasedly estimable, then there exists a unique function $g(\nu, \theta)$ such that

$$E_{\nu|\mu}[g(\nu, \theta)] = h(\mu, \theta) \qquad \text{for all } \mu, \theta \qquad (11.6)$$

and any UE $\delta(X)$ of $h(\mu, \theta)$ satisfies the condition

$$E_{X|\nu, \theta}[\delta(X)] = g(\nu, \theta) \qquad \text{for all } \nu, \theta. \qquad (11.7)$$

Thus, all unbiased estimators of $h(\mu, \theta)$ for an NHPP-I model are also unbiased estimators of a related (and unique) quantity $g(\nu, \theta)$ in the underlying GOS model. The converse is obviously true. In particular, the classes of unbiased estimators for θ for the two models are the same and the classes of unbiased estimators of μ and ν are the same.

Equations (11.6) and (11.7) also imply that for any UE δ of $h(\mu, \theta)$,

$$E_{X|\mu, \theta}[\{\delta(X) - g(\nu, \theta)\}\{g(\nu, \theta) - h(\mu, \theta)\}]$$
$$= E_{\nu|\mu}[\{g(\nu, \theta) - h(\mu, \theta)\}E_{X|\nu, \mu}\{\delta(X) - g(\nu, \theta)\}] = 0$$

and hence

$$\text{MSE}(\delta; \mu, \theta) = E_{X|\mu,\theta}[\delta(X) - h(\mu, \theta)]^2$$
$$= E_{\nu|\mu}E_{X|\nu,\theta}[\delta(X) - g(\nu, \theta)]^2 + E_{\nu|\mu}[g(\nu, \theta) - h(\mu, \theta)]^2. \quad (11.8)$$

Note that the first term in the MSE decomposition (11.8) is the expectation [with respect to the Poisson (μ) distribution of ν] of the MSE of δ as an estimator of $g(\nu, \theta)$ under the GOS model. The second term does not involve the observations and does not depend on the estimator δ as long as it is unbiased. This has two implications. The first is that among all unbiased estimators of $h(\mu, \theta)$ [or equivalently of $g(\nu, \theta)$ as noted earlier], if there exists δ that minimizes $E_{X|\nu,\theta}[\delta(X) - g(\nu, \theta)]^2$ for all ν and θ, then it has the smallest MSE as an estimator of $h(\mu, \theta)$. In other words, if δ is the best UE of $g(\nu, \theta)$, then it is also the best UE of $h(\mu, \theta)$.

The second implication is that the MSE of any UE δ of $h(\mu, \theta)$ is larger than the average [with respect to the Poisson (μ) distribution of ν] MSE of δ for estimating $g(\nu, \theta)$, unless $g(\nu, \theta) \equiv h(\mu, \theta)$; that is, $h(\mu, \theta)$ is a function only of θ. We may expect this phenomenon to hold more generally, especially for slightly biased estimators. Note that if $h(\mu, \theta) = \theta$ then $g(\nu, \theta) = \theta$ and the second term of (11.8) is 0. This suggests that an estimator of θ derived under one of the two models would perform about equally well for the other model. If $h(\mu, \theta) = \mu$ then $g(\nu, \theta) = \nu$, in which case the second term of (11.8) equals μ and we would expect an estimator of μ to have larger variation than its variation as an estimator of ν. We may also note that the second term of (11.8), $E_{\nu|\mu}[g(\nu, \theta) - h(\mu, \theta)]^2$, provides a lower bound of the MSE of any UE of $h(\mu, \theta)$. If the quantity $E_{\nu|\mu}[g(\nu, \theta) - h(\mu, \theta)]^2$ is difficult to calculate, one can bound it below by the Cramer–Rao lower bound, which equals $\mu[\partial/\partial\mu h(\mu, \theta)]^2$, assuming the derivative exists.

We have argued in the previous section that when an NHPP-I model is assumed, in essence the data come from a GOS process and hence GOS models should be used for analyzing software failure data. In this section we have shown that according to likelihood comparison the underlying GOS model is preferable to the NHPP-I model and that for estimating features of an NHPP-I process it is sensible to estimate actually as closely as possible, related features of the underlying GOS process. The next section presents results of simulations that investigate this issue and the behavior of certain estimators.

11.4   Simulation Results

The probabilistic and inferential connections between an NHPP-I model and its underlying GOS model make us wonder if the estimates of μ and θ under an NHPP-I model are close to the estimates of ν and θ under the corresponding

GOS model. In particular, we want to know how well the estimators of ν and θ under a GOS model estimate the parameters μ and θ of the corresponding NHPP-I model. Another question of natural interest is: how similar are the reliability estimates under the two models? We conducted a simulation study to investigate these questions for the Goel–Okumoto and Jelinski–Moranda pair of models. The G–O model is the most commonly used NHPP-I model, and its failure rate function is $\lambda(t) = \mu\theta \exp(-\theta t)$. The J–M model is the most commonly used GOS model and it underlies the G–O model; the G–O likelihood is a Poisson mixture of J–M likelihoods. We examined the MLEs of the model parameters and of the reliability measure $\gamma_1(k)$, whose theoretical expressions under the G–O and the J–M models, respectively, are:

$$\gamma_{1\{GO\}}(k) = \exp[-\mu(e^{-\theta\tau} - e^{-\theta(\tau+k)})], \qquad (11.9)$$

$$\gamma_{1\{JM\}}(k) = \exp[-\theta k(\nu - R)]. \qquad (11.10)$$

We investigated properties of the estimators under both models, that is, by separately generating data from each of the two models. For the G–O model, we experimented with various values of μ, τ, and k. As the likelihoods for both G–O and J–M models depend on θ and τ only through $\tau\theta$, we decided to hold θ fixed at 0.01 and vary τ. For each μ and τ we generated 10,000 samples and for each sample we calculated the MLEs $\hat{\mu}, \hat{\theta}_{\{GO\}}$, and $\hat{\gamma}_{1\{GO\}}(k)$ assuming the G–O model, and the MLEs $\hat{\nu}, \hat{\theta}_{\{JM\}}$ and $\hat{\gamma}_{1\{JM\}}(k)$ assuming the J–M model. We should note that the MLEs of μ and ν may not exist and both can be infinite; see Hossain and Dahiya (1993) for $\hat{\mu}$ and Blumenthal and Marcus (1975) and Littlewood and Verrall (1981) for $\hat{\nu}$. If $\hat{\mu} = \infty$ for the G–O model (or, $\hat{\nu} = \infty$ for the J–M model), the MLEs of θ and $\gamma_1(k)$ are 0. For sample generation we exploited the mixture representation of the G–O model. First we generate a ν from the Poisson (μ) distribution and then we generated ν failure times (observations) from the exponential distribution with pdf $f(t) = \theta e^{-\theta t}$. The failure times falling in the interval $(0, \tau]$ constituted one sample.

Table 11.1 presents summary results for $\hat{\mu}$ and $\hat{\nu}$ for $\mu = 20, 60$, and 100 and $\tau = 75, 150$, and 300. In the context of the J–M model, the probability of detecting any specific error [i.e., $F_\theta(\tau)$] with $\tau = 75, 150$, and 300 are: 0.5276, 0.7769, and 0.9502, respectively. As both $\hat{\nu}$ and $\hat{\mu}$ are ∞ for some samples, we report the quartiles [Q_1, median (Me), and Q_3] of their simulated distributions. We also present the fraction of times $\hat{\mu}$ and $\hat{\nu}$ equal infinity, under the $P(\hat{\mu} = \infty)$ and $P(\hat{\nu} = \infty)$ columns, respectively. Those numbers show that: (i) for both models the probability that the estimate is ∞ decreases as μ and/or τ increases and (ii) $P(\hat{\mu} = \infty)$ is much larger than $P(\hat{\nu} = \infty)$ unless both are very small. One criticism of the J–M model is that the maximum likelihood method may fail to estimate its parameters [see, e.g., Forman and Singpurwalla (1977)]. As

Table 11.1. Empirical performance of the MLE of model parameters

	Estimates based on G–O model				Estimates based on J–M model			
μ		$\hat{\mu}$				$\hat{\nu}$		
	$P(\hat{\mu} = \infty)$	Q_1	Me	Q_3	$P(\hat{\nu} = \infty)$	Q_1	Me	Q_3
			$\tau = 75,$	$F_\theta(\tau) = 0.5276$				
20	0.241	13.29	21.44	397.64	0.105	11	16	25
60	0.109	45.11	61.46	112.55	0.065	42	54	81
100	0.060	79.45	101.41	150.99	0.039	75	92	127
			$\tau = 150,$	$F_\theta(\tau) = 0.7769$				
20	0.051	16.48	21.16	28.89	0.018	15	19	25
60	0.004	52.91	61.12	71.53	0.002	52	59	68
100	0.000	90.82	101.09	113.79	0.000	89	99	111
			$\tau = 300,$	$F_\theta(\tau) = 0.9502$				
20	0.001	17.19	20.35	23.73	0.000	17	20	23
60	0.000	54.73	60.17	65.76	0.000	55	60	66
100	0.000	93.12	100.30	107.63	0.000	93	100	108

our results show, that situation occurs even more frequently for the G–O model. We believe this phenomenon holds more generally for other pairs of NHPP-I and GOS models.

We now discuss behavior of $\hat{\mu}$ and $\hat{\nu}$. Because $\hat{\nu}$ is integer-valued, its quartiles are also integers. This is not so for $\hat{\mu}$. For $\tau = 300$, all three quartiles of $\hat{\nu}$ are very close to those of $\hat{\mu}$ for all values of μ reported in Table 11.1. Also, the medians of $\hat{\mu}$ and $\hat{\nu}$ are very close to the true value of μ. For $\tau = 75$, $\hat{\mu}$ has a larger interquartile range (IQR) than $\hat{\nu}$. Although $\hat{\mu}$ is approximately median unbiased in all cases, $\hat{\nu}$ has negative median bias (for estimating μ). Table 11.1 also shows that the differences in the behavior of $\hat{\mu}$ and $\hat{\nu}$ diminish gradually as τ and/or μ increases. In summary, for small μ and small τ neither $\hat{\mu}$ nor $\hat{\nu}$ is a satisfactory estimator of μ. For large μ and large τ the two estimators are equally good. For other cases, one may prefer $\hat{\nu}$ to $\hat{\mu}$ (for estimating μ) as $\hat{\nu}$ has smaller sampling variation and lower probability of being ∞.

Table 11.2 gives summary results for the MLE of θ under the G–O and the J–M models, when the true value of θ is 0.01. In all cases, the two estimators differ very little in their means and standard deviations. For small τ and small μ both estimators are positively biased and have large standard deviations. The bias and variance of the two estimators decrease as τ and/or μ increase.

Table 11.3 gives a summary of certain performance characteristics of the reliability estimators $\hat{\gamma}_{1\{GO\}}(k)$ and $\hat{\gamma}_{1\{JM\}}(k)$. As $\gamma_1(k)$ depends also on k, for each μ and τ, we present results for three different values of k. For each setting,

Table 11.2. Empirical performance of the MLEs of θ

		Based on G–O Model		Based on J–M model	
τ	μ	Mean	SD	Mean	SD
	20	0.018	0.014	0.021	0.016
75	60	0.012	0.007	0.013	0.008
	100	0.011	0.006	0.012	0.006
	20	0.011	0.006	0.014	0.007
150	60	0.010	0.004	0.011	0.004
	100	0.010	0.003	0.011	0.003
	20	0.011	0.004	0.012	0.003
300	60	0.010	0.002	0.011	0.002
	100	0.010	0.001	0.010	0.002

the true value of $\gamma_1(k)$ for the G–O model is given in the third column. For each estimator, we report its mean and the three quartiles. We may recall that $\hat{\gamma}_{1\{JM\}}(k)$ estimates $\gamma_{1\{JM\}}(k)$ in (11.10) assuming that the data come from a J–M process. However, we assess how well it estimates $\gamma_{1\{GO\}}(k)$ in (11.9), denoted subsequently by γ_1. The upper and lower quartiles show that both estimators have large sampling variation, and in most cases $\hat{\gamma}_{1\{JM\}}(k)$ has larger IQR than $\hat{\gamma}_{1\{GO\}}(k)$. Both estimators are quite unreliable when the true value of γ_1 is small. The median (Me) of $\hat{\gamma}_{1\{GO\}}(k)$ is usually close to the true value of γ_1. For $\mu = 20$, $\hat{\gamma}_{1\{JM\}}(k)$ overestimates γ_1, and as μ increases, the bias decreases. For each of the two estimators, the mean and median differ noticeably in many cases, indicating skewness. To give an idea about the correlation between the estimators, in Figure 11.1 we plotted $\hat{\gamma}_{1\{JM\}}(k)$ against $\hat{\gamma}_{1\{GO\}}(k)$ along with the 45-degree line for two settings of μ, τ, and k. In the scatterplots, each point displays the two estimates for one sample. We may note that if $\hat{\nu} = r$ then $\hat{\gamma}_{1\{JM\}}(k) = 1$, and if $\hat{\mu} = \infty$ then $\hat{\gamma}_{1\{GO\}}(k) = 0$. Excluding those cases, which occur considerably often in the case of $\mu = 20, \tau = 150$ but not in the case of $\mu = 60, \tau = 200$, we see a strong linear relationship between the two estimators. It is generally believed that reliability estimates based on the J–M model are larger (and more optimistic) than those based on the G–O model [see, e.g., Goel and Okumoto (1979) and Musa et al. (1987)]. However, that is not always true as Figure 11.1 shows.

We also examined properties of the estimators by simulating data from the J–M model. We kept θ fixed at 0.01 and varied ν and τ. For each sample we computed parameter and reliability estimates assuming the G–O and the J–M model, respectively. For each setup, the summary results were calculated from 5000 simulated samples. In Figure 11.2, we show the quartiles of $\hat{\mu}$ and $\hat{\nu}$ for $\tau = 200$ and 300 for different values of ν. The plots show good agreement

Table 11.3. Empirical performance of reliability estimators

			$\hat{\gamma}_{1\{GO\}}(k)$				$\hat{\gamma}_{1\{JM\}}(k)$			
τ	k	γ_1	Mean	Q_1	Me	Q_3	Mean	Q_1	Me	Q_3
					$\mu = 20$					
	5	0.631	0.528	0.367	0.631	0.771	0.671	0.585	0.724	0.835
75	10	0.407	0.389	0.116	0.407	0.605	0.525	0.342	0.524	0.693
	20	0.180	0.251	0.020	0.185	0.404	0.366	0.119	0.276	0.484
	10	0.654	0.631	0.532	0.659	0.776	0.701	0.596	0.705	0.813
150	20	0.445	0.457	0.292	0.453	0.624	0.530	0.354	0.498	0.664
	40	0.230	0.288	0.097	0.235	0.434	0.344	0.125	0.247	0.424
	10	0.910	0.900	0.864	0.913	0.950	0.934	0.862	1.000	1.000
300	20	0.835	0.820	0.757	0.841	0.907	0.877	0.744	1.000	1.000
	40	0.720	0.707	0.594	0.733	0.843	0.793	0.554	1.000	1.000
					$\mu = 60$					
	5	0.251	0.259	0.161	0.251	0.357	0.293	0.193	0.285	0.391
75	10	0.067	0.103	0.029	0.071	0.145	0.114	0.039	0.085	0.161
	20	0.006	0.027	0.001	0.006	0.026	0.023	0.001	0.007	0.025
	10	0.280	0.297	0.198	0.282	0.381	0.306	0.210	0.294	0.387
150	20	0.088	0.119	0.045	0.091	0.164	0.110	0.045	0.087	0.153
	40	0.012	0.033	0.003	0.013	0.040	0.020	0.002	0.007	0.024
	10	0.753	0.748	0.691	0.755	0.813	0.738	0.686	0.740	0.795
300	20	0.582	0.583	0.492	0.586	0.678	0.552	0.471	0.547	0.632
	40	0.374	0.388	0.270	0.377	0.497	0.321	0.221	0.299	0.399
					$\mu = 100$					
	5	0.100	0.118	0.060	0.101	0.160	0.129	0.069	0.112	0.172
75	10	0.011	0.023	0.004	0.011	0.029	0.024	0.005	0.012	0.030
	20	0.000	0.003	0.000	0.000	0.001	0.002	0.000	0.000	0.001
	5	0.337	0.345	0.271	0.339	0.412	0.353	0.281	0.348	0.420
150	10	0.120	0.138	0.079	0.121	0.182	0.136	0.080	0.121	0.179
	20	0.018	0.030	0.007	0.018	0.039	0.024	0.006	0.015	0.031
	10	0.623	0.623	0.559	0.627	0.693	0.607	0.548	0.608	0.662
300	20	0.406	0.411	0.326	0.406	0.491	0.373	0.296	0.367	0.434
	40	0.194	0.213	0.126	0.196	0.281	0.151	0.087	0.135	0.190

between the quartiles of the two estimators and they change almost linearly with ν. It seems that $\hat{\mu}$ is estimating the parameter ν of the J–M model. These plots also provide additional information on the behavior of $\hat{\mu}$ for estimating μ. For example, if $\mu = 60$, the distribution of ν is centered around 60, and the interval [52, 68] has approximate probability 0.95. Figure 11.2a shows that $\hat{\mu}$

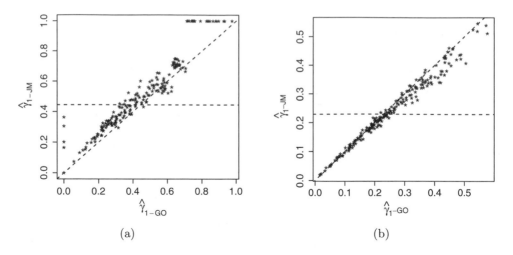

(a)   (b)

Figure 11.1. Comparison of $\hat{\gamma}_{1\{GO\}}(k)$ and $\hat{\gamma}_{1\{JM\}}(k)$ for (a) $\mu = 20, \tau = 150$, $k = 20$, and (b) $\mu = 60, \tau = 200, k = 20$. Horizontal broken line represents the true value of $\gamma_{1\{GO\}}(k)$.

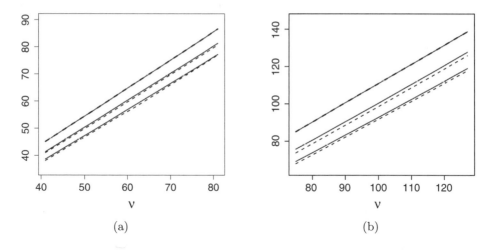

(a)   (b)

Figure 11.2. Quartiles of $\hat{\mu}$ (solid line) and $\hat{\nu}$ (broken line) under the J–M model for (a) $\tau = 200$, and (b) $\tau = 300$.

under- (over)estimates μ if ν is smaller (larger) than $\mu = 60$ and the bias grows with $|\mu - \nu|$.

Our discussion in Section 11.3 suggests that an estimator of $h(\mu, \theta)$ for the G–O model may actually be an estimator of a related parametric function $g(\nu, \theta)$ for the J–M model. We explored this aspect for $\hat{\gamma}_{1\{GO\}}(k)$. We suspected that $\hat{\gamma}_{1\{GO\}}(k)$ would be in closer agreement with

$$g(\nu, \theta) = \exp[-\nu(e^{-\theta\tau} - e^{-\theta(\tau+k)})], \tag{11.11}$$

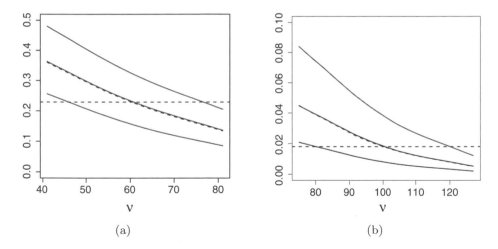

Figure 11.3. Quartiles of $\hat{\gamma}_{1\{GO\}}(k)$ (solid curves) and $g(\nu, \theta)$ (broken curve) for (a) $\tau = 200$, $k = 20$, and (b) $\tau = 300$, $k = 40$. Horizontal broken line represents true $\gamma_{1\{GO\}}(k)$ for $\mu = 60$ in plot (a) and for $\mu = 100$ in plot (b).

which is obtained by replacing μ by ν in the expression of $\gamma_{1\{GO\}}(k)$ in (11.9), than $\gamma_{1\{GO\}}(k)$. In other words, we felt it may be more appropriate to think of $\hat{\gamma}_{1\{GO\}}(k)$ as an estimator of $g(\nu, \theta)$ in (11.11) rather than of $\gamma_{1\{GO\}}(k)$. To explore this, we plot the quartiles of $\hat{\gamma}_{1\{GO\}}(k)$ and $g(\nu, \theta)$ for $\tau = 200, k = 20$ and for $\tau = 300, k = 40$ in Figure 11.3. We also show the true value of $\gamma_{1\{GO\}}(k)$ for $\mu = 60$ in plot (a) and for $\mu = 100$ in plot (b). Note that the ranges of ν values displayed in the two plots are compatible with the Poisson (μ) distribution of ν with $\mu = 60$ and 100, respectively. The plots show that in both cases, the median of $\hat{\gamma}_{1\{GO\}}(k)$ is very close to $g(\nu, \theta)$ and the IQR decreases as ν increases. Performance of $\hat{\gamma}_{1\{GO\}}(k)$ for estimating $\gamma_{1\{GO\}}(k)$ depends substantially on ν. It overestimates the reliability for ν smaller than μ and underestimates for ν larger than μ. Also, the bias increases as the difference between μ and ν increases. The graphs also illustrate the two sources of variation for estimating a parametric function for an NHPP-I model, discussed in Section 11.3. Specifically, Figure 11.3 displays the variation of $\hat{\gamma}_{1\{GO\}}(k)$ around $g(\nu, \theta)$ and the variation of $g(\nu, \theta)$ around $\gamma_{1\{GO\}}(k)$.

11.5 Discussion

The assumptions of perfect debugging and iid error detection times of the J–M model, and more generally of the GOS models, have been criticized as unrealistic. However, Nayak (1986) showed that if one assumes perfect debugging, then the assumption that the detection times of the errors are identically distributed is harmless. The NHPP models, most of which are NHPP-I, were proposed as better models for analyzing software failure data. However, our results cast further doubt on that suggestion. We showed that the principle of likelihood maximization prefers the underlying GOS model, the probability of getting an infinite estimate for an NHPP-I model is higher than that for the underlying GOS model, and inferences derived under an NHPP-I model may be more unreliable than those derived assuming the underlying GOS model. We also identified important connections between estimation of parametric functions under the two models.

Some logical implications of NHPP assumptions also raise concerns about suitability of nonhomogeneous Poisson processes for modeling software reliability. The NHPP-I models assume independence of the failure process in nonoverlapping intervals, but one would expect debugging activities at any time to affect the failure process subsequent to that time. One implication of this is that the reliability of a program does not depend on past failures and associated debugging activities. Logically, software reliability changes only when changes are made in the code, for example, by detecting and fixing bugs. In between such changes, the reliability does not change. Let M denote the total number of failures in $[0, \infty)$; that is, $M = \lim_{t \to \infty} M(t)$. Then, M has Poisson distribution with mean μ (which is the same as the mixing distribution of ν). Because M is unbounded for all values of the parameters μ and θ, NHPP-I models implicitly assume imperfect debugging. Also, $P(M = 0) = \exp(-\mu) > 0$; that is, the probability of observing no failures in infinite testing is positive. Another drawback of NHPP-I models is that their parameters cannot be estimated consistently as the testing time τ goes to infinity [see, e.g., Zhao and Xie (1996) and Nayak *et al.* (2008)]. The assumptions of GOS models may be unrealistic and faulty but it is dubious that NHPP-I models offer any improvement.

References

1. Blumenthal, S. and Marcus, R. (1975). Estimating population size with exponential failure, *Journal of the American Statistical Association*, **70**, 913–921.

2. Duran, J. W. and Wiorkowski, J. J. (1981). Capture-recapture sampling for estimating software error content, *IEEE Transactions on Software Engineering*, **SE-7**, 147–148.

3. Forman, E. H. and Singpurwalla, N. D. (1977). An empirical stopping rule for debugging and testing computer software, *Journal of the American Statistical Association*, **72**, 750–757.

4. Goel, A. L. (1985). Software reliability models: Assumptions, limitations, and applicability, *IEEE Transactions on Software Engineering*, **11**, 1411–1423.

5. Goel, A. L. and Okumoto, K. (1979). Time-dependent error detection rate model for software reliability and other performance measures, *IEEE Transactions on Reliability*, **28**, 206–211.

6. Hossain, S. A. and Dahiya, R. C. (1993). Estimating the parameters of a non-homogeneous Poisson process model for software reliability, *IEEE Transactions on Reliability*, **42**, 604–612.

7. Jelinski, Z. and Moranda, P.M. (1972). Software reliability research, In *Statistical Computer Performance Evaluation* (Ed., W. Freiberger), pp. 465–484, Academic Press, New York.

8. Kuo, L. and Yang, T. Y. (1996). Bayesian computation for nonhomogeneous Poisson processes in software reliability, *Journal of the American Statistical Association*, **91**, 763–773.

9. Langberg, N. and Singpurwalla, N. D. (1985). A unification of some software reliability models, *SIAM Journal of Science and Statistical Computing*, **6**, 781–790.

10. Littlewood, B. (1984). Rationale for a modified Duane model, *IEEE Transactions on Reliability*, **R-33**, 157–159.

11. Littlewood, B. and Verrall, J. L. (1981). Likelihood function of a debugging model for computer software reliability, *IEEE Transactions on Reliability*, **30**, 145–148.

12. Miller, D. R. (1986). Exponential order statistic model of software reliability growth, *IEEE Transactions on Software Engineering*, **12**, 12–24.

13. Musa, J. D., Iannino, A., and Okumoto, K. (1987). *Software Reliability: Measurement, Prediction, Application*, McGraw-Hill, New York.

14. Nayak, T. K. (1986). Software reliability: Statistical modeling and estimation, *IEEE Transactions on Reliability*, **35**, 566–570.

15. Nayak, T. K. (1988). Estimating population size by recapture debugging, *Biometrika*, **75**, 113–120.

16. Nayak, T. K. (1991). Estimating the number of component processes of a superimposed process, *Biometrika*, **78**, 75–81.

17. Nayak, T. K., Bose, S., and Kundu, S. (2008). On inconsistency of estimators of parameters of non-homogeneous Poisson process models for software reliability, *Statistics and Probability Letters* (to appear).

18. Pham, H. (2000). *Software Reliability*, Springer-Verlag, New York.

19. Raftery, A. E. (1987). Inference and prediction for a general order statistic model with unknown population size, *Journal of the American Statistical Association*, **82**, 1163–1168.

20. Singpurwalla, N. D. and Wilson, S. P. (1999). *Statistical Methods in Software Engineering: Reliability and Risk*, Springer-Verlag, New York.

21. Xie, M. (1991). *Software Reliability Modelling*, World Scientific, Singapore.

22. Zhao, M. and Xie, M. (1996). On maximum likelihood estimation for a general non-homogeneous Poisson process, *Scandinavian Journal of Statistics*, **23**, 597–607.

12

Multistate System Reliability Assessment by Using the Markov Reward Model

Anatoly Lisnianski,[1,2] **Ilia Frenkel,**[2] **Lev Khvatskin,**[2] **and Yi Ding**[2]

[1] *The Israel Electric Corporation Ltd., Haifa, Israel*
[2] *Center for Reliability and Risk Management, Sami Shamoon College of Engineering, Beer Sheva, Israel*

Abstract: The chapter considers reliability measures for a multistate system where the system and its components can have different performance levels, ranging from perfect functioning up to complete failure. The general approach is suggested for computation of commonly used reliability measures. According to the approach, the general Markov reward model should be built, so that different reliability measures can be calculated by the corresponding reward matrix determination. A numerical example is presented in order to illustrate this approach.

Keywords and Phrases: Multistate system, reliability measure, Markov reward model, demand

12.1 Introduction

Traditional binary-state reliability models allow for a system and its components only two possible states: perfect functionality (up) and complete failure (down). However, many real-world systems are composed of multistate components, which have different performance levels and for which one cannot formulate an "all or nothing" type of failure criterion. Failures of some system elements lead, in these cases, only to performance degradation. Such systems are called multistate systems (MSS). Traditional reliability theory, which is based on a binary approach, has recently been extended by allowing components and systems to have an arbitrary finite number of states. According to the generic multistate system model [Lisnianski and Levitin (2003)], any system element $j \in \{1, 2, \ldots, n\}$ can have k_j different states corresponding to the performance rates, represented by the set $g_j = \{g_{j1}, g_{j2}, \ldots, g_{jk}\}$, where g_{ji} is the performance rate of element j in the state i, $i \in \{1, 2, \ldots, k_j\}$. The performance rate $G_j(t)$ of element j at any instant $t \geq 0$ is a discrete-state continuous-time stochastic process that takes its values from $g_j : G(t) \in g_j$. The system structure function $G(t) = \phi(G_1(t), \ldots, G_n(t))$ produces the stochastic process corresponding to the output performance of the entire MSS. In practice, a desired level of system performance (demand) also can be represented by a discrete-state continuous-time stochastic process $W(t)$. The relation between the MSS output performance and the demand represented by two corresponding stochastic processes should be studied in order to define reliability measures for the entire MSS. In practice the most commonly used MSS reliability measures are probability of failure-free operation during time interval $[0, t]$ or MSS reliability function $R(t)$, MSS availability, mean time to MSS failure, mean accumulated performance deficiency for a fixed time interval $[0, t]$, and so on. In this chapter, a generalized approach for the computation of main MSS reliability measures has been suggested. This approach is based on the application of the Markov reward model. The main MSS reliability measures can be found by corresponding reward matrix definitions for this model and then by using a standard procedure for finding expected accumulated rewards during a time interval $[0, t]$ as a solution of system of differential equations.

12.2   Model Description

12.2.1   Generalized MSS reliability measure

The MSS behavior is characterized by its evolution in the space of states. The entire set of possible system states can be divided into two disjoint subsets corresponding to acceptable and unacceptable system functioning. MSS entrance into the subset of unacceptable states constitutes a failure. The system state acceptability depends on the relation between the MSS output performance and the desired level of this performance—demand $W(t)$—that is determined outside the system. Often the demand $W(t)$ is also a random process that can take discrete values from the set $w = \{w_1, \ldots, w_M\}$. The desired relation between the system performance and the demand at any time instant t can be expressed by the acceptability function $\Phi(G(t), W(t))$. In many practical cases, the MSS performance should be equal to or exceed the demand. So, in such cases the acceptability function takes the following form

$$\Phi(G(t), W(t)) = G(t) - W(t) \tag{12.1}$$

and the criterion of state acceptability can be expressed as $\Phi(G(t), W(t)) \geq 0$. A general expression defining MSS reliability measures can be written in the following form,

$$R = E\{F[\Phi(G(t), W(t))]\}, \tag{12.2}$$

where E = expectation symbol, F = functional that determines corresponding type of reliability measure, and Φ = acceptability function. Many important MSS reliability measures can be derived from the expression (12.2) depending on the functional F that may be determined in different ways. It may be a probability $\Pr\{\Phi\left(G\left(t\right),W\left(t\right)\right) \geq 0\}$ that within specified time interval $[0,t]$ the acceptability function (12.1) will be nonnegative. This probability characterizes MSS availability. It may be also a time up to MSS first entrance into the set of unacceptable states, where $\Phi\left(G\left(t\right),W\left(t\right)\right) < 0$, a number of such entrances within time interval $[0,t]$ and so on. If the acceptability function is defined as

$$F\left[\Phi\left(G\left(t\right),W\left(t\right)\right)\right] = \left\{ \begin{array}{ll} W\left(t\right) - G\left(t\right), & \text{if } W\left(t\right) > G\left(t\right) \\ 0, & \text{if } W\left(t\right) \leq G\left(t\right) \end{array} \right.$$

a functional $F\left[\Phi\left(G\left(t\right),W\left(t\right)\right)\right] = \int_0^T \Phi\left(G\left(t\right),W\left(t\right)\right)dt$ will characterize an accumulated performance deficiency during time interval $[0,t]$.

In this chapter a generalized approach for main reliability measures computation is considered.

12.2.2 Markov reward model: General description

The general Markov reward model was introduced by Howard (1960). It considers the continuous-time Markov chain with a set of states $\{1,\ldots,k\}$ and a transition intensity matrix $a = |a_{ij}|$, $i,j = 1,\ldots,k$. It is assumed that while the process is in any state i during any time unit, some money r_{ii} should be paid. It is also assumed that if there is a transition from state i to state j the amount r_{ij} will be paid. The amounts r_{ii} and r_{ij} are called rewards. They can be negative while representing a loss or penalty. The main problem is to find the total expected reward accumulated up to time instant T under specific initial conditions. Let $V_i\left(t\right)$ be the total expected reward accumulated up to time t at state i. According to Howard (1960), the following system of differential equations must be solved under initial conditions $V_i\left(0\right) = 0$, $i = 1,\ldots,k$ in order to find the total expected reward.

$$\frac{dV_i\left(t\right)}{dt} = r_{ii} + \sum_{j=1,j\neq i}^{k} a_{ij}r_{ij} + \sum_{j=1}^{k} a_{ij}V_j\left(t\right), \qquad i = 1,\ldots,k. \qquad (12.3)$$

Markov reward models are widely used in financial calculations and operations research [Hiller and Lieberman (1995)]. General Markov reward models for system dependability and performability analysis one can find in Carrasco (2003), Sahner *et al.* (1996), and Lisnianski *et al.* (2006). Here we present the new approach where the main MSS reliability measures can be found by determination of the corresponding reward matrix. Such an idea was primarily introduced for a binary-state system and constant demand in Volik *et al.* (1988).

In this chapter, we extend the approach for multistate systems and variable demand.

12.2.3   Rewards determination for MSS reliability computation

MSS instantaneous (point) availability $A(t)$ is the probability that the MSS at instant $t > 0$ is in one of the acceptable states: $A(t) = \Pr\{\Phi(G(t), W(t)) \geq 0\}$.

The MSS average availability $\overline{A}(T)$ is defined in Modarres *et al.* (1999) as a mean fraction of time when the system resides in the set of acceptable states during the time interval $[0, T]$, $\overline{A}(T) = (1/T)\int_0^T A(t)\, dt$.

In order to assess $\overline{A}(T)$ for MSS the rewards in matrix r for the MSS model should be determined in the following manner.

- The rewards associated with all acceptable states should be defined as one.

- The rewards associated with all unacceptable states should be zeroed as well as all rewards associated with all transitions.

The mean reward $V_i(T)$ accumulated during interval $[0, T]$ will define a time that MSS will be in the set of acceptable states in the case when the state i is the initial state. This reward should be found as a solution of a system (12.3). After solving (12.3) and finding $V_i(t)$, MSS average availability can be obtained for every initial state $i = 1, \ldots, k$, $\overline{A}_i(T) = (V_i(T))/T$.

Usually, the initial state is assumed as the best state.

Mean number $N_f(t)$ *of MSS failures during time interval* $[0, t]$. This measure can be treated as the mean number of MSS entrances to the set of unacceptable states during time interval $[0, t]$. For its computation the rewards associated with each transition from the set of acceptable states to the set of unacceptable states should be defined as one. All other rewards should be zeroed. In this case mean accumulated reward $V_i(t)$ will define the mean number of entrances in the unacceptable area during time interval $[0, t]$: $N_{fi}(t) = V_i(t)$.

Mean time to failure (MTTF) is the mean time up to the instant when the MSS enters the subset of unacceptable states for the first time. For its computation the combined performance-demand model should be transformed; all transitions that return MSS from unacceptable states should be forbidden, because for this case all unacceptable states should be treated as absorbing states. In order to assess MTTF for MSS the rewards in matrix r for the transformed performance-demand model should be determined in the following manner.

- The rewards associated with all acceptable states should be defined as one.

- The reward associated with unacceptable (absorbing) states should be zeroed as well as all rewards associated with transitions.

In this case mean accumulated reward $V_i(t)$ will define the mean time accumulated up to the first entrance into the subset of unacceptable states or MTTF.

Probability of MSS failure during time interval $[0, t]$. The model should be transformed as in the previous case: all unacceptable states should be treated as absorbing states and, therefore, all transitions that return MSS from unacceptable states should be forbidden. Rewards associated with all transitions to the absorbing state should be defined as one. All other rewards should be zeroed. Mean accumulated reward $V_i(t)$ will define for this case probability of MSS failure during time interval $[0, t]$ if the state i is the initial state. Therefore, the MSS reliability function can be obtained as $R_i(t) = 1 - V_i(t)$, where $i = 1, \ldots, k$.

12.3   Numerical Example

Consider the air-conditioning system used in one Israeli hospital. The system consists of two main online air conditioners and one air conditioner in cold reserve. The reserve conditioner begins to work only when one of the main conditioners has failed. Air conditioner failure rates are: $\lambda = 3$ year^{-1} for the main conditioner and $\lambda^* = 10$ year^{-1} for the conditioner in cold reserve ($\lambda^* > \lambda$, because the reserve conditioner is usually a secondhand device). The repair rates for the main and reserve conditioners are the same, $\mu = \mu^*$. Repair rate depends on the repair team and may be changed from 6 hours^{-1} to 7 days^{-1}. Demand is a discrete-state continuous-time Markov process with two levels: peak and low. The mean duration of the peak-demand period is $\overline{T}_d = 7$ hours. The mean duration of the low-demand period is equal to $\overline{T}_N = 24 - \overline{T}_d = 17$ hours. The state–space diagram for this system is presented in Figure 12.1.

There are 12 states. States from 1 to 6 are associated with the peak demand period, states from 7 to 12 are associated with the low-demand period. States 6 and 12 indicate both main air conditioners are online and the reserve air conditioner is available. The system performance is $g_6 = g_{12} = 2$. States 5 and 11 indicate one of the main air conditioners failed and is replaced by the reserve air conditioner. The system performance is $g_5 = g_{11} = 2$. States 4 and 10 indicate the second main air conditioner failed; only the reserve air conditioner is online. The system performance is $g_4 = g_{10} = 1$. States 3 and 9 indicate that the reserve air conditioner failed; only one main air conditioner is online. The system performance is $g_3 = g_9 = 1$. States 2 and 8 indicate the reserve air conditioner failed and two main air conditioners are online. The system performance is $g_2 = g_8 = 2$. State 1 indicates full system failure. The system performance is $g_1 = g_7 = 0$. If in the peak-demand period the required

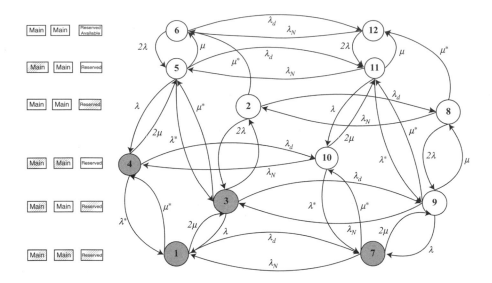

Figure 12.1. System with two online conditioners and one conditioner in cold reserve.

demand level is $w = 2$ and in the low-demand period the required demand level is $w = 1$, then there are eight acceptable states: 12, 11, 10, 9, 8, 6, 5, and 2. States 7, 4, 3, and 1 are unacceptable. The transitions from state 6 to state 5, from state 2 to state 3, from state 12 to state 11, and from state 9 to state 8 are associated with the failure of one of the main air conditioners and have an intensity of 2λ. The transitions from state 5 to state 4, from state 3 to state 1, from state 11 to state 10, and from state 9 to state 7 are associated with failure of the second main air conditioner and have an intensity of λ.

The transitions from state 5 to state 3, from state 4 to state 1, from state 11 to state 9, and from state 10 to state 7 are associated with failure of the reserve air conditioner and have an intensity of λ^*. The transitions from state 4 to state 5 and from state 1 to state 3, from state 10 to state 11 and from state 7 to state 9 are associated with repair of one of the main air conditioners and have an intensity of 2μ. The transitions from state 5 to state 6 and from state 3 to state 2, from state 11 to state 12 and from state 9 to state 8 are associated with failure of the main air conditioner and have an intensity of μ. The transitions from state 3 to state 5, from state 2 to state 6 and from state 1 to state 4 and from state 9 to state 11, from state 8 to state 12 and from state 7 to state 10 are associated with repair of the reserve air conditioner and have an intensity of μ^*.

The transitions from state 6 to state 12, from state 5 to state 11, from state 4 to state 10, from state 3 to state 9, from state 2 to state 8, and from state 1 to state 7 are associated with a variable demand and have an intensity of

$\lambda_d = 1/\overline{T}_d$. The transitions from state 12 to state 6, from state 11 to state 5, from state 10 to state 4, from state 9 to state 3, from state 8 to state 2, and from state 7 to state 1 are associated with a variable demand and have an intensity of $\lambda_N = 1/\overline{T}_N = 1/(24 - \overline{T}_d)$.

In order to find the MSS average availability $\overline{A}(T)$ we should present the reward matrix r_A in the following form.

$$r_A = |r_{ij}| = \begin{vmatrix} 0 & 0 & 0 & 0 & 0 & 0 & 0 & 0 & 0 & 0 & 0 & 0 \\ 0 & 1 & 0 & 0 & 0 & 0 & 0 & 0 & 0 & 0 & 0 & 0 \\ 0 & 0 & 0 & 0 & 0 & 0 & 0 & 0 & 0 & 0 & 0 & 0 \\ 0 & 0 & 0 & 0 & 0 & 0 & 0 & 0 & 0 & 0 & 0 & 0 \\ 0 & 0 & 0 & 0 & 1 & 0 & 0 & 0 & 0 & 0 & 0 & 0 \\ 0 & 0 & 0 & 0 & 0 & 1 & 0 & 0 & 0 & 0 & 0 & 0 \\ 0 & 0 & 0 & 0 & 0 & 0 & 0 & 0 & 0 & 0 & 0 & 0 \\ 0 & 0 & 0 & 0 & 0 & 0 & 0 & 1 & 0 & 0 & 0 & 0 \\ 0 & 0 & 0 & 0 & 0 & 0 & 0 & 0 & 1 & 0 & 0 & 0 \\ 0 & 0 & 0 & 0 & 0 & 0 & 0 & 0 & 0 & 1 & 0 & 0 \\ 0 & 0 & 0 & 0 & 0 & 0 & 0 & 0 & 0 & 0 & 1 & 0 \\ 0 & 0 & 0 & 0 & 0 & 0 & 0 & 0 & 0 & 0 & 0 & 1 \end{vmatrix}. \tag{12.4}$$

In this matrix, rewards associated with all acceptable states are defined as one and rewards associated with all unacceptable states are zeroed as well as all rewards associated with all transitions.

The system of differential equations (12.5) can be written in order to find the expected total rewards $V_i(t)$, $i = 1, \ldots, 12$. The initial conditions are $V_i(0) = 0$, $i = 1, \ldots, 12$.

After solving this system and finding $V_i(t)$, MSS average availability can be obtained as follows. $A(t) = V_6(t)/t$, where the sixth state is the initial state.

$$\begin{cases} \frac{dV_1(t)}{dt} = -C_1 V_1(t) + 2\mu V_3(t) + \mu^* V_4(t) + \lambda_d V_7(t) \\ \frac{dV_2(t)}{dt} = 1 - C_2 V_2(t) + 2\lambda V_3(t) + \mu^* V_6(t) + \lambda_d V_8(t) \\ \frac{dV_3(t)}{dt} = \lambda V_1(t) + \mu V_2(t) - C_3 V_3(t) + \mu^* V_5(t) + \lambda_d V_9(t) \\ \frac{dV_4(t)}{dt} = \lambda^* V_1(t) - C_4 V_4(t) + 2\mu V_5(t) + \lambda_d V_{10}(t) \\ \frac{dV_5(t)}{dt} = 1 + \lambda^* V_3(t) + \lambda V_4(t) - C_5 V_5(t) + \mu V_6(t) + \lambda_d V_{11}(t) \\ \frac{dV_6(t)}{dt} = 1 + 2\lambda V_5(t) - C_6 V_6(t) + \lambda_d V_{12}(t) \\ \frac{dV_7(t)}{dt} = \lambda_N V_1(t) - C_7 V_7(t) + 2\mu V_9(t) + \mu^* V_{10}(t) \\ \frac{dV_8(t)}{dt} = 1 + \lambda_N V_2(t) - C_8 V_8(t) + 2\lambda V_9(t) + \mu^* V_{10}(t) \\ \frac{dV_9(t)}{dt} = 1 + \lambda_N V_3(t) + \lambda V_7(t) + \mu V_8(t) - C_9 V_9(t) + \mu^* V_{11}(t) \\ \frac{dV_{10}(t)}{dt} = 1 + \lambda_N V_4(t) + \lambda^* V_7(t) - C_{10} V_{10}(t) + 2\mu V_{11}(t) \\ \frac{dV_{11}(t)}{dt} = 1 + \lambda_N V_5(t) + \lambda^* V_9(t) + \lambda V_{10}(t) - C_{11} V_{11}(t) + \mu V_{12}(t) \\ \frac{dV_{12}(t)}{dt} = 1 + \lambda_N V_6(t) + 2\lambda V_{11}(t) - C_{12} V_{12}(t), \end{cases} \tag{12.5}$$

where

$$
\begin{aligned}
C_1 &= 2\mu + \mu^* + \lambda_d & C_7 &= 2\mu + \mu^* + \lambda_N \\
C_2 &= 2\lambda + \mu^* + \lambda_d & C_8 &= 2\lambda + \mu^* + \lambda_N \\
C_3 &= \lambda + \mu + \mu^* + \lambda_d & C_9 &= \lambda + \mu + \mu^* + \lambda_N \\
C_4 &= \lambda^* + 2\mu + \lambda_d & C_{10} &= \lambda^* + 2\mu + \lambda_N \\
C_5 &= \lambda + \lambda^* + \mu + \lambda_d & C_{11} &= \lambda + \lambda^* + \mu + \lambda_N \\
C_5 &= 2\lambda + \lambda_d & C_5 &= 2\lambda + \lambda_N.
\end{aligned}
\tag{12.6}
$$

The results of the calculations are presented in Figures 12.2 and 12.3.

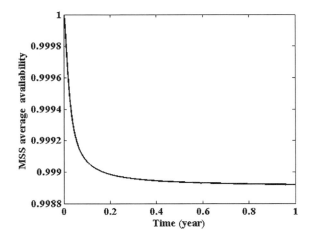

Figure 12.2. Calculation of the MSS average availability $\left(\mu = 100 \text{ year}^{-1}\right)$.

The curve in Figure 12.3 supports the engineering decision making and determines the area where required reliability/availability level of the air-conditioner system can be provided. For example, from this figure we can conclude that the system can provide the required average availability level (0.999), if mean time to repair is less than 3.6 days $(\mu > 120 \text{ year}^{-1})$

In order to find the *mean total number of system failures* $N_f(t)$ we should present the reward matrix r_N in the form (12.7). In this matrix the rewards associated with each transition from the set of acceptable states to the set

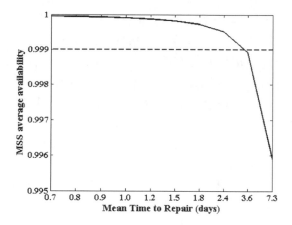

Figure 12.3. MSS average availability dependent on mean time to repair.

of unacceptable states should be defined as one. All other rewards should be zeroed.

$$r_A = |r_{ij}| = \begin{vmatrix} 0 & 0 & 0 & 0 & 0 & 0 & 0 & 0 & 0 & 0 & 0 & 0 \\ 0 & 0 & 1 & 0 & 0 & 0 & 0 & 0 & 0 & 0 & 0 & 0 \\ 0 & 0 & 0 & 0 & 0 & 0 & 0 & 0 & 0 & 0 & 0 & 0 \\ 0 & 0 & 0 & 0 & 0 & 0 & 0 & 0 & 0 & 0 & 0 & 0 \\ 0 & 0 & 1 & 1 & 0 & 0 & 0 & 0 & 0 & 0 & 0 & 0 \\ 0 & 0 & 0 & 0 & 0 & 0 & 0 & 0 & 0 & 0 & 0 & 0 \\ 0 & 0 & 0 & 0 & 0 & 0 & 0 & 0 & 0 & 0 & 0 & 0 \\ 0 & 0 & 0 & 0 & 0 & 0 & 0 & 0 & 0 & 0 & 0 & 0 \\ 0 & 0 & 1 & 0 & 0 & 0 & 1 & 0 & 0 & 0 & 0 & 0 \\ 0 & 0 & 0 & 1 & 0 & 0 & 1 & 0 & 0 & 0 & 0 & 0 \\ 0 & 0 & 0 & 0 & 0 & 0 & 0 & 0 & 0 & 0 & 0 & 0 \\ 0 & 0 & 0 & 0 & 0 & 0 & 0 & 0 & 0 & 0 & 0 & 0 \end{vmatrix}. \qquad (12.7)$$

The following system of differential equations (12.8) can be written in order to find the expected total rewards $V_i(t)$, $i = 1, \ldots, 12$.

$$\begin{cases} \frac{dV_1(t)}{dt} = -C_1V_1(t) + 2\mu V_3(t) + \mu^* V_4(t) + \lambda_d V_7(t) \\ \frac{dV_2(t)}{dt} = 2\lambda - C_2V_2(t) + 2\lambda V_3(t) + \mu^* V_6(t) + \lambda_d V_8(t) \\ \frac{dV_3(t)}{dt} = \lambda V_1(t) + \mu V_2(t) - C_3V_3(t) + \mu^* V_5(t) + \lambda_d V_9(t) \\ \frac{dV_4(t)}{dt} = \lambda^* V_1(t) - C_4V_4(t) + 2\mu V_5(t) + \lambda_d V_{10}(t) \\ \frac{dV_5(t)}{dt} = \lambda + \lambda^* + \lambda^* V_3(t) + \lambda V_4(t) - C_5V_5(t) + \mu V_6(t) + \lambda_d V_{11}(t) \\ \frac{dV_6(t)}{dt} = 2\lambda V_5(t) - C_6V_6(t) + \lambda_d V_{12}(t) \\ \frac{dV_7(t)}{dt} = \lambda_N V_1(t) - C_7V_7(t) + 2\mu V_9(t) + \mu^* V_{10}(t) \\ \frac{dV_8(t)}{dt} = \lambda_N V_2(t) - C_8V_8(t) + 2\lambda V_9(t) + \mu^* V_{10}(t) \\ \frac{dV_9(t)}{dt} = \lambda_N + \lambda + \lambda_N V_3(t) + \lambda V_7(t) + \mu V_8(t) - C_9V_9(t) + \mu^* V_{11}(t) \\ \frac{dV_{10}(t)}{dt} = \lambda_N + \lambda^* + \lambda_N V_4(t) + \lambda^* V_7(t) - C_{10}V_{10}(t) + 2\mu V_{11}(t) \\ \frac{dV_{11}(t)}{dt} = \lambda_N V_5(t) + \lambda^* V_9(t) + \lambda V_{10}(t) - C_{11}V_{11}(t) + \mu V_{12}(t) \\ \frac{dV_{12}(t)}{dt} = \lambda_N V_6(t) + 2\lambda V_{11}(t) - C_{12}V_{12}(t). \end{cases}$$

$$(12.8)$$

Here C_1–C_{12} are calculated via formulas (12.6).

The initial conditions are $V_i(0) = 0$, $i = 1, \ldots, 12$ After solving this system and finding $V_i(t)$, the mean total number of system failures $N_f(t)$ can be obtained as follows: $N_f(t) = V_6(t)$, where the sixth state is the initial state.

The results of the calculations are presented in Figures 12.4 and 12.5.

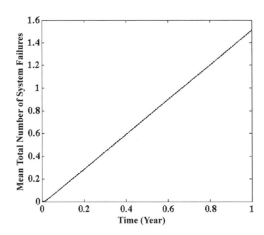

Figure 12.4. Calculation of the mean total number of system failures $\left(\mu = 100 \text{ year}^{-1}\right)$.

In order to calculate mean time to failure (MTTF), the initial model should be transformed; all transitions that return MSS from unacceptable states should be forbidden and all unacceptable states should be treated as absorbing states. The transformed model is shown on Figure 12.6.

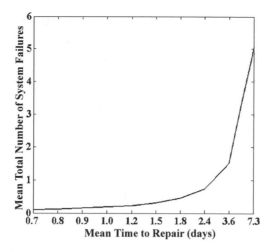

Figure 12.5. Mean total number of system failures dependent on mean time to repair.

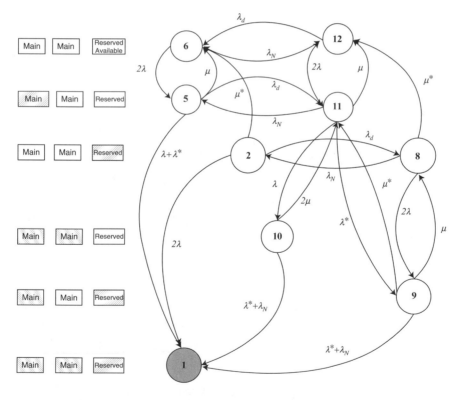

Figure 12.6. The state–space diagram for the transformed system with two online air conditioners and one in cold reserve with absorbing state.

In order to assess MTTF for MSS, the rewards in matrix r for the transformed model should be determined in the following manner. The rewards associated with all acceptable states should be defined as one and the rewards associated with unacceptable (absorbing) states should be zeroed as well as all rewards associated with transitions.

The reward matrix for the system with two online conditioners and one in cold reserve is as follows.

$$
r = |r_{ij}| = \begin{vmatrix} 0 & 0 & 0 & 0 & 0 & 0 & 0 & 0 & 0 \\ 0 & 1 & 0 & 0 & 0 & 0 & 0 & 0 & 0 \\ 0 & 0 & 1 & 0 & 0 & 0 & 0 & 0 & 0 \\ 0 & 0 & 0 & 1 & 0 & 0 & 0 & 0 & 0 \\ 0 & 0 & 0 & 0 & 1 & 0 & 0 & 0 & 0 \\ 0 & 0 & 0 & 0 & 0 & 1 & 0 & 0 & 0 \\ 0 & 0 & 0 & 0 & 0 & 0 & 1 & 0 & 0 \\ 0 & 0 & 0 & 0 & 0 & 0 & 0 & 1 & 0 \\ 0 & 0 & 0 & 0 & 0 & 0 & 0 & 0 & 1 \end{vmatrix}. \tag{12.9}
$$

The following system of differential equations can be written in order to find the expected total rewards $V_i(t)$, $i = 0, 2, 5, 6, 8, 9, 10, 11, 12$.

$$
\begin{cases}
\frac{dV_0(t)}{dt} = 0 \\
\frac{dV_2(t)}{dt} = 1 + 2\lambda V_0(t) - C_2 V_2(t) + \mu^* V_6(t) + \lambda_d V_8(t) \\
\frac{dV_5(t)}{dt} = 1 + (\lambda + \lambda^*) V_0(t) - C_5 V_5(t) + \mu V_6(t) + \lambda_d V_{11}(t) \\
\frac{dV_6(t)}{dt} = 1 + 2\lambda V_5(t) - C_6 V_6(t) + \lambda_d V_{12}(t) \\
\frac{dV_8(t)}{dt} = 1 + \lambda_N V_2(t) - C_8 V_8(t) + 2\lambda V_9(t) + \mu^* V_{10}(t) \\
\frac{dV_9(t)}{dt} = 1 + (\lambda + \lambda_N) V_0(t) + \mu V_8(t) - C_9 V_9(t) + \mu^* V_{11}(t) \\
\frac{dV_{10}(t)}{dt} = 1 + (\lambda^* + \lambda_N) V_0(t) - C_{10} V_{10}(t) + 2\mu V_{11}(t) \\
\frac{dV_{11}(t)}{dt} = 1 + \lambda_N V_5(t) + \lambda^* V_9(t) + \lambda V_{10}(t) - C_{11} V_{11}(t) + \mu V_{12}(t) \\
\frac{dV_{12}(t)}{dt} = 1 + \lambda_N V_6(t) + 2\lambda V_{11}(t) - C_{12} V_{12}(t),
\end{cases} \tag{12.10}
$$

where

$$
\begin{aligned}
C_2 &= 2\lambda + \mu^* + \lambda_d & C_9 &= \lambda + \mu + \mu^* + \lambda_N \\
C_5 &= \lambda + \lambda^* + \mu + \lambda_d & C_{10} &= \lambda^* + 2\mu + \lambda_N \\
C_6 &= 2\lambda + \lambda_d & C_{11} &= \lambda + \lambda^* + \mu + \lambda_N \\
C_8 &= 2\lambda + \mu^* + \lambda_N & C_{12} &= 2\lambda + \lambda_N.
\end{aligned} \tag{12.11}
$$

The initial conditions are $V_i(0) = 0$, $i = 0, 2, 5, 6, 8, 9, 10, 11, 12$.

After solving this system and finding $V_i(t)$, the MTTF for MSS can be obtained as $V_6(t)$, where the sixth state is the initial state. The results of the calculations are presented in Figures 12.7 and 12.8.

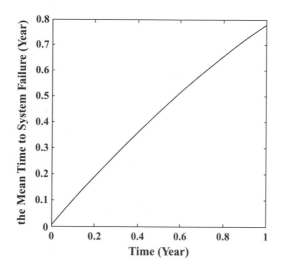

Figure 12.7. Calculation of the mean time to system failure $\left(\mu = 100 \text{ year}^{-1}\right)$.

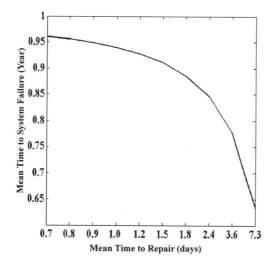

Figure 12.8. Mean time to system failure dependent on mean time to repair.

To calculate the probability of MSS failure during time interval $[0, t]$ the model should be transformed as in the previous case: all unacceptable states should be treated as absorbing states and, therefore, all transitions that return MSS from unacceptable states should be forbidden. Rewards associated with all transitions to the absorbing state should be defined as one. All other rewards should be zeroed.

The reward matrix for the system with two online conditioners and one in cold reserve will be as follows.

$$r = |r_{ij}| = \begin{vmatrix} 0 & 0 & 0 & 0 & 0 & 0 & 0 & 0 & 0 \\ 1 & 0 & 0 & 0 & 0 & 0 & 0 & 0 & 0 \\ 1 & 0 & 0 & 0 & 0 & 0 & 0 & 0 & 0 \\ 0 & 0 & 0 & 0 & 0 & 0 & 0 & 0 & 0 \\ 0 & 0 & 0 & 0 & 0 & 0 & 0 & 0 & 0 \\ 1 & 0 & 0 & 0 & 0 & 0 & 0 & 0 & 0 \\ 1 & 0 & 0 & 0 & 0 & 0 & 0 & 0 & 0 \\ 0 & 0 & 0 & 0 & 0 & 0 & 0 & 0 & 0 \\ 0 & 0 & 0 & 0 & 0 & 0 & 0 & 0 & 0 \end{vmatrix}. \tag{12.12}$$

Mean accumulated reward $V_i(t)$ will define the probability $Q(t)$ of MSS failure during time interval $[0, t]$.

The following system of differential equations can be written in order to find the expected total rewards $V_i(t)$, $i = 0, 2, 5, 6, 8, 9, 10, 11, 12$.

$$\begin{cases} \frac{dV_0(t)}{dt} = 0 \\ \frac{dV_2(t)}{dt} = 2\lambda + 2\lambda V_0(t) - C_2 V_2(t) + \mu^* V_6(t) + \lambda_d V_8(t) \\ \frac{dV_5(t)}{dt} = \lambda + \lambda^* + (\lambda + \lambda^*) V_0(t) - C_5 V_5(t) + \mu V_6(t) + \lambda_d V_{11}(t) \\ \frac{dV_6(t)}{dt} = 2\lambda V_5(t) - C_6 V_6(t) + \lambda_d V_{12}(t) \\ \frac{dV_8(t)}{dt} = \lambda_N V_2(t) - C_8 V_8(t) + 2\lambda V_9(t) + \mu^* V_{10}(t) \\ \frac{dV_9(t)}{dt} = \lambda + \lambda_N + (\lambda + \lambda_N) V_0(t) + \mu V_8(t) - C_9 V_9(t) + \mu^* V_{11}(t) \\ \frac{dV_{10}(t)}{dt} = \lambda^* + \lambda_N + (\lambda^* + \lambda_N) V_0(t) - C_{10} V_{10}(t) + 2\mu V_{11}(t) \\ \frac{dV_{11}(t)}{dt} = \lambda_N V_5(t) + \lambda^* V_9(t) + \lambda V_{10}(t) - C_{11} V_{11}(t) + \mu V_{12}(t) \\ \frac{dV_{12}(t)}{dt} = \lambda_N V_6(t) + 2\lambda V_{11}(t) - C_{12} V_{12}(t). \end{cases} \tag{12.13}$$

Here C_i, $i = 2, 5, 6, 8, 9, 10, 11, 12$ are calculated via formulas (12.11). The initial conditions are $V_i(0) = 0$, $i = 0, 2, 5, 6, 8, 9, 10, 11, 12$.

After solving this system and finding $V_i(t)$, MSS reliability function can be obtained as $R(t) = 1 - V_6(t)$, where the sixth state is the initial state. The results of the calculation are presented in Figure 12.9.

12.4   Conclusions

1. A generalized reliability measure for MSS that is an expectation of the functional from two stochastic processes—MSS output performance $G(t)$ and demand $W(t)$—was suggested in this chapter. Many MSS reliability measures usually used in practice can be easily derived from this generalized measure.

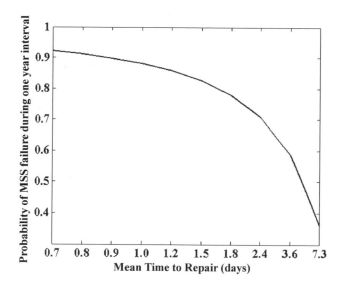

Figure 12.9. Probability of MSS failure during one-year time interval depends on mean time to repair.

2. The general method was suggested to compute main MSS reliability measures. The method is based on determination of different reward matrices for the MSS model. Such a model is interpreted as a Markov reward model.

3. The approach suggested is well formalized and suitable for practical applications in reliability engineering.

4. The numerical example is presented in order to illustrate the suggested approach.

References

1. Carrasco, J. (2003). Markovian dependability/performability modeling of fault-tolerant systems, In *Handbook of Reliability Engineering*, (Ed., H. Pham), Springer-Verlag, New York.

2. Hiller, F. and Lieberman, G. (1995). *Introduction to Operation Research*, McGraw-Hill, New York.

3. Howard, R. (1960). *Dynamic Programming and Markov Processes*, MIT Press, Cambridge, MA.

4. Lisnianski, A. and Levitin, G. (2003). *Multi-state System Reliability. Assessment, Optimization and Applications*, World-Scientific, Singapore.

5. Lisnianski, A., Frenkel, I., and Khvatskin, L. (2006). Markov reward models for reliability assessment of air conditioning systems, In *Safety and Reliability for Managing Risk* (Eds. G. Soares and E. Zio), pp. 2337–2341, Taylor Francis, London.

6. Modarres, M., Kaminskiy, M., and Krivtsov, V. (1999). *Reliability Engineering and Risk Analysis. A Practical Guide*, Marcel Dekker, New York.

7. Sahner, R., Trivedi, K., and Poliafito, A. (1996). *Performance and Reliability Analysis of Computer Systems. An Example-based Approach Using the SHARPE Software Package*, Kluwer Academic, Boston.

8. Volik, B. G., Buyanov, B. B., Lubkov, N. V., Maximov, V. I., and Stepanyants A. S. (1988). *Methods of Analysis and Synthesis of Control Systems Structures*, Moscow, Energoatomizdat (in Russian).

PART III
Inferential Analysis

13

Asymptotic Certainty Bands for Kernel Density Estimators Based upon a Bootstrap Resampling Scheme

Paul Deheuvels[1] **and Gérard Derzko**[2]

[1]*LSTA, Université Paris VI, Bourg-la-Reine, France*
[2]*Sanofi-Aventis Recherche, Montpellier, France*

Abstract: In this chapter, we show that a single bootstrap suffices to construct sharp uniform asymptotic certainty (or asymptotically almost sure confidence) bands for nonparametric kernel-type density estimators.

Keywords and Phrases: Kernel density estimators, nonparametric functional estimation, bootstrap and resampling, confidence bands

13.1 Introduction and Results

Let $X_1, X_2, \ldots$ be a sequence of independent random replicæ of a random variable X with distribution function $F(x) = \mathbb{P}(X \leq x)$ for $x \in \mathbb{R}$. We are concerned with the estimation of the density $f(x) = (d/dx)F(x)$ of X, assumed to be continuous and positive on the interval $J = [c', d']$, where c' and d' are two constants such that $-\infty < c' < d' < \infty$. We consider here the classical Akaike–Parzen–Rosenblatt [refer to Akaike (1954), Rosenblatt (1956), and Parzen (1962)] kernel estimator defined as follows. We first pick a kernel $K(\cdot)$, defined as a function of bounded variation on $\mathbb{R}$ such that

$$(i) \quad K(t) = 0 \quad \text{for} \quad |t| \geq \tfrac{1}{2} \quad \text{and} \quad (ii) \quad \int_{\mathbb{R}} K(t)dt = 1. \qquad (13.1)$$

We then select a bandswidth $h > 0$, and estimate $f(x)$ by the statistic

$$f_{n,h}(x) = \frac{1}{nh} \sum_{i=1}^{n} K\left(\frac{x - X_i}{h}\right).$$

In the forthcoming Section 13.2, we also consider a discretized version $\widehat{f}_{n,h}(\cdot)$ of $f_{n,h}(\cdot)$, which is defined, later on, in (13.23). We are concerned with the limiting behavior of $f_{n,h}(x)$, uniformly over $x \in I = [c,d] \subset J = [c',d']$, where c,d are specified constants such that $-\infty < c' < c < d < d' < \infty$. Setting $h_0 = \{c - c'\} \wedge \{d' - d\}$, we assume, unless otherwise specified, that $h = h_n$ is a sequence depending upon n, and taking values within the interval $(0, h_0]$. At times, we work under the variant, denoted by (H.b), of the above set of hypotheses, denoted hereafter by (H.a). Under (H.b), we let $K(\cdot)$ fulfill $(13.1)(ii)$ only, and make the additional assumption on the distribution $F(x)$ of X, that there exists a version of the density $f(x) = (d/dx)F(x)$, bounded on $\mathbb{R}$ [recall that $f(\cdot)$ is only defined uniquely up to an a.e. equivalence].

The study of the uniform consistency of $f_{n,h}(x)$ to $f(x)$ on I makes use of the decomposition of $f_{n,h}(x) - f(x)$ into two components. The first one captures the *bias part*

$$\mathbb{E}f_{n,h}(x) - f(x) = \int_{\mathbb{R}} \{f(x - hu) - f(x)\}K(u), \qquad (13.2)$$

which is independent of the sample size $n \geq 1$, and, under either (H.a) or (H.b), converging uniformly to 0 over $x \in I$, as $h \to 0$. The corresponding rate of convergence is a purely analytic problem, depending upon regularity assumptions on f, which are not considered here, except in the application, presented in the forthcoming Section 13.2 [refer to Deheuvels (2000), and Deheuvels and Mason (2004), for details and references on this question]. We concentrate our interest on the *random part*

$$f_{n,h}(x) - \mathbb{E}f_{n,h}(x),$$

and investigate its limiting behavior over $x \in I$. We seek *sharp uniform asymptotic certainty bands*, defined as statistics $\theta_n = \theta_n(X_1, \ldots, X_n) \geq 0$, assumed to be nonnegative measurable functions of $n \geq 1$, and of the sample $X_1, \ldots, X_n$, such that, for each $\varepsilon \in (0,1)$, as $n \to \infty$,

$$P\left(\sup_{x \in I} |f_{n,h}(x) - \mathbb{E}f_{n,h}(x)| \leq \theta_n(1 + \varepsilon) + \varepsilon \right) \to 1, \qquad (13.3)$$

and

$$P\left(\sup_{x \in I} |f_{n,h}(x) - \mathbb{E}f_{n,h}(x)| \leq \theta_n(1 - \varepsilon) - \varepsilon \right) \to 0. \qquad (13.4)$$

Following a suggestion of D. M. Mason, we use, for these upper and lower functional bounds for $\mathbb{E}f_{n,h}(x)$, the qualification of *certainty bands*, rather than that of *confidence bands*, because there is here no preassigned confidence level $\alpha \in (0,1)$. Some authors [see, e.g., Härdle and Marron (1991)] have used the alternate concept of *simultaneous error bars*, which is not quite equivalent to the present definitions. Our approach differs, in particular, from that initiated by

Bickel and Rosenblatt (1973), and giving rise to some recent refinements in Giné *et al.* (2004) (see also the list of references of this last article). These authors evaluate limiting distributions for weighted sup-norms of $|f_{n,h}(x) - \mathbb{E}f_{n,h}(x)|$. As mentioned in their paper, the convergence of such statistics to their limit laws is so slow as to render their use difficult for small sample sizes. The methodology we follow here should appear, therefore, less refined, but more applicable to the usual statistical datasets. The practical interest of our asymptotic certainty bands appears through the plots of the functions $(f_{n,h}(x) - \theta_n) \vee 0$ and $(f_{n,h}(x) + \theta_n) \vee 0$ on the interval $I = [c, d]$. Some examples of the kind are provided in Figures 13.1 to 13.3, in the forthcoming Section 13.2. Assuming that the order of uniform convergence to 0 of the bias part (13.2) is negligible, with respect to the order of uniform convergence to 0 of θ_n, the asymptotic certainty bands turn out to give a useful visual insight on the behavior of the exact density $f(\cdot)$ on I. This density $f(x)$ should then, with probability tending to 1, be in between or close to (in the sense of (13.3)–(13.4)) the *lower certainty bound* $(f_{n,h}(x) - \theta_n) \vee 0$, and the *upper certainty bound* $(f_{n,h}(x) + \theta_n) \vee 0$. We refer to Deheuvels and Mason (2004) for additional details and references on this methodology. Note here that our assumptions allow $K(u)$ to be negative for some values of $u \in \mathbb{R}$, so that $f_{n,h}(x)$, or $f_{n,h}(x) \pm \theta_n$, may be negative for some values of $n \geq 1$ and $x \in \mathbb{R}$. This explains why we use $(f_{n,h}(x) \pm \theta_n) \vee 0$ instead of $f_{n,h}(x) \pm \theta_n$.

Set $\log_+ u = \log(u \vee e)$ for $u \in \mathbb{R}$. The limit law, stated in Fact 13.1.1 below, is due to Deheuvels and Einmahl (2000) and Deheuvels (2000) [see also Stute

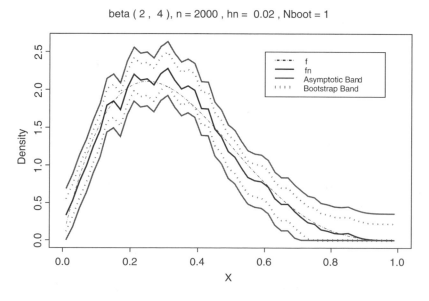

Figure 13.1. Certainty bands $\beta(2, 4)$, $n = 2000$, 1 bootstrap.

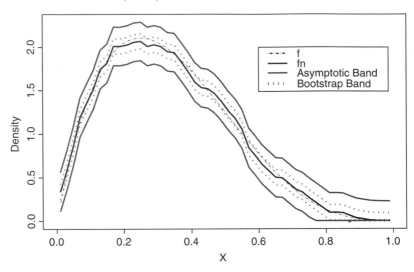

Figure 13.2. Certainty bands $\beta(2,4)$, $n = 5000$, 1 bootstrap.

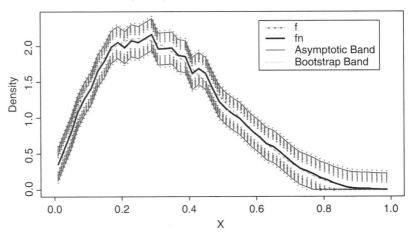

Figure 13.3. Repeated bootstrap bands $\beta(2,4)$, $n = 5000$.

(1982), Deheuvels (1992), and Deheuvels and Mason (1992), and the references therein]. It shows that a possible choice for θ_n in (13.3)–(13.4) is given by

$$\theta_n = \theta_{n,0} := \Big\{ \frac{2\log_+(1/h_n)}{nh_n} \Big(\sup_{x \in I} f(x)\Big) \int_{\mathbb{R}} K^2(t)dt \Big\}^{1/2}. \qquad (13.5)$$

Fact 13.1.1 *Let* $\{h_n : n \geq 1\}$ *be a sequence such that, as* $n \to \infty$,

(H.c) $h_n \to 0$ *and* $nh_n/\log n \to \infty$.

Then, under either (H.a) or (H.b), as $n \to \infty$,

$$\sup_{x \in I} \pm \left\{ f_{n,h_n}(x) - \mathbb{E}f_{n,h_n}(x) \right\} \tag{13.6}$$

$$= (1 + o_{\mathbb{P}}(1)) \left\{ \frac{2\log_+(1/h_n)}{nh_n} \left(\sup_{x \in I} f(x) \right) \int_{\mathbb{R}} K^2(t)dt \right\}^{1/2}.$$

The choice of $\theta_n = \theta_{n,0}$, given by (13.5), is not very useful to construct limiting asymptotic certainty bands for $\sup_{x \in I} \pm \{f_{n,h_n}(x) - \mathbb{E}f_{n,h_n}(x)\}$ of practical interest. The fact that $\theta_{n,0}$ depends upon the unknown density $f(\cdot)$ is a minor problem, because, as shown in Deheuvels (2000), and Deheuvels and Mason (2004), an application of Slutsky's lemma allows us to replace, without loss of generality, this quantity by $f_{n,h_n}(x)$ (or by any other estimator of $f(x)$ which is uniformly consistent on I), thus yielding

$$\theta_n = \theta_{n,1} := \left\{ \frac{2\log_+(1/h_n)}{nh_n} \left(\left\{ \sup_{x \in I} f_{n,h_n}(x) \right\} \vee 0 \right) \int_{\mathbb{R}} K^2(t)dt \right\}^{1/2}. \tag{13.7}$$

The difficulty, in the practical use of setting either $\theta_n = \theta_{n,0}$ or $\theta_n = \theta_{n,1}$ in (13.3)–(13.4), is due to the factor $\log_+(1/h_n)$, in (13.5) and (13.7), which is *scale-dependent*. Consider the change of scale replacing, respectively, h_n by λh_n, and $\{X_i : 1 \le i \le n\}$, by $\{\lambda X_i + \mu : 1 \le i \le n\}$, for some constants $\lambda > 0$ and μ. This transformation leaves unchanged f_{n,h_n}, whereas $\theta_{n,0}$ and $\theta_{n,1}$ are each multiplied by the factor $\{(\log_+(1/(\lambda h_n)))/(\log_+(1/h_n))\}^{1/2}$. Thus, the logarithmic terms in $\theta_{n,0}$ and $\theta_{n,1}$, which should be tending to infinity, are truncated, and hence, unrealistic, when the above factor λ is chosen such that $\lambda h_n > 1$.

The main purpose of the present chapter is to propose a simple and practical way, based upon a *resampling (or bootstrap) methodology*, to override the above-mentioned difficulty. There is a huge literature on the application of the bootstrap methodology to nonparametric kernel density and regression estimation. We refer, in particular to Härdle and Bowman (1988), Hall (1992), Härdle and Marron (1991), Li and Datta (2001), and the references therein. Our method is based on the introduction of random weights $\{W_{i,n} : 1 \le i \le n\}$ defined, via one of the following alternate resampling schemes, denoted hereafter by (RS.1) and (RS.2).

Resampling Scheme 1 [(RS.1)] This is a version of the Mason–Newton bootstrap [see, e.g., Mason and Newton (1992), and the references therein]. We start by the introduction [on the original probability space $(\Omega, \mathcal{A}, \mathbb{P})$ carrying the dataset $X_1, \ldots, X_n$, and, eventually, enlarged by products] of a sequence $\{Z_n : n \ge 1\}$ of independent and identically distributed random replicæ of a random variable Z. We assume that $\{X_n : n \ge 1\}$ and $\{Z_n : n \ge 1\}$ are independent, and let the following additional conditions be satisfied.

(A.1) $\mathbb{E}(Z) = 1; \quad \mathbb{E}(Z^2) = 2$ [or, equivalently, $\text{Var}(Z) = 1$].

(A.2)   For some $\epsilon > 0$, $\mathbb{E}(e^{tZ}) < \infty$ for all $|t| \le \epsilon$.

We denote by $T_n = Z_1 + \cdots + Z_n$ the partial sum of order $n \ge 1$ of these random variables, and denote by $\mathcal{E}_n = \{T_n > 0\}$ the event that $T_n > 0$. We note for further use that $\mathbb{P}(\mathcal{E}_n) \to 1$ as $n \to \infty$ [the LLN in combination with (A.1) implies that $n^{-1}T_n \to 1$ a.s.]. We define, further, the random weights, for $i = 1, \ldots, n$,

$$
W_{i,n} = \begin{cases} \dfrac{Z_i}{T_n} = \dfrac{Z_i}{\sum_{j=1}^n Z_j} & \text{when} \quad T_n > 0, \\ \dfrac{1}{n} & \text{when} \quad T_n \le 0. \end{cases} \tag{13.8}
$$

Resampling Scheme 2 [(RS.2)] This corresponds to the classical Efron (or multinomial) bootstrap [see, e.g., Efron (1979)]. We let $(Y_1, \ldots, Y_n)$ follow a multinomial $\text{Mult}(1/n, \ldots, 1/n; n)$ distribution. Namely, for each n-tuple of integers $k_1 \ge 0, \ldots, k_n \ge 0$, with $k_1 + \cdots + k_n = n$, we let

$$
\mathbb{P}(Y_1 = k_1, \ldots, Y_n = k_n) = \frac{n^{-n} n!}{k_1! \ldots k_n!}. \tag{13.9}
$$

We then define the random weights $\{W_{i,n} : 1 \le i \le n\}$, via

$$
W_{i,n} = \frac{Y_i}{n} = \frac{Y_i}{\sum_{j=1}^n Y_j} \quad \text{for} \quad i = 1, \ldots, n. \tag{13.10}
$$

Under either (RS.1) or (RS.2), we define a *resampled*, or *bootstrapped*, version of $f_{n,h}(\cdot)$ by setting, for each $h > 0$ and $x \in \mathbb{R}$,

$$
f_{n,h}^*(x) = \frac{1}{h} \sum_{i=1}^n W_{i,n} K\left(\frac{x - X_i}{h}\right). \tag{13.11}
$$

The following main result of the present chapter turns out to provide a solution to our problem of constructing *scale-free* sharp uniform asymptotic certainty bands for $f(\cdot)$.

Theorem 13.1.1 *Let either (H.a) or (H.b) hold. Then, under (H.c) and (A.1–A.2), we have, as $n \to \infty$,*

$$
\sup_{x \in I} \pm \left\{ f_{n,h_n}^*(x) - f_{n,h_n}(x) \right\} \tag{13.12}
$$

$$
= (1 + o_\mathbb{P}(1)) \left\{ \frac{2 \log_+(1/h_n)}{n h_n} \left(\sup_{x \in I} f(x) \right) \int_\mathbb{R} K^2(t) dt \right\}^{1/2}.
$$

A straightforward consequence of Theorem 13.1.1 and Fact 13.1.1 is stated in Corollary 13.1.1 below.

Corollary 13.1.1 *Let either (H.a) or (H.b) hold. Then, under (H.c) and (A.1–A.2), for any choice of $\epsilon_1 = \pm 1$ or $\epsilon_2 = \pm 1$, we have, as $n \to \infty$,*

$$\frac{\sup_{x \in I} \epsilon_1 \left\{ f_{n,h_n}(x) - \mathbb{E} f_{n,h_n}(x) \right\}}{\sup_{x \in I} \epsilon_2 \left\{ f^*_{n,h_n}(x) - f_{n,h_n}(x) \right\}} = 1 + o_{\mathbb{P}}(1). \tag{13.13}$$

PROOF. Observe that the factors on the RHS of (13.6) and (13.12) are identical. ∎

As follows from (13.13), we may choose θ_n in (13.3)–(13.4), by setting either

$$\theta_n = \theta_{n,2} := \sup_{x \in I} \pm \left\{ f^*_{n,h_n}(x) - f_{n,h_n}(x) \right\}, \tag{13.14}$$

or, preferably,

$$\theta_n = \theta_{n,3} := \sup_{x \in I} \left| f^*_{n,h_n}(x) - f_{n,h_n}(x) \right|. \tag{13.15}$$

Corollary 13.1.1 implies that *a single bootstrap suffices* to obtain, via (13.14) or (13.15), *sharp asymptotic certainty bands* fulfilling (13.3)–(13.4). Moreover, the above-defined choices of $\theta_n = \theta_{n,2}$, or $\theta_n = \theta_{n,3}$, are, obviously, scale-free, and improve upon $\theta_{n,0}$ and $\theta_{n,1}$ with respect to this property.

The remainder of our chapter is organized as follows. In Section 13.2, we present an application of our results based upon simulated data. These results give some empirical evidence of the practical interest of our methods. The general ideas underlying our proofs are given in Section 13.3, the completion of which will be published elsewhere.

13.2 An Example of Application

In this section we provide plots of density estimators corresponding to the $\beta(2,4)$ distribution. We assume, therefore, and unless otherwise specified, that $f(x)$ is the $\beta(2,4)$ density, given by

$$f(x) = \begin{cases} \frac{1}{\beta(2,4)} x(1-x)^3 = 20\, x(1-x)^3 & \text{when} \quad 0 \le x \le 1, \\ 0 & \text{otherwise.} \end{cases} \tag{13.16}$$

Because the density $f(x)$ in (13.16) is polynomial on its support $[0,1]$, it has bounded derivatives of all orders, so that the Taylor expansions of f and its derivatives, which we use later on, will hold uniformly on this interval. This property is used implicitly in the sequel. For numerical purposes, we work on a discretized, binned version $\widetilde{f}_h(x)$ of $f(x)$, defined, for each choice of the bandwidth $h > 0$, and of the index $j \in \mathbb{Z}$, by

$$\widetilde{f}_h(x) = \frac{1}{h} \int_{(j-1)h}^{jh} f(t)dt \quad \text{for} \quad x \in ((j-1)h, jh]. \tag{13.17}$$

We work on the following intervals. We set throughout this section $I = [0.2, 0.8]$ and $J = [0.1, 0.9]$. Some calculus based upon (13.16) shows that, for $0 < x < 1$,

$$f'(x) = 20(1-x)^2(1-4x) \quad \text{and} \quad \sup_{x \in I} |f'(x)| = 5, \tag{13.18}$$

$$f''(x) = 120(1-x)(2x-1) \quad \text{and} \quad \sup_{x \in [0,1]} |f''(x)| = 120. \tag{13.19}$$

By Taylor's formula and (13.18), it is readily checked that, when $h \to 0$,

$$\sup_{x \in I} |f(x) - \widetilde{f}_h(x)| = (1 + o(1))\frac{h}{2} \sup_{x \in I} |f'(x)| = (1 + o(1))\frac{5h}{2}. \tag{13.20}$$

By combining Taylor's formula with (13.17)–(13.19), we get that, for each specified $\ell \in \mathbb{Z}$, uniformly over $j \in \mathbb{Z}$ with $jh \in I$, as $h \to 0$,

$$\widetilde{f}_h(jh - \ell h) - \widetilde{f}_h(jh) = \frac{1}{h} \int_0^h \left\{ f(jh - t - \ell h) - f(jh - t) \right\} dt$$
$$= -\ell f'(jh) + \ell^2 h^2 f''(jh) + O(h^3). \tag{13.21}$$

in the forthcoming Figures 13.1 to 13.3, the *kernel smoothed histogram* $\widehat{f}_{n,h}(x)$, defined below as a discretized version of the kernel estimator $f_{n,h}(x)$, is plotted. The *kernel smoothed histogram* [KSH] was introduced by Derzko (1998), and further investigated by Deheuvels *et al.* (2004). Given a choice of the bandwidth $h > 0$, we first estimate $\widetilde{f}_h(x)$, out of the sample $X_1, \ldots, X_n$, by a classical *histogram* $\widetilde{f}_{n,h}(x)$, defined by setting

$$\widetilde{f}_{n,h}(x) = (nh)^{-1} \sum_{i=1}^{n} \mathbb{1}_{\{X_i \in ((j-1)h, jh]\}}$$
$$\text{for} \quad x \in ((j-1)h, jh] \quad \text{and} \quad j \in \mathbb{N}. \tag{13.22}$$

Next, we smooth $\widetilde{f}_{n,h}(\cdot)$, to obtain the *kernel smoothed histogram* [KSH] [see, e.g., Derzko (1998), and Derzko and Deheuvels (2002)], defined by

$$\widehat{f}_{n,h}(x) = \sum_{\ell=-\infty}^{\infty} \mathcal{K}(\ell)\widetilde{f}_{n,h}(x - \ell h), \tag{13.23}$$

where $\mathcal{K}(t)$ is a *discrete kernel*, constant on the intervals $(\ell - \frac{1}{2}, \ell + \frac{1}{2}]$ for $\ell \in \mathbb{Z}$, and defined by setting, for each $\ell \in \mathbb{Z}$,

$$
\begin{aligned}
\mathcal{K}(t) \;=\; \mathcal{K}(\ell) &:= \frac{1}{2} \int_0^{1/2} \frac{x^{|\ell|} dx}{(1-x)^2} \\
&= \frac{1}{2^{|\ell|+2}} \sum_{k=0}^{\infty} \frac{k+1}{(|\ell|+k+1)2^k} \quad \text{for} \quad t \in (\ell - \tfrac{1}{2}, \ell + \tfrac{1}{2}].
\end{aligned}
\tag{13.24}
$$

It is noteworthy that $K(t) = \mathcal{K}(t)$, as defined by (13.24) for $t \in \mathbb{R}$, is a kernel in the usual sense, being of bounded variation on $\mathbb{R}$ and fulfilling (13.1)(ii). This follows from the identity

$$
\begin{aligned}
\int_{\mathbb{R}} \mathcal{K}(t) dt &= \sum_{\ell \in \mathbb{Z}} \mathcal{K}(\ell) \\
&= \frac{1}{2} \int_0^{1/2} \frac{dx}{(1-x)^2} + \sum_{\ell=1}^{\infty} \int_0^{1/2} \frac{x^{|\ell|} dx}{(1-x)^2} \\
&= 1 + \int_0^{1/2} \frac{dx}{(1-x)^3} - \int_0^{1/2} \frac{dx}{(1-x)^2} = 1.
\end{aligned}
\tag{13.25}
$$

Likewise, it is readily checked that the *discrete kernel* $\mathcal{K}(\cdot)$ fulfills

$$
\int_{\mathbb{R}} t\mathcal{K}(t) dt = \sum_{\ell \in \mathbb{Z}} \mathcal{K}(\ell) \int_{\ell - 1/2}^{\ell + 1/2} t \, dt = \sum_{\ell \in \mathbb{Z}} \ell \mathcal{K}(\ell) = 0,
\tag{13.26}
$$

and

$$
\int_{\mathbb{R}} t^2 \mathcal{K}(t) dt - \tfrac{1}{12} = \sum_{\ell \in \mathbb{Z}} \ell^2 \mathcal{K}(\ell) = 2.
\tag{13.27}
$$

We infer from (13.21), (13.23), (13.24), (13.26), (13.27), and the observations at the beginning of the present section, that, uniformly over $j \in \mathbb{Z}$, as $h \to 0$,

$$
\begin{aligned}
\mathbb{E}\widehat{f}_{n,h}(jh) &- \widetilde{f}_h(jh) \\
&= \sum_{\ell=-\infty}^{\infty} \mathcal{K}(\ell)\{\widetilde{f}_h(jh - \ell h) - \widetilde{f}_h(jh)\} \\
&= h^2 f''(jh) \sum_{\ell=-\infty}^{\infty} \ell^2 \mathcal{K}(\ell) + O(h^3) = 2h^2 f''(jh) + O(h^3).
\end{aligned}
\tag{13.28}
$$

By combining (13.19) and (13.28) with the triangle inequality, we see that the bias part of the estimator $\widehat{f}_{n,h}(x)$ of $f(x)$ fulfills, as $h \to 0$,

$$\left| \sup_{x \in I} |\mathbb{E}\widehat{f}_{n,h}(x) - f(x)| - \sup_{x \in I} |\widetilde{f}_h(x) - f(x)| \right|$$
$$\leq \sup_{x \in [0,1]} |\mathbb{E}\widehat{f}_{n,h}(x) - \widetilde{f}_h(x)| = (1 + o(1))2h^2 \sup_{x \in [0,1]} |f''(x)|$$
$$= (1 + o(1))240h^2.$$

In view of (13.20), this, in turn, implies that, as $h \to 0$,

$$\sup_{x \in I} |\mathbb{E}\widehat{f}_{n,h}(x) - f(x)| = (1 + o(1))\frac{5h}{2}. \tag{13.29}$$

In the forthcoming estimators of $f(\cdot)$, we make use of the bandwidth $h = h_n = 0.02$, for which the above evaluation of the bias term yields

$$\sup_{x \in I} |\mathbb{E}\widehat{f}_{n,h}(x) - f(x)| \simeq \frac{5h_n}{2} = 0.05, \tag{13.30}$$

which turns out to introduce a relatively small, and practically negligible, error in the estimation process we consider (e.g., we show below in the example considered in Figure 13.1, with a sample size of $n = 2000$, that the "right" choice of θ_n is close to $\theta_n \simeq 0.35$, so that the maximal bias of 0.05 remains small with respect to this factor). We limit ourselves to the (relatively large) sample sizes of $n = 2000$ (Figure 13.1) and $n = 5000$ (Figure 13.2). These are chosen as to render meaningful the asymptotic formulæ, stated in Fact 13.2.1.

The bootstrapped version, $\widehat{f}^*_{n,h}(x)$, of $\widehat{f}_{n,h}(x)$, is obtained by similar steps, as in (13.22)–(13.23), making use of Resampling Scheme 1, with Z following a Poisson distribution with mean 1 [denoted by $Z \overset{d}{=} \mathrm{Po}(1)$]. Namely, we simulate, independently of the sample $X_1, \ldots, X_n$, a sequence of independent $\mathrm{Po}(1)$ Poisson random variables $Z_1, \ldots, Z_n$, with, independently of $i = 1, \ldots, n$,

$$\mathbb{P}(Z_i = m) = \frac{e^{-1}}{m!} \quad \text{for} \quad m \in \mathbb{N}. \tag{13.31}$$

Second, we define random weights $W_i = Z_i / \sum_{j=1}^{n} Z_j$, for $i = 1, \ldots, n$, as in (13.8). We then set

$$\widetilde{f}^*_{n,h}(x) = \left(h \sum_{i=1}^{n} Z_i \right)^{-1} \sum_{i=1}^{n} Z_i \mathbb{1}_{\{X_i \in ((j-1)h, jh]\}} \tag{13.32}$$
$$\text{for} \quad x \in ((j-1)h, jh] \quad \text{and} \quad j \in \mathbb{N},$$

and, with $\mathcal{K}(\cdot)$ defined by (13.24), for each $x \in \mathbb{R}$,

$$\widehat{f}^*_{n,h}(x) = \sum_{\ell=-\infty}^{\infty} \mathcal{K}(\ell)\widetilde{f}^*_{n,h}(x - \ell h). \tag{13.33}$$

The versions of (13.4) and (13.12) holding for the discretized versions $\widehat{f}_{n,h}(x)$ and $\widehat{f}^*_{n,h}(x)$ of the kernel estimators $f_{n,h}$ and $f^*_{n,h}$, are established by the same arguments as Fact 13.1.1 and Theorem 13.1.1 [see Theorem 1 in Derzko (1998), and, e.g., Deheuvels *et al.* (2004)]. The details are given elsewhere. We thus obtain the following fact.

Fact 13.2.1 *Under (H.c) and, either (H.a) or (H.b), as $n \to \infty$,*

$$\sup_{x \in I} \pm \left\{ \widehat{f}_{n,h_n}(x) - \mathbb{E}\widehat{f}_{n,h_n}(x) \right\}$$

$$= (1 + o_{\mathbb{P}}(1)) \left\{ \frac{2 \log_+(1/h_n)}{nh_n} \left(\sup_{x \in I} f(x) \right) \sum_{\ell=-\infty}^{\infty} \mathcal{K}^2(\ell) \right\}^{1/2} \quad (13.34)$$

and

$$\sup_{x \in I} \pm \left\{ \widehat{f}^*_{n,h_n}(x) - \widehat{f}_{n,h_n}(x) \right\}$$

$$= (1 + o_{\mathbb{P}}(1)) \left\{ \frac{2 \log_+(1/h_n)}{nh_n} \left(\sup_{x \in I} f(x) \right) \sum_{\ell=-\infty}^{\infty} \mathcal{K}^2(\ell) \right\}^{1/2}.$$

$$(13.35)$$

We readily obtain the following corollary of Fact 13.2.1.

Corollary 13.2.1 *Let either (H.a) or (H.b) hold. Then, under (H.c) and (A.1– A.2), for any choice of $\epsilon_1 = \pm 1$ or $\epsilon_2 = \pm 1$, we have, as $n \to \infty$,*

$$\frac{\sup_{x \in I} \epsilon_1 \left\{ \widehat{f}_{n,h_n}(x) - \mathbb{E}\widehat{f}_{n,h_n}(x) \right\}}{\sup_{x \in I} \epsilon_2 \left\{ \widehat{f}^*_{n,h_n}(x) - \widehat{f}_{n,h_n}(x) \right\}} = 1 + o_{\mathbb{P}}(1). \quad (13.36)$$

A numerical evaluation of the constants in the right-hand sides of (13.34) and (13.35) is easily achieved (e.g., by a direct use of any one among the available numerical mathematical software). We thus obtain that

$$\sum_{\ell=-\infty}^{\infty} \mathcal{K}^2(\ell) \simeq 0.304806 \,. \quad (13.37)$$

Moreover, by choosing $I = [0, 1]$, and for $f(\cdot)$ as in (13.16), we get

$$\sup_{x \in I} f(x) = 20 \times \tfrac{1}{4} \left(1 - \tfrac{1}{4} \right)^3 \simeq 2.10938. \quad (13.38)$$

In Figures 13.1 and 13.2 we plot, over $x \in [0, 1]$, the estimator, $f_n(x) = f_{n,h_n}(x)$, the exact density $f(x)$, the *asymptotic bounds*, $(f_n(x) - \theta_{n,4}) \vee 0$

and $(f_n(x) + \theta_{n,4}) \vee 0$, in combination with the asymptotic *bootstrap bounds*, $(f_n(x) - \theta_{n,5}) \vee 0$ and $(f_n(x) + \theta_{n,5}) \vee 0$, where

$$\theta_n = \theta_{n,4} \; := \; \left\{ \frac{2 \log(1/h_n)}{n h_n} \left(\sup_{x \in I} f(x) \right) \sum_{\ell=-\infty}^{\infty} \mathcal{K}^2(\ell) \right\}^{1/2},$$

and

$$\theta_n = \theta_{n,5} \; := \; \sup_{x \in I} \left| \widehat{f}^*_{n,h_n}(x) - \widehat{f}_{n,h_n}(x) \right|.$$

At this point, we note that the restriction, made to fit in the framework of our assumptions, of studying our estimators on $I = [0.2, 0.8] \subset J = [0.1, 0.9]$, appears too restrictive. Our results seem to be unaffected if we plot the graphs in Figures 13.1 to 13.3, on $I = [0, 1]$, so that we have kept this choice. The numerical values of $\theta_n = \theta_{n,4}$ are (up to a precision of 10^{-4}) $\theta_n = 0.3546$ for $n = 2000$, and $\theta_n = 0.2243$ for $n = 5000$. The *bootstrap asymptotic certainty bands* in Figures 13.1 and 13.2 are obtained by using a single bootstrap, so that the number of resamplings is set to Nboot $= 1$. In Figure 13.3, we plot, for $n = 5000$, the variation of the *bootstrap asymptotic certainty bands* observed when several bootstraps are used. The number of bootstraps is here chosen equal to Nboot $= 20$.

Figures 13.1 to 13.3 give some empirical evidence to the fact that the *bootstrap asymptotic certainty bands* $\theta_{n,5}$ appear to behave in a quite satisfactory way, with respect to the nonrandom "exact" *asymptotic certainty bands* $\theta_{n,4}$, based upon the asymptotic formulæ, making use of the exact knowledge of $f(\cdot)$. Of course, when the underlying density is unknown, the derivation of $\theta_{n,4}$ is more problematic, so that the bootstrap asymptotic certainty bands turn out, in this case, to be easier to implement than the "exact" asymptotic ones. In practice, for obvious reasons, when several bootstraps are available, the recommended value of θ_n should be taken as the median of the θ_n's obtained for these different resampled estimates.

13.3 Proofs

13.3.1 Proof of Theorem 13.1.1

We assume below that $(K.a)$ is satisfied, and that the assumptions of the Resampling Scheme (RS.1) hold. We limit ourselves to this case, and the details concerning (RS.2) are given elsewhere. Namely, we let $W_{i,n}$ be defined, for $i = 1, \ldots, n$, by (13.8). In this case, the proof of Theorem 13.1.1 relies on a version of Theorem 3.1 and Corollary 3.1 of Deheuvels and Mason (2004). A simplified version of these results, adapted to the present assumptions, is stated in Lemma 13.3.1 below. For the statement of this result, we need the following notation. Denote by $G(z) = \mathbb{P}(Z \leq z)$ the distribution function of the random variable Z in (A.1–A.2), and let $H(u) = \inf\{z : G(z) \geq u\}$, for $u \in (0,1)$ denote the corresponding quantile function. Without loss of generality, it is possible to enlarge the probability space $(\Omega, \mathcal{A}, \mathbb{P})$ on which $\{X_n : n \geq 1\}$ is defined, in order to carry a sequence $\{V_n : n \geq 1\}$ of independent and identically distributed random variables, with a uniform distribution on $(0,1)$, independent of $\{X_n : n \geq 1\}$, and such that $Z_n = H(V_n)$ for $n \geq 1$. It is noteworthy that $(X,V) := (X_1, V_1)$ has then a joint continuous density $f_{X,V}(x,v) = f(x)1\!\mathrm{I}_{[0,1]}(v)$ on $J \times [0,1]$. This is not quite sufficient for (X,V) to fulfill the assumptions of Deheuvels and Mason (2004). For this, we use the following trick. We denote by $\Phi(y) = (2\pi)^{-1/2} \int_{-\infty}^{\infty} \varphi(t)dt$ [resp., $\varphi(t) = e^{-t^2/2}$], the standard normal $N(0,1)$ distribution (resp., density) function. The corresponding quantile function is $\Phi^{-1}(t) := \inf\{y : \Phi(y) \geq t\}$ for $t \in (0,1)$. We then set, for $n \geq 1$, $Y_n = \Phi^{-1}(V_n)$, and observe that $Z_n - 1 = \psi(Y_n) = H(\Phi(Y_n)) - 1$, where $\psi(y) := H(\Phi(y)) - 1$ for $y \in \mathbb{R}$. By all this, we see that $(X,Y) := (X_1, Y_1)$ has a joint continuous density $f_{X,Y}(x,y) = f(x)\varphi(y)$ on $J \times \mathbb{R}$, fulfilling the assumptions (F.1) and (F.2), on p. 226 in Deheuvels and Mason [DM] (2004). We see also that our assumption (A.2) is tailored to ensure that Assumption (F.4), on p. 226 in [DM] (2004) is fulfilled, with the choice of $\mathcal{M}(s) = e^{\epsilon s}$. Making use of the notation of [DM] (2004), we see that under (A.1), for each $x \in J$,

$$m_\psi(x) := \mathbb{E}(\psi(Y)|X = x) = \mathbb{E}(Z) - 1 = 0, \tag{13.39}$$

and

$$\sigma_\psi^2(x) := \mathrm{Var}(\psi(Y)|X = x) = \mathrm{Var}(Z) = 1. \tag{13.40}$$

Set now, for each $n \geq 1$ and $h > 0$,

$$\widehat{r}_{n,h}(x) := \frac{1}{nh} \sum_{i=1}^{n} \psi(Y_i) K\left(\frac{x - X_i}{h}\right)$$

$$= \frac{1}{nh} \sum_{i=1}^{n} Z_i K\left(\frac{x - X_i}{h}\right) - f_{n,h}(x) = \left\{\frac{1}{n} \sum_{j=1}^{n} Z_i\right\} f_{n,h}^*(x) - f_{n,h}(x), \tag{13.41}$$

which holds on the event $\mathcal{E}_n$ of (13.8). Observe that, under (A.1),

$$r_{n,h}(x) \quad := \quad \mathbb{E}\widehat{r}_{n,h}(x) = 0. \tag{13.42}$$

Given the above notation, we may now cite in the following lemma the version of Corollary 3.1, p. 248 in DM (2004), which is adapted to our setup. This corollary is taken with $\lambda_1 = \lambda_2 = 1$.

Lemma 13.3.1 *Under (H.1), (K.a), and (A.1–2), we have, as $n \to \infty$,*

$$\left\{\frac{nh_n}{2\log(1/h_n)}\right\}^{1/2} \sup_{x\in I} \pm\{\widehat{r}_{n,h_n}(x) - r_{n,h_n}(x)\}$$
$$= \left\{\sup_{x\in I}\left(\sigma_\psi^2(x)f(x)\right)\int_{\mathbb{R}} K^2(t)dt\right\}^{1/2} + o_{\mathbb{P}}(1). \qquad (13.43)$$

PROOF OF THEOREM 13.1.1. As an application of (13.41), and (13.42)–(13.43), we obtain that, under the assumptions of Fact 13.3.1, we have, on the event $\mathcal{E}_n$ of (13.8), as $n \to \infty$,

$$\left\{\frac{nh_n}{2\log(1/h_n)}\right\}^{1/2} \sup_{x\in I} \pm\left\{\left\{\frac{1}{n}\sum_{j=1}^n Z_i\right\}f_{n,h_n}^*(x) - f_{n,h_n}(x)\right\}$$
$$= \left\{\sup_{x\in I} f(x)\int_{\mathbb{R}} K^2(t)dt\right\}^{1/2} + o_{\mathbb{P}}(1). \qquad (13.44)$$

Next, we repeat the arguments above, with the formal change of $\psi(\cdot)$ into $\psi(\cdot)+1$, so that $\psi(Y_n) = Z_n$. We thus obtain, likewise, that, under the assumptions of Fact 13.3.1, we have, as $n \to \infty$,

$$\left\{\frac{nh_n}{2\log(1/h_n)}\right\}^{1/2} \sup_{x\in I} \pm\left\{\left\{\frac{1}{n}\sum_{j=1}^n Z_i\right\}f_{n,h_n}^*(x) - \mathbb{E}f_{n,h_n}(x)\right\}$$
$$= \left\{\sup_{x\in I} f(x)\int_{\mathbb{R}} K^2(t)dt\right\}^{1/2} + o_{\mathbb{P}}(1). \qquad (13.45)$$

By combining (A.1) with the central limit theorem, we see that, as $n \to \infty$,

$$\left|\frac{1}{n}\sum_{j=1}^n Z_i - 1\right| = O_{\mathbb{P}}(n^{-1/2}). \qquad (13.46)$$

Thus, by Slutsky's lemma and the uniform convergence of $\mathbb{E}f_{n,h}(x)$ to $f(x)$ on I, and making use of the observation that $\mathbb{P}(\mathcal{E}_n) \to 1$, we obtain that

$$\sup_{x\in I} f_{n,h_n}^*(x) = (1+o_{\mathbb{P}}(1))\sup_{x\in I} f(x),$$

hence, by (13.46) and (H.1), as $n \to \infty$,

$$\sup_{x\in I}\left|\left\{\frac{1}{n}\sum_{j=1}^n Z_i\right\}f_{n,h_n}^*(x) - f_{n,h_n}^*(x)\right| = O_{\mathbb{P}}(n^{-1/2})$$
$$= o_{\mathbb{P}}\left(\left\{\frac{2\log(1/h_n)}{nh_n}\right\}^{1/2}\right).$$

This, when combined with (13.44), entails that, as $n \to \infty$,

$$\left\{ \frac{nh_n}{2\log(1/h_n)} \right\}^{1/2} \sup_{x \in I} \pm \left\{ f^*_{n,h_n}(x) - f_{n,h_n}(x) \right\} \qquad (13.47)$$
$$= \left\{ \sup_{x \in I} f(x) \int_{\mathbb{R}} K^2(t)dt \right\}^{1/2} + o_{\mathbb{P}}(1).$$

We thus obtain (13.12), as sought. The proof of the remaining parts of the theorem are obtained by similar arguments, and are omitted. ∎

Remark 13.3.1 The same arguments, in a slightly more involved setup, allow us to derive bootstrap-based asymptotic certainty bands for the Nadaraya–Watson regression estimators. The results are in the spirit of those given in Deheuvels and Mason (2004). Likewise, we may apply this methodology to randomly censored observations. This will be considered elsewhere.

References

1. Akaike, H. (1954). An approximation of the density function, *Annals of the Institute of Statistical Mathematics*, **6**, 127–132.

2. Bickel, P. J. and Rosenblatt, M. (1973). On some global measures of the deviations of density functions estimates, *Annals of Statistics*, **1**, 1071–1095.

3. Deheuvels, P. (1992). Functional laws of the iterated logarithm for large increments of empirical and quantile processes, *Stochastic Processes and Their Applications*, **43**, 133–163.

4. Deheuvels, P. (2000). Limit laws for kernel density estimators for kernels with unbounded supports, In *Asymptotics in Statistics and Probability*, (Ed., M. L. Puri), V.S.P., Amsterdam.

5. Deheuvels, P. and Einmahl, J. H. J. (2000). Functional limit laws for the increments of Kaplan–Meier product-limit processes and applications, *Annals of Probability*, **28**, 1301–1335.

6. Deheuvels, P. and Mason, D. M. (1992). Functional laws of the iterated logarithm for the increments of empirical and quantile processes, *Annals of Probability*, **20**, 1248–1287.

7. Deheuvels, P. and Mason, D. M. (2004). General asymptotic confidence bands based upon kernel-type function estimators, *Statistical Inference for Stochastic Processes*, **7**, 225–277.

8. Deheuvels, P., Derzko, G., and Devroye, L. (2004). Kernel smoothed histograms, In *Longevity, Aging and Degradation Models*, (Eds., V. Antonov, C. Huber, M. Nikulin, and V. Polishook), Vol. 2, pp. 68–82, St. Petersburg University Press, Russia.

9. Derzko, G. (1998). Une approche intrinsèque de l'estimation non paramétrique de la densité, *Comptes Rendus de l'Académie des Sciences. Série I. Mathématique*, **327**, 985–988.

10. Derzko, G. and Deheuvels, P. (2002). Estimation non-paramétrique de la régression dichotomique - Application biomédicale, *Comptes Rendus de l'Académie des Sciences. Série I. Mathématique*, **334**, 59–63.

11. Efron, B. (1979). Bootstrap methods: Another look at the jackknife, *Annals of Mathematics and Statistics*, **7**, 1–26.

12. Giné, E., Koltchinskii, V., and Sakhanenko, L. (2004). Kernel density estimators: convergence in distribution for weighted sup-norms, *Probability Theory and Related Fields*, **130**, 167–198.

13. Hall, P. (1992). *The Bootstrap and Edgeworth Expansion*, Springer-Verlag, New York.

14. Härdle, W. and Bowman, A. W. (1988). Bootstrapping in nonparametric regression: Local adaptative smoothing and confidence bands, *Journal of the American Statistical Association*, **83**, 102–110.

15. Härdle, W. and Marron, J. S. (1991). Bootstrap simultaneous error bars for nonparametric regression, *Annals of Statistics*, **19**, 778–796.

16. Li, G. and Datta, S. (2001). A bootstrap approach to nonparametric regression for right censored data, *Annals of the Institute of Statistical Mathematics*, **53**, 708–729.

17. Mason, D. M. and Newton, M. A. (1992). A rank statistic approach to the consistency of a general bootstrap, *Annals of Statistics*, **20**, 1611–1624.

18. Parzen, E. (1962). On the estimation of probability density and mode. *Annals of Mathematics and Statistics*, **33**, 1065–1076.

19. Rosenblatt, M. (1956). *Annals of Mathematics and Statistics*, **27**, 832–837.

20. Stute, W. (1982). The oscillation behavior of empirical processes, *Annals of Probability*, **10**, 414–422.

14

Estimation of Rescaled Distribution

H. Läuter,[1] **M. Nikulin,**[2] **and V. Solev**[3]

[1] *Institut für Mathematik, Universität Potsdam, Potsdam, Germany*
[2] *Statistique Mathématique et Applications, Université Victor Segalen Bordeaux 2, Bordeaux, France*
[3] *St.-Petersburg Department of the Steklov Mathematical Institute, St. Petersburg, Russia*

Abstract: In this chapter we propose a minimum distance estimator for rescaled density from a totally bounded class and prove that the rate of convergence depends only on Kolmogorov's entropy of the class.

Keywords and Phrases: Nonparametric statistics, skeleton estimates, rescaled observations, transportation metric, concentration inequality

14.1 Introduction

Let $Z = (X, Y)$ be a random vector, P_Z be the distribution of Z, and P^X, P^Y be the distributions of X, Y correspondingly. We consider the product measure

$$P_Z^\times = P_X \times P_Y.$$

We assume that the measure P_Z is absolutely continuous with respect to the measure $P_Z^\times$ and set

$$p(x, y) = \frac{dP_Z}{dP_Z^\times}(x, y).$$

We suppose that there exists the density function $f(x, y)$ of the distribution P_Z with respect to the Lebesgue measure. The density function f can be represented in the form:

$$f(x, y) = p(x, y) f_X(x) f_Y(x), \tag{14.1}$$

where f_X, f_Y are density functions of random variables X, Y.

We denote by F^X, F^Y the distribution functions of random variables X, Y and put

$$q(x, y) = p\left(\left(F^X\right)^{-1}(x), \left(F^Y\right)^{-1}(y) \right), \tag{14.2}$$

where F^{-1} is the notation for the inverse function. The function $q(x, y)$ is the density function on $[0, 1] \times [0, 1]$. It is the density function of the rescaled random vector

$$U = (X^*, Y^*) = \left(F^X(X), F^Y(Y)\right). \tag{14.3}$$

The distribution of the vector U is denoted by Q. It is clear that the random variables X^*, Y^* are uniformly distributed on $[0, 1]$. The density function $q(x, y)$ is called a copula density and is responsible for the type of dependence of coordinates of vector Z.

So, we have

$$f(x, y) = q\left(F^X(x), F^Y(y)\right) f_X(x) f_Y(y), \tag{14.4}$$

Let $Z_1 = (X_1, Y_1), \ldots, Z_n = (X_n, Y_n)$ be i.i.d. random vectors with common distribution P_Z, P_n^X and P_n^Y be empirical measures constructed on samples $X_1 \ldots, X_n$ and $Y_1 \ldots, Y_n$, correspondingly,

$$P_n^X\{A\} = \frac{1}{n}\sum_{j=1}^{n} \mathbb{I}_A(X_j), \qquad P_n^Y\{A\} = \frac{1}{n}\sum_{j=1}^{n} \mathbb{I}_A(Y_j),$$

and F_n^X, F_n^Y be the corresponding empirical distribution functions. Denote

$$U_j = \left(F^X(X_j), F^Y(Y_j)\right), \qquad U_{n,j} = \left(F_n^X(X_j), F_n^Y(Y_j)\right), \tag{14.5}$$

and set

$$Q_n\{A\} = \frac{1}{n}\sum_{j=1}^{n} \mathbb{I}_A(U_j) \quad \text{and} \quad \widetilde{Q}_n\{A\} = \frac{1}{n}\sum_{j=1}^{n} \mathbb{I}_A\left(U_{n,j}\right).$$

Suppose we observe the sample $Z_1, \ldots, Z_n$. If distributions of X and Y are unknown, then it is impossible to construct the empirical measure Q_n on observations $Z_1, \ldots, Z_n$. There are many reasons to think [see, for example, Rüschendorf (1976)] that the observable empirical measure $\widetilde{Q}_n$ is close (in a certain sense) for large n to Q_n.

14.2   Transportation Metric

Let $(\mathfrak{X}, \rho)$ be a compact metric space. We consider the Kantorovich metric (one of the most-used Vasserstein metrics) $\kappa(\mu_1, \mu_2)$ [see Kantorovich (1942)],

$$\kappa(\mu_1, \mu_2) = \inf_{\mu} \iint_{\mathfrak{X} \times \mathfrak{X}} \rho(x, y)\, \mu(dx, dy),$$

where μ runs over all probability measures on $\mathfrak{X} \times \mathfrak{X}$ with marginal measures μ_1 and μ_1. In the case which is considered in this work $\mathfrak{X} = [0,1] \times [0,1]$ and $x = (x_1, x_2), y = (y_1, y_2), \rho(x, y) = |x_1 - y_1| \vee |x_1 - y_1|$.

A function ψ is said to be C-Lipschitz if

$$\|\psi\|_{Lip} = \sup_{x \neq y} \frac{|\psi(x) - \psi(y)|}{\rho(x, y)} \leq C,$$

where the supremum is taken over all $x, y \in \mathfrak{X}, x \neq y$. We assume in this case: $\psi \in$ C-*Lip*. The Kantorovich–Rubinstein theorem states that

$$\kappa(\mu_1, \mu_2) = \sup_{\varphi \in 1\text{-}Lip} \int_{\mathfrak{X}} \varphi \, d(\mu_1 - \mu_2).$$

Here and further integrals without the limits mean the integral over all space.

For two probability distributions μ_1 and μ_2 with densities f_1, f_2 with respect to the measure $\nu = \mu_1 + \mu_2$ we use the notation $|\mu_1 - \mu_2|$ for the measure

$$|\mu_1 - \mu_2| \{A\} = \int_A |f_1 - f_2| \, d\nu.$$

For a collection $\mathfrak{C}$ of functions, which is defined on a set $\mathfrak{X}$, we set

$$\kappa_{\mathfrak{C}}(\mu_1, \mu_2) = \sup_{\varphi \in \mathfrak{C}} \int \varphi \, d(\mu_1 - \mu_2),$$

where we assume that $\varphi \in L^1(d|\mu_1 - \mu_2|)$ for all $\varphi \in \mathfrak{C}$.

14.3   Entropy, Duality of Metric Entropy

In a Banach space $(\mathfrak{Y}, \| \cdot \|)$ we denote by $V_\varepsilon(h)$ the ball of radius ε with center in the point h. For a set $\mathfrak{D} \subset \mathfrak{X}$ the covering number $N = N(\varepsilon) = N(\varepsilon, \mathfrak{D}, \| \cdot \|)$ is the minimum number N such that

$$\mathfrak{D} \subset \bigcup_{j=1}^{N} V_\varepsilon(h_j), \quad \text{where } h_j \in \mathfrak{D}, \ j = 1, \dots, N.$$

The value $H(\varepsilon) = H(\varepsilon, \mathfrak{D}, \| \cdot \|) = \log N(\varepsilon, \mathfrak{D}, \| \cdot \|)$ is called the entropy of $\mathfrak{D}$.

For $\beta > 0$ denote by $r = r(\beta)$ the largest integer which is less than β and $\alpha = \alpha(\beta) = \beta - r(\beta)$. Thus

$$\beta = r + \alpha, \qquad 0 < \alpha \leq 1.$$

For any vector $m = (m_1, \ldots, m_d)$ of d integers denote $|m| = m_1 + \cdots + m_d$, consider the differential operator

$$D^m = \frac{\partial^{|m|}}{\partial^{m_1} \ldots \partial^{m_d}},$$

set $G \subset \mathbb{R}^d$, and put

$$\|h\|_{(\beta)} = \max_{|m| \le r} \sup_x D^m h(x) + \max_{|m| \le r} \sup_{x \ne y} \frac{|D^m h(x) - D^m h(y)|}{\|x - y\|^\alpha}, \qquad (14.6)$$

where the supremum is taken over all x, y in the interior of G, $x \ne y$. Let $\mathbf{C}_C^\beta = \mathbf{C}_C^\beta(G)$ be the set of all continuous functions h with $\|h\|_{(\beta)} \le C$.

Theorem 14.3.1 [Kolmogorov and Tihomirov (1959)] *Let G be a bounded, convex subset of $\mathbb{R}^d$ with nonempty interior. Then for a constant $\mathfrak{K} = \mathfrak{K}(G, \beta, d)$,*

$$H\left(\varepsilon, \mathbf{C}_1^\beta(G), \|\cdot\|_\infty\right) \le \mathfrak{K}(G, \beta, d) \left(\frac{1}{\varepsilon}\right)^{\frac{d}{\beta}}, \qquad (14.7)$$

For two convex bodies K and T in $\mathbb{R}^n$, the covering number $N(K, T)$ is defined as the minimal number of translates of T needed to cover K,

$$N(K, T) = \min\{N : \exists x_1, \ldots, x_N \in \mathbb{R}^n, K \subset \bigcup_{j=1}^n \{T + x_j\}. \qquad (14.8)$$

Denote by K^0 the polar body of K,

$$K^0 = \left\{ x : \sup_{y \in K}(x, y) \le 1 \right\}.$$

Here (x, y) is the scalar product in $\mathbb{R}^n$. Let V be the unit ball in $\mathbb{R}^n$.

Theorem 14.3.2 [Artstein et al. (2004)] *There exist two universal constants α and β such that for any n, $\varepsilon > 0$, and any centrosymmetric convex body $K \in \mathbb{R}^n$ one has*

$$N\left(V, \frac{\varepsilon}{\alpha} K^0\right)^{1/\beta} \le N(K, \varepsilon V) \le N\left(V, \alpha \varepsilon K^0\right)^\beta. \qquad (14.9)$$

Let us consider the case as in $\mathfrak{X} = [0, 1] \times [0, 1]$, $x = (x_1, x_2), y = (y_1, y_2)$, $\rho(x, y) = |x_1 - y_1| \vee |x_1 - y_1|$,

$$\mathfrak{C} = \{\varphi : \|\varphi\|_{Lip} \le 1\}.$$

Let $\mathfrak{P}$ be a set of probability distributions P on $\mathfrak{X}$ with densities $f = \theta(P)$ with respect to a σ-finite measure μ. We set

$$\mathfrak{F} = \{f : f = \theta(P) \text{ for some } P \in \mathfrak{P}\},$$
$$\mathfrak{F}_* = \{g : g = f_1 - f_2 \text{ for some } f_1, f_2 \in \mathfrak{F}\}.$$

We suppose that $\mathfrak{F} \in L^2(d\mu)$ and denote by K the smallest convex centrosymmetric body, which contains $\mathfrak{F}$. Introduce the following semi-norm, generated by K

$$\|\varphi\|_{\mathfrak{P}} = \sup_{h \in K} \int \varphi h \, d\mu. \tag{14.10}$$

Let $V_r(\mathbf{h})$ be the ball in the space $L^2(d\mu)$ of radius $r > 0$ and with center in a point h. We would compare the entropy $H(\varepsilon, \mathfrak{C}, \|\cdot\|_{\mathfrak{P}})$ and the entropy $H(\varepsilon, \mathfrak{P}, \|\cdot\|_{L^2(d\mu)})$. From the Artstein et al. theorem we obtain

Proposition 14.3.1 *Suppose that* $\mathfrak{C} \subset V_r(\mathbf{h})$*; then there exist two universal constants* $c > 0$ *and* $C > 0$ *such that for any* n*,* $\varepsilon > 0$

$$H\left(cr\varepsilon, \mathfrak{C}, \|\cdot\|_{\mathfrak{P}}\right) \leq CH\left(\varepsilon, \mathfrak{F}, \|\cdot\|_{L^2(d\mu)}\right). \tag{14.11}$$

14.4 Expectation of $\kappa_{\mathfrak{C}}(P, P_n)$

For a centrosymmetric set $\mathfrak{C}$ and two probability measures P and Q we use the notation

$$\kappa_{\mathfrak{C}}(P, Q) = \sup_{\varphi \in \mathfrak{C}} \int \varphi \, d(P - Q).$$

Here we assume that $\varphi \in L^1(d|P - Q|)$.

Furthermore, for a set A we denote by $|A|$ the cardinality of A. We set

$$\mathbf{E}_P \psi = \int \psi(x) \, P(dx).$$

Let $X_1, \ldots, X_n$ be i.i.d. elements with values in $\mathfrak{X}$ and common distribution $P \in \mathfrak{P}$, and P_n be the empirical distribution:

$$P_n\{A\} = \frac{1}{n} \sum_{j=1}^{n} \mathbb{I}_A(X_j).$$

Suppose that there exists a semi-metric d such that for all $\varphi \in \mathfrak{C}$,

$$|\varphi(x) - \varphi(y)| \leq d(x, y), \tag{14.12}$$

and for all $P \in \mathfrak{P}$,

$$\iint d(x,y)^2 P(dx)P(dy) \leq \mathfrak{L}(\mathfrak{P}, \mathfrak{C}). \tag{14.13}$$

We use the following well-known lemma [see Massart (2000)].

Lemma 14.4.1 *Let A be some finite subset of $\mathbb{R}^n$ of cardinality N, and $\varepsilon_1, \ldots, \varepsilon_n$ be independent Rademacher variables such that $P\{\varepsilon_1 = 1\} = P\{\varepsilon_1 = -1\} = 1/2$, $a = (a_1, \ldots, a_n) \in \mathbb{R}^n$,*

$$R = \sup_{a \in A} \|a\| = \sqrt{\sup_{a \in A} \sum_{j=1}^n a_j^2}.$$

Then

$$\mathbf{E} \sup_{a \in A} \sum_{j=1}^n a_j \varepsilon_j \leq R\sqrt{2 \ln N}. \tag{14.14}$$

Proposition 14.4.1 *Suppose $|\mathfrak{C}| = N$; then under conditions (14.12) and (14.13),*

$$\mathbf{E}_P \kappa_{\mathfrak{C}}(P, P_n) \leq \sqrt{\mathfrak{L}(\mathfrak{P}, \mathfrak{C})} \sqrt{\frac{2 \ln N}{n}}. \tag{14.15}$$

PROOF.

First step: Symmetrization.

Let $X_1^\bullet, \ldots, X_n^\bullet$ be an independent copy of $X_1, \ldots, X_n$. It is well known [see Devroye and Lugosi (2001)] that

$$\mathbf{E}_P \kappa_{\mathfrak{C}}(P, P_n) = \mathbf{E}_P \sup_{\varphi \in \mathfrak{C}} \frac{1}{n} \sum_{j=1}^n (\varphi(X_j) - \mathbf{E}_P\varphi(X_j))$$

$$\leq \mathbf{E}_P \sup_{\varphi \in \mathfrak{C}} \frac{1}{n} \sum_{j=1}^n (\varphi(X_j) - \varphi(X_j^\bullet)). \tag{14.16}$$

Second step: Rademacher variables.

Now we take n i.i.d. Rademacher variables $\varepsilon_1, \ldots, \varepsilon_n$ independent of $X_1, \ldots, X_n, X_1^\bullet, \ldots, X_n^\bullet$ such that $P\{\varepsilon_1 = 1\} = P\{\varepsilon_1 = -1\} = 1/2$. It is clear that

$$\mathbf{E}_P \sup_{\varphi \in \mathfrak{C}} \frac{1}{n} \sum_{j=1}^n (\varphi(X_j) - \varphi(X_j^\bullet)) = \mathbf{E}_P \sup_{\varphi \in \mathfrak{C}} \frac{1}{n} \sum_{j=1}^n \varepsilon_j (\varphi(X_j) - \varphi(X_j^\bullet)).$$

$$\tag{14.17}$$

Third step: We use Lemma 14.4.1.

We set

$$a_j = a_j(\varphi) = \frac{1}{n}\left(\varphi(X_j) - \varphi(X_j^\bullet)\right), \quad A = \{a_\varphi = (a_1(\varphi), \dots, a_n(\varphi)), \varphi \in \mathfrak{C}\}.$$

Under conditions (14.12) and (14.13) we obtain

$$\mathbf{E}_P R \le \sqrt{\mathbf{E}_P R^2} \le \sqrt{\frac{1}{n}\mathbf{E}_P d^2(X_1, X_1^\bullet)} \le \sqrt{\frac{\mathfrak{L}(\mathfrak{P}, \mathfrak{C})}{n}}. \tag{14.18}$$

Thus, (14.15) follows from Lemma 14.4.1. ∎

14.5 Minimum Distance Estimator

Let $Z = (X, Y)$, $Z_1 = (X_1, Y_1), \dots, Z_n = (X_n, Y_n), \dots$ be a sequence of independent, identically distributed random vectors with common distribution $P_Z \in \mathfrak{P}_Z$ and density $f_Z \in \mathfrak{F}_Z$. We assume that functions $f_Z \in \mathfrak{F}_Z$ may be represented in the form

$$f(x, y) = q\left(F^X(x), F^Y(y)\right) f_X(x) f_Y(y). \tag{14.19}$$

Here F^X, F^Y are the distribution functions, and $f_X(x)f_Y(y)$ are density functions of random variables X, Y. So $q(x, y)$ is the density function of the rescaled random vector

$$U = (X^*, Y^*) = \left(F^X(X), F^Y(Y)\right).$$

We denoted by Q the distribution of U. It is clear that $Q = \vartheta(P_Z)$ for appropriately chosen function ϑ. In the following we use the notation

$$\mathfrak{P}_U = \{Q : Q = \vartheta(P_Z) \text{ for some } P_Z \in \mathfrak{P}_Z\},$$

$$\mathfrak{F}_U = \left\{q : q = \frac{dQ}{du} \text{ for some } Q \in \mathfrak{P}_U\right\},$$

where du is the Lebesgue measure on $[0, 1] \times [0, 1]$. We construct an estimator $\widehat{q}_n$ of $q \in \mathfrak{F}_U$ on observations $Z_1 = (X_1, Y_1), \dots, Z_n = (X_n, Y_n)$. We use the notation $\widehat{Q}_n$ for the probability measure with density $\widehat{q}_n$.

Recall the notation $\widetilde{Q}_n$ for the observable empirical measure

$$\widetilde{Q}_n\{A\} = \frac{1}{n}\sum_{j=1}^{n} \mathbb{I}_A\left(U_{n,j}\right),$$

and Q_n for the nonobservable empirical measure

$$Q_n\{A\} = \frac{1}{n}\sum_{j=1}^{n} \mathbb{I}_A(U_j).$$

Here

$$U_j = \left(F^X(X_j), F^Y(Y_j)\right), \qquad U_{n,j} = \left(F_n^X(X_j), F_n^Y(Y_j)\right).$$

Let $\widehat{q}_n \in \mathfrak{F}_U$ be the minimum distance estimator of q,

$$\kappa_{\mathfrak{C}}(\widehat{Q}_n, \widetilde{Q}_n) \leq \kappa_{\mathfrak{C}}(Q, \widetilde{Q}_n), \qquad Q \in \mathfrak{F}_U.$$

Here for a centrosymmetric set $\mathfrak{C}$ of functions φ, which is defined on $[0,1]\times[0,1]$,

$$\kappa_{\mathfrak{C}}(P, Q) = \sup_{\varphi \in \mathfrak{C}} \int \varphi\, du.$$

Then from the triangle inequality for $Q \in \mathfrak{P}_U$,

$$\begin{aligned}
\kappa_{\mathfrak{C}}(Q, \widehat{Q}_n) &\leq & \kappa_{\mathfrak{C}}(Q, \widetilde{Q}_n) + \kappa_{\mathfrak{C}}(\widehat{Q}_n, \widetilde{Q}_n) \leq 2\kappa_{\mathfrak{C}}(Q, \widetilde{Q}_n) \\
&\leq & 2\kappa_{\mathfrak{C}}(Q, Q_n) + 2\kappa_{\mathfrak{C}}(\widetilde{Q}_n, Q_n).
\end{aligned} \tag{14.20}$$

So, in order to control the deviation of the estimated measure $\widehat{Q}_n$ from the unknown true distribution Q we need to control the distribution of $\kappa_{\mathfrak{C}}(Q, Q_n)$ and $\kappa_{\mathfrak{C}}(\widetilde{Q}_n, Q_n)$.

Lemma 14.5.1 *Suppose that* $\mathfrak{C} \subset C\text{-}Lip$. *Then*

$$P\left\{\kappa_{\mathfrak{C}}(\widetilde{Q}_n, Q_n) > t\right\} \leq 4e^{-\frac{2nt^2}{C^2}}. \tag{14.21}$$

PROOF. By definitions of $\widetilde{Q}_n$ and Q_n

$$\kappa_{\mathfrak{C}}(\widetilde{Q}_n, Q_n) = \sup_{\varphi \in \mathfrak{C}} \frac{1}{n}\sum_{j=1}^{n}\left(\varphi\left(F_n^X(X_j), F_n^Y(Y_j)\right) - \varphi\left(F^X(X_j), F^Y(Y_j)\right)\right).$$

$$\tag{14.22}$$

Because $\varphi \in C\text{-}Lip$, then

$$|\varphi(x_1, x_2) - \varphi(y_1, y_2)| \leq C\left\{|x_1 - y_1| \vee |x_2 - y_2|\right\}.$$

Therefore,

$$\kappa_{\mathfrak{C}}(\widetilde{Q}_n, Q_n) \leq C\left\{\sup_x |F_n^X(x) - F^X(x)|\right\} \vee \left\{\sup_y |F_n^Y(y) - F^Y(y)|\right\}. \tag{14.23}$$

So, we conclude

$$P\left\{\kappa_{\mathfrak{C}}(\widetilde{Q}_n, Q_n) \geq t\right\} \;\leq\; P\left\{\sup_x |F_n^X(x) - F^X(x)| > t/C\right\}$$
$$+ P\left\{\sup_y |F_n^Y(y) - F^Y(y)| > t/C\right\}. \quad (14.24)$$

Finally, from the Dvoretzky–Kiefer–Wolfowitz inequality [see Massart (1990)]

$$P\left\{\sup_x |F_n(x) - F(x)| \geq t\right\} \leq 2e^{-2nt^2}$$

we obtain the statement of Lemma 14.5.1. ∎

14.6 Empirical Process, Concentration Inequality

Let $U_1, \ldots, U_n$ be i.i.d. random elements with values in $\mathfrak{X} = [0,1] \times [0,1]$, with common distribution $Q \in \mathfrak{P}_U$ and density $q \in \mathfrak{F}_U$. For appropriately chosen centrosymmetric set $\mathfrak{C}$ consider the empirical process $\xi_n(\varphi), \varphi \in \mathfrak{C}$,

$$\xi_n(\varphi) = \frac{1}{n}\sum_{j=1}^{n}\left(\varphi(U_j) - \int \varphi \, dQ\right). \quad (14.25)$$

We use the following result.

Lemma 14.6.1 [Massart (2003)] *Let $\Omega^n = \prod_{j=1}^{n} \Omega_j$, where, for all j, (Ω_j, d_j) is a metric space with diameter c_j. Let P be some product measure and ψ be some 1-Lip function:$\Omega_n \to \mathbb{R}^1$,*

$$|\psi(x) - \psi(y)| \leq \sum_{j=1}^{n} d_j(x_j, y_j).$$

Then, for any $x > 0$

$$P\left\{\psi - \mathbf{E}_P\psi > x\right\} \leq \exp\left\{-\frac{2x^2}{\sum_{j=1}^{n} c_j^2}\right\}. \quad (14.26)$$

Proposition 14.6.1 *Suppose that $\mathfrak{C} \subset C\text{-Lip}$. Then*

$$P\left\{\sup_{\varphi \in \mathfrak{C}} \xi(\varphi) - \mathbf{E}\sup_{\varphi \in \mathfrak{C}} \xi(\varphi) > x\right\} \leq e^{-2nx^2/C^2}. \quad (14.27)$$

PROOF. For $u = (u^1, \ldots, u^n) \in \mathfrak{X}^n$ we denote

$$\psi(u) = \frac{1}{C} \sup_{\varphi \in \mathfrak{C}} \sum_{j=1}^{n} \left(\varphi(u_j) - \int \varphi \, dQ \right).$$

We suppose that $\mathfrak{C} \subset C\text{-}Lip$:

$$|\varphi(x_1, x_2) - \varphi(y_1, y_2)| \leq C|x_1 - y_1| \vee |x_2 - y_2|.$$

So, if $u^j = (x_1^j, x_2^j), v^j = (y_1^j, y_2^j)$, then

$$d_j(u^j, v^j) = d(u^j, v^j) = |x_1 - y_1| \vee |x_2 - y_2|,$$

and

$$
\begin{aligned}
\psi(u) &= \frac{1}{C} \sup_{\varphi \in \mathfrak{C}} \left\{ \sum_{j=1}^{n} \left(\varphi(v_j) - \int \varphi \, dQ \right) + \sum_{j=1}^{n} (\varphi(u_j) - \varphi(v_j)) \right\} \\
&\leq \psi(v) + \sum_{j=1}^{n} d(u^j, v^j).
\end{aligned}
$$

From Lemma 14.6.1 we obtain

$$P\{\psi - \mathbf{E}_P \psi > x\} \leq \exp\left\{ -\frac{2x^2}{n} \right\}. \tag{14.28}$$

From (14.28) we obtain (14.27). $\blacksquare$

14.7 The Main Result

Let $Z = (X, Y), Z_1 = (X_1, Y_1), \ldots, Z_n = (X_n, Y_n), \ldots$ be a sequence of independent, identically distributed random vectors with common distribution $P_Z \in \mathfrak{P}_Z$ and density $f_Z \in \mathfrak{F}_Z$. We assume that the functions $f_Z \in \mathfrak{F}_Z$ may be represented in the form

$$f(x, y) = q\left(F^X(x), F^Y(y)\right) f_X(x) f_Y(y). \tag{14.29}$$

Here F^X, F^Y are the distribution functions, and $f_X(x) f_Y(y)$ are density functions of random variables X, Y. So $q(x, y)$ is the density function of the rescaled random vector

$$U = (X^*, Y^*) = \left(F^X(X), F^Y(Y)\right).$$

We suppose that $q \in \mathfrak{F}_U$. Denote by $\vartheta(q)$ the probability distribution on $\mathfrak{X} = [0,1] \times [0,1]$ with density q and set

$$\mathfrak{Q} = \{Q : Q = \vartheta(q) \text{ for some } q \in \mathfrak{F}_U\}.$$

We have to estimate q from observations $Z_1, \ldots, Z_n$. We denote by $\widehat{q}_n$ the minimum distance estimator,

$$\kappa_{\mathfrak{C}}(\widetilde{Q}_n, \vartheta(\widehat{q}_n)) \leq \kappa_{\mathfrak{C}}(\widetilde{Q}_n, Q) \quad \text{for all } Q \in \mathfrak{Q}. \tag{14.30}$$

Here $\kappa_{\mathfrak{C}}(P, Q)$ is defined by

$$\kappa_{\mathfrak{C}}(P, Q) = \sup_{\varphi \in \mathfrak{C}} \int \varphi \, d(P - Q),$$

$\widetilde{Q}_n$ is the observable empirical measure,

$$\widetilde{Q}_n \{A\} = \frac{1}{n} \sum_{j=1}^{n} \mathbb{I}_A(U_{n,j}), \qquad U_{n,j} = \left(F_n^X(X_j), F_n^Y(Y_j)\right).$$

It is necessary to notice that these estimators are a version of the well-known skeleton estimates of Yatracos (1985). Let $\mathfrak{C} = \mathfrak{C}_N \subset 1\text{-}Lip$ be a centrosymmetric collection of functions φ of cardinality N. Suppose that $\mathfrak{C}$ is optimal ε-net in $1\text{-}Lip$. That is,

$$N = N(\varepsilon, 1\text{-}Lip, L^2), \tag{14.31}$$

and

$$1\text{-}Lip \subset \bigcup_{j=1}^{N} V_\varepsilon(\varphi_j), \tag{14.32}$$

where

$$\mathfrak{C} = \{\varphi_1, \ldots, \varphi_N\}, \qquad V_\varepsilon(\varphi) = \{g : \|\varphi - g\|_{\mathfrak{P}}\}.$$

Clearly, for any $\varphi \in \mathfrak{C}$ there exists an element $\varphi_* \in \mathfrak{C}_N$ such that $\|\varphi - \varphi_*\|_{\mathfrak{P}} \leq \varepsilon$. Therefore, for any $P, Q \in \mathfrak{P}$,

$$\kappa_{\mathfrak{C}}(P, Q) \leq \varepsilon + \kappa_{\mathfrak{C}_N}(P, Q). \tag{14.33}$$

Suppose that there exist a function G on $\mathfrak{X} = [0,1] \times [01]$ and a density q_*, $\beta > 1$ such that

$$\int G^2 \, dx_1 dx_2 < \infty, \tag{14.34}$$

for any $q \in \mathfrak{F}_u$

$$q = Gg + q_*, \quad \text{where } g \in \mathfrak{C}_L^\beta. \tag{14.35}$$

Theorem 14.7.1 *Suppose that the parametric set $\mathfrak{F}_U$ satisfies the conditions* (14.34) *and* (14.35). *Then*

$$\mathbf{E}_Q \|\widehat{q} - q\|_2 \leq \mathfrak{L}(\mathfrak{F}_U) \, n^{-\frac{\beta}{2\beta+2}}.$$

Acknowledgements

The investigation was supported in part by RFBR grants 05-01-00920, NSH–4222.2006.1, and RFBR–DFG 04-01-0400.

References

1. Artstein, S., Milman, V., and Szarek, S. J. (2004). Duality of metric entropy, *Annals of Math.*, **159**(3), 1313–1328.

2. Devroye, L. and Lugosi, G. (2001). *Combinatorial Methods in Density Estimation*, Springer-Verlag, New York.

3. Kantorovich, L. V. (1942). On the translation of masses, *Dokl. Acad. Nauk SSSR*, **37**, 227–229.

4. Kantorovich, L. V. and Rubinstein, G. Sh. (1958). On the space of totally additive functions, *Vestn. Lening. Univ.*, **13**, 52–59.

5. Kolmogorov, A. N. and Tihomirov, V. M. (1959) . The epsilon-entropy and epsilon-capacity of scts in functional spaces, *Usp. Mat. Nauk.*, **86**, 3–86.

6. Massart, P. (1990). The tight constant in the Dvorettzky–Kiefer–Wolfowitz inequality, *Annals of Probability*, **18**, 1269–1283.

7. Massart, P. (2000). Some applications of concentration inequality, *Annales de la faculté des science de Toulouse, 6 serie*, **9**, 245–303.

8. Massart, P. (2003). *Concentration Inequality and Model Selection. Ecole d'Eté de Probabilités de Saint-Fleur XXXIII – 2003*, Springer-Verlag, New York.

9. Rüschendorf, L. (1976). Asymptotic distributions of multivariate rank order statistics, *Annals of Statistics*, **4**, 912–923.

10. Yatracos, Y. G. (1985). Rates of convergence of minimum distance estimators and Kolmogorov's entropy, *Annals of Statistics*, **13**, 768–774.

15

Nested Plans for Sequential Change Point Detection—The Parametric Case

Paul Feigin,[1] **Gregory Gurevich,**[2] **and Yan Lumelskii**[1]

[1] *Technion–Israel Institute of Technology, Haifa, Israel*
[2] *Shamoon College of Engineering, Beer Sheva, Israel*

Abstract: We consider the problem of sequential quality control and propose nested plans for the early detection, with low false alarm rate, of a change in a stochastic system. The nested plan includes two phases: a variable plan and an attributes plan. For the proposed specific nested plan we present exact (nonasymptotic) expressions for the mean and for the standard deviation of the run length, both for the in-control (time to false alarm) and out-of-control (time to change detection) cases. We assume that the initial and the final distributions come from an exponential family of distributions and show the existence of optimal nested plans in the one-parameter case and for the multivariate normal case.

Keywords and Phrases: Nested plan, change detection, exponential family of distributions, multivariate normal distribution, average run length, optimal nested plan

15.1   Introduction and Notation

There are extensive references in the statistics and engineering literature on the subject of early detection, with low false alarm rate, of parameter changes in stochastic systems on the basis of sequential observations from the system. Such problems are very important in the context of quality assurance [see Gordon and Pollak (1994), Lai (1995), and Zacks (1991)]. In this chapter we consider nested plans for the early detection of a parameter change within the context of an exponential family. We continue research which began in articles by Feigin *et al.* (2005), Lumelskii and Feigin (2005), and Lumelskii *et al.* (2006).

Often instead of individual observations $X_1, X_2, \ldots$ one has a sequence of samples, each of n observations. We assume that the process under investigation yields independent samples, each consisting of n independent observations $(X_{11}, \ldots, X_{1n})$, $(X_{21}, \ldots X_{2n})$, ... Initially these observations follow a distribution $F(x \mid \theta_1)$. At m, an unknown point in time, something happens to the process, causing the distribution of the sample's observations to change to $F(x \mid \theta_2)$; $F(x \mid \theta_1) \neq F(x \mid \theta_2)$. In this chapter we assume that the distribution $F(x \mid \theta)$ is of exponential family form.

A common performance measure for an inspection scheme (or *stopping rule*) is the average run length (*ARL*). Let T be the time when the scheme signals that the process is out of control (i.e., that the distribution of the observations has changed). The *in-control* or *false alarm ARL* is defined to be $\mathrm{E}_{F(x\mid\theta_1)}T$ where we define $\mathrm{E}_{F(x\mid\theta_h)}T \equiv \mathrm{E}(T \mid \theta_h)$ to be the expectation of the stopping time T under the assumption that the observations come from the distribution $F(x \mid \theta_h)$.

Clearly, one wants $\mathrm{E}(T \mid \theta_1)$ to be large and the *out-of-control* ARL $\mathrm{E}(T \mid \theta_2)$ to be small. There are known optimal CUSUM and Shiryaev–Roberts control charts which rapidly detect a change in distribution among all procedures with a bounded in-control ARL. However, the practical design of such charts is not simple because there are no simple explicit expressions for the in-control and out-of-control ARLs [$\mathrm{E}(T \mid \theta_h)$ for $h = 1, 2$, respectively]. As a result, these schemes are geared toward detecting small changes, whereas for large changes Shewhart control charts are typically preferred.

15.2 Definitions and Characteristics of Nested Plans

We propose nested plans, denoted $\prod_{nes}(\Pi^{G_1} \mid \Pi^{G_2})$, for the quick detection of a change in the distribution of observations. A nested plan consists of two steps, Π^{G_1} and Π^{G_2}, where Π^{G_1} is a variables plan and Π^{G_2} is an attributes plan [see Feigin *et al.* (2005)].

We consider the first step of the nested plan with parameters n and C (n is the sample size; C is a real constant). Using sequential observations $(X_{11}, \ldots, X_{1n})$, $(X_{21}, \ldots, X_{2n})$, ... with distribution $F(x \mid \theta_h)$, the first step of the nested plan is defined by

$$Y_i(\theta_1, \theta_2) = \ln \prod_{j=1}^{n} \frac{f(X_{ij} \mid \theta_2)}{f(X_{ij} \mid \theta_1)} \ , \qquad i = 1, 2, \ldots \qquad (15.1)$$

and

$$Z_i = \begin{cases} 1, & \text{if } Y_i(\theta_1, \theta_2) > C, \\ 0, & \text{if } Y_i(\theta_1, \theta_2) \leq C. \end{cases} \qquad (15.2)$$

Defining

$$P_h \equiv P(Z_i = 0 \mid \theta_h) \equiv P(Y_i(\theta_1, \theta_2) \leq C \mid \theta_h), \qquad Q_h = P(Z_i = 1 \mid \theta_h), \tag{15.3}$$

we have a binary sequence of observations $Z_1, Z_2, \ldots$ with probability of zero equal to P_h.

The second step is an attributes plan Π^{G_2}, which is based on $Z_i = 0$ or $Z_i = 1$, $i = 1, 2, \ldots$. We consider the plan $\Pi^2(d; 2)$ for which the stopping rule is defined as $T = \min\{n : Z_{n-d+1} + \cdots + Z_n = 2\}$; that is, the first time that 2 ones appear among the last d observations. For nested sampling plans it is possible to evaluate exact expressions for the ARLs. We demonstrate such calculations for the multinormal case, and show that for this example the speed of detection of a change is close to that of the CUSUM procedure.

The following results were obtained by Hald (1981, p. 291) and Lumelskii and Chichagov (1983) for a different problem.

Theorem 15.2.1 *For* $\Pi^2(d; 2)$ *the expectation* $E(T \mid \Pi^2(d; 2); \; \theta_h) \equiv E_h(T)$ *and standard deviation* $\sigma(T \mid \Pi^2(d; 2); \; \theta_h) \equiv \sigma_h(T)$ *of the stopping time* T *are given by*

$$E_h(T) = \frac{n\left(2 - P_h^{d-1}\right)}{Q_h\left(1 - P_h^{d-1}\right)}, \tag{15.4}$$

$$\sigma_h(T) = \frac{n\left[2P_h + P_h^{2d-1} + P_h^{d-1}((2d+1)Q_h - 2)\right]^{0.5}}{Q_h\left(1 - P_h^{d-1}\right)}. \tag{15.5}$$

From Theorem 15.2.1 we immediately obtain that if $P_h \to 0$ then

$$E_h(T) \to 2n, \qquad \sigma_h(T) \to 0 \quad \text{for all } d \geq 2.$$

15.3 Multivariate Normal Distributions and Optimal Nested Plans

We consider a situation where the observations $(X_{i1}, \ldots X_{in})$, $i = 1, 2, \ldots$ have a k-variate normal distribution with means μ_1 and μ_2 and covariance matrices Σ_1 and Σ_2. If $\Sigma_1 = \Sigma_2 \equiv \Sigma$ then the logarithm of the likelihood ratio [from (15.1)] is given by

$$Y_i(\mu_1, \mu_2, \Sigma) = n(\mu_2 - \mu_1)'\Sigma^{-1}\bar{X}_i - 0.5n(\mu_2 + \mu_1)'\Sigma^{-1}(\mu_2 - \mu_1), \tag{15.6}$$

where $\bar{X}_i = \frac{1}{n}\sum_{j=1}^n X_{ij}$.

Theorem 15.3.1 *Let μ_1, μ_2, and Σ be known. Then for any μ_h the probability (15.3) is given by the following formula.*

$$P_h = P(Z_i = 0 \mid \mu_h) = \Phi\left(\frac{C + 0.5n(\mu_2 - \mu_1)'\Sigma^{-1}(\mu_2 + \mu_1 - 2\mu_h)}{\sqrt{nR^2}}\right). \quad (15.7)$$

Here $R^2 = (\mu_2 - \mu_1)'\Sigma^{-1}(\mu_2 - \mu_1)$ and $\Phi(x)$ is the cumulative distribution function of the standard normal distribution.

PROOF. By using (15.1) and (15.6) we obtain

$$P_h = P(n(\mu_2 - \mu_1)'\Sigma^{-1}\bar{X}_i \leq C + 0.5n(\mu_2 + \mu_1)'\Sigma^{-1}(\mu_2 - \mu_1) \mid \mu_h). \quad (15.8)$$

If the X_{ij} have mean vector μ_h then the random variable

$$\xi_{hi} \equiv n(\mu_2 - \mu_1)'\Sigma^{-1}\bar{X}_i$$

has a normal distribution with the following expectation and variance [see Anderson (1958)],

$$\mathrm{E}(\xi_{hi}) = n(\mu_2 - \mu_1)'\Sigma^{-1}\mu_h \; ; \; \sigma^2(\xi_{hi}) = n(\mu_2 - \mu_1)'\Sigma^{-1}(\mu_2 - \mu_1) \equiv nR^2.$$

That is,

$$\frac{\xi_{hi} - \mathrm{E}(\xi_{hi})}{\sigma(\xi_{hi})}$$

has a standard normal distribution and the result follows.   ■

Corollary 15.3.1

$$P_1 = \Phi\left(\frac{C}{\sqrt{nR^2}} + 0.5\sqrt{nR^2}\right), \qquad P_2 = \Phi\left(\frac{C}{\sqrt{nR^2}} - 0.5\sqrt{nR^2}\right). \quad (15.9)$$

Note that the probabilities P_1 and P_2 only depend on the parameters (μ_1, μ_2, Σ) through R^2. If $\mu_h \neq \mu_1$ and $\mu_h \neq \mu_2$ then according to (15.7) P_h depends on all the parameters μ_h, μ_1, μ_2, and Σ.

Obviously, for each given n (individual sample size) and for known parameters μ_1, μ_2, μ_h, Σ, the probability P_h is specified by the value of the threshold C. Therefore, the choice of the threshold C for the first step of the nested plan determines the in-control and out-of-control means $(E(T \mid \mu_h))$, and standard deviations $(\sigma(T \mid \mu_h))$ of the run length (when $h = 1, 2$, respectively). Moreover the exact expressions (15.4) allow the a priori determination of any desirable in-control or out-of-control ARL, by choosing the appropriate threshold value C at the first step of the nested plan. More precisely, in order to attain a given value of the in-control ARL for given parameters (n and d) of the nested plan and for a given value of R, we solve the equation (15.4) to find the appropriate value of the probability P_1. Then, using (15.9) we may obtain the appropriate value of the threshold C. Finally, from (15.9) we evaluate P_2 and by (15.4) the value of the out-of-control ARL $E(T \mid \mu_2)$.

The following theorem guarantees the possibility of an optimal choice of the parameters n and d for a nested plan with any given in-control ARL (W) and value of R, in order to minimize the out-of-control ARL.

Theorem 15.3.2 *Consider the multivariate normal case with fixed R^2 and in-control ARL $W = E(T \mid \mu_1) > 2$. Then there exists an optimal nested plan with parameters n and d, which minimizes the out-of-control ARL $E(T \mid \mu_2)$. The parameters n and d are bounded:*

$$1 \le n \le W/2, \tag{15.10}$$

and there exists $\delta > 0$ depending on W (see the proof) such that

$$2 \le d(n) < \frac{\log\left[\frac{\delta W - 2n}{\delta W - n}\right]}{\log(1 - \delta)} + 1. \tag{15.11}$$

PROOF. Because n and d are natural numbers, for the proof of existence of the optimal nested plan it is enough to prove that they are bounded.

From (15.4) we rewrite

$$\frac{\mathrm{E}(T|P, s)}{n} = f(P, s) = \frac{1}{1 - P}\left(1 + \frac{1}{1 - P^s}\right),$$

where $s \equiv d - 1 \ge 1$. Let $w_n = W/n$ for any $1 \le n$. Note that $f(P, s)$ is increasing in P and decreasing in s. In order to meet the in-control requirement $f(P_1, s) = w_n$, P_1 must satisfy $\lim_{s \to \infty} f(P_1, s) = 2/(1 - P_1) \le w_n$, which in turn implies that $w_n > 2$ for all n. Therefore we have $1 \le n < W/2$ and because n is integral and W finite $n \le n_0 < W/2$ and there exists $\epsilon > 0$ such that $2 + \epsilon < w_n < W$.

Now fix n in the permitted (finite) range $1 \le n \le n_0 < W/2$. Writing $w = w_n$, denote the solution of

$$f(P, s) = w \tag{15.12}$$

for given s by $P(s, w)$ and note that $P(s, w)$ is increasing in $s \ge 1$. It can be shown that

$$0 < 1 - \frac{1 + \sqrt{1 + 4w}}{2w} = P(1, w) \le P(s, w) < P(\infty, w) = 1 - 2/w. \tag{15.13}$$

Having established bounds for $P(s, w)$ and for w, we can conclude that there exists $\delta > 0$ such that $\delta < P(s, w) < 1 - \delta$ for all $(s, w = w_n); 1 \le n \le n_0$: namely, choose

$$0 < \delta < \min\left(1 - \frac{1 + \sqrt{1 + 4(2 + \epsilon)}}{2(2 + \epsilon)}, \frac{2}{W}\right). \tag{15.14}$$

Returning to Equation (15.12), now consider the solution $s(P, w)$ for s for given P. This function is increasing in P for fixed n (implying fixed $w = w_n$). [The latter follows from the monotonicity properties of $f(P, s)$.] In fact, one can write:

$$s(P, w) = \frac{\log\left[\frac{(1-P)w-1}{(1-P)w-2}\right]}{\log(1/P)} \leq \frac{\log\left[\frac{\delta w-2}{\delta w-1}\right]}{\log(1-\delta)}. \tag{15.15}$$

Thus we have shown that $1 \leq n \leq n_0$ and for each n, taking $w = W/n$, $d = s+1$ is bounded between 2 and

$$\left[\log\left(\frac{\delta w - 2}{\delta w - 1}\right)\Big/\log(1-\delta)\right] + 1. \qquad\blacksquare$$

15.4   Nested Plans for One-Parameter Exponential Distributions

We consider also the one-parameter exponential families of distributions with density function

$$f(x \mid \theta) = u(x)\exp\{a(\theta)s(x) + b(\theta)\}. \tag{15.16}$$

Here $a(\theta)$ and $b(\theta)$ are continuous functions of the parameter θ, $\theta \in \Theta \subset \mathbf{R}^1$, $x \in \mathbf{A} \subset \mathbf{R}^1$. Normal, Rayleigh, Pareto, Weibull, and other one-parameter families of distributions have density functions of the form given in (15.16).

According to Equation (15.1) in this case

$$Y_i(\theta_1, \theta_2) = \ln\prod_{j=1}^{n}\frac{f(X_{ij} \mid \theta_2)}{f(X_{ij} \mid \theta_1)} = S_i(n)[a(\theta_2) - a(\theta_1)] + n[b(\theta_2) - b(\theta_1)], \tag{15.17}$$

where $S_i(n) = \sum_{j=1}^{n} s(X_{ij})$ is the sufficient statistic for the family of distributions (15.17).

Using the distribution function $(G_{S_i}(z) = P(S_i(n) < z \mid \theta_h))$ or the density function $(g(z \mid \theta_h))$ of the sufficient statistic $S_i(n)$, the probability (15.3) has the form

$$P_h = P\left(S_i(n)[a(\theta_2) - a(\theta_1)] + n[b(\theta_2) - b(\theta_1)] \leq C \mid \theta_h\right). \tag{15.18}$$

We now present an extension of Theorem 15.3.2 to the one-parameter exponential case.

Theorem 15.4.1 *Consider the one-parameter exponential family case with fixed θ_1 and θ_2 and desired in-control ARL $W = E(T \mid \theta_1) > 2$. Then there exists an optimal nested plan with parameters n and d, which minimizes the out-of-control ARL $E(T \mid \theta_2)$. The parameters n and d are bounded:*

$$1 \leq n \leq W/2, \tag{15.19}$$

and there exists $\delta > 0$ depending on W such that

$$2 \le d(n) < \frac{\log\left[\frac{\delta W - 2n}{\delta W - n}\right]}{\log(1 - \delta)} + 1. \tag{15.20}$$

PROOF. The first part of the proof follows exactly that of Theorem 15.3.2. Assume that $a(\theta_2) > a(\theta_1)$; this can always be achieved by defining $S_i(n)$ appropriately. As long as the support of $S_i(n)$ does not depend on θ—a property of the exponential family of (15.16)—then we can still define the required δ as in (15.14) and there will exist C such that

$$B(n) = \frac{C - n[b(\theta_2) - b(\theta_1)]}{a(\theta_2) - a(\theta_1)} \tag{15.21}$$

will satisfy $\delta < P_1 = \Pr(S_i(n) < B(n)|\theta_1) < 1 - \delta$. The remainder of the proof follows as before. ∎

Example 15.4.1 Let the random variable X_{ij} have the gamma distribution [gamma(α, θ), α known] with the density function

$$f(x|\theta) = \frac{x^{\alpha-1}}{\Gamma(\alpha)\theta^\alpha} \exp\{-\frac{x}{\theta}\}; \qquad x \ge 0, \qquad \theta > 0, \qquad \alpha > 0, \tag{15.22}$$

where $\Gamma(a) = \int_o^\infty t^{a-1}e^{-t}dt$ is the gamma function. Here $a(\theta) = -1/\theta$ is increasing in θ. In this case the sufficient statistic $S_i(n) = \sum_{j=1}^n X_{ij}$ has the gamma$(n\alpha,\theta)$ distribution. If $\theta_1 < \theta_2$ then the probability (15.18) has the form

$$P_h = P\left(S_i(n) < B(n) \mid \theta_h\right); \quad B(n) = \frac{C - n\alpha \ln(\theta_1\theta_2^{-1})}{\theta_1^{-1} - \theta_2^{-1}}.$$

We obtain finally:

$$P_h = G\left(\frac{B(n)}{\theta_h}\right). \tag{15.23}$$

Here $G(z)$ is the cumulative distribution function of the gamma$(n\alpha, 1)$ distribution.

Example 15.4.2 Let the random variable X_{ij} have the one-parameter Pareto distribution (λ is known) with density function

$$f(x|\theta) = \frac{\theta \lambda^\theta}{x^{\theta+1}} = \frac{1}{x} \exp\{-\theta \ln x + \ln(\theta\lambda^\theta)\}; \qquad x \ge \lambda > 0; \qquad \theta > 0. \tag{15.24}$$

In this case the sufficient statistic $S_i(n) = \sum_{j=1}^n \ln(X_{ij})$ has the density function

$$g(z \mid \theta_h) = \frac{\theta_h{}^n}{\Gamma(n)}(z - n\ln\lambda)^{n-1} \exp\{-\theta_h(z - n\ln\lambda)\} ; \qquad z > n\ln\lambda.$$

If $\theta_1 > \theta_2$ then the probability (15.18) can be written in the form

$$P_h = G\left(\theta_h\left([C + n\ln(\theta_1\theta_2{}^{-1}\lambda^{\theta_1-\theta_2})](\theta_1 - \theta_2)^{-1} - n\ln\lambda\right)\right). \qquad (15.25)$$

Here $G(z)$ is the cumulative distribution function of the gamma$(n, 1)$ distribution.

15.5   Numerical Examples and Comparisons

Example 15.5.1 Consider the nested plan with $n = 4$, $d = 3$, and the X_{ij} having a trivariate normal distribution with in-control and out-of-control means μ_1, μ_2, respectively, and covariance matrix Σ given by:

$$\mu_1 = (0, 0.5, 0.7)'; \qquad \mu_2 = (0.8, 1.7, 1.5)'; \qquad \Sigma = \mathrm{diag}(2, 4, 2).$$

We thus obtain

$$R^2 = (\mu_2 - \mu_1)'\Sigma^{-1}(\mu_2 - \mu_1) = \frac{0.8^2}{2} + \frac{1.2^2}{4} + \frac{0.8^2}{2} = 1.$$

For example, for setting the ARL at $E_1(T) \equiv E_{F(x|\mu_1, \Sigma)}(T) = 1000$, we use (15.4) and $n = 4$, $d = 3$ to obtain

$$\frac{4\left(2 - P_1{}^2\right)}{Q_1P_1\left(1 - P_1{}^2\right)} = 1000,$$

and hence $P_1 = 0.95270$. By (15.8) we get $C = 1.343152$ and $P_2 = 0.37130$. According to the formulas (15.4) and (15.5) $E_2(T) = 13.74$, $\sigma_1(T) = 992.52$, and $\sigma_2(T) = 7.67$. If $\mu_3 = (1.4\ 2.6\ 2.1)'$ then from (15.7) the probability P_3 is

$$P_3 = \Phi\left(\frac{1.343152 + 2(0.8\ 1.2\ 0.8)'\Sigma^{-1}(-2\ -3\ -2)}{2}\right) \simeq \Phi(-1.83) = 0.034.$$

In Table 15.1 we provide the results of computing, using (15.4), (15.5), and (15.8), some values for the out-of-control mean and the standard deviation of the run length for different (given) values of in-control ARL and for various values of d, n, and R. From Table 15.1 we conclude that for a given value of in-control ARL the influence of d on the out-of-control ARL is smaller than the influence of n. Obviously, increasing R yields a decrease in the out-of-control ARL. In addition, it is possible to see that, for small values of R, large values of n are required in order to decrease the out-of-control ARL. We conclude also

Table 15.1. Out-of-control mean and standard deviation of the run length of nested plans when the initial and the final distributions are multivariate normal with known different means and the same covariance matrix

$E_1(T)$	d	R	n	$E_2(T)$	P_1	C	P_2	$\sigma_1(T)$	$\sigma_2(T)$
1000	3	0.5	8	40.58	0.9315	1.1032	0.5291	985.42	28.53
1000	3	0.5	12	40.17	0.9146	0.8723	0.3585	978.53	21.92
1000	3	0.5	16	43.12	0.8999	0.5618	0.2360	971.79	18.01
1000	4	0.5	6	43.56	0.9511	1.2773	0.6666	986.56	33.22
1000	4	0.5	8	40.83	0.9427	1.2313	0.5650	982.35	27.42
1000	4	0.5	12	40.86	0.9281	1.0324	0.3936	974.17	21.07
1000	3	1.0	2	16.66	0.9671	1.6018	0.6648	996.19	13.58
1000	3	1.0	4	13.74	0.9527	1.3432	0.3713	992.52	7.67
1000	3	1.0	6	15.06	0.9413	0.8359	0.1885	988.94	5.46
1000	4	1.0	2	16.41	0.9728	1.7206	0.6948	995.32	12.93
1000	4	1.0	4	13.92	0.9607	1.5178	0.4047	990.87	7.32
1000	4	1.0	6	15.33	0.9511	1.0545	0.2135	986.56	5.32
1000	3	2.0	1	4.64	0.9770	1.9909	0.4982	998.07	3.14
1000	3	2.0	2	4.83	0.9671	1.2036	0.1614	996.19	1.59
1000	3	2.0	4	8.08	0.9527	−1.3137	0.0099	992.52	0.58
1000	4	2.0	1	4.63	0.9811	2.1524	0.5304	997.61	2.97
1000	4	2.0	2	4.91	0.9728	1.4411	0.1828	995.32	1.55
1000	4	2.0	4	8.10	0.9607	−0.9644	0.0125	990.87	0.64
2000	3	0.5	8	51.54	0.9527	1.3640	0.6016	1985.05	39.39
2000	3	0.5	12	47.33	0.9413	1.2124	0.4341	1977.88	29.25
2000	3	0.5	16	48.32	0.9315	0.9744	0.3040	1970.84	23.71
2000	4	0.5	6	57.72	0.9663	1.4901	0.7272	1986.15	47.09
2000	4	0.5	8	51.35	0.9607	1.4874	0.6348	1981.74	37.71
2000	4	0.5	12	47.84	0.9511	1.3670	0.4694	1973.11	27.98
2000	3	1.0	2	21.91	0.9770	1.8220	0.7195	1996.14	18.77
2000	3	1.0	4	15.86	0.9671	1.6795	0.4363	1992.38	9.84
2000	3	1.0	6	16.27	0.9593	1.2697	0.2400	1988.69	6.87
2000	4	1.0	2	21.34	0.9811	1.9362	0.7460	1995.23	17.76
2000	4	1.0	4	15.95	0.9728	1.8475	0.4696	1990.63	9.34
2000	4	1.0	6	16.54	0.9663	1.4802	0.2675	1986.15	6.59
2000	3	2.0	1	5.52	0.9839	2.2825	0.5562	1998.05	4.01
2000	3	2.0	2	5.12	0.9770	1.6440	0.2024	1996.14	1.94
2000	3	2.0	4	8.13	0.9671	−0.6410	0.0154	1992.38	0.73
2000	4	2.0	1	5.45	0.9868	2.4377	0.5866	1997.58	3.77
2000	4	2.0	2	5.20	0.9811	1.8723	0.2260	1995.23	1.87
2000	4	2.0	4	8.15	0.9728	−0.3051	0.0189	1990.63	0.79

that the standard deviation of the in-control run length is a little smaller than the corresponding mean run length but, roughly, the values are quite similar.

The change point problem for multivariate normal observations was also considered by Crosier (1988) in the context of the CUSUM procedure. We compare in Table 15.2 the nested plan and the multivariate CUSUM procedure [see Crosier (1988)] for detecting a change in the mean of the bivariate normal distribution, assuming all parameters (μ_1, μ_2, and Σ) are known. From Table 15.2 it turns out that for the considered situation the speed of detection of a change for the proposed nested plan is approximately the same as for the multivariate CUSUM chart. For the situation where the dimension of the observations is greater than two ($k > 2$), the nested plan may be preferable to the multivariate CUSUM procedure presented in Crosier (1988) [see Lumelskii *et al.* (2006)].

Table 15.2. Out-of-control ARL of the multivariate CUSUM parametric procedures (by simulation) and those of the proposed nested plan for detecting a change in the mean of the bivariate normal distribution

R	$E_1(T)$	Rule	$E_2(T)$
1	200	CUSUM	9.35
1	200	$\prod_{nes}(n = 2; d = 3)$	9.43
2	200	CUSUM	3.48
2	200	$\prod_{nes}(n = 1; d = 3)$	3.29
3	200	CUSUM	1.69
3	200	$\prod_{nes}(n = 1; d = 3)$	2.19

Example 15.5.2 Consider the choice of the optimal nested plan for the multivariate normal distributions when $E(T \mid \mu_1) = 1000$, $R = 1$. In Table 15.3 we present values of the out-of-control ARL of the proposed nested plan for this example for different values of the parameters n and d. Note that the minimum value of the out-of control ARL is $E(T \mid \mu_2) = 2n$. Therefore one can infer from Table 15.3 that it is sufficient to consider only $n < 7$ because for $n \geq 7$ we get an out-of-control ARL $E(T \mid \mu_2) \geq 14$ which exceeds 13.74. By examination of all possibilities we find that optimal nested plan is attained for $n = 4$ and $d = 3$.

Example 15.5.3 Consider the nested plan where the observations X_{ij} are univariate normal and parameters are given by: $\mu_1 = 0$, $\mu_2 = 1$ and $\sigma^2 = 1$. For this situation it is known that the CUSUM procedure provides a minimal out-of-control ARL among all procedures with the same prescribed in-control ARL.

Table 15.3. Comparison of out-of-control ARLs for nested plans for multivariate normal distribution for different values of parameters n and d: in-control ARL $= 1000$, $R = 1$

	d				
n	**2**	**3**	**4**	**5**	**6**
1	30.69	27.55	26.48	26.05	25.90
2	18.10	16.66	16.41	16.49	16.69
3	15.02	14.17	14.21	14.45	14.75
4	14.29	**13.74**	13.92	14.23	14.55
5	14.53	14.17	14.41	14.74	15.05
6	15.29	15.06	15.33	15.64	15.91

It is interesting to compare the proposed nested plan with an optimal CUSUM chart. In Table 15.4 we provide the results of such a comparison for which the CUSUM procedure is tuned to the normal shift case of detecting a change from $\mu_1 = 0$ to $\mu_2 = 1$. The table presents values for the out-of control ARL for various true drifts R. For the normal parametric CUSUM procedure the tabulated values were obtained by simulation using 10,000 replicated samples. The values for the nested plan are exact. All procedures have critical values selected so as to yield a nominal in-control ARL equal to 1000. The critical values of the CUSUM procedure are evaluated by simulations. For the nested plan all values are obtained by our explicit results for the in-control and out-of-control ARL. From Table 15.4 it turns out that for this univariate normal example the speed of detection of a change for the proposed nested plan is about 20–25 percent worse than that of the optimal CUSUM procedure.

Example 15.5.4 Consider the nested plan with $n = 9$, $d = 4$, and univariate observations X_{ij} having a Pareto(θ, λ) distribution, where $\theta_1 = 3$, $\theta_2 = 2$, $\lambda = 1$. For this case we compare the out-of control ARL of the CUSUM parametric procedure with those of the proposed nested plan. In Table 15.5 we provide the results of such a comparison for which the CUSUM procedure is tuned to the case of detecting a change from Pareto$(3, 1)$ to Pareto$(2, 1)$. Table 15.5 provides values for the out-of control ARL for various values of θ. For the parametric CUSUM procedure the tabulated values were obtained by simulation using 10,000 replicated samples of T. The values for the nested plan are exact. All procedures have critical values selected so as to yield a nominal in-control ARL equal to 1000. The critical values of the CUSUM procedure are evaluated by simulation. For the nested plan all values are obtained by our explicit results for the in-control and out-of-control ARL.

Table 15.4. Out-of-control expectation and standard deviation of the run length of the CUSUM parametric procedures (by simulation) and those of the proposed nested plan (exact) for detecting univariate normal shifts

μ_h	Rule	$E_{\mu_h}(T)$	$\sigma_{\mu_h}(T)$
0.00	CUSUM	1005.08	995.19
0.00	$\prod_{nes}(n = 4; d = 3)$	1000.00	992.52
0.25	CUSUM	146.59	138.93
0.25	$\prod_{nes}(n = 4; d = 3)$	179.28	172.36
0.50	CUSUM	38.24	30.78
0.50	$\prod_{nes}(n = 4; d = 3)$	52.26	45.91
0.75	CUSUM	17.31	11.30
0.75	$\prod_{nes}(n = 4; d = 3)$	22.94	16.89
1.00	CUSUM	10.60	5.50
1.00	$\prod_{nes}(n = 4; d = 3)$	13.74	7.67
1.25	CUSUM	7.50	3.28
1.25	$\prod_{nes}(n = 4; d = 3)$	10.26	3.91

Table 15.5. Out-of-control expectation and standard deviation of the run length of the CUSUM parametric procedures (by simulation) and those of the proposed nested plan (exact) for detecting a change in the parameter of the Pareto (θ, λ) distribution

θ_h	Rule	$E_{\theta_h}(T)$	$\sigma_{\theta_h}(T)$
3.0	CUSUM	1018.24	998.11
3.0	$\prod_{nes}(n = 9; d = 4)$	1000.00	980.28
2.5	CUSUM	130.32	115.13
2.5	$\prod_{nes}(n = 9; d = 4)$	166.73	149.67
2.0	CUSUM	36.78	24.49
2.0	$\prod_{nes}(n = 9; d = 4)$	49.55	34.39
1.5	CUSUM	16.16	9.29
1.5	$\prod_{nes}(n = 9; d = 4)$	25.01	10.09

From Table 15.5 it turns out that these comparisons are rather similar to the same comparisons of the previous example for the univariate normal observations. That is, the speed of detection of a change for the proposed nested plan is about 20–25 percent worse than those of the optimal CUSUM procedure.

References

1. Anderson, T. W. (1958). *An Introduction to Multivariate Statistical Analysis*, John Wiley & Sons, New York, London.

2. Crosier, R. B. (1988). Multivariate generalizations of cumulative sum quality-control Schemes, *Technometrics, 30*, 291–303.

3. Feigin, P., Gurevich, G., and Lumelskii, Ya. (2005). Nested plans and the sequential change point problems, In *Proceedings of the International Symposium on Stochastic Models in Reliability, Safety Security and Logistics*, pp. 107–110, Beer Sheva, Israel.

4. Gordon, L. and Pollak, M. (1994). An efficient sequential nonparametric scheme for detecting a change of distribution, *Annals of Statistics, 22*, 763–804.

5. Hald, A. (1981). *Statistical Theory of Sampling Inspection by Attributes*, Academic Press, London.

6. Lai, T. L. (1995). Sequential changepoint detection in quality control and dynamical systems, *Journal of the Royal Statistical Society, Series B, 57*, 1–33.

7. Lumelskii, Ya. P. and Chichagov, V. V. (1983). A testing stopping rule, *Reliability and Quality Control, 3*, 22–28 (in Russian).

8. Lumelskii, Ya. P. and Feigin, P. D. (2005). Embedded polynomial plans of random walks and their applications, *Journal of Mathematical Sciences, 127*, 2103–2113.

9. Lumelskii, Ya., Gurevich, G., and Feigin, P. D. (2006). Nested plans as sequential quality control schemes for detecting change in multivariate normal distribution, *Quality Technology and Quantitative Management, 3*, 493–512.

10. Zacks, S. (1991). Detection and change-point problems, In *Handbook of Sequential Analysis* (Eds., B. K. Ghosh and P. K. Sen), pp. 531–562, Marcel Dekker, New York.

16

Sampling in Survival Analysis and Estimation with Unknown Selection Bias and Censoring

Agathe Guilloux

LSTA, Université Pierre et Marie Curie, Paris, France

Abstract: In a population of individuals, where the random variable (r.v.) σ denotes the birth time and X the lifetime, we consider that an individual can be observed only if its life-line $\mathcal{L}(\sigma, X) = \{(\sigma + y, y), 0 \leq y \leq X\}$ intersects a general Borel set $\mathcal{S}$ in $\mathbb{R} \times \mathbb{R}_+$. Denoting by $\sigma_{\mathcal{S}}$ and $X_{\mathcal{S}}$ the birth time and lifetime for the observed individuals, we point out that the distribution function (d.f.) $F_{\mathcal{S}}$ of the r.v. $X_{\mathcal{S}}$ suffers from a selection bias in the sense that $F_{\mathcal{S}} = \int w dF / \mu_{\mathcal{S}}$, where w and $\mu_{\mathcal{S}}$ depend only on the distribution of σ and F is the d.f. of X. Considering in addition that the r.v. $X_{\mathcal{S}}$ is randomly right-censored, as soon as the individual is selected, we construct a product-limit estimator $\hat{F}_{\mathcal{S}}$ for the d.f. $F_{\mathcal{S}}$ and a nonparametric estimator $\hat{w}$ for the weighting function w. We investigate the behavior of these estimators through a simulation study.

Keywords and Phrases: Lexis diagram, nonparametric inference, right-censored data, selection-bias, weighting or biasing function

16.1   Introduction

Consider a population of individuals $i \in I$. Let the random variable (r.v.) σ_i be the birth date of individual i and the nonnegative r.v. X_i its lifetime. As described by Keiding (1990) and Lund (2000), such a population can be represented in the following way. Consider a coordinate system with the calendar time as abscissa and the age as ordinate, which is referred to as the Lexis diagram [Lexis (1875)]. In this diagram, a life-line $\mathcal{L}(\sigma, X)$ is defined by:

$$\mathcal{L}(\sigma, X) = \{(\sigma + y, y), 0 \leq y \leq X\}.$$

Hence the life-line $\mathcal{L}(\sigma, X)$ is a segment with slope 1 joining the point $(\sigma, 0)$ of birth and the point $(\sigma + X, X)$ of death. The population I is then represented in the Lexis diagram as the set of all life-lines $\mathcal{L}(\sigma_i, X_i)$ for $i \in I$; see Figure 16.1.

In classical survival analysis, one would consider that an i.i.d. sample (possibly censored) could be drawn from population I and then would estimate the distribution of X on the basis of this i.i.d. sample. In practice, however, it may happen that the way individuals are chosen for the study prevents observation of an i.i.d. sample directly from population I.

As carefully described by Lund (2000), most of the sampling patterns in survival analysis can be described as follows. Let $\mathcal{S}$ be a deterministic Borel set in the Lexis diagram. Consider now that only the individuals whose life-lines intersect the Borel set $\mathcal{S}$ can be included in the study, that is, the individuals with a pair (σ, X) such that $\mathcal{L}(\sigma, X) \cap \mathcal{S} \neq \emptyset$. In Figure 16.1 only the individual with bold life-lines is included in the study.

Let $\sigma_{\mathcal{S}}$ denote the birth time and $X_{\mathcal{S}}$ the lifetime for the included individuals. From now on, the pair $(\sigma_{\mathcal{S}}, X_{\mathcal{S}})$ is referred to as the observable r.v. as opposed to the unobservable pair (σ, X). Straightforwardly, we have for all $s \in \mathbb{R}$ and $t \geq 0$:

$$\mathbb{P}(\sigma_{\mathcal{S}} \leq s, X_{\mathcal{S}} \leq t) = \mathbb{P}\left(\sigma \leq s, X \leq t | \mathcal{L}(\sigma, X) \cap \mathcal{S} \neq \emptyset\right) \neq \mathbb{P}(\sigma \leq s, X \leq t).$$

More precisely, we show in Section 16.2 that, under some condition on the collection $(\sigma_i)_{i \in I}$, we have, for all $t \geq 0$:

$$F_{\mathcal{S}}(t) = \mathbb{P}\left(X_{\mathcal{S}} \leq t\right) = \frac{\int_{[0,t]} w(v) dF(v)}{\mu_{\mathcal{S}}}, \tag{16.1}$$

where F is the distribution function (d.f.) of the r.v. X and w is a nonnegative weight function, which depends only on the distribution of the r.v. σ and $\mu_{\mathcal{S}} = \int_0^\infty w(v) dF(v)$.

The r.v. $X_{\mathcal{S}}$ with d.f. $F_{\mathcal{S}}$ given in Equation (16.1) is usually said to suffer from a selection bias. In the case where the weight function w is known, the problem of estimating the cumulative distribution function (d.f.) F of X given an i.i.d. biased sample $X_{\mathcal{S},1}, \ldots, X_{\mathcal{S},n}$ has received a lot of attention. We refer to Gill et al. (1988), Efromovich (2004), and de Uña-Àlvarez (2004a) for theoretical results in the general case. The special case where $w(x) = x$ for all $x > 0$, called "length-biased sampling," has received particular attention, see Vardi (1982), de Uña-Àlvarez (2002), Asgharian et al. (2002), and de Uña-Àlvarez and Saavedra (2004). Unfortunately these results cannot be applied here as w is not assumed to be known.

On the other hand, Winter and Földes (1988) have constructed and studied a product-limit type estimator of the d.f. F on the basis of a censored biased sample of (σ_S, X_S), without assuming that w is known. They still considered the particular case where $S = \{(t_0, y), y \geq 0\}$ and the censoring times are deterministic.

Selection-biased data can also be considered as a special form of truncated data, as (σ, X) is observed conditionally on $\mathcal{L}(\sigma, X) \cap S \neq \emptyset$. There is an extensive literature on nonparametric estimation for the cumulative distribution function under left truncation. We refer to Woodroofe (1985), Wang *et al.* (1986), and Chen *et al.* (1995) among others.

The problem addressed here is to estimate the d.f. F of the r.v. X as well as the weight function w on the basis of an i.i.d. censored (in a way defined later) sample of (σ_S, X_S). The outline of this chapter is as follows. In Section 16.2, the relations between the distributions of (σ, X) and (σ_S, X_S) for a general set S are derived and the form of the censoring is introduced. An uniformly consistent product-limit estimator for the d.f. F of the r.v. X is developed in Section 16.3 on the basis of a selection-biased sample and under censoring. Section 16.4 is dedicated to the estimation of the weight function w and a consistency result is stated. A simulation study is conducted in Section 16.5.

16.2   Sampling in the Lexis Diagram

16.2.1   Modeling the Lexis diagram

Consider the Lexis diagram for a population of individuals $i \in I$ as described in Section 16.1 and a Borel set S in $\mathcal{B}_{\mathbb{R} \times \mathbb{R}_+}$ (the Borel σ-algebra on $\mathbb{R} \times \mathbb{R}_+$) describing the sampling pattern (see Figure 16.1). As mentioned earlier, an individual i in the population, with birth date σ_i and lifetime X_i, is included in the sample if its life-line $\mathcal{L}(\sigma_i, X_i)$ intersects the Borel set S.

Let the age $a_S(s)$ at inclusion for the birth time s in $\mathbb{R}$ be defined as

$$\left\{ \begin{array}{l} a_S(s) = \inf\{y \geq 0, (s + y, y) \in S\} \\ a_S(s) = \infty \text{ if the infimum does not exist.} \end{array} \right.$$

The individual i with birth date σ_i and lifetime X_i is then included in the sample if:

$$\mathcal{L}(\sigma_i, X_i) \cap S \neq \emptyset \Leftrightarrow a_S(\sigma_i) < \infty \quad \text{and} \quad X_i \geq a_S(\sigma_i). \tag{16.2}$$

See indeed in Figure 16.1 that individual 1 is included in the sample; individual 2 could have been included but he died before its inclusion $x_2 < a_S(s_2)$, whereas individual 3 is not included because $a_S(s_3) = \infty$.

We assume that the point process $\eta = \sum_{i \in I} \varepsilon_{\sigma_i}$, with the collection of birth times as occurrence times, is a nonhomogeneous Poisson process on $\mathbb{R}$ with

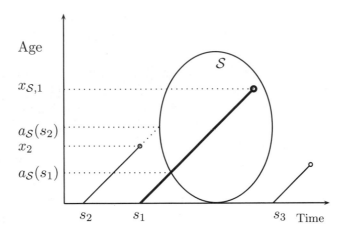

Figure 16.1. Age at inclusion.

intensity φ (where ε_a is the Dirac measure at point a), and that the lifetimes X_i, for $i \in I$, are i.i.d. with common probability density function (p.d.f.) f.

As a consequence and from Equation (16.2), we have, for all $s \in \mathbb{R}$ and $t \in \mathbb{R}_+$:

$$\mathbb{P}\left(\sigma_{\mathcal{S}} \leq s, X_{\mathcal{S}} \leq t\right) = \frac{\int\int_{]-\infty,s]\times[0,t]} I\left((u,v) \in \mathcal{S}\right)\varphi(u)f(v)dudv}{\int\int_{\mathbb{R}\times\mathbb{R}_+} I\left((u,v) \in \mathcal{S}\right)\varphi(u)f(v)dudv}$$

$$= \frac{\int\int_{]-\infty,s]\times[0,t]} I\left(\{a_{\mathcal{S}}(u) < \infty\}\right) I\left(\{a_{\mathcal{S}}(u) \leq v\}\right)\varphi(u)f(v)dudv}{\mu_{\mathcal{S}}},$$

where

$$\mu_{\mathcal{S}} = \int\int_{\mathbb{R}\times\mathbb{R}_+} I\left(\{a_{\mathcal{S}}(u) < \infty\}\right) I\left(\{a_{\mathcal{S}}(u) \leq v\}\right)\varphi(u)f(v)dudv.$$

Hence the marginal distribution of the r.v. $X_{\mathcal{S}}$ is given, for all $t \in \mathbb{R}_+$, by:

$$\begin{aligned} F_{\mathcal{S}}(t) &= \mathbb{P}\left(X_{\mathcal{S}} \leq t\right) = \frac{1}{\mu_{\mathcal{S}}} \int_0^t w(s)f(s)ds \\ &= \frac{1}{\mu_{\mathcal{S}}} \int_{\mathbb{R}} I\left(\{a_{\mathcal{S}}(u) \leq t\}\right)\varphi(u)\{1 - F(a_{\mathcal{S}}(u))\}du - \frac{1}{\mu_{\mathcal{S}}}w(t)(1 - F(t)), \end{aligned}$$

with

$$\begin{aligned} w(t) &= \int_{-\infty}^{\infty} I\left(\{a_{\mathcal{S}}(u) < \infty\}\right) I\left(\{a_{\mathcal{S}}(u) \leq t\}\right)\varphi(u)du \qquad (16.3) \\ &= \int_{-\infty}^{\infty} I\left(\{a_{\mathcal{S}}(u) \leq t\}\right)\varphi(u)du. \end{aligned}$$

On the other hand, the marginal distribution of the r.v. σ_S is given, for all $s \in \mathbb{R}$, by:

$$\Phi_S(s) = \mathbb{P}(\sigma_S \leq s) = \frac{1}{\mu_S} \int_{-\infty}^{s} \varphi(u) \bar{F}(a_S(u)) du, \qquad (16.4)$$

where $\bar{F} = 1 - F$. Our aim is then to estimate the functions F and w on the basis of a biased (censored) sample from (σ_S, X_S).

16.2.2 Censored observations

Now only the individuals whose life-lines intersect the Borel set S are included in the study. For included individual i, with birth date $\sigma_{S,i}$ and lifetime $X_{S,i}$, we assume that its age at inclusion $a_S(\sigma_{S,i})$ is observable. The lifetime $X_{S,i}$ can straightforwardly be written as follows.

$$X_{S,i} \quad = \quad \underbrace{a_S(\sigma_{S,i})}_{\text{age at inclusion}} \quad + \quad \underbrace{(X_{S,i} - a_S(\sigma_{S,i}))}_{\text{time spent in the study}}.$$

As the time spent in the study is given by $X_{S,i} - a_S(\sigma_{S,i})$, we assume that this time can be censored. It would indeed be the case, for example, if individual i leaves the study before its death. We follow here Asgharian (2003) and Winter and Földes (1988).

For that matter, we introduce a nonnegative r.v. C with d.f. H and independent of X_S and $a_S(\sigma_S)$, such that the observable time for individual i is

$$Z_i = a_S(\sigma_{S,i}) \quad + \quad (X_{S,i} - a_S(\sigma_{S,i})) \wedge C_i.$$

As usual, we assume furthermore that the r.v. $I\left(\{X_{S,i} - a_S(\sigma_{S,i}) \leq C\}\right)$ [where $I(.)$ is the indicator function] is observable. As a consequence, the available data are i.i.d. replications of:

$$\begin{cases} \sigma_{S,i} \\ Z_i = a_S(\sigma_{S,i}) + (X_{S,i} - a_S(\sigma_{S,i})) \wedge C_i \\ \delta_i = I\left(\{X_{S,i} - a_S(\sigma_{S,i}) \leq C_i\}\right) \end{cases}$$

for $i = 1, \ldots, n$.

We seek to estimate the d.f. F of the unbiased r.v. X as well as the weight function w defined in Equation (16.3) with the data described above. Remark that the data described above are close to the left-truncated and right-censored data or interval-censored data, however, with some modifications. First of all, individuals with $a_S(\sigma) = \infty$ are totally ineligible to enter the study irrespective of the duration of their lifetimes. Moreover the particular form of censoring considered here is strictly adapted to the selection mechanism.

16.3   Inference for the Distribution of the r.v. X

Considering the situation of interest described in Section 16.2, we now introduce the counting process D defined, for all $t \geq 0$, as follows.

$$D(t) = \sum_{i=1}^{n} I\left(\{Z_i \leq t, X_{\mathcal{S},i} - a_{\mathcal{S}}(\sigma_{\mathcal{S},i}) \leq C_i\}\right). \tag{16.5}$$

Notice that, for $t \geq 0$, the r.v. $D(t)$ is the "number of observed deaths before age t" in the sample. Let, furthermore, the process O be defined, for all $t \geq 0$, by:

$$
\begin{aligned}
O(t) &= \sum_{i=1}^{n} I\left(\{a_{\mathcal{S}}(\sigma_{\mathcal{S},i}) \leq t \leq Z_i\}\right) \\
&= \sum_{i=1}^{n} I\left(\{a_{\mathcal{S}}(\sigma_{\mathcal{S},i}) \leq t \leq X_{\mathcal{S},i}, t \leq a_{\mathcal{S}}(\sigma_{\mathcal{S},i}) + C_i\}\right). \tag{16.6}
\end{aligned}
$$

The r.v. $O(t)$ represents the "number of individuals at risk at age t." In the sampling situation considered here, to be at risk at age t for an individual means that it was included in the study at an age less than t and it did not experience death nor censoring before age t.

We are now in a position to define the estimator $\widehat{F}_n$ for the d.f. F of the r.v. X. Mimicking the construction of the Kaplan–Meier estimator in classical survival analysis, we define, for all $t \geq 0$:

$$\widehat{F}_n(t) = 1 - \prod_{i:Z_{(i)} \leq t} \left(1 - \frac{I\left(\{X_{\mathcal{S},i} - a_{\mathcal{S}}(\sigma_{\mathcal{S},i}) \leq C_i\}\right)}{O(Z_{(i)}) + n\epsilon_n}\right), \tag{16.7}$$

where $Z_{(1)}, \ldots, Z_{(n)}$ are the ordered statistics of the sample $Z_1, \ldots, Z_n$ and $(\epsilon_n)_{n \geq 1}$ is a sequence of positive numbers such that $\epsilon_n \to 0$ as $n \to \infty$. Notice indeed that the process O is not a monotone process and may be null for some s less than the largest observed $Z_{(n)}$. However, we have $O(Z_i) \geq 1$ for all $i = 1, \ldots, n$ by definition. Consequently, to avoid the problem of multiplying by zero in the estimator [it would be the case when $O(Z_i) = 1$], it is necessary to introduce the sequence $n\epsilon_n$ in the denominator. Such a slight modification will not affect the asymptotic properties of the estimator.

Even though the construction of $\widehat{F}_n$ presented above is closely related to the one of the product-limit type estimator introduced by Winter and Földes (1988), our estimator generalizes theirs in the following ways. We consider here a general sampling set $\mathcal{S}$, an nonhomogeneous Poisson process, and a nondeterministic censoring r.v. C or, equivalently, a unknown weight function w and a nondeterministic censoring r.v. C.

The following theorem states the uniform consistency of $\widehat{F}_n$; see Guilloux (2006) for a proof.

Theorem 16.3.1 *Let τ be defined as $\tau = \sup\{t > 0, (1 - F(t))(1 - H(t)) > 0\}$ and assume that, for all $t \geq 0$, we have $w_1 \leq w(t)$. The following convergence holds, for all $\tau' < \tau$, as n goes to infinity:*

$$\sup_{t \leq \tau'} |\widehat{F}_n(t) - F(t)| \xrightarrow{\mathbb{P}} 0.$$

Remark. If the interior of $\mathcal{S} \cap \{(x, 0), x \in \mathbb{R}\}$ is nonempty, the bound w_1 exists. This is, in particular, the case for the time-window and cohort studies when $t_1 \neq t_2$. The condition $w_1 \leq w(t)$ could be replaced by $\int_0^\infty dF(w)/w(x) < \infty$, as in de Uña-Àlvarez (2004b), which is uncheckable in practice.

16.4   Inference for the Weight Function w

The weighting function w has been defined, for all $t \geq 0$, by:

$$w(t) = \int_{-\infty}^{\infty} I\left(\{a_{\mathcal{S}}(u) \leq t\}\right) \varphi(u) du.$$

From Equation (16.4), we have, for all $t \geq 0$:

$$\frac{w(t)}{\mu_{\mathcal{S}}} = \int_{-\infty}^{\infty} \frac{I\left(\{a_{\mathcal{S}}(u) \leq t\}\right)}{(1 - F)(a_{\mathcal{S}}(u))} d\Phi_{\mathcal{S}}(u).$$

A natural estimator for the function $w/\mu_{\mathcal{S}}$ based on the i.i.d. sample described in Section 16.2.2 is then given by:

$$\frac{\widehat{w(t)}}{\mu_{\mathcal{S}}} = \frac{1}{n} \sum_{i=1}^{n} \frac{I\left(\{a_{\mathcal{S}}(\sigma_{\mathcal{S},i}) \leq t\}\right)}{1 - \widehat{F}_n(a_{\mathcal{S}}(\sigma_{\mathcal{S},i}))}, \tag{16.8}$$

where $\widehat{F}_n$ has been defined in Equation (16.7) of Section 16.3. From the construction of $\widehat{F}_n$, it follows that, for all $t \geq 0$, we have:

$$(1 - F_n(t)) \geq \left(1 - \frac{1}{1 + n\epsilon_n}\right)^n = \frac{1}{\kappa_n}. \tag{16.9}$$

Because $\mathbb{P}(a_{\mathcal{S}}(\sigma_{\mathcal{S},i}) < X_{\mathcal{S},i}) = 1$, the estimator $\widehat{w/\mu_{\mathcal{S}}}$ is bounded. Equation (16.8) is straightforwardly equivalent to:

$$\frac{\widehat{w(t)}}{\mu_{\mathcal{S}}} = \int \frac{I\{a_{\mathcal{S}}(s) \leq t\}}{1 - \widehat{F}_n(a_{\mathcal{S}}(s))} d\left(\widehat{\Phi}_{\mathcal{S},n}(s)\right) \quad \text{for all } t \geq 0,$$

where, for all $s \geq 0$:

$$\widehat{\Phi}_{\mathcal{S},n}(s) = \frac{1}{n} \sum_{i=1}^{n} I\left(\{\sigma_{\mathcal{S},i} \leq s\}\right)$$

is the empirical counterpart of $\mathbb{P}\left(\sigma_{\mathcal{S}} \leq s\right)$.

The following theorem is then a consequence of the Glivenko–Cantelli theorem and the consistency of Theorem 16.3.1.

Theorem 16.4.1 *Let τ be defined as $\tau = \sup\{t > 0, (1 - F(t))(1 - H(t)) > 0\}$. The following convergence holds, for all $\tau' \leq \tau$, as n goes to infinity,*

$$\sup_{t \leq \tau'} \left| \frac{\widehat{w(t)}}{\mu_{\mathcal{S}}} - \frac{w(t)}{\mu_{\mathcal{S}}} \right| \xrightarrow{\mathbb{P}} 0.$$

16.5   Simulation Study

We present here an example of a sampling pattern, which can be described through a Borel set in $\mathcal{B}_{\mathbb{R} \times \mathbb{R}_+}$: the time-window study. The individuals alive at time t_1 as well as those born between t_1 and t_2 are included in the study, where t_1 and t_2 are fixed in advance; see Figure 16.2. In this case, the Borel set to be considered is:

$$\mathcal{S}_{tw} = \{(s, y), s \leq t_2, s + y \geq t_1\}.$$

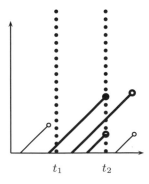

Figure 16.2. Time-window study.

The age $a_{\mathcal{S}_{tw}}$ at inclusion is then given by:

$$\begin{cases} a_{\mathcal{S}_{tw}}(\sigma) = t_1 - \sigma & \text{if} \quad -\infty < \sigma \le t_1 \\ a_{\mathcal{S}_{tw}}(\sigma) = 0 & \text{if} \quad t_1 < \sigma \le t_2 \\ a_{\mathcal{S}_{tw}}(\sigma) = +\infty & \text{if} \quad \sigma > t_2 \end{cases}$$

and finally the weight function w is given, for $t \ge 0$, by:

$$w(t) = \int_{t_1-t}^{t_2} \varphi(u)du.$$

In the particular case where $t_1 = t_2$ and φ is a constant, such a sample is referred to as a "length-biased sample;" see Asgharian *et al.* (2002) and de Uña-Àlvarez (2002). We refer to Lund (2000) for an extensive review of studies described via the Lexis diagram.

We now have to build an n-sample of $(\sigma_{\mathcal{S}}, Z, \delta)$ and for this purpose, the steps are the following:

1. Given $t_1, t_2 > 0$ with $t_1 < t_2$, draw N birth-times $(\sigma_i)_{i=1,\dots,N}$ on $\mathbb{R}^+$ as realizations of a Poisson process with given intensity $\varphi(s) \propto s^{-2/3}$ (inhomogeneous Poisson process) resulting in a power bias (denoted by PB) $w(t) \propto t^{1/3}$. For the simulations of an inhomogeneous Poisson process, we refer to Devroye (1986). Moreover, the intensity φ is "calibrated" in functions of the values t_1 and t_2 such that the generated birth-times satisfy both conditions: with probability near 1, at least n lifetimes X_is fall in the time-window $[t_1, t_2]$ and the largest simulated birth-time σ_N would exceed t_2. Notice that N is much greater than n.

2. For each birth-time σ_i, draw the associated lifetime X_i with given d.f F.

3. Inclusion in the study: the age at inclusion $a_{\mathcal{S}}(\sigma_{\mathcal{S},i})$ in the study is given by $a_{\mathcal{S}}(\sigma_{\mathcal{S},i}) = t_1 - \sigma_i$ if $\sigma_i \le t_1$ and $a_{\mathcal{S}}(\sigma_{\mathcal{S},i}) = 0$ if $t_1 \le \sigma_i \le t_2$. So, choose the $X_i = X_{\mathcal{S},i}$ such that $a_{\mathcal{S}}(\sigma_{\mathcal{S},i}) \le t_1$ and $X_i \ge a_{\mathcal{S}}(\sigma_{\mathcal{S},i})$. This mechanism of inclusion in the study involves a bias selection and we keep only selected couples $(a_{\mathcal{S}}(\sigma_{\mathcal{S},i}), X_{\mathcal{S},i})$.

4. Draw an n-sample $(\sigma_{\mathcal{S},1}, X_{\mathcal{S},1}), \dots, (\sigma_{\mathcal{S},n}, X_{\mathcal{S},n})$ by uniform random sampling among all the individuals falling in the time-window and selected in Step 3.

5. Draw the censoring variables $C_1, \dots, C_n$ with exponential d.f. $\mathcal{E}(c)$ for several values of $c > 0$ involving different censoring proportions.

6. Put $Z_i = (t_1 - \sigma_{\mathcal{S},i}) + (X_{\mathcal{S},i} - (t_1 - \sigma_{\mathcal{S},i})) \wedge C_i$ if $\sigma_{\mathcal{S},i} \le t_1$ and $Z_i = X_{\mathcal{S},i} \wedge C_i$ if $t_1 \le \sigma_{\mathcal{S},i} \le t_2$.

We consider two distributions for the initial lifetime X: the gamma distributions with parameters, respectively, $\Gamma(1, 0.5)$ and $\Gamma(1, 1.5)$. We conduct the study for three sample sizes $n = 50, 100, 150$ and three levels of censoring, approximatively 0%, 25%, and 50%. The values of $\sup_{[0,\infty]} |\hat{F}_n - F|$ are reported in

Table 16.1. $X \sim \Gamma(1, 0.5)$

n	Generalized W&F	K&M Censoring	Forward Censoring	Usual
	0.1400	0.1216	0	0
50	0.1366	0.1221	0.1968	0.2516
	0.1669	0.1654	0.5044	0.4544
	0.0961	0.0857	0	0
100	0.1083	0.0908	0.2069	0.2583
	0.1143	0.1223	0.5035	0.4492
	0.0786	0.0690	0	0
150	0.0835	0.1030	0.1958	0.2605
	0.0992	0.0993	0.5035	0.4563

Table 16.2. $X \sim \Gamma(1, 1.5)$

n	Generalized W&F	K&M Censoring	Forward Censoring	Usual
	0.1489	0.1212	0	0
50	0.1531	0.1340	0.1798	0.2250
	0.1658	0.1736	0.5020	0.5014
	0.1016	0.0829	0	0
100	0.1045	0.0874	0.1786	0.2317
	0.1234	0.1369	0.4942	0.5128
	0.0796	0.0686	0	0
150	0.0853	0.0685	0.1786	0.2291
	0.0991	0.1136	0.5025	0.5107

Tables 16.1 and 16.2, as well as the level of censoring, for each sample size. We compare the deviation $\sup_{[0,\infty]} |\hat{F}_n - F|$ with the one obtained for the Kaplan–Meier estimator in a standard situation, that is, without selection bias. We called our estimator "generalized W&F" and the censoring in this situation "forward censoring," referring to Winter and Földes (1988). The Kaplan–Meier estimator is referred to as "K&M" and the censoring as "usual censoring."

In this biased case with censoring, we get very conforming results to those obtained in the usual case, that is, with independent censoring and the Kaplan–Meier estimator. Indeed, in the gamma case studied therein, the two deviation measures are of the same order in each case studied. Besides, the censoring effect degrades the deviation measures in both cases. This confirms the theoretical results stated above, in the sense that our estimator is accurate even in the presence of selection bias.

References

1. Asgharian, M. (2003). Biased sampling with right censoring: A note on Sun, Cui & Tiwari (2002), *Canadian Journal of Statistics*, **30**, 475–490.

2. Asgharian, M., M'Lan, C. E., and Wolfson, D. B. (2002). Length-biased sampling with right censoring: An unconditional approach, *Journal of the American Statistical Association*, **97**, 201–209.

3. Chen, K., Chao, M.-T., and Lo, S.-H. (1995). On strong uniform consistency of the Lynden-Bell estimator for truncated data, *Annals of Statistics*, **23**, 440–449.

4. Devroye, L. (1986). *Non-Uniform Random Variate Generation*, Springer-Verlag, New York.

5. Efromovich, S. (2004). Distribution estimation for biased data, *Journal of Statistical Planning and Inference*, **124**, 1–43.

6. Gill, R.D., Vardi, Y., and Wellner, J. A. (1988). Large sample theory of empirical distributions in biased sampling models, *Annals of Statistics*, **16**, 1069–1172.

7. Guilloux, A. (2006). Non-parametric estimation for censored lifetimes suffering from an unknown selection bias. Submitted and prepublication of the LSTA 2006-04, Université Pierre et Marie Curie Paris VI, France.

8. Keiding, N. (1990). Statistical inference for the Lexis diagram, *The Royal Society of London. Philosophical Transactions. Series A. Mathematical, Physical and Engineering Sciences*, **332**, 487–509.

9. Lexis, W. (1875). Einleitung in die Theorie der Bevölkerung-Statistik, In *Mathematical Demography* (Eds., D. Smith and N. Keyfitz), *Biomathematics*, **6**, 39–41 (1977). Springer-Verlag, Berlin.

10. Lund, J. (2000). Sampling bias in population studies - How to use the Lexis diagram, *Scandinavian Journal of Statistics*, **27**, 589–604.

11. de Uña-Àlvarez, J. (2002). Product-limit estimation for length-biased censored data, *Test*, **11**, 109–125.

12. de Uña-Álvarez, J. (2004a). Nonparametric estimation under length-biased sampling and type I censoring: A moment based approach, *Annals of the Institute of Statistical Mathematics*, **56**, 667–681.

13. de Uña-Álvarez, J. (2004b). Nelson-Aalen and product-limit estimation in selection bias models for censored populations, *Journal of Nonparametric Statistics*, **16**, 761–777.

14. de Uña-Álvarez, J. and Saavedra, Á. (2004). Bias and variance of the nonparametric MLE under length-biased censored sampling: A simulation study. *Communications in Statistics—Simulation and Computation*, **33**, 397–413.

15. Vardi, Y. (1982). Nonparametric estimation in presence of length bias, *Annals of Statitics*, **10**, 616–620.

16. Wang, M-C., Jewell, N. P., and Tsai, W. Y. (1986). Asymptotic properties of the product limit estimate under random truncation, *Annals of Statistics*, **14**, 1597–1605.

17. Winter, B. B. and Földes, A. (1988) A product-limit estimator for use with length-biased data, *Canadian Journal of Statistics*, **16**, 337–355.

18. Woodroofe, M. (1985). Estimating a distribution function with truncated data, *Annals of Statistics*, **13**, 163–177.

17

Testing the Acceleration Function in Lifetime Models

Hannelore Liero[1] and Matthias Liero[2]

[1]*Institute of Mathematics, University of Potsdam, Potsdam, Germany*
[2]*Institute of Mathematics, Humboldt–University of Berlin, Berlin, Germany*

Abstract: The accelerated lifetime model is considered. First, test procedures for testing the parameter of a parametric acceleration function are investigated; this is done under the assumption of parametric and nonparametric baseline distribution. Furthermore, based on nonparametric estimators for regression functions, tests are proposed for checking whether a parametric acceleration function is appropriate to model the influence of the covariates. Resampling procedures are discussed for the realization of these methods. Simulations complete the considerations.

Keywords and Phrases: Accelerated lifetime model, parametric regression, nonparametric regression estimation, L_2-type test, resampling, simulation

17.1 Introduction

Let T be a random lifetime that depends on some explanatory variable X; examples for X are the dose of a drug, temperature, or stress. To describe the influence of the covariate X on the lifetime there are several proposals. A well-known model is the accelerated lifetime model (ALT), which is intensively studied in Bagdonavičius and Nikulin (2001). In distinction from the models studied by these authors we assume throughout the chapter that the covariate does not depend on time. We suppose that the covariate X reduces a basic lifetime, say T_0, by a factor $\psi(X)$ and write the lifetime T as

$$T = \frac{T_0}{\psi(X)}.$$

The conditional survival function of T given $X = x$ is defined by

$$S(t|x) = \mathsf{P}(T > t|X = x) = S_0(t\psi(x)),$$

where $S_0(\cdot) = \mathsf{P}(T_0 > \cdot)$ is the survival function of the baseline lifetime T_0. The distribution function is denoted by F_0. It is assumed that T is an absolute continuous random variable.

In the present chapter we study the problem of testing the acceleration function ψ. Different assumptions on the baseline distribution and the considered class of acceleration functions require different test methods. We study these different constellations of the underlying model. Given independent copies (T_i, X_i), $i = 1, \ldots, n$ of the pair (T, X) we propose test statistics and consider their limit distributions under the hypotheses. Test procedures formulated on the basis of these limit statements are only *asymptotic* α-tests. Thus it seems to be useful to discuss some resampling methods for the realization of these tests in practice. We complete these discussions by simulations. The program files (written in the R-language) for these simulations can be found on our Web site http://www.mathematik.hu-berlin.de/liero/.

17.2   The Parametric ALT Model

We start with the simplest model, namely the completely parametric model, where it is assumed that both the survival function S_0 and the acceleration function ψ belong to a known parametric class of functions. That is, there exist parameters $\nu \in \mathbb{R}^k$ and $\beta \in \mathbb{R}^d$ such that

$$S_0(t) = S_0(t; \nu) \quad \text{and} \quad \psi(x) = \psi(x; \beta),$$

where the functions $S_0(\cdot; \nu)$ and $\psi(\cdot; \beta)$ are known except the parameters ν and β. A hypothesis about the function ψ is then a hypothesis about the parameter β, and we consider the test problem

$$\mathcal{H} : \beta = \beta_0 \quad \text{against} \quad \mathcal{K} : \beta \neq \beta_0$$

for some $\beta_0 \in \mathbb{R}^d$.

The classical way for the construction of a test procedure is to estimate β by the maximum likelihood estimator (m.l.e.) and to use the likelihood ratio statistic (or a modification such as the Rao score statistic or the Wald statistic) for checking $\mathcal{H}$. In Bagdonavičius and Nikulin (2001) this approach is carried out for several distributions, for $\psi(x; \beta) = \exp(-x^T \beta)$, and for censored data.

Another possibility is to take the logarithm of the lifetime $Y = \log T$. Then with

$$m(x; \vartheta) = \mu - \log \psi(x; \beta) \qquad \vartheta = (\mu, \beta)$$

we obtain the parametric regression model

$$Y_i = m(X_i; \vartheta) + \varepsilon_i \tag{17.1}$$

with

$$\mu = \mathsf{E} \log T_0 = \mu(\nu) \qquad \text{and} \qquad \mathsf{E}\varepsilon_i = 0.$$

Assuming $\psi(0; \beta) = 1$ the parameter β can be estimated by the least squares estimator (l.s.e.).

In the case that T_0 is distributed according to the log normal distribution the resulting regression model is the normal model. Then the maximum likelihood estimator and the least squares estimator coincide. Furthermore, assuming $\psi(x; \beta) = \exp(-x^T \beta)$ we have the linear regression, and for testing $\mathcal{H}$ we apply the F-test, which is exact in this case.

Now, suppose that $\log T$ is not normally distributed. Then it is well known that under regularity conditions the m.l.e. for β is asymptotically normal, and an asymptotic α- test is provided by critical values derived from the corresponding limit distribution.

Let us propose another method, a resampling method, to determine critical values. We restrict our considerations here to the maximum likelihood method; the regression approach is discussed in detail in the following section. For simplicity of presentation we consider the case $d = 1$.

1. On the basis of the (original) data (t_i, x_i), $i = 1, \ldots, n$, compute the maximum likelihood estimates for ν and β, say $\hat{\nu}$ and $\hat{\beta}$.

2. For $r = 1, \ldots, R$

   (a) Generate

   $$t_i^* = \frac{t_{0i}^*}{\psi(x_i; \hat{\beta})} \qquad \text{where} \qquad t_{0i}^* \sim F_0(\cdot; \hat{\nu})$$

   (b) Compute the m.l.e. $\hat{\beta}^{*(r)}$ for each sample.

3. (a) *Naive approach.* Take the quantiles of the empirical distribution of these $\hat{\beta}^{*(r)}$s as critical values; that is, let $\hat{\beta}^{*[1]}, \hat{\beta}^{*[2]}, \ldots, \hat{\beta}^{*[R]}$ be the ordered estimates, then reject the hypothesis $\mathcal{H}$ if

   $$\beta_0 < \hat{\beta}^{*[R\alpha/2]} \quad \text{or} \quad \beta_0 > \hat{\beta}^{*[R(1-\alpha/2)]}.$$

   (The number R is chosen such that $R\alpha/2$ is an integer.)

   (b) *Corrected normal approach.* Estimate the bias and the variance of the estimator by

   $$b_R = \overline{\beta^*} - \hat{\beta}, \qquad v_R = \frac{1}{R-1} \sum_{r=1}^{R} (\hat{\beta}^{*(r)} - \overline{\beta^*})^2,$$

   where $\overline{\beta^*} = \frac{1}{R} \sum_{r=1}^{R} \hat{\beta}^{*(r)}$ and accept the hypothesis $\mathcal{H}$ if β_0 belongs to the interval

   $$[\hat{\beta} - b_R - \sqrt{v_R}\, u_{1-\alpha/2}\,, \ \hat{\beta} - b_R + \sqrt{v_R}\, u_{1-\alpha/2}].$$

Here $u_{1-\alpha/2}$ is the $1 - \alpha/2$-quantile of the standard normal distribution.

(c) *Basic bootstrap.* As estimator for the quantiles of the distribution of $\hat{\beta} - \beta$ take $\hat{\beta}^{*[R\alpha/2]} - \hat{\beta}$ and $\hat{\beta}^{*[R(1-\alpha/2)]} - \hat{\beta}$, respectively. Thus, accept $\mathcal{H}$ if β_0 belongs to

$$\left[\hat{\beta} - (\hat{\beta}^{*[R(1-\alpha/2)]} - \hat{\beta}), \, \hat{\beta} - (\hat{\beta}^{*[R\alpha/2]} - \hat{\beta})\right].$$

To demonstrate this proposal we have carried out the following **simulations:** As the baseline distribution we have chosen the exponential distribution, the covariates are uniformly distributed, and for computational simplicity the acceleration function has the form $\psi(x; \beta) = \exp(-x\beta)$.

We generated n realizations (t_i, x_i) of random variables (T_i, X_i). The X_is are uniformly distributed over $[2, 4]$; the T_is have the survival function

$$S(t|x_i) = \exp(-t\psi(x_i; \beta_0)/\nu) \quad \text{with} \quad \psi(x; \beta_0) = \exp(-x\beta_0)$$

for the parameters
$$n = 12, \qquad \beta_0 = 2, \qquad \nu = 2.$$

As values of the m.l.e. we obtained $\hat{\beta} = 1.82$ and $\hat{\nu} = 3.42$. The asymptotic confidence interval based on the asymptotic normality of the m.l.e. was:

$$[0.839, 2.800].$$

With $R - 1000$ resamples constructed by the methods given above we obtained as confidence intervals ($\alpha = 0.05$) for β:

Method	Lower Bound	Upper Bound
Naive approach	0.550	2.973
Corrected normal	0.681	2.979
Basic bootstrap	0.666	3.089

Figure 17.1 shows a histogram of the $\hat{\beta}^{*(r)}$s. In this case the true parameter $\beta_0 = 2$ is covered by all intervals, also by that based on the limit distribution. Moreover, this interval is shorter. We repeated this approach $M = 1000$ times. The number of cases, where the true parameter was not covered, say w, was counted. Here are the results.

Method	w
Asymptotic distribution	87
Naive approach	48
Corrected normal	50
Basic bootstrap	49

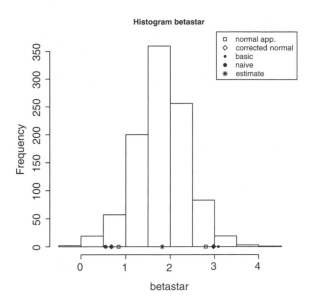

Figure 17.1. Histogram of the resampled betas.

Thus, the price for the shortness of the interval based on the normal approximation is that the coverage probability is not preserved. Furthermore, the results show no difference between the proposed resampling methods.

17.3 The ALT Model with Nonparametric Baseline Distribution

Consider the situation that the acceleration function ψ still has a known parametric form $\psi(\cdot; \beta)$, $\beta \in \mathbb{R}^d$ but the underlying distribution of the baseline lifetime is completely unknown. Thus we have an infinite-dimensional nuisance parameter and the application of the maximum likelihood method is not possible. We use the regression approach to estimate and to test the parameter β. Using the asymptotic normality of the l.s.e. in the regression model, often confidence intervals or tests for β are based on the quantiles of the normal ($d = 1$) or χ^2-distribution ($d > 1$). For large n the results will turn out satisfactorily. But for small n this asymptotic approach is not justified. Here one can use resampling procedures for regression; see, for example, Davison and Hinkley (1997) or Efron and Tibshirani (1993).

For simplicity we consider the problem of testing a single component β_j. In our simulation study we compared the following methods.

1. On the basis of the regression model (17.1) with the original data compute the l.s.e. $\hat{\mu}$ and $\hat{\beta}$ for μ and β, respectively. Derive the residuals e_i and let

$$r_i = \frac{e_i}{\sqrt{(1 - h_i)}} = \frac{y_i - \hat{y}_i}{\sqrt{(1 - h_i)}}$$

   be the modified residuals. Here the $\hat{y}_i$s are the fitted values $m(x_i; \hat{\mu}, \hat{\beta})$, and the h_is are the leverages.

   Let V be a variance estimator for the $\mathsf{Var}\hat{\beta}$.

2. For $r = 1, \ldots, R$,

   1. (a) *Model-based resampling*
           For $i = 1, \ldots, n$
           i. Set $x_i^* = x_i$.
           ii. Randomly sample ε_i^* from the centered modified residuals $r_1 - \overline{r}, \ldots, r_n - \overline{r}$.
           iii. Set $y_i^* = m(x_i^*; \hat{\mu}, \hat{\beta}) + \varepsilon_i^*$.
      (b) *Resampling cases*
           i. Sample $l_1^*, \ldots, l_n^*$ randomly with replacement from the index set $\{1, \ldots, n\}$.
           ii. For $i = 1, \ldots, n$ set $x_i^* = x_{l_i^*}$ and $y_i^* = y_{l_i^*}$.

   2. Derive the l.s.e. $\hat{\beta}^{*(r)}$ and the variance estimator $V^{*(r)}$ based on the observations (y_i^*, x_i^*).

   3. Compute the standardized

   $$z_j^{*(r)} = \frac{\hat{\beta}_j^{*(r)} - \hat{\beta}_j}{\sqrt{V_{jj}^{*(r)}}}.$$

3. A confidence interval for the component β_j is given by

$$\left[\hat{\beta}_j - \sqrt{V_{jj}}\, z_j^{*[R(1-\alpha/2)]} , \ \hat{\beta}_j - \sqrt{V_{jj}}\, z_j^{*[R\alpha/2]} \right].$$

For our simulation study we took the same parameter constellation as before. As estimator for the variance we used

$$V = \frac{\sum e_i^2}{n \sum (x_i - \overline{x})^2}.$$

Again this approach was repeated M times. In the following table confidence intervals constructed by the methods above ($R = 1000$, $M = 1$) are given; in the last column are the number of cases out of $M = 1000$, where the true parameter is not covered.

Method	Lower Bound	Upper Bound	w
Asymptotic normality	0.641	3.536	106
Model-based resampling	0.389	3.808	50
Resampling cases	0.752	4.00	58

We see that the resampling methods lead to much better results than the approach based on the limiting distribution.

17.4 The ALT Model with Parametric Baseline Distribution and Nonparametric Acceleration Function

Now, consider an ALT model where it is not assumed that the acceleration function has a parametric form, but we wish to check whether a prespecified parametric function $\psi(\cdot; \beta)$ fits the influence of the covariates. In this section we assume that the baseline distribution is known, except a finite-dimensional parameter ν. The test problem can be formulated in the following way:

$$\mathcal{H} : S \in \mathcal{A}_{\text{par}} \quad \text{against} \quad \mathcal{K} : S \in \mathcal{A}, \tag{17.2}$$

with

$$\mathcal{A}_{\text{par}} = \{S \mid S(t|x) = S_0(t\psi(x; \beta); \nu) \ \ \beta \in \mathbb{R}^d, \ \nu \in \mathbb{R}^k\}$$

and

$$\mathcal{A} = \{S \mid S(t|x) = S_0(t\psi(x); \nu) \ \ \psi \in \Psi, \ \nu \in \mathbb{R}^k\},$$

where Ψ is a nonparametric class of acceleration functions.

A possible solution for this test problem is to apply a goodness-of-fit test similar to the classical Kolmogorov test or the Cramér–von Mises test. The conditional survival function S can be estimated by a conditional empirical survival function $\hat{S}$, which is a special case of the so-called U-statistics considered by Stute (1991) and Liero (1999). Such a test would compare $\hat{S}$ with $S_0(\cdot \psi(\cdot; \hat{\beta}); \hat{\nu})$. But this approach seems to be inadequate. Namely the alternative does not consist of "all conditional survival functions," but of functions defined by $\mathcal{A}$, and $\hat{S}$ is an estimator, which is "good for all conditional survival functions."

So we follow the regression approach. Instead of (17.2) we consider model (17.1) and the test problem

$$\mathcal{H} : m \in \mathcal{M} \quad \text{against} \quad \mathcal{K} : m \notin \mathcal{M},$$

where

$$\mathcal{M} = \{m \mid m(x) = m(x; \vartheta) = \mu - \log \psi(x; \beta), \ \beta \in \mathbb{R}^d, \mu \in \mathbb{R}\}.$$

Again, for simplicity we consider $d = 1$, and as test statistic we propose an L_2-type distance between a good estimator for all possible regression functions m, that is, a nonparametric estimator, and a good approximation for the hypothetical $m \in \mathcal{M}$. The general form of a nonparametric estimator is the weighted average of the response variables

$$\hat{m}_n(x) = \sum_{i=1}^{n} W_{b_n i}(x, X_1, \ldots, X_n) Y_i,$$

where $W_{b_n i}$ are weights depending on a smoothing parameter b_n. The hypothetical regression function can be estimated by $m(\cdot; \hat{\beta}, \hat{\mu})$, where $\hat{\beta}$ and $\hat{\mu}$ are estimators under the hypothesis. It is well known that nonparametric estimators are biased; they are a result of smoothing. So it seems to be appropriate to compare $\hat{m}_n$ not with $m(\cdot; \hat{\beta}, \hat{\mu})$, but with the smoothed parametric estimator

$$\tilde{m}_n(x) = \sum_{i=1}^{n} W_{b_n i}(x, X_1, \ldots, X_n) m(X_i; \hat{\beta}, \hat{\mu}).$$

A suitable quantity to measure the distance between the functions $\hat{m}_n$ and $\tilde{m}_n$ is the L_2-distance

$$\begin{aligned} Q_n &= \int \left(\hat{m}_n(x) - \tilde{m}_n(x) \right)^2 a(x) \, \mathrm{d}x \\ &= \int \left(\sum_{i=1}^{n} W_{b_n i}(x, X_1, \ldots, X_n)(Y_i - m(X_i; \hat{\beta}, \hat{\mu})) \right)^2 a(x) \, \mathrm{d}x. \end{aligned}$$

Here a is a known weight function, which is introduced to control the region of integration. The limit distribution of (properly standardized) integrated squared distances is considered by several authors; we mention Collomb (1976), Liero (1992), and Härdle and Mammen (1993). Under appropriate conditions asymptotic normality can be proved.

For the presentation here let us consider kernel weights; that is, m is estimated nonparametrically by

$$\hat{m}_n(x) = \frac{\sum_{i=1}^{n} K_{b_n}(x - X_i) Y_i}{\sum_{i=1}^{n} K_{b_n}(x - X_i)},$$

where $K : \mathbb{R} \to \mathbb{R}$ is the kernel function, $K_b(x) = K(x/b)/b$, and b_n is a sequence of smoothing parameters. To formulate the limit statement for Q_n let us briefly summarize the assumptions.[1]

1. Regularity conditions on kernel K and conditions on the limiting behavior of b_n

2. Smoothness of the regression function m and the marginal density g of the X_is

3. Conditions ensuring the $\sqrt{n}$-consistency of the parameter estimators $\hat{\beta}$ and $\hat{\mu}$

If these assumptions are satisfied we have under $\mathcal{H}$,

$$nb_n^{1/2} \left(Q_n - e_n \right) \xrightarrow{\mathcal{D}} \mathrm{N}(0, \tau^2)$$

with

$$e_n = (nb_n)^{-1} \sigma^2 \kappa_1 \int g^{-1}(x)\, a(x)\, \mathrm{d}x \qquad \tau^2 = 2\sigma^4 \kappa_2 \int g^{-2}(x) a^2(x)\, \mathrm{d}x,$$

where

$$\kappa_1 = \int K^2(x)\, \mathrm{d}x \quad \text{and} \quad \kappa_2 = \int (K * K)^2(x)\, \mathrm{d}x$$

and

$$\sigma^2 = \sigma^2(\nu) = \mathsf{Var}(\log T_0).$$

On the basis of this limit theorem we can derive an asymptotic α-test: Reject the hypothesis $\mathcal{H}$ if

$$Q_n \geq (nb_n^{1/2})^{-1} \hat{\tau}_n z_\alpha + \hat{e}_n,$$

where $\hat{e}_n$ and $\hat{\tau}_n$ are appropriate estimators of the unknown constants e_n and τ^2, and $z\alpha$ is the $(1 - \alpha)$-quantile of the standard normal distribution. Note that the unknown variance σ^2 depends only on the parameter ν of the underlying baseline distribution. A simple estimator is $\hat{\sigma}^2 = \sigma^2(\hat{\nu})$. The density g is assumed to be known or can be estimated by the kernel method.

To demonstrate this approach we have carried out the following **simulations**. First we simulated the behavior under $\mathcal{H}$. We generated $M = 1000$ samples (t_i, x_i), $i = 1, \ldots, n$, with $t_i = t_{0i} \exp(x_i\beta)$, where the t_{0i}s are values of exponentially distributed random variables with expectation ν (β and ν as before). The sample size was $n = 100$, because the application of nonparametric curve estimation always requires a large sample size. In each sample the m.l.e.s $\hat{\beta}$ and $\hat{\nu}$ and the nonparametric kernel estimate were determined. To evaluate

---

[1]The detailed conditions can be found in Liero (1999).

the nonparametric estimates we used the normal kernel and an adaptive procedure for choosing b_n. Based on these estimators Q_n was computed. As weight function a we took the indicator of the interval $[2.25, 3.75]$; so problems with the estimation at boundaries were avoided. Note that in this case the variance σ^2 is known. It is $\sigma^2 = \pi^2/6$, independent of ν. Thus, in our simple simulation example it is not necessary to estimate e_n and τ. The result of the simulations was that $\mathcal{H}$ was rejected only once.

The error that occurs by approximating the distribution of the test statistic by the standard normal distribution depends not only on the sample size n but also on the smoothing parameter. Thus it can happen that this approximation is not good enough, even when n is large. So we considered the following resampling procedures.

Carry out Steps 1 and 2(a) described in Section 17.2. Continue with:

3. Based on the resampled (y_i^*, x_i), $y_i^* = \log(t_i^*)$ compute for $r = 1, \ldots, R$ the nonparametric estimates $\hat{m}_n^{*(r)}$ and the smoothed estimated hypothetical regression $\tilde{m}_n^{*(r)}$.

   (a) *Resampling Q_n*
       Evaluate the distances $Q_n^{*(1)}, Q_n^{*(2)}, \ldots, Q_n^{*(R)}$.

   (b) *Resampling T_n*
       Compute
       $$T_n^{*(r)} = n b_n^{(r)\,1/2} \left(Q_n^{*(r)} - \hat{e}_n^{*(r)} \right) / \hat{\tau}_n^{*(r)}.$$

4. From the ordered distances a critical value is given by $Q_n^{*[(1-\alpha)R]}$, and the hypothesis $\mathcal{H}$ is rejected if

$$Q_n > Q_n^{*[(1-\alpha)R]}.$$

Or, based on the $T_n^{*(r)}$s we obtain: the hypothesis $\mathcal{H}$ is rejected if

$$n b_n^{1/2} \left(Q_n - \hat{e}_n \right) / \hat{\tau}_n = T_n > T_n^{*[(1-\alpha)R]}.$$

Histograms of resampled $Q_n^{*(r)}$s and $T_n^{*(r)}$s for our chosen simulation parameters and $R = 1000$ are shown in Figure 17.2. We repeated this resampling procedure also M times. The numbers of rejections are given in the second column of the following table.

Method	Hypothesis True	Hypothesis Wrong
Normal distribution	39	349
Resampling Q_n	64	488
Resampling T_n	64	488

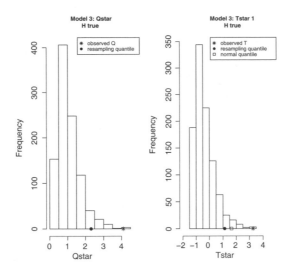

Figure 17.2. Resampling under $\mathcal{H}$, $R = 1000$.

Furthermore, we repeated the whole approach to demonstrate the behavior under an alternative. That means, our original data (t_i, x_i) satisfy the model

$$t_i = t_{0i} \exp(x_i\beta + \sin(\pi * x_i/2)),$$

where the baseline times t_{0i} are as above. The numbers of rejections in this simulation are also given in the table above. It turns out that the test based on the asymptotic distribution already leads to satisfactory results. The significance level $\alpha = 0.05$ is not preserved by the tests based on resampling; the power of the resampling procedures under the considered alternative is higher.

Furthermore, Figure 17.3 shows the simulation results for one resampling procedure ($M = 1$). In the left figure you see the R resampled nonparametric curve estimates (thin lines) and the $\hat{m}_n$ based on the original data (bold line). The right figure shows the same, but here the nonparametric estimates are resampled under the (wrong) hypothetical model, and the bold line is the nonparametric estimate based on the original data from the alternative model.

Note that our simulations under the alternative are only for illustration. A further investigation of the power of these test procedures under alternatives is necessary.

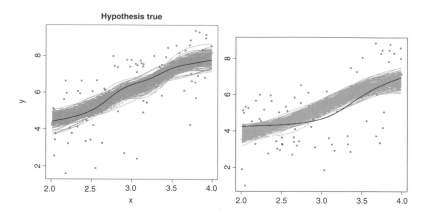

Figure 17.3. Resampled nonparametric regression estimates under the hypothesis and an alternative.

17.5   The Nonparametric ALT Model

Let us consider the same test problem as in the previous section, but with the difference that we do not suppose the baseline distribution is parametric. Thus, the underlying model is a completely nonparametric one. The test problem has the form

$$\mathcal{H} \,:\, S \in \mathcal{C}_{\mathrm{par}} \qquad \text{against} \qquad \mathcal{K} \,:\, S \in \mathcal{C},$$

with

$$\mathcal{C}_{\mathrm{par}} \,=\, \{S \mid S(t|x) \,=\, S_0(t\psi(x;\beta)) \;\; \beta \in \mathbb{R}^d, \; S_0 \in \mathcal{S}\}$$

and

$$\mathcal{C} \,=\, \{S \mid S(t|x) \,=\, S_0(t\psi(x)) \;\; \psi \in \Psi, \; S_0 \in \mathcal{S}\},$$

where $\mathcal{S}$ is a nonparametric class of survival functions.

We apply the same idea of testing. The only difference is that the variance σ^2 in the standardizing terms e_n and τ^2 has to be estimated nonparametrically. The limit theorem gives the distribution under the hypothesis, thus σ^2 can be estimated by the usual variance estimator in the parametric regression model.

Furthermore, resampling methods for the determination of the empirical critical values must take into account the lack of knowledge of the underlying distribution in the hypothetical model. Thus we combine the methods described in Section 17.3 with those from the previous section.

1. The parameter $\vartheta = (\mu, \beta)$ is estimated by the least squares method.

2. (a) Based on the modified residuals r_i, construct R samples of pairs (y_i^*, x_i^*), $i = 1, \ldots, n$, by *model-based resampling*.

(b) Generate R samples of pairs (y_i^*, x_i^*) by the method *"resampling cases."*

3. Use these data to construct the nonparametric estimates $\hat{m}_n^{*(r)}$ and the smoothed estimated regression $\tilde{m}_n^{*(r)}$.

4. Evaluate the distances $Q_n^{*(r)}$ and $T_n^{*(r)}$. Reject the hypothesis as described before on the basis of the ordered $Q_n^{*[r]}$ and $T_n^{*[r]}$.

Using these procedures we obtained the following numbers of rejections.

Method	Hypothesis True	Hypothesis Wrong
Normal distribution	23	155
model-based resampling Q_n	55	438
Resampling cases Q_n	0	0
Model-based resampling T_n	66	458
Resampling cases T_n	0	0

The results concerning the "resampling cases" can be explained as follows: If $\mathcal{H}$ is true Q_n is small; the same holds for the resampled $Q_n^{*(r)}$s. And under the alternative Q_n is large, and again, the same holds for the $Q_n^{*(r)}$s. That is, with this resampling method we do not mimic the behavior under the hypothesis. Thus, this resampling method is not appropriate.

Moreover, we compare these results with those obtained in the previous section. It turns out that the test in the completely nonparametric model distinguishes worse between hypothesis and alternative than in the model with parametric baseline distribution.

A histogram for a simulation under the alternative is given in Figure 17.4. Here we see that the values of the $Q_n^{*(r)}$s are much larger for "resampling cases."

Final remark. The resampling methods presented here are only first intuitive ideas. The proposed methods were demonstrated by very simple examples; this was done to avoid computational difficulties. But, nevertheless, the results show that resampling can be a useful tool for testing the acceleration function. Of course it is necessary to find a deeper theoretic insight into the methods. In that sense our results are a starting point for further investigations.

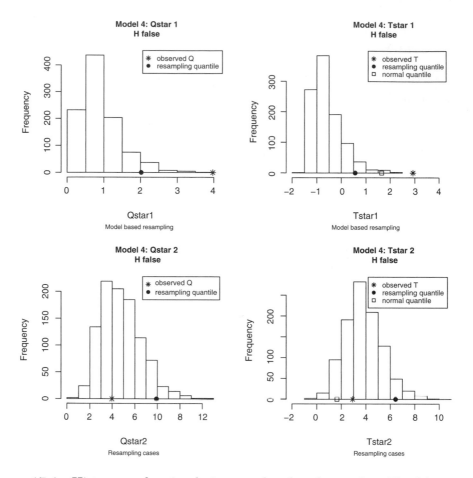

Figure 17.4. Histogram for simulations under the alternative. The histograms in the bottom show the results for "resampling cases."

References

1. Bagdonavičius, V. and Nikulin, M. (2001). *Accelerated Life Models*, Chapman & Hall, Boca Raton, FL.

2. Collomb, G. (1976). Estimation non paramétrique, de la régression par la méthode du noyau, *Thèse*, Université Paul Sabatier, Toulouse.

3. Davison, A. C. and Hinkley, D. V. (1997). *Bootstrap Methods and Their Application*, Cambridge University Press, Cambridge.

4. Efron, B. and Tibshirani, R. J. (1993). *An Introduction to the Bootstrap*, Chapman & Hall, Boca Raton, FL.

5. Härdle, W. and Mammen, E. (1993). Comparing nonparametric versus parametric regression fits, *Annals of Statistics*, **21**, 1926–1947.

6. Liero, H. (1992). Asymptotic normality of a weighted integrated square error of kernel regression estimates with data-dependent bandwidth, *Journal Statistical Planning and Inference*, **30**, 307–325.

7. Liero, H. (1999). Global measures of deviation of nonparametric curve estimators, *Habilitationsschrift, Mathematisch-Naturwissenschaftliche Fakultät der Universität Potsdam*.

8. Stute, W. (1991). Conditional U-statistics, *Annals of Probability*, **19**, 812–825.

18

Recent Achievements in Modified Chi-Squared Goodness-of-Fit Testing

Vassilly Voinov,[1] **Roza Alloyarova,**[2] **and Natalie Pya**[1]

[1]*Kazakhstan Institute of Management, Economics and Strategic Research, Almaty, Kazakhstan*
[2]*Halyk Savings Bank of Kazakhstan, Almaty, Kazakhstan*

Abstract: Milestones of the theory and applications of modified chi-squared tests are briefly discussed. Recent achievements in the theory and applications (in particular in reliability and survival analysis) are considered.

Keywords and Phrases: Pearson's chi-squared test, modified chi-squared tests, maximum likelihood and moment type estimators, structure and power of modified chi-squared tests, reliability and survival analysis

18.1 Introduction

The famous chi-squared goodness-of-fit test was discovered by Karl Pearson in 1900 [Pearson (1900)]. Today we know that his fantastically remarkable result is true only for a simple null hypothesis when the hypothetical distribution (a form of the distribution and parameters) is defined uniquely. The limit distribution of Pearson's sum would not be chi-squared if the parameters were unknown and were estimated by a sample [Fisher (1924)]. Moreover, this limit distribution essentially depends on the method of estimation of the parameters. In particular, if parameters are estimated by minimizing a chi-squared sum for grouped data (MCSE) or by some other asymptotically equivalent method, then the limit distribution will again be chi-squared but the number of degrees of freedom should be reduced by the number of estimated parameters. Chernoff and Lehmann (1954) showed that replacing unknown parameters by, say, their maximum likelihood estimates (MLEs) obtained by ungrouped data would dramatically change the limit distribution of Pearson's sum. In this case it will follow a distribution which depends on unknown parameters and strictly speaking may not be used for testing. Chernoff and Lehmann derived their result considering grouping cells to be fixed. Roy (1956) and Watson (1959) extended this result to the case of random grouping cells. A problem of obtaining a test statistic, the limit distribution of which would not depend on parameters, arose. Dahiya and Gurland (1972) showed that for location and scale families with properly chosen random cells the limit distribution of Pearson's sum may not depend on unknown parameter but instead depend on the null hypothesis.

Another possible way is to modify Pearson's sum to make the modification chi-squared distributed independent from the parameters in the limit. The first officially unpublished evidence of solving this problem for a family of exponential distributions appeared in 1971 in a doctoral thesis [Rao (1971); see citations in Moore and Spruill (1975) and Moore (1977)]). A published version of the result appeared in Rao and Robson (1974). In the above-mentioned unpublished doctoral thesis of Rao the author proposed a modification for Pearson's sum, which for the exponential family of distributions follows in the limit the chi-squared probability distribution and does not depend on unknown parameters. A first officially published result valid for any continuous probability distribution (under some regularity conditions) was obtained by Nikulin (1973). Nikulin's result is formally the same as in Rao (1971) but it was obtained in a much more general and universal way. Now this test is known as the Rao–Robson–Nikulin (RRN) statistic [Drost (1988) and Van Der Vaart (1998)].

Nikulin (1973) thought that his general result would be true if an unknown parameter were replaced by any consistent estimate obtained by ungrouped data (e.g., by MLE), but in 1976 Hsuan and Robson (1976) showed that the resulting modified statistic would be quite different in the case of moment-type estimates (MME). Hsuan and Robson succeeded in deriving the limit covariance matrix of generalized frequencies and proving the theorem that a corresponding quadratic form will follow in the limit the chi-squared distribution, but were unable to derive an explicit form of the modified test. Mirvaliev succeeded in deriving the explicit form in 2001 [Mirvaliev (2001)]. In 1974 Dzhaparidze and Nikulin (1974) proposed a modified chi-squared test, which possesses the limiting chi-squared probability distribution for any square root of n consistent estimates of unknown parameters based on ungrouped data. Later McCulloch (1985) for the MLE case and Mirvaliev (2001) for the general case showed that the Dzhaparidze–Nikulin (DN) statistic is an important independent part of any modified chi-squared test. Later we show see that the power of the DN test would essentially depend on the manner of constructing grouping intervals. Roy (1956), Moore (1971), and Chibisov (1971) obtained a very important result, which shows that the limit distribution of a vector of generalized grouped frequencies with any $\sqrt{n}$-consistent estimator instead of unknown parameter, would be multivariate normal and not depend on the fact that boundaries of grouping intervals are fixed or random based on any consistent estimator of unknown parameter. It is this result which was used by Nikulin (1973) to construct a modified test.

Moore and Spruill (1975) and Moore (1977) systemized all results concerning construction of modified tests known by that date. In particular he showed that all modified chi-squared tests can be derived using a modification of Wald's (1943) approach [see, e.g., Greenwood and Nikulin (1996)]. Actually this approach was first used by Nikulin (1973). Moore (1977) also emphasized that an explicit form of a modified Wald's quadratic form (not only its limit probability distribution) will not depend on the manner of obtaining a generalized, not necessarily unique, matrix inverse [Moore (1977, p. 132)].

The next very important input to the theory of modified chi-squared goodness-of-fit tests was done by Mirvaliev. He [Mirvaliev (2000, 2001)] thoroughly considered two types of a decomposition of chi-squared tests. The first is a decomposition of a Pearson's statistic on a sum of DN and another quadratic form being asymptotically independent of DN in the case of MLEs, and asymptotically correlated in the case of MMEs. The second way decomposes a modified test statistic on a sum of a classical Pearson's test and a correcting term, which makes it chi-squared distributed in the limit, and independent on unknown parameters. The second case was first described by McCulloch (1985), but only for MLEs. The case of MMEs was first investigated by Mirvaliev (2001). The decomposition of a modified chi-squared test on a sum of DN and an additional term is of importance because later it was shown [see, e.g., Voinov and Pya (2004)] that the DN part is in many cases insensitive to an alternative hypothesis in the case of equiprobable cells and would be sensitive to it for example, for nonequiprobable two Neyman–Pearson classes [Voinov *et al.* (2006a)]. The second way also clearly shows that a correcting term takes into account the Fisher's information lost while grouping the data [McCulloch (1985), Mirvaliev (2001), Voinov (2006)]. Mirvaliev has also derived explicitly a modified chi-squared goodness-of-fit test, which can be used for any square root of n moment type estimator. His result disproves the common opinion that only efficient MLEs may be used when constructing modified chi-squared tests. Because Hsuan and Robson first showed the validity of this fact, we suggest calling this test a Hsuan–Robson–Mirvaliev (HRM) statistic. Recently [Voinov and Pya (2004)] it has been shown that for the exponential family of distributions the HRM modified statistic identically equals that of RRN. This is a consequence of the well-known fact that MLEs coincide with MMEs for this family of distributions [Dzhaparidze and Nikulin (1992)].

Many other interesting results concerning chi-squared testing have been obtained during recent years, but, because they are beyond the scope of this chapter, we would simply attract readers' attention by listing some of the most interesting from our point of view [Singh (1986), McLaren *et al.* (1994), Anderson (1994), Zhang (1999), Lemeshko *et al.* (2001), and Boero *et al.* (2004).

In Section 18.2 we briefly consider a contemporary status of the theory of modified chi-squared goodness-of-fit tests. Section 18.3 is devoted to a consideration of some examples which illustrate the theory and applications.

In Section 18.4 we summarize results obtained and give recommendations on implementations of modified chi-squared goodness-of-fit tests.

18.2 A Contemporary Status of the Theory of Modified Chi-Squared Tests

Let $X_1, \ldots, X_n$ be i.i.d. random variables. Consider the problem of testing a simple hypothesis H_0, according to which a probability distribution function of the X_i is supposed to be $F(x)$. Denote by $f(x)$ the density of the hypothetical probability distribution function $F(x)$ with respect to a certain σ-finite measure μ. Let $N_j^{(n)} = \text{Card}\{i : X_i \in \Delta_j, i = 1, \ldots, n\}$, $p_j = \int_{\Delta_j} dF(x)$, $j = 1, \ldots, r$, where Δ_j are nonintersecting fixed grouping intervals such that $\Delta_1 \cup \cdots \cup \Delta_r = \mathbf{R}^1$, $\Delta_i \cap \Delta_j = \emptyset$, $i \neq j$. Denote by $\mathbf{V}^{(n)}$ a column r-vector of a standardized cell frequency with components $v_i^{(n)} = (np_i)^{-1/2}(N_i^{(n)} - np_i)$, $i = 1, \ldots, r$. Under these notations the standard Pearson's chi-squared statistic X_n^2 for a simple null hypothesis H_0 can be written as

$$X_n^2 = \mathbf{V}^{(n)T}\mathbf{V}^{(n)} = \sum_{i=1}^{r} \frac{[N_i^{(n)} - np_i]^2}{np_i}. \tag{18.1}$$

Since Pearson (1900) it has been known that for a sufficiently large sample size n $\mathbf{P}\{X_n^2 \geq x | H_0\} \approx \mathbf{P}\{\chi_{r-1}^2 \geq x\}$, where χ_{r-1}^2 is a continuous random variable possessing the chi-squared probability distribution with $r - 1$ degrees of freedom.

In almost all practical situations a hypothetical distribution $F(x)$ is not known uniquely. In this case one has to test a composite null hypothesis according to which a distribution of the X_i is a member of a parametric family $\mathbf{P}\{X_i \leq x \mid H_0\} = F(x; \boldsymbol{\theta})$, $\boldsymbol{\theta} = (\theta_1, \ldots, \theta_s)^T \in \Theta \subset \mathbf{R}^s$, $x \in \mathbf{R}^1$, where Θ is an open set. Denote by $f(x; \boldsymbol{\theta})$ the density of the probability distribution function $F(x; \boldsymbol{\theta})$. In this case the probability to fall into an interval Δ_j, components of a r-vector of standardized grouped frequencies, and Pearson's sum X_n^2 should be written as $p_j(\boldsymbol{\theta}) = \int_{\Delta_j} dF(x; \boldsymbol{\theta})$, $j = 1, \ldots, r$, $v_i^{(n)}(\boldsymbol{\theta}) = [np_i(\boldsymbol{\theta})]^{-1/2}(N_i^{(n)} - np_i(\boldsymbol{\theta}))$, $i = 1, \ldots, r$, and

$$X_n^2(\boldsymbol{\theta}) = \mathbf{V}^{(n)T}(\boldsymbol{\theta})\mathbf{V}^{(n)}(\boldsymbol{\theta}) = \sum_{i=1}^{r} \frac{[N_i^{(n)} - np_i(\boldsymbol{\theta})]^2}{np_i(\boldsymbol{\theta})} \tag{18.2}$$

correspondingly. For any composite null hypothesis a parameter $\boldsymbol{\theta}$ is considered to be unknown.

Suppose that $\tilde{\boldsymbol{\theta}}_n$ is an estimator of $\boldsymbol{\theta}$ based on grouped data, which minimizes the chi-squared sum (18.2). Fisher (1928) showed that the distribution of

$X_n^2(\tilde{\boldsymbol{\theta}}_n)$ possesses in the limit the chi-squared probability distribution χ_{r-s-1}^2 with $r - s - 1$ degrees of freedom, where s is the number of estimating parameters. Later it was shown [McCulloch (1985)] that the limit distribution of the Pearson–Fisher (PF) statistic based on grouped data is the same as that of the DN test based on ungrouped data. Recently Voinov and Pya (2004) have shown that in many particular cases PF and DN tests have no power with respect to an alternative for equiprobable fixed or random cells and may even be biased.

Up to 1954 statisticians thought that estimating parameters by the well-known method of maximum likelihood based on ungrouped data would give the χ^2 limit distribution of (18.2) with $r - s - 1$ degrees of freedom. Maximum likelihood estimators (MLEs) are asymptotically normally distributed and efficient. Despite these remarkable features of MLEs Chernoff and Lehmann (1954) [see also LeCam *et al.* (1983)] proved that under some regularity conditions for fixed classes

$$\lim_{n\to\infty} \mathbf{P}\{X_n^2(\hat{\boldsymbol{\theta}}_n) \geq x \mid H_0\} = \mathbf{P}\{\chi_{r-s-1}^2 + \sum_{i=1}^{s} \lambda_i(\boldsymbol{\theta})\xi_i^2 \geq x\}, \qquad (18.3)$$

where $\hat{\boldsymbol{\theta}}_n$ is the MLE of $\boldsymbol{\theta}$, $\chi_{r-s-1}^2, \xi_1, \ldots, \xi_s$ are independent, $\xi_i \sim N(0, 1)$, and $0 < \lambda_i(\boldsymbol{\theta}) < 1$, $i = 1, 2, \ldots, s$. From (18.3) we see that the limit distribution of (18.2) with $\boldsymbol{\theta}$ replaced by the MLE $\hat{\boldsymbol{\theta}}_n$ does depend on unknown parameter $\boldsymbol{\theta}$ and, strictly speaking, is inapplicable for hypotheses testing.

Watson (1957) considered χ^2 tests for normality with random boundaries depending on consistent estimators of parameters. He showed that in this case the limit distribution of (18.2) coincides with that of (18.3). Later on Watson (1958, 1959) generalized this result for arbitrary continuous distributions. Chibisov (1971) and Moore (1971) generalized Watson's result for the multivariate case and gave a rigorous proof that standardized cell frequencies

$$v_i^{(n)}(\tilde{\boldsymbol{\theta}}_n) = [np_i(\tilde{\boldsymbol{\theta}}_n)]^{-1/2}(N_i^{(n)} - np_i(\tilde{\boldsymbol{\theta}}_n)), \qquad i = 1, \ldots, r, \qquad (18.4)$$

where $\tilde{\boldsymbol{\theta}}_n$ is any consistent estimator of $\boldsymbol{\theta}$, are asymptotically normally distributed. From this result it follows that the limit distribution of (18.2) with $\tilde{\boldsymbol{\theta}}_n$ instead of $\boldsymbol{\theta}$ will be the same if one used grouping intervals with fixed or random boundaries. But again the limit distribution of the Pearson's test will depend on the unknown parameter $\boldsymbol{\theta}$ and may not be used for testing.

Let $\{\mathbf{V}^{(n)T}(\tilde{\boldsymbol{\theta}}_n)\}$ be a sequence of statistics such that $\mathbf{V}^{(n)T}(\tilde{\boldsymbol{\theta}}_n)$ converges in distribution to $N_r(\mathbf{0}, \boldsymbol{\Sigma})$, where $\boldsymbol{\Sigma}$ is of rank r. If $\{\boldsymbol{\Sigma}_n\}$ is a sequence of consistent estimators of $\boldsymbol{\Sigma}$, then asymptotically $(n \to \infty)$ [Wald (1943)]

$$\mathbf{V}^{(n)T}(\tilde{\boldsymbol{\theta}}_n)\boldsymbol{\Sigma}_n^{-1}\mathbf{V}^{(n)}(\tilde{\boldsymbol{\theta}}_n) \xrightarrow{D} \chi_r^2. \qquad (18.5)$$

Nikulin (1973) [see also Moore (1977) and Hadi and Wells (1990)] generalized this result for the case when $\boldsymbol{\Sigma}$ is singular with a rank $k < r$. Moore (1977) noted that $\boldsymbol{\Sigma}_n^{-1}$ in (18.5) can be replaced by an estimate $\boldsymbol{\Sigma}_n^-$ of any generalized $\boldsymbol{\Sigma}^-$ matrix inverse of $\boldsymbol{\Sigma}$ and that the limit distribution of the quadratic form

$$\mathbf{V}^{(n)T}(\tilde{\boldsymbol{\theta}}_n)\boldsymbol{\Sigma}_n^-\mathbf{V}^{(n)}(\tilde{\boldsymbol{\theta}}_n) \tag{18.6}$$

will follow χ_k^2 regardless of how matrix $\boldsymbol{\Sigma}$ is inverted. Moore (1971) showed that the limit covariance matrix of standardized frequencies (18.4) with $\tilde{\boldsymbol{\theta}}_n = \hat{\boldsymbol{\theta}}_n$ is

$$\boldsymbol{\Sigma} = \mathbf{I} - \mathbf{q}\mathbf{q}^T - \mathbf{B}\mathbf{J}^{-1}\mathbf{B}^T, \tag{18.7}$$

where $\mathbf{q} = ((p_1(\boldsymbol{\theta}))^{1/2}, \ldots, (p_r(\boldsymbol{\theta}))^{1/2})^T$, and $\mathbf{B} = \mathbf{B}(\boldsymbol{\theta})$ is an $r \times s$ matrix with elements

$$\frac{1}{\sqrt{p_i(\boldsymbol{\theta})}} \frac{\partial p_i(\boldsymbol{\theta})}{\partial \theta_j}, \qquad i = 1, 2, \ldots, r, \qquad j = 1, 2, \ldots, s. \tag{18.8}$$

Using formula (18.7) Nikulin (1973) derived the generalized $\boldsymbol{\Sigma}^-$ matrix inverse of $\boldsymbol{\Sigma}$ as

$$\boldsymbol{\Sigma}^- = \mathbf{I} + \mathbf{B}(\mathbf{J} - \mathbf{J}_g)^{-1}\mathbf{B}^T, \tag{18.9}$$

where $\mathbf{J}$ is the information matrix of $F(x; \boldsymbol{\theta})$ and $\mathbf{J}_g = \mathbf{B}^T\mathbf{B}$ is Fisher's information matrix for grouped data. Nikulin presented his modified chi-squared test for a continuous null hypothetical probability distribution in the case of the efficient MLE as

$$Y1_n^2(\hat{\boldsymbol{\theta}}_n) = X_n^2(\hat{\boldsymbol{\theta}}_n) + \mathbf{V}^{(n)T}(\hat{\boldsymbol{\theta}}_n)\mathbf{B}(\mathbf{J}_n - \mathbf{J}_{gn})^{-1}\mathbf{B}^T\mathbf{V}^{(n)}(\hat{\boldsymbol{\theta}}_n), \tag{18.10}$$

where $\mathbf{J}_n$ and $\mathbf{J}_{gn}$ in (18.10) are MLEs of the corresponding matrices.

The matrix inverse (18.9) can be presented identically as [Moore and Spruill (1975)] $\boldsymbol{\Sigma}^- = (\mathbf{I} - \mathbf{B}\mathbf{J}^{-1}\mathbf{B}^T)^{-1}$, but this representation has much less value for the theory of modified chi-squared tests than the result (18.9) of Nikulin (see a discussion of this below). Note also that the generalized Wald's method is universal. It may be used even for deriving the classical Pearson's test [see, e.g., Greenwood and Nikulin (1996, p. 14)].

From the trivial orthogonal decomposition of the r-dimensional identity matrix $\mathbf{I} = \mathbf{q}\mathbf{q}^T + \mathbf{B}(\mathbf{B}^T\mathbf{B})^-\mathbf{B}^T + [\mathbf{I} - \mathbf{q}\mathbf{q}^T - \mathbf{B}(\mathbf{B}^T\mathbf{B})^-\mathbf{B}^T]$ and the relation $\mathbf{q}\mathbf{q}^T\mathbf{V}^{(n)} = \mathbf{0}$ it follows [Mirvaliev (2001)] that $\mathbf{V}^{(n)} = \mathbf{U}^{(n)}(\boldsymbol{\theta}) + \mathbf{W}^{(n)}(\boldsymbol{\theta})$, where $\mathbf{U}^{(n)}(\boldsymbol{\theta}) = [\mathbf{I} - \mathbf{q}\mathbf{q}^T - \mathbf{B}(\mathbf{B}^T\mathbf{B})^-\mathbf{B}^T]\mathbf{V}^{(n)}$ and $\mathbf{W}^{(n)}(\boldsymbol{\theta}) = \mathbf{B}(\mathbf{B}^T\mathbf{B})^-\mathbf{B}^T\mathbf{V}^{(n)}$. From this one gets the following decomposition of Pearson's sum

$$X_n^2(\tilde{\boldsymbol{\theta}}_n) = U_n^2(\tilde{\boldsymbol{\theta}}_n) + W_n^2(\tilde{\boldsymbol{\theta}}_n), \tag{18.11}$$

where $U_n^2(\tilde{\boldsymbol{\theta}}_n) = \mathbf{V}^{(n)T}(\tilde{\boldsymbol{\theta}}_n)[\mathbf{I} - \mathbf{B}_n(\mathbf{B}_n^T\mathbf{B}_n)^-\mathbf{B}_n^T]\mathbf{V}^{(n)}(\tilde{\boldsymbol{\theta}}_n)$ is the well-known Dzhaparidze and Nikulin (1974) (DN) statistic,

$$W_n^2(\tilde{\boldsymbol{\theta}}_n) = \mathbf{V}^{(n)T}(\tilde{\boldsymbol{\theta}}_n)\mathbf{B}_n(\mathbf{B}_n^T\mathbf{B}_n)^-\mathbf{B}_n^T\mathbf{V}^{(n)}(\tilde{\boldsymbol{\theta}}_n),$$

and $\mathbf{B}_n = \mathbf{B}_n(\tilde{\boldsymbol{\theta}}_n)$ is the estimate of $\mathbf{B}$. The idempotent quadratic forms $U_n^2(\tilde{\boldsymbol{\theta}}_n)$ and $W_n^2(\tilde{\boldsymbol{\theta}}_n)$ are generalized chi-squared type statistics, which are invariant with respect to how matrix $\mathbf{J}_g = \mathbf{B}^{\mathbf{T}}\mathbf{B}$ is inverted. If an estimator $\tilde{\boldsymbol{\theta}}_n$ is efficient (e.g., MLE), then statistics $U_n^2(\hat{\boldsymbol{\theta}}_n)$ and $W_n^2(\hat{\boldsymbol{\theta}}_n)$ will be asymptotically independent. Otherwise (if, e.g., $\tilde{\boldsymbol{\theta}}_n$ is MME $\bar{\boldsymbol{\theta}}_n$) they will be asymptotically correlated [Mirvaliev (2001)]. Note also that for any $\sqrt{n}$-consistent estimator $\tilde{\boldsymbol{\theta}}_n$ of $\boldsymbol{\theta}$ obtained by ungrouped data the DN statistic will be distributed in the limit as χ_{r-s-1}^2. From this we see that the DN test is asymptotically equivalent to the Pearson–Fisher test, when the parameter $\boldsymbol{\theta}$ is estimated by grouped data [see also McCulloch (1985) and Mirvaliev (2001)].

From (18.10) and (18.11) it follows that the Rao–Robson–Nikulin statistic can be written down as

$$Y1_n^2(\hat{\boldsymbol{\theta}}_n) = U_n^2(\hat{\boldsymbol{\theta}}_n) + W_n^2(\hat{\boldsymbol{\theta}}_n) + P_n^2(\hat{\boldsymbol{\theta}}_n) = X_n^2(\tilde{\boldsymbol{\theta}}_n) + P_n^2(\hat{\boldsymbol{\theta}}_n), \qquad (18.12)$$

where $P_n^2(\hat{\boldsymbol{\theta}}_n) = \mathbf{V}^{(n)T}(\hat{\boldsymbol{\theta}}_n)\mathbf{B}_n(\mathbf{J}_n - \mathbf{J}_{gn})^{-1}\mathbf{B}_n^T\mathbf{V}^{(n)}(\hat{\boldsymbol{\theta}}_n)$. The quadratic forms $U_n^2(\hat{\boldsymbol{\theta}}_n)$ and $W_n^2(\hat{\boldsymbol{\theta}}_n) + P_n^2(\hat{\boldsymbol{\theta}}_n)$ of (18.12) are statistically independent in the limit and can be used as test statistics independently [McCulloch (1985) and Mirvaliev (2001)]. Because $U_n^2(\hat{\boldsymbol{\theta}}_n)$ based on ungrouped data is asymptotically distributed as χ_{r-s-1}^2 like Pearson–Fisher's test based on grouped data, the sum $W_n^2(\hat{\boldsymbol{\theta}}_n) + P_n^2(\hat{\boldsymbol{\theta}}_n)$ can be considered as a correcting term, which takes into account the information lost while data grouping.

Consider now the case of MMEs. Let $\mathbf{K} = \mathbf{K}(\boldsymbol{\theta})$ be an s×s matrix with elements

$$\int x^i \frac{\partial f(x;\boldsymbol{\theta})}{\partial \theta_j} dx \qquad i,j = 1,\ldots,s. \qquad (18.13)$$

Let also

$$\mathbf{V} = \mathbf{V}(\boldsymbol{\theta}) = (m_{ij} - m_i m_j), \qquad (18.14)$$

where $m_i = E[\mathbf{X}^i]$, $m_{ij} = E[\mathbf{X}^{i+j}]$, $i,j = 1,\ldots,s$, and $\mathbf{C} = \mathbf{C}(\boldsymbol{\theta})$ is an $r \times s$ matrix with elements

$$p_i^{-1/2}(\boldsymbol{\theta})\left(\int_{\Delta_i} x^j f(x;\boldsymbol{\theta})dx - p_i(\boldsymbol{\theta})m_j(\boldsymbol{\theta})\right), \qquad i = 1,\ldots,r, \qquad j = 1,\ldots,s.$$
$$(18.15)$$

Denote $\mathbf{A} = \mathbf{I} - \mathbf{q}\mathbf{q}^T + \mathbf{C}(\mathbf{V} - \mathbf{C}^T\mathbf{C})^{-1}\mathbf{C}^T$, and $\mathbf{L} = \mathbf{V} + (\mathbf{C} - \mathbf{B}\mathbf{K}^{-1}\mathbf{V})^T\mathbf{A}(\mathbf{C} - \mathbf{B}\mathbf{K}^{-1}\mathbf{V})$, where elements of matrices $\mathbf{K}$ and $\mathbf{C}$ are defined by formulas (18.13), (18.15) and the elements of the s×s matrix $\mathbf{V}$ by (18.14), respectively, and $\mathbf{B} \equiv \mathbf{B}(\boldsymbol{\theta})$.

Hsuan and Robson (1976) showed that if one replaced $\boldsymbol{\theta}$ in (18.2) by a $\sqrt{n}$-consistent MME $\bar{\boldsymbol{\theta}}_n$, then under the proper regularity conditions, $\lim_{n\to\infty} \mathbf{P}\{\mathbf{X}_n^2(\bar{\boldsymbol{\theta}}_n) \geq x \mid H_0\} = \mathbf{P}\{\sum_{j=1}^{r-1}\lambda_j(\boldsymbol{\theta})\chi_j^2 \geq x\}$, where $\lambda_j(\boldsymbol{\theta})$ are nonzero characteristic roots of the limit covariance matrix

$$\boldsymbol{\Sigma}_1 = \mathbf{I} - \mathbf{q}\mathbf{q}^T + \mathbf{B}\mathbf{K}^{-1}\mathbf{V}(\mathbf{K}^{-1})^T\mathbf{B}^T - \mathbf{C}(\mathbf{K}^{-1})^T\mathbf{B}^T - \mathbf{B}\mathbf{K}^{-1}\mathbf{C}^T \qquad (18.16)$$

of standardized cell frequencies (18.4) with $\tilde{\boldsymbol{\theta}}_n = \bar{\boldsymbol{\theta}}_n$, χ_j^2 being independent central χ_1^2 random variables. Hsuan and Robson (1976) proved also that if one substituted $\boldsymbol{\Sigma}_n^-$ in (18.6) by a $\sqrt{n}$-consistent MME of any generalized matrix inverse of $\boldsymbol{\Sigma}_1$, then the corresponding modified chi-squared test would follow a χ_{r-1}^2 limit distribution under H_0. Unfortunately, they did not give the explicit expression for $\boldsymbol{\Sigma}_1^-$.

Mirvaliev (2001) derived the Moore–Penrose matrix inverse $\boldsymbol{\Sigma}_1^-$ of $\boldsymbol{\Sigma}_1$ as

$$\boldsymbol{\Sigma}_1^- = \mathbf{A} - \mathbf{A}(\mathbf{C} - \mathbf{B}\mathbf{K}^{-1}\mathbf{V})\mathbf{L}^{-1}(\mathbf{C} - \mathbf{B}\mathbf{K}^{-1}\mathbf{V})^T\mathbf{A}. \tag{18.17}$$

Taking into account (18.6), (18.17), and the fact that $\mathbf{q}\mathbf{q}^T\mathbf{V}^{(n)}(\bar{\boldsymbol{\theta}}_n) = \mathbf{0}$ the HRM modified chi-squared test can be written as

$$Y2_n^2(\bar{\boldsymbol{\theta}}_n) = X_n^2(\bar{\boldsymbol{\theta}}_n) + R_n^2(\bar{\boldsymbol{\theta}}_n) - Q_n^2(\bar{\boldsymbol{\theta}}_n), \tag{18.18}$$

or

$$Y2_n^2(\bar{\boldsymbol{\theta}}_n) = U_n^2(\bar{\boldsymbol{\theta}}_n) + W_n^2(\bar{\boldsymbol{\theta}}_n) + R_n^2(\bar{\boldsymbol{\theta}}_n) - Q_n^2(\bar{\boldsymbol{\theta}}_n), \tag{18.19}$$

where $R_n^2(\bar{\boldsymbol{\theta}}_n) = \mathbf{V}^{(n)T}(\bar{\boldsymbol{\theta}}_n)\mathbf{C}_n(\mathbf{V}_n - \mathbf{C}_n^T\mathbf{C}_n)^{-1}\mathbf{C}_n^T\mathbf{V}_n^{(n)}(\bar{\boldsymbol{\theta}}_n)$, $Q_n^2(\bar{\boldsymbol{\theta}}_n) = \mathbf{V}_n^{(n)T}(\bar{\boldsymbol{\theta}}_n)\mathbf{A}_n$ $(\mathbf{C}_n - \mathbf{B}_n\mathbf{K}_n^{-1}\mathbf{V}_n)\mathbf{L}_n^{-1}(\mathbf{C}_n - \mathbf{B}_n\mathbf{K}_n^{-1}\mathbf{V}_n)^T\mathbf{A}_n\mathbf{V}^{(n)}(\bar{\boldsymbol{\theta}}_n)$, $\mathbf{K}_n = \mathbf{K}(\bar{\boldsymbol{\theta}}_n)$, $\mathbf{V}_n = \mathbf{V}(\bar{\boldsymbol{\theta}}_n)$, $\mathbf{C}_n = \mathbf{C}(\bar{\boldsymbol{\theta}}_n)$, and $\mathbf{A}_n$ and $\mathbf{L}_n$ are the corresponding MMEs of $\mathbf{A}$ and $\mathbf{L}$. Under rather general conditions the statistic $Y_n^2(\bar{\boldsymbol{\theta}}_n)$ will possess in the limit the chi-squared probability distribution χ_{r-1}^2, the sum $W_n^2(\bar{\boldsymbol{\theta}}_n) + R_n^2(\bar{\boldsymbol{\theta}}_n) - Q_n^2(\bar{\boldsymbol{\theta}}_n)$ being asymptotically independent on $U_n^2(\bar{\boldsymbol{\theta}}_n)$ and distributed as χ_s^2 [Mirvaliev (2001)]. For the same reason as above, the statistic $W_n^2(\bar{\boldsymbol{\theta}}_n) + R_n^2(\bar{\boldsymbol{\theta}}_n) - Q_n^2(\bar{\boldsymbol{\theta}}_n)$ can be considered as a correcting statistic, which recovers the information lost in estimating $\boldsymbol{\theta}$ by grouped data instead of the MME based on the initial ungrouped data. It is clear that due to the limit independence of $Y2_n^2(\bar{\boldsymbol{\theta}}) - U_n^2(\bar{\boldsymbol{\theta}}) = W_n^2(\bar{\boldsymbol{\theta}}_n) + R_n^2(\bar{\boldsymbol{\theta}}_n) - Q_n^2(\bar{\boldsymbol{\theta}}_n)$ on $U_n^2(\bar{\boldsymbol{\theta}}_n)$ it can be considered as a test, which may be used separately from Dzhaparidze–Nikulin's $U_n^2(\bar{\boldsymbol{\theta}}_n)$. It is worth noting that the limit distribution of $Y2_n^2(\bar{\boldsymbol{\theta}})$ will be the same if one uses cells with random boundaries. Note also that for the exponential family of distributions $Y2_n^2(\tilde{\boldsymbol{\theta}}_n) \equiv Y1_n^2(\tilde{\boldsymbol{\theta}}_n)$ [Voinov and Pya (2004)].

18.3 Some Recent Results

18.3.1 Testing for normality

Rao and Robson (1974) and McCulloch (1985) used Monte Carlo simulation and showed that the power of the Rao–Robson–Nikulin statistic $Y1_n^2$ [Nikulin (1973b)] is significantly higher than that of the Dzhaparidze–Nikulin U_n^2. A more detailed simulation study [Voinov (2006b)] shows that:

(a) If one uses equiprobable random cells, then the power of U_n^2 is indeed smaller or even much smaller than that of $Y1_n^2$ against the logistic, uniform, triangular, and Laplace (double-exponential) alternatives in a rather wide range of the number of cells r.

(b) The Dzhaparidze–Nikulin U_n^2 can be biased and, hence, inapplicable when testing for normality against uniform and triangular alternatives.

(c) Among all modified tests considered, the test $Y1_n^2 - U_n^2$ is the most powerful when testing for normality against the above-mentioned alternatives.

(d) The power of both $Y1_n^2$ and $Y1_n^2 - U_n^2$ is the largest for alternatives considered if one uses $r \in [10, 14]$ equiprobable fixed or random cells.

(e) The power of $Y1_n^2 - U_n^2$ becomes very small for four Neyman–Pearson-type classes. At the same time the power of U_n^2 based on the same four classes is slightly less or greater (depending on an alternative) than the power of $Y1_n^2$ for two Neyman–Pearson classes and is significantly higher than the maximal power of $Y1_n^2 - U_n^2$ for equiprobable cells.

18.3.2 Testing for the logistic probability distribution

Aguirre and Nikulin (1994) constructed the RRN test $Y1_n^2$ based on an approximate solution of the maximum likelihood equations proposed by Harter and Moore (1967). They gave the explicit form of the $Y1_n^2$ but have not investigated the power of their test. Voinov *et al.* (2003) [see also Voinov *et al.* (2006b)] constructed in explicit form and investigated the power of the HRM $Y2_n^2$ test based on MMEs. Explicit expressions for elements of matrices $\mathbf{B}, \mathbf{C}, \mathbf{K}$, and $\mathbf{V}$ needed to evaluate the test statistic (18.19) are given in the appendix.

(a) The HRM test $Y2_n^2$ based on inefficient but $\sqrt{n}$-consistent MMEs and equiprobable random or fixed cells performs well. As in the case of normal null the test $Y2_n^2 - U_n^2$ is the most powerful for those cells against the normal alternative. Under the same conditions the DN test U_n^2 does not work (see Figure 18.1). The same results are observed for the triangular and Laplace alternative hypotheses [Voinov *et al.* (2006b)].

(b) The power of $Y2_n^2 - U_n^2$ becomes very small for four Neyman–Pearson-type classes. At the same time the power of U_n^2 based on the same four classes is slightly less or greater (w.r.t. the normal alternative) than the power of $Y2_n^2$ for two Neyman–Pearson classes and is significantly more than maximal power of $Y2_n^2 - U_n^2$ for equiprobable cells (see Table 18.1).

Table 18.1. Power of $Y2_n^2$, U_n^2, and $Y2_n^2 - U_n^2$ for two and four Neyman–Pearson classes

Power of $Y2_n^2$	Power of $Y2_n^2$	Power of U_n^2	Power of $Y2_n^2 - U_n^2$
$(r = 2)$	$(r = 4)$	$(r = 4)$	$(r = 4)$
0.334	0.204	0.357 ± 0.013	0.034

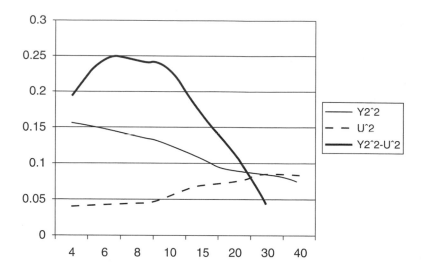

Figure 18.1. Estimated powers as functions of the number of equiprobable cells r of $Y2_n^2$, U_n^2, and $Y2_n^2 - U_n^2$ tests versus the normal alternative. Sample size $n = 200$, type one error $\alpha = 0.05$.

18.3.3   Testing for the three-parameter Weibull null hypothesis

Consider the three-parameter Weibull family with the probability density function

$$f(x; \theta, \mu, p) = \frac{p}{\theta} \left(\frac{x - \mu}{\theta} \right)^{p-1} \exp \left\{ - \left(\frac{x - \mu}{\theta} \right)^p \right\},$$

$$x > \mu, \theta > 0, \quad p > 0, \quad \mu \in R^1.$$

It is well known that sometimes there are serious problems with obtaining MLEs for this probability distribution. If all three parameters are unknown, the likelihood can be infinite. For some datasets there is no local maximum for the likelihood [Lockhart and Stephens (1994)]. It has to be mentioned also that Fisher's information matrix for this probability distribution does not exist for infinitely many values of the parameter p, namely for $p = 1/2 + k$ and $p = 2/1 + k$, where $k = 0, 1, \ldots$. Because of this one can hardly implement the RRN test.

Alternatively, one may use the HRM test $Y2_n^2$ based on inefficient MMEs, because for this test it is enough if estimates are $\sqrt{n}$-consistent [Hsuan and Robson (1976)]. Such a test was developed in Voinov *et al.* (2006a).

The HRM test $Y2_n^2$ based on MMEs and equiprobable random or fixed cells performs well. Under the same conditions the DN test U_n^2 does not work and the power of the test $Y2_n^2 - U_n^2$ is essentially higher than that of $Y2_n^2$. A typical example of these facts is presented in Figure 18.2. The same picture is observed when testing for the three-parameter Weibull family against the

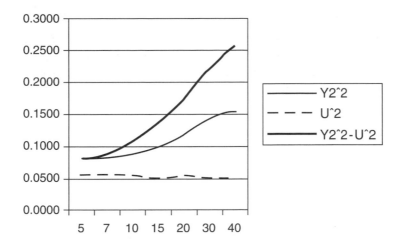

Figure 18.2. Estimated powers as functions of the number of equiprobable cells r of $Y2_n^2$, U_n^2, and $Y2_n^2 - U_n^2$ tests versus exponentiated Weibull alternative $F(x) = \left[1 - \exp(-(x/\alpha)^\beta)\right]^\gamma$, $x, \alpha, \beta, \gamma > 0$, of Mudholkar *et al.* (1995). Sample size $n = 200$, type one error $\alpha = 0.05$.

power-generalized Weibull alternative of Bagdonavičius and Nikulin (2002). It is worth noting that the power of $Y2_n^2 - U_n^2$ is not very high w.r.t. these closed-form alternatives and is very high versus alternatives of quite different form, such as the generalized Weibull distribution of Mudholkar *et al.* (1996) [see Voinov *et al.* (2006a)].

As in the case of testing for the logistic null hypothesis the power of the test $Y2_n^2$ based on two Neyman–Pearson classes is higher than that of $Y2_n^2 - U_n^2$ (See Table 18.2).

18.3.4 Testing for the power-generalized Weibull family

Bagdonavičius and Nikulin (2002) proposed a very nice family of the power-generalized Weibull distributions to be used in survival analysis especially in accelerated life studies. Depending on parameter values, the hazard rate for the family can be constant, monotone increasing or decreasing, $\cap$-shaped, and $\cup$-shaped. If all three parameters of the proposed distribution function

$$F(x; \theta, \nu, \gamma) = 1 - \exp\left\{1 - \left[1 + \left(\frac{x}{\theta}\right)^\nu\right]^{1/\gamma}\right\}, \qquad x, \theta, \nu, \gamma > 0.$$

Table 18.2. Power of HRM test for two Neyman–Pearson classes

	W-PGW	ExpW	GWeib
$\alpha = 0.05$	0.141	0.294 ± 0.015	1.000

are unknown, MLEs and MMEs would be inconsistent. Considering the shape parameter γ to be fixed and using inefficient but $\sqrt{n}$-consistent MMEs, Alloyarova *et al.* (2006) constructed and analyzed the HRM test for this family. It has been shown that the HRM test $Y2_n^2$ based on MMEs and equiprobable random or fixed cells performs well but the test $Y2_n^2 - U_n^2$ as in all previously considered examples is the best one.

18.4   Conclusion

Some important new results obtained during the last 20 years can be summarized as follows.

(a) The structure of Pearson's sum and modified chi-squared goodness-of-fit tests was thoroughly investigated. It was shown that both proposed decompositions include as an essential part the DN statistic, which possesses in the limit the same χ_{r-s-1}^2 distribution as the PF test based on grouped data. The decomposition of modified tests and the last fact permit us to understand that all modified tests are sums of the DN statistic and a correcting term, which takes into account the Fisher's information lost while grouping the data.

(b) A modified chi-squared test $Y2_n^2$ based on inefficient $\sqrt{n}$-consistent MMEs has been derived explicitly. This result shows that not only efficient MLEs may be used for constructing tests. It does not mean that one should necessarily use MMEs if there are problems with obtaining MLEs. Those inefficient MMEs can be made efficient with the use of Fisher's technique [Fisher (1925), and Dzhaparidze (1983)] and, after that improvement, one may use the RRN $Y1_n^2$ statistic [Voinov *et al.* (2006b)].

(c) The $Y1_n^2 - U_n^2$ and $Y2_n^2 - U_n^2$ statistics when testing for the normal and the logistic null hypotheses are the most powerful for equiprobable cells because they recover the largest part of Fisher's information lost while grouping the data. Under the same conditions the DN test does not work. On the contrary, the DN test based on four Neyman–Pearson-type classes when testing for the normal and the logistic nulls performs well and possesses even more power compared to the highest power of $Y1_n^2 - U_n^2$ or $Y2_n^2 - U_n^2$. This is explained by the fact that for two or four Neyman–Pearson-type classes there is almost no loss of Fisher's information.

(d) Implementation of the modified chi-squared tests considered in the chapter shows that shapes of the power generalized Weibull (PGW), exponentiated Weibull (EW), and the three-parameter Weibull (W3) distributions are very close to each other, although their hazard rate functions can be essentially different. Thus, to select one of these models for a survival analysis one needs to have a test that will compare their hazard rate functions directly. At the same time to discriminate between different-shaped generalized Weibull (GW) models [Mudholkar *et al.* (1996)] and three models mentioned above, any test $Y2_n^2$, $Y2_n^2 - U_n^2$ and even insensitive U^2 can be used, because the power of all those tests is very close to one. This suggests renaming the GW model as not belonging to a Weibull family.

Acknowledgments

The authors would like to thank Professor M. Nikulin for his many valuable comments and suggestions that helped us in improving the presentation. The authors are grateful also to Professor N. Balakrishnan for his comments concerning the power of tests with respect to the three-parameter Weibull alternative.

Appendix

Let $b_0 = -\infty$, $b_i, i = 1, 2, \ldots, r-1$, $b_r = +\infty$ be the borders of grouping intervals; then the probabilities to fall into each interval are

$$p_i = \left(1 + \exp\left(-\frac{\pi(b_i - \theta_1)}{\sqrt{3}\theta_2}\right)\right)^{-1} - \left(1 + \exp\left(-\frac{\pi(b_{i-1} - \theta_1)}{\sqrt{3}\theta_2}\right)\right)^{-1}, \quad i = 1, \ldots, r.$$

Elements of $r \times 2$ matrix $\mathbf{B}$ for $i = 1, \ldots, r$ are

$$B_{i1} = \frac{\pi}{\sqrt{3}p_i\theta_2}\left[\frac{\exp\left(-\frac{\pi(b_{i-1} - \theta_1)}{\sqrt{3}\theta_2}\right)}{\left(1 + \exp\left(-\frac{\pi(b_{i-1} - \theta_1)}{\sqrt{3}\theta_2}\right)\right)^2} - \frac{\exp\left(-\frac{\pi(b_i - \theta_1)}{\sqrt{3}\theta_2}\right)}{\left(1 + \exp\left(-\frac{\pi(b_i - \theta_1)}{\sqrt{3}\theta_2}\right)\right)^2}\right]$$

and

$$B_{i2} = \frac{\pi}{\sqrt{3}p_i\theta_2^2}\left[\frac{(b_{i-1} - \theta_1)\exp\left(-\frac{\pi(b_{i-1} - \theta_1)}{\sqrt{3}\theta_2}\right)}{\left(1 + \exp\left(-\frac{\pi(b_{i-1} - \theta_1)}{\sqrt{3}\theta_2}\right)\right)^2} - \frac{(b_i - \theta_1)\exp\left(-\frac{\pi(b_i - \theta_1)}{\sqrt{3}\theta_2}\right)}{\left(1 + \exp\left(-\frac{\pi(b_i - \theta_1)}{\sqrt{3}\theta_2}\right)\right)^2}\right].$$

Elements of the $r \times 2$ matrix $\mathbf{C}$ are

$$C_{11} = -\frac{(b_1 - \theta_1)}{\sqrt{p_1}\left(1 + \exp\left(\frac{\pi(b_1 - \theta_1)}{\sqrt{3}\theta_2}\right)\right)} - \frac{\sqrt{3}\theta_2}{\sqrt{p_1}\pi}\ln\left(1 + \exp\left(-\frac{\pi(b_1 - \theta_1)}{\sqrt{3}\theta_2}\right)\right),$$

$$C_{i1} = \frac{(b_{i-1} - \theta_1)}{\sqrt{p_i}\left(1 + \exp\left(\frac{\pi(b_{i-1} - \theta_1)}{\sqrt{3}\theta_2}\right)\right)} - \frac{(b_i - \theta_1)}{\sqrt{p_i}\left(1 + \exp\left(\frac{\pi(b_i - \theta_1)}{\sqrt{3}\theta_2}\right)\right)}$$

$$+ \frac{\sqrt{3}\theta_2}{\pi\sqrt{p_i}}\ln\frac{\left(1 + \exp\left(-\frac{\pi(b_{i-1} - \theta_1)}{\sqrt{3}\theta_2}\right)\right)}{\left(1 + \exp\left(-\frac{\pi(b_i - \theta_1)}{\sqrt{3}\theta_2}\right)\right)}, \quad i = 2, \ldots, r-1,$$

$$C_{r1} = \frac{(b_{r-1} - \theta_1)}{\sqrt{p_r}\left(1 + \exp\left(\frac{\pi(b_{r-1}-\theta_1)}{\sqrt{3}\theta_2}\right)\right)} + \frac{\sqrt{3}\theta_2}{\sqrt{p_r}\pi}\ln\left(1 + \exp\left(-\frac{\pi(b_{r-1}-\theta_1)}{\sqrt{3}\theta_2}\right)\right),$$

$$C_{12} = \frac{(b_1^2 - \theta_1^2 - \theta_2^2)}{\sqrt{p_1}\left(1 + \exp\left(-\frac{\pi(b_1-\theta_1)}{\sqrt{3}\theta_2}\right)\right)} - \frac{2\sqrt{3}\theta_2 b_1}{\pi\sqrt{p_1}}\ln\left(1 + \exp\left(\frac{\pi(b_1-\theta_1)}{\sqrt{3}\theta_2}\right)\right)$$

$$- \frac{6\theta_2^2}{\pi^2\sqrt{p_1}}\mathrm{Li}_2\left(-\exp\left(\frac{\pi(b_1-\theta_1)}{\sqrt{3}\theta_2}\right)\right),$$

$$
\begin{aligned}
C_{i2} = {}& -\frac{b_i^2 - \theta_1^2}{\sqrt{p_i}\left(1 + \exp\left(\frac{\pi(b_i-\theta_1)}{\sqrt{3}\theta_2}\right)\right)} + \frac{b_{i-1}^2 - \theta_1^2}{\sqrt{p_i}\left(1 + \exp\left(\frac{\pi(b_{i-1}-\theta_1)}{\sqrt{3}\theta_2}\right)\right)} \\
& + \frac{2\sqrt{3}\theta_2}{\pi\sqrt{p_i}}\ln\left[\frac{\left(1 + \exp\left(-\frac{\pi(b_{i-1}-\theta_1)}{\sqrt{3}\theta_2}\right)\right)^{b_{i-1}}}{\left(1 + \exp\left(-\frac{\pi(b_i-\theta_1)}{\sqrt{3}\theta_2}\right)\right)^{b_i}}\right] \\
& + \frac{6\theta_2^2}{\pi^2\sqrt{p_i}}\mathrm{Li}_2\left(-\exp\left(-\frac{\pi(b_i-\theta_1)}{\sqrt{3}\theta_2}\right)\right) \\
& - \frac{6\theta_2^2}{\pi^2\sqrt{p_i}}\mathrm{Li}_2\left(-\exp\left(-\frac{\pi(b_{i-1}-\theta_1)}{\sqrt{3}\theta_2}\right)\right) \\
& + \frac{\theta_2^2}{\sqrt{p_i}\left(1 + \exp\left(-\frac{\pi(b_{i-1}-\theta_1)}{\sqrt{3}\theta_2}\right)\right)} - \frac{\theta_2^2}{\sqrt{p_i}\left(1 + \exp\left(-\frac{\pi(b_i-\theta_1)}{\sqrt{3}\theta_2}\right)\right)}, \\
& \hspace{8cm} i = 2, \ldots, r-1,
\end{aligned}
$$

$$C_{r2} = \frac{(b_{r-1}^2 - \theta_1^2 - \theta_2^2)}{\sqrt{p_r}\left(1 + \exp\left(-\frac{\pi(b_{r-1}-\theta_1)}{\sqrt{3}\theta_2}\right)\right)} + \frac{2\sqrt{3}\theta_2 b_{r-1}}{\pi\sqrt{p_r}}\ln\left(1 + \exp\left(\frac{\pi(b_{r-1}-\theta_1)}{\sqrt{3}\theta_2}\right)\right)$$

$$- \frac{6\theta_2^2}{\pi^2\sqrt{p_r}}\mathrm{Li}_2\left(-\exp\left(\frac{\pi(b_{r-1}-\theta_1)}{\sqrt{3}\theta_2}\right)\right),$$

where $\mathrm{Li}_2(-x)$ is Euler's dilogarithm, which can be evaluated by the series expansion

$$\mathrm{Li}_2(-x) = \sum_{k=1}^{\infty} \frac{(-x)^k}{k^2}$$

for $x \leq (\sqrt{5} - 1)/2$ and by formula

$$\mathrm{Li}_2(-x) = \sum_{k=1}^{\infty} \frac{1}{k^2(1+x)^k} + \frac{1}{2}\ln^2(1+x) - \ln x \ln(1+x) - \frac{\pi^2}{6}$$

for $x > (\sqrt{5} - 1)/2$ [Prudnikov *et al.* (1986)].

Matrices $\mathbf{K}$ and $\mathbf{V}$ are

$$\mathbf{K} = \left(\begin{array}{cc} 1 & 0 \\ 2\theta_1 & 2\theta_2 \end{array} \right) \quad \text{and} \quad \mathbf{V} = \left(\begin{array}{cc} \theta_2^2 & 2\theta_1\theta_2^2 \\ 2\theta_1\theta_2^2 & 4\theta_1^2\theta_2^2 + \frac{16}{5}\theta_2^4 \end{array} \right),$$

respectively.

References

1. Aguirre, N. and Nikulin, M. S. (1994). Chi-squared goodness-of-fit test for the family of logistic distributions, *Kybernetika*, **30**, 214–222.

2. Alloyarova, R., Nikulin, M., Pya, N., and Voinov, V. (2006). The power-generalized Webull probability distribution and its use in survival analysis, In *Proceedings of the International Conference on Statistical Methods for Biomedical and Technical Systems*, pp. 189–194. Limassol, Cyprus.

3. Anderson, G. (1994). Simple tests of distributional form, *Journal of Econometrics*, **62**, 265–276.

4. Bagdonavicius, V. and Nikulin, M. (2002). *Accelerated life models*, Chapman & Hall/CRC, Boca Raton.

5. Boero, G., Smith, J., and Wallis, K. F. (2004). Decompositions of Pearson's chi-squared test, *Journal of Econometrics*, **123**, 189–193.

6. Chernoff, H., and Lehmann, E. L. (1954). The use of maximum likelihood estimates in χ^2 tests for goodness of fit, *Annals of Mathematical Statistics*, **25**, 579–586.

7. Chibisov, D. M. (1971). On asymptotic power of goodness-of-fit tests for approaching alternatives, *Theory of Probability and Applications*, **10**, 3–20 (in Russian).

8. Dahiya, R.C. and Gurland, J. (1972). Pearson chi-square test-of-fit with random intervals, *Biometrika*, **59**, 147–153.

9. Drost, F. (1988). *Asymptotics for Generalized Chi-Square Goodness-of-Fit Tests*, Amsterdam, Center for Mathematics and Computer Sciences, CWI Tracts, V. 48.

10. Dzhaparidze, K. O. (1983). On iterative procedures of asymptotic inference, *Statistica Neerlandica*, **37**, 181–189.

11. Dzhaparidze, K. O. and Nikulin, M. S. (1974). On a modification of the standard statistic of Pearson, *Theory of Probability and Its Applications*, **19**, 851–852.

12. Dzhaparidze, K. O. and Nikulin, M. S. (1992). On calculating chi-squared type statistics, *Problems of the theory of probability distributions*, **12**, 1–17, Nauka, St. Petersburg, Russia.

13. Fisher, R. A. (1924). The condition under which χ^2 measures the discrepancy between observation and hypothesis, *Journal of the Royal Statistical Society*, **87**, 442–450.

14. Fisher, R. A. (1925). Theory of statistical estimation, *Proceedings of the Cambridge Philosophical Society*, **22**, 700–725.

15. Fisher, R. (1928) On a property connecting the chi-square measure of discrepancy with the method of maximum likelihood. *Atti de Congresso Internazionale di Mathematici*, Bologna, **6**, 95–100.

16. Greenwood, P. S. and Nikulin, M. (1996). *A Guide to Chi-Squared Testing*, John Wiley & Sons, New York.

17. Hadi, A. S. and Wells, M. T. (1990). A note on generalized Wald's method, *Metrika*, **37**, 309–315.

18. Harter, H. L. and Moore, A. H. (1967). Maximum likelihood estimation, from censored samples, of the parameters of a logistic distribution, *Journal of the American Statistical Association*, **62**, 675–684.

19. Hsuan, T. A. and Robson, D.S. (1976). The χ^2 goodness-of-fit tests with moment type estimators, *Communications in Statistics—Theory and Methods*, **16**, 1509–1519.

20. LeCam, L., Mahan, C., and Singh, A. (1983). An extension of a theorem of H. Chernoff and E. L. Lehmann, In *Recent Advances in Statistics*, pp. 303–332, Academic Press, Orlando, FL.

21. Lemeshko, B. Yu., Postovalov, S. N., and Chimitova, E. V. (2001). On the distribution and power of Nikulin's chi-squared test, *Industrial laboratory*, **67**, 52–58 (in Russian).

22. Lockhart, R.A. and Stephens, A. (1994). Estimation and tests of fit for the three-parameter Weibull distribution, *Journal of the Royal Statistical Society*, **56**, 491–500.

23. McCulloch, Ch. E. (1985). Relationships among some chi-squared goodness of fit statistics, *Communications in Statistics—Theory and Methods*, **14**, 593–603.

24. McLaren, C. E., Legler, J. M., and Brittenham, G. M. (1994). The generalized χ^2 goodness-of-fit test, *The Statistician*, **43**, 247–258.

25. Mirvaliev, M. (2000). Invariant generalized chi-squared type statistics in problems of homogeneity, *O'Zbekiston Respublikasi Fanlar Akademiyasining Ma'Ruzalari*, **2**, 6–10.

26. Mirvaliev, M. (2001). An investigation of generalized chi-squared type statistics, *Ph.D. Thesis*, Academy of Science, Republic of Uzbekistan, Tashkent.

27. Moore, D. S. (1971). A chi-square statistic with random sell boundaries, *Annals of Mathematical Statistics*, **42**, 147–156.

28. Moore, D. S. (1977). Generalized inverses, Wald's method and the construction of chi-squared tests of fit, *Journal of the American Statistical Association*, **72**, 131–137.

29. Moore, D. S. and Spruill, M. C. (1975). Unified large-sample theory of general chi-squared statistics for tests of fit, *Annals of Statistics*, **3**, 599–616.

30. Mudholkar, G. S., Srivastava, D. K., and Freimer, M. (1995). The exponentiated Weibull family: A reanalysis of the bus-motor-failure data, *Technometrics*, **37**, 436–445.

31. Mudholkar, G. S. Srivastava, D. K., and Kollia, G.D. (1996). A generalization of the Weibull distribution with application to the analysis of survival data, *Journal of the American Statistical Association*, **91**, 1575–1583.

32. Nikulin, M. S. (1973). On a chi-square test for continuous distributions, *Theory of Probability and Its Applications*, **18**, 638–639 (in Russian).

33. Nikulin, M. S. (1973b). Chi-square test for continuous distributions with shift and scale parameters, *Theory of Probability and Its Applications*, **18**, 559–568.

34. Pearson, K. (1900). On the criterion that a given system of deviations from the probable in the case of a correlated system of variables is such that it can be reasonably supposed to have arisen from random sampling, *Philosophical Magazine*, **5**, 157–175.

35. Prudnikov, A. P., Brychkov, Y. A., and Marichev, O. I. (1986). *Integrals and Series. Additional Chapters*, Moscow, Nauka.

36. Rao, K. C. (1971). A chi-squared statistic for goodness-of-fit tests, *unpublished Ph.D. dissertation, Biometrics Unit*, Cornell University.

37. Rao, K. C. and Robson, D. S. (1974). A chi-square statistic for goodness-of-fit tests within the exponential family, *Communications in Statistics*, **3**, 1139–1153.

38. Roy, A. R. (1956). On χ^2- statistics with variable intervals, *Technical Report N1, Stanford University*, Statistics Department, Palo Alto, CA.

39. Singh, A. C. (1986). Categorical data analysis for simple random samples, *Proceedings of the Survey Research Methods Section*, ASA, 659–664.

40. Van Der Vaart, A. W. (1998). *Asymptotic Statistics. Cambridge Series in Statistical and Probabilistic Mathematics*, Cambridge University Press, Cambridge, UK.

41. Voinov, V. and Pya, N. (2004). On the power of modified chi-squared goodness-of-fit tests for the family of logistic and normal distributions, In *Proceedings of the Seventh Iranian Statistical Conference*, pp. 385–403, Allameh Tabatabaie University, Tehran, Iran.

42. Voinov, V., Alloyarova, R., and Pya, N. (2006a). A modified chi-squared test for the three-parameter Weibull distribution and its applications in reliability, In *Proceedings Of the International Conference on Degradation, Damage, Fatigue and Accelerated Life Models in Reliability Testing*, pp. 82–88, Angers, France.

43. Voinov, V., Naumov, A., and Pya, N. (2003). Some recent advances in chi-squared testing, In *Proceedings of the Internatinal Conference on Advances in Statistical Inferential Methods*, pp. 233–247, KIMEP, Almaty, Kazakhstan.

44. Voinov, V., Pya, N., and Alloyarova, R. (2006b). A comparative study of some modified chi-squared tests, Submitted to *Communications in Statistics— Simulation and Computation*.

45. Voinov, V. G. (2006). On optimalty of Rao-Robson-Nikulin test, *Industrial Laboratory*, **72**, 65-70 (in Russian).

46. Wald, A. (1943). Tests of statistical hypotheses concerning several parameters when the number of observations is large, *Transactions of the American Mathematical Society*, **54**, 426–482.

47. Watson, G. S. (1957). The chi-squared goodness-of-fit test for normal distributions, *JRSSB*, **19**, 262–267.

48. Watson, G. S. (1958). On chi-square goodness-of-fit tests for continuous distributions, *JPSSB*, **20**, 44–61.

49. Watson, G. S. (1959). Some resent results in χ^2 goodness-of-fit tests, *Biometrics*, **15**, 440–468.

50. Zhang, B. (1999). A chi-squared goodness-of-fit test for logistic regression models based on case-control data, *Biometrika*, **86**, 531–539.

19

Goodness-of-Fit Tests for Pareto Distribution

Sneh Gulati and Samuel Shapiro

Department of Statistics, Florida International University, Miami, FL, USA

Abstract: The Pareto distribution can serve to model several types of datasets, especially those arising in the insurance industry. In this chapter, we present methods to test the hypothesis that the underlying data come from a Pareto distribution. The tests presented for both the type I and type II Pareto distributions are based on the regression test of Brain and Shapiro (1983) for the exponential distribution. Power comparisons of the tests are carried out via simulations.

Keywords and Phrases: Type I Pareto distribution, type II Pareto distribution, regression tests, extreme values

19.1 Introduction

Statisticians and engineers have been expanding the types of models used in the analysis of measurement data. Initially the normal distribution was used for most problems. Presently however, distributions such as the exponential, Weibull, lognormal, gamma, and Pareto, have been used in the search for models that more closely match the phenomenon under study. Because the choice of a model can significantly affect the results of the analysis of a dataset, testing model assumptions plays an important role. This chapter presents simplified composite tests for the assumption that a set of data comes from type I and type II Pareto populations. The test statistic for type I uses a chi-squared two degree of freedom (exponential) as the null distribution, and the null distribution for the test statistic for type II has a chi-squared one degree of freedom, in other words, the square of the standard normal random variable distribution. These null distributions are approximately independent of the unknown parameters when n is large enough.

The Pareto distribution originates from the work of Pareto (1897) and has been used in many applications including modeling income distributions, hydrology, insurance claims, and in general populations representing extreme occurrences. Arnold (1983) stated that this model is useful for approximating data that arise from distributions with "fat tails." A comprehensive discussion of the Pareto distribution can be found in this reference. Various modifications have been made to the classical distribution proposed by Pareto. In Arnold's book he has labeled these as type I, type II, type III, and type IV.

This chapter discusses distributional tests for the first two of these. The estimation of the Pareto parameters using the maximum likelihood method results in biased estimators for the type I Pareto and is not straightforward for the other types. Several authors have presented simplified corrections for the bias of the maximum likelihood estimators for the type I model [see, e.g., Saksena (1978), Baxter (1980), and Cook and Mumme (1981)]. Harris (1968) and Arnold and Laguna (1977) proposed the technique of matching of moments for type II, and maximum likelihood estimation and other alternative methods of estimation of parameters were studied by Hosking and Wallis (1987) and Grimshaw (1993) among others. Voinov and Nikulin (1993) also present unbiased estimators for the Pareto distribution in addition to citing other references.

The classical or type I Pareto distribution is defined by the density function,

$$f(x) = \frac{\alpha \sigma^\alpha}{x^{\alpha+1}}, \qquad x \geq \sigma > 0, \qquad \alpha > 0. \tag{19.1}$$

The parameter α is the shape parameter and σ is the scale parameter. Note that the minimum value of X is equal to σ. It is easy to see that if X has a type I Pareto distribution, then $T = \ln(X/\sigma)$ has an exponential distribution with a mean of $1/\alpha$.

One reparametrization of the type II Pareto distribution which is used in this chapter is defined by the distribution function

$$F(x) = 1 - (1 + \theta x)^{-1/k}, \qquad x \geq 0, \qquad \theta \geq 0, \qquad k > 0. \tag{19.2}$$

If one assumes that k < 1, then the distribution has a finite first moment. Also note that $T = \ln(1 + X)$ has an exponential distribution with mean k.

Unlike other distributions there are few tests to assess whether it is reasonable to use the Pareto model with a given set of data when the two parameters are unknown. When the parameters are known it is a simple matter to transform the data to an exponential distribution and use one of the many tests for the exponential. In the composite case, when there are no specific tests known to the general public the classical chi-squared goodness-of-fit procedure using maximum likelihood estimates of the parameters is often used; however, this procedure results in a test statistic that does not have a central chi-square distribution and is only approximated by one [see Chernoff and

Lehmann (1954) and Greenwood and Nikulin (1996)]. Moreover, the procedure also has poor power properties for continuous distributions and small sample sizes. Choulakian and Stephens (2001) developed two composite hypothesis tests for a generalized Pareto distribution based on the Anderson–Darling and the Cramér–von Mises statistics. Their generalized Pareto is a type II distribution that has been reparametrized and where the parameter k can be negative. These tests require using the maximum likelihood estimators for the two parameters. Using this test one estimates the parameters, applies the probability integral transformation and uses either of the two tests to assess whether the transformed data could have been sampled from a uniform distribution. The critical value of the test statistic is compared to a table that is used to assess whether the Pareto model fits the data. The null critical values depend on the estimated parameters.

Beirlant et al. (2006) also proposed a test for the Pareto distribution. In this procedure the data are transformed to an exponential distribution and a modified Jackson (1967) statistic is used to test for the exponential distribution. They then used a bootstrapping procedure to get the null distribution. This chapter proposes a composite hypothesis test for the type I and type II Pareto models that is based on transforming the data to an exponential distribution and uses a modification of a test of exponentiality devised by Brain and Shapiro (1983). The Brain and Shapiro test procedure has in the limit a chi-squared distribution with two degrees of freedom and requires a correction factor that is a function of the sample size. Simulation studies have indicated that the null distribution of the proposed test statistic for the Pareto I distribution can be approximated by the chi-squared two-degree distribution (exponential) for sample sizes as small as 10 without use of the correction. For the type II distribution simulation results indicate that the null percentiles for the test statistic have an approximate chi-square distribution with one degree of freedom square of a standard normal random variable, are independent of the scale parameter, for all practical purposes are independent of the shape parameter for samples sizes of 30 or higher, and are not strongly dependent on the sample size. Because tests of distributional assumptions for models with an unknown shape parameter have low power for small sample sizes the limitation of samples of size 30 is not critical. Thus the advantages of the proposed procedure are that a p value can be obtained directly without any special tables.

Section 19.2 discusses estimation of the parameters of the Pareto type I, evaluates the bias and mean square error (MSE), describes the estimation procedure, and how the shape parameter affects these quantities. The third section describes the test for the exponential distribution proposed by Brain and Shapiro (1983) and gives the results of a study when using this with the Pareto type I distribution, and demonstrates how the null distribution is affected by estimating the Pareto shape parameter. The fourth section contains the results of a simulation study of the power of the procedure with a comparison to the results using the standard chi-square goodness-of-fit procedure. Sections 19.5 through 19.7 give the corresponding procedures and comparisons for the type II Pareto test. The final sections contain examples to illustrate the calculations using actual examples with real insurance claim data, an example analyzed by Choulakian and Stephens (2001), and some concluding remarks.

19.2   Type I Pareto Distribution

The first step in testing for either the type I or the type II Pareto distribution is the estimation of the parameters. Maximum likelihood estimates for the type I Pareto are easy to compute and are given by:

$$\sigma_{mle} = X_{(1)} = \text{the smallest observation} \tag{19.3}$$

$$\alpha_{mle} = \frac{n}{\sum_{i=1}^{n} \ln\left(\frac{X_{(i)}}{X_{(1)}}\right)} . \tag{19.4}$$

where $X_{(1)} \leq X_{(2)} \leq \cdots \leq X_{(n)}$. The estimator of α is biased which can be corrected by multiplying by $(n-2)/n$. Both these estimators are consistent and mutually independent and their sampling distributions are given in Malik (1970). A simulation study of the mean square error for the shape and scale parameters shows that the MSEs are usually quite small (below 0.01 in most cases) indicating that using the scale parameter estimate to transform the data to an exponential distribution should yield satisfactory results. The simulation was based on 10,000 trials using sample sizes between 10 and 100, a scale parameter of 1.0, and shape parameters between 0.5 and 6.0. The meansquare errors decrease for increasing sample size and increase for increasing value of the shape parameter. Because the major concern in this study is the power of the test procedure these results are quite adequate for the purpose of transforming the data for use in the testing procedure.

The data are transformed as follows for use in the test procedure,

$$T = \ln(X/X_{(1)}) \tag{19.5}$$

which is described in the next section.

19.3   Test for the Type I Pareto Distribution

Brain and Shapiro (1983) introduced a test procedure for assessing whether a set of data could have come from an exponential distribution. The test was based on using the Laplace test, a procedure suggested by Cox and Lewis (1966,

p. 53), for assessing whether the failure rate function was constant in order to assess whether a sample was drawn from an exponential distribution. The procedure uses the ordered weighted spacings and regresses these versus the order number using first- and second-degree orthogonal polynomials. It then tests whether the linear and/or quadratic terms are significantly different from zero for each polynomial. Because the regression uses orthogonal polynomials, the test statistics for each term are independent. Each statistic has an approximate standard normal distribution. The test statistic for assessing the distributional assumption uses the sum of the squares of the two individual test statistics and hence the null distribution for the exponential test has in the limit a chi-squared two degree of freedom distribution. The authors provided equations for correcting the critical values for finite sample sizes.

Using the notation from Brain and Shapiro (1983) let n be the sample size and denote the ordered statistics as $X_{(1)} \leq X_{(2)} \leq \cdots \leq X_{(n)}$. Let the ith weighted spacing be given by $Y_i = (n - i + 1)(X_{(i)} - X_{(i-1)})$; $(i = 1, 2, \ldots, n)$ and $X_0 = 0$. The n observations will generate n spacings. Let $TY_i = \sum_{j=1}^{i} Y_j$, $i = 1, 2, \ldots, n$ and $U_i = TY_i / TY_n$, $i = 1, 2, \ldots, n - 1$; then the test statistic for the linear component is given by:

$$Z_1 = \sqrt{\frac{12}{n-1}} (\bar{U} - 1/2) \tag{19.6}$$

where

$$\bar{U} = \sum_{i=1}^{n-1} \frac{U_i}{n-1}.$$

Similarly, Z_2, the test statistic for the quadratic component is given by:

$$Z_2 = \sqrt{\frac{5}{4(n+2)(n-1)(n-2)}} * \left(n - 2 + 6n\bar{U} - 12 \sum_{i=1}^{n-1} \frac{iU_i}{n-1} \right). \tag{19.7}$$

The test statistic is

$$Z_0 = Z_1^2 + Z_2^2. \tag{19.8}$$

The null distribution of Z_0 is in the limit a chi-squared distribution with two degrees of freedom. This is an upper-tail test with a critical region of $Z_0 > \chi_{2,\alpha}^2$ for an α-level test. It is also simply an exponential distribution with a mean of 2.0 and thus the p-value is given by

$$p = e^{-Z_0/2}. \tag{19.9}$$

A Monte Carlo analysis was conducted to assess the null distribution of Z_0 to determine the effect of using estimates in the transformation process. Values of the shape parameter from 0.1 to 6.0 were used for sample sizes from 10 to 100. Critical values of $\alpha = 0.025, 0.05$, and 0.10 were used. The simulation was based on a sample of 10,000 for each combination of sample size and shape parameter. A review of these results indicates that there was no systematic change in the critical values as a function of either sample size or value of the shape parameter. The empirical critical values fluctuated around the theoretical values for a chi-squared two degree of freedom distribution deviating in most cases by less than 3σ from the theoretical value. Here $\sigma = \sqrt{pq/N}$ where $N = 10,000$. A further analysis of the type I error of Z_0 using the chi-squared distribution with two degrees of freedom was conducted using simulations. Empirical type I errors for Z_0 were generated with $\alpha = 0.025, 0.05$, and 0.10 for sample sizes from 10 to 100 and values of the shape parameter between 0.1 and 6.0 as before. Once again the results indicated that the differences between the results and the nominal values were trivial and did not vary as a function of parameter nor sample size.

Thus a test for the type I Pareto distribution is obtained via the following steps.

1. Obtain the estimate of the scale parameter using the maximum likelihood estimator from (19.3).
2. Transform the data to $T = \ln(X/X_1)$ where X_1 is the smallest data value. Note that this transformation converts the shape parameter to a scale parameter and the scale parameter to the origin parameter of zero. As pointed out in Section 19.1, the transformed data will be exponential with origin of zero and a scale parameter of α.
3. Compute Z_1 from (19.6) and Z_2 from (19.7) using the ordered T_i's for the ordered X's to obtain the Y_i's, TY_i's, and the U_i's in these equations.
4. Compute Z_0 from (19.8).
5. Reject the null hypothesis of a Pareto type I distribution if $Z_0 > \chi^2_{2,\alpha}$ for an α-level test. The critical values of the chi-squared distribution with two degrees of freedom for $\alpha = 0.025, 0.05$, and 0.10 are 4.605, 5.991, and 7.378. Note this is an upper-tail test and that this procedure is a modification of the Brain and Shapiro (1983) procedure where a correction for sample size was needed. In the Pareto test the origin parameter is known to be zero and this places a constraint on the test statistic possibly resulting in eliminating the need for the correction and increasing the power of the procedure.
6. The p-value for the test is obtained from (19.9).

19.4   Power Study

The measure of the value of a test procedure is how well it performs when used with a variety of alternative distributions. In order to assess the proposed procedure a Monte Carlo study of the power of the test was conducted. The study was based on 10,000 Monte Carlo runs for each sample size and alternative distribution. The following alternative distributions were used.

1. Weibull shape parameters 0.25, 0.5, 0.75, and 2.0
2. Half-normal $\sigma = 1.0$
3. Gamma shape parameter 0.5
4. Lognormal shape parameter 1.0

The results of the power study for these distributions are given in Table 19.1 for $\alpha = 0.05$ which show that the power was more than 0.90 for samples of size 20 and higher except in the case of the lognormal distribution where the power was only 0.70 for a sample size of 20. The power reached 0.90 for the lognormal for samples of 30 or higher.

The power of the chi-squared test was compared with the above procedure in the following manner.

1. A sample of size n was generated from the alternate distribution.
2. The two parameters σ and α were estimated using Equations (19.3) and (19.4) and the unbiased estimator of α was obtained by multiplying by $n/(n-2)$.
3. The intervals $(0, L_1), (L_1, L_2), \ldots, (L_7, \infty)$ were calculated, where

$$L_i = \frac{\sigma_{mle}}{(1 - 0.125i)^{\frac{1}{\sigma_{mle}}}} \; .$$

Thus the expected number for each interval is $0.125 * n$.
4. These intervals are constructed so that probability of being in each interval is the same. The probability of observing a value in each interval is $0.125n$ under the null hypothesis.
5. The chi-square test using five degrees of freedom was used.

The power study for the chi-square test was limited to samples of 40 or higher in order to ensure that the expected number per cell was at least five. The power of the two procedures was comparable (see Tables 19.1 and 19.2); however, the proposed test can be used for smaller sample sizes and does not require dividing the data into cells where the results may depend on the number of cells chosen.

19.5   Type II Pareto Distribution

The first step in testing for the type II Pareto distribution involves the estimation of the underlying parameters θ and k. The maximum likelihood estimates of the parameters are obtained by solving the nonlinear equation for θ given below:

Table 19.1. Power of the Pareto test for various alternate distributions, type I error = 0.05

N	WE(0.25)	WE(0.5)	WE(0.75)	WE(2)	G(0.5)	HN	LN
20	0.9391	0.9408	0.9403	0.9383	0.9737	0.9707	0.7034
30	0.9971	0.9980	0.9998	0.9984	0.9993	0.9996	0.9515
40	0.9998	0.9999	1.000	1.000	1.000	1.000	0.9952
50	1.000	1.000	1.000	1.000	1.000	1.000	0.9992
60	1.000	1.000	1.000	1.000	1.000	1.000	1.000
70	1.000	1.000	1.000	1.000	1.000	1.000	1.000
80	1.000	1.000	1.000	1.000	1.000	1.000	1.000
90	1.000	1.000	1.000	1.000	1.000	1.000	1.000
100	1.000	1.000	1.000	1.000	1.000	1.000	1.000

$WE(\eta) =$ Weibull with shape parameter η.
$G(\eta) =$ gamma shape parameter η.
$HN =$ half-normal $\sigma = 1$.
$LN =$ log-normal $\sigma = 1$.

Table 19.2. Power of the chi-square test for various alternate distributions, type I error = 0.05

N	WE(0.25)	WE(0.5)	WE(0.75)	WE(2)	G(0.5)	HN	LN
40	0.9997	0.9997	0.9997	0.9999	1.000	1.000	0.9851
50	1.000	1.000	1.000	1.000	1.000	1.000	0.9968
60	1.000	1.000	1.000	1.000	1.000	1.000	0.9995
70	1.000	1.000	1.000	1.000	1.000	1.000	1.000
80	1.000	1.000	1.000	1.000	1.000	1.000	1.000
90	1.000	1.000	1.000	1.000	1.000	1.000	1.000
100	1.000	1.000	1.000	1.000	1.000	1.000	1.000

$WE(\eta) =$ Weibull with shape parameter η.
$G(\eta) =$ gamma shape parameter η.
$HN =$ half-normal $\sigma = 1$.
$LN =$ log-normal $\sigma = 1$.

$$f(\hat{\theta}) = \left(1 + (1/n)\sum_{i=1}^{n}\ln(1 + \theta X_i)\right) \star \left((1/n)\sum_{i=1}^{n}(1 + \theta X_i)^{-1}\right) = 0. \quad (19.10)$$

Using $\hat{\theta}$, the estimator of k, $\hat{k}$ is given by:

$$\hat{k} = \frac{\sum_{i=1}^{n}\ln(1 + \hat{\theta}X_i)}{n}. \quad (19.11)$$

To solve Equation (19.10), we used the iterative method proposed by Grimshaw (1993). In some cases the procedure did not converge. In these cases we switched to using a probability weighted moment procedure developed by Hosking and Wallis (1987). In these cases the model was reparametrized to model (19.12). (The initial parameterization is given in Section 19.2.)

$$F(x) = 1 - \left(1 + \frac{k}{\alpha} x\right)^{1/k}. \tag{19.12}$$

The estimators for this model are

$$\hat{\alpha} = \frac{2\alpha_0 \alpha_1}{\alpha_0 - 2\alpha_1} \tag{19.13}$$

$$\hat{k} = \frac{\alpha_0}{\alpha_0 - 2\alpha_1} - 2, \tag{19.14}$$

where

$$\alpha_0 = \bar{X}$$

$$\alpha_1 = \frac{1}{n} \sum_{j=1}^{n} (1 - p_{(j)}) X_{(j)}; \qquad X_{(1)} \le X_{(2)} \le \cdots \le X_{(n)}$$

and

$$p_j = \frac{j - 0.35}{n}.$$

Thus the estimated parameters in terms of the original model (19.2) are given by:

$$\hat{k} = -\hat{k}^* \quad \text{and} \quad \hat{\theta} = \frac{\hat{k}}{\hat{\alpha}}.$$

These estimators exist provided that $0 < k < 1$ This assumption is not overly restrictive because according to Hosking and Wallis (1987) values of $k > 1/2$ rarely occur in practice.

The estimation procedure goes as follows.

1. Set θ equal to 1 to start. Hosking and Wallis (1987) indicate that the estimation procedure is not affected by the initial value of θ.
2. Generate the Xs from the type II Pareto distribution.
3. Using the MLE procedure for model (19.2) estimate θ and k.
4. If the MLE does not exist use the probability weighted moment procedure with (19.12).
5. In the case where the estimator of k using the method of Hosking and Wallis is negative we set $\hat{k} = 0.005$ and let $\hat{\theta} = 0.005/\hat{\alpha}$.
6. Transform the data using

$$T_i = \ln(1 + \hat{\theta} X_i); \qquad i = 1, 2, \ldots n.$$

7. Use the Ts as input to the test procedure as shown in Section 19.3 substituting the Ts for the Xs in that section.

8. The p-value can be obtained as described in Section 19.6.

As in the case of the type I Pareto, a simulation study was conducted to assess the performance of these estimators. Biases and mean square errors of the estimators were computed for a total of 10,000 simulation runs. In all the runs, the scale parameter was set at 1.0 and the shape parameter varied from $k = 1$ down to $k = 0.2$ for samples ranging from 30 to 100. Note that the only statistic of interest in this study is the estimator of the shape parameter because the distributional test statistic is scale invariant.

The estimators for the shape parameter k were quite good with the highest errors arising when $k = 1$; the maximum MSE was less than 0.15 when $n = 30$ and less than 0.11 for higher values of n. The maximum value of the MSE for values of k of 0.5 or less was less than 0.07 and dropped to less than 0.02 for $k = 0.2$. The proportion of cases where the MLE did not converge and the probability weighted moment estimators had to be used was also recorded. This proportion was low when $k = 1$, less than 0.01, but increased as k decreased to $k = 0.2$; reaching up to 0.3 in some cases. The proportion decreased with increasing sample size.

In this study the important concern is not so much the MSE of the estimators but how the estimation procedure affects the power of the test of the distributional assumption. This effect on the power is investigated in Section 19.7.

19.6   Null Distribution of the Proposed Procedure and Power Study

A simulation of 10,000 runs was used to determine the null distribution of the Shapiro–Brain statistic Z_0 for values of n between 30 and 100 and k between 1.0 and 0.2. The scale parameter was set at 1.0. Critical values corresponding to 0.01, 0.075, 0.05, and 0.025 were determined. There was no systematic change in the critical values as a function of either n or k. As a further check a regression function for each of the critical values as a function of n and k showed little relationship between them and the critical value. Therefore the critical values for each value of n and k were averaged together to determine the critical values of Z_0 for each of the levels of the test. Unlike the results for the type I case, these averages were closely approximated by a one degree of freedom chi-squared distribution. In order to check on this supposition the critical values from this distribution were used to compute the simulated critical values for test levels of 0.1, 0.05, 0.025, and 0.01 for samples of size 30 to 100 and k from

1.0 to 0.2. Once again the variation of the simulated critical values in the range investigated is nominal and thus the approximation for the null distribution is adequate. Note that the chi-squared distribution with one degree of freedom is the square of a standard normal distribuiton and so the p-value of the test can be obtained directly from normal tables.

19.7 Power of the Proposed Procedure

The power of the procedure for type II Pareto was studied against a variety of alternative distributions. The study was based on 10,000 Monte Carlo runs for each sample size and alternative distribution. The following alternative distributions were used.

Weibull shape parameters 0.25–2.0 (0.25)
Half-normal $\sigma = 1.0$
Gamma shape parameters 0.25–2.0 (0.25)
Lognormal shape parameters 0.50–2.0 (0.25)

The results of the power study for these distributions are given in Tables 19.3–19.5 for $\alpha = 0.05$.

For both the Weibull and the gamma distributions the power was extremely high for values of the shape parameter far away from 1.0, reaching 1 for a number of cases. For shape parameters of 0.75 and 1.25, the power dropped down considerably ranging from 0.1555 (gamma, shape 0.75, $n = 30$) to 0.4760 (gamma, shape $= 1.25$, $n = 100$). In all these cases, the power for the Weibull distribution was generally higher than that for the gamma. For shape parameter equal to 1 (the case of the exponential distribution), the power was low for both cases (staying between 0.095 to 0.1004 for all sample sizes). This is not unexpected because in the limit as $k \to 0$, the Pareto distribution approaches

Table 19.3. Power of the Pareto II test for the Weibull, type I error = 0.05

N	WE(0.25)	WE(0.5)	WE(0.75)	WE(1)	WE(1.25)	WE(1.5)	WE(2.0)
30	0.9121	0.5387	0.1555	0.0951	0.3790	0.7968	0.9975
40	0.9750	0.6915	0.2030	0.0957	0.4777	0.8949	0.9999
50	0.9935	0.8002	0.2480	0.0957	0.5604	0.9562	1.000
60	0.9989	0.8816	0.2920	0.0977	0.6253	0.9800	1.000
70	0.9996	0.9253	0.3432	0.0980	0.6873	0.9922	1.000
80	1.000	0.9557	0.3837	0.0977	0.7493	0.9966	1.000
90	1.000	0.9745	0.4283	0.1004	0.7984	0.9987	1.000
100	1.000	0.9854	0.4676	0.0965	0.8383	0.9988	1.000

$WE(\eta)$ = Weibull with shape parameter η.

Table 19.4. Power of the Pareto II test for the gamma, type I error = 0.05

N	$G(0.25)$	$G(0.5)$	$G(0.75)$	$G(1.25)$	$G(1.5)$	$G(2.0)$
30	0.9500	0.4658	0.1298	0.2201	0.4399	0.8270
40	0.9871	0.6009	0.1564	0.2573	0.5314	0.9222
50	0.9964	0.7147	0.1881	0.2906	0.6256	0.9677
60	0.9993	0.7989	0.2129	0.3298	0.6998	0.9847
70	1.000	0.8567	0.2476	0.3699	0.7636	0.9955
80	1.000	0.9039	0.2863	0.4038	0.8134	0.9973
90	1.000	0.9353	0.3048	0.4419	0.8502	0.9995
100	1.000	0.9534	0.3336	0.4761	0.8849	0.9998

$G(\eta) =$ Gamma shape parameter η.

Table 19.5. Power of the Pareto II test for the half-normal and log-normal, type I error = 0.05

N	HN	$LN(0.5)$	$LN(1.0)$	$LN(1.5)$
30	0.4449	1.000	0.3636	0.0360
40	0.5528	1.000	0.4586	0.0388
50	0.6515	1.000	0.5474	0.0363
60	0.7348	1.000	0.6287	0.0403
70	0.8027	1.000	0.7015	0.0377
80	0.8563	1.000	0.7561	0.0376
90	0.8928	1.000	0.8024	0.0397
100	0.9238	1.000	0.8445	0.0375

$LN(\eta) =$ Lognormal with shape η.

$HN =$ Half-normal distribution.

the exponential distribution.

In the case of the half-normal distribution, the power ranged from 0.4449 ($n = 30$) to 0.9238 ($n = 100$). Finally, for the lognormal, the power was extremely low for values of σ greater than 1; ranging from 0.0360 ($n = 30$, $\sigma = 1.5$) to 0.2933 ($n = 100$, $\sigma = 2$). For values of σ below 1, the power increased rapidly reaching almost 1 for almost all sample sizes for $\sigma = 0.5$. The results are not surprising because the lognormal distribution becomes more heavily skewed as σ increases making it very hard to differentiate between the two models.

19.8   Examples

A random sample of 55 payments made by a reinsurance agency that pays insurance companies the excess losses they suffered from their payout of claims was used to investigate the tests described in Sections 19.3 and 19.5. The data consist of payments made between 1990 and 1993 and include payments made for pension actuaries and property and liability actuaries [see Tables 1.3 and 1.4 in Klugman *et al.* (1998)]. It was of interest to find out whether one could use one Pareto model for both pension and property and liability claims. The following steps illustrate the calculations necessary for testing the composite hypothesis that the data came from a type I distribution with unspecified parameters.

1. The estimate of the scale parameter $\sigma = X_1 = 189$ which is the smallest payout.

2. Transform the data using $T = \ln[X/189]$.

3. Using (19.6) and (19.7) $Z_1 = 5.813$ and $Z_2 = 2.497$.

4. From (19.8) $Z_0 = 40.0267$ and from (19.9) the p-value is close to zero.

5. Thus it is highly improbable that a type I Pareto distribution can be used to model this dataset. The data cannot be combined or another model must be found.

The type II model was also tested for use with the combined dataset. The maximum likelihood equations converged and the estimates of k and θ were 2.8278 and 0.0001, respectively. This yielded a value of Z_0 of 10.55 resulting in a p-value close to zero. Thus a single Pareto model cannot be used to describe this dataset.

In Choulakian and Stephens (2001) a dataset consisting of 72 exceedances of flood peaks of the Wheatan River in the Yukon Territory, Canada was analyzed to determine if a generalized Pareto model could be used to model the data. They applied both of the two procedures given in that paper and obtained $p < 0.025$ from one and $p < 0.01$ for the other. Using these data for the proposed test, it was found that the maximum likelihood procedures did not converge and hence the probability weighted moments were employed. This resulted in estimates of k and θ of 0.10257 and 0.009358 yielding a value of Z_0 of 6.4968. The p-value was 0.0108. Thus the results agreed closely with those in the cited paper without use of special tables.

19.9 Conclusions

This chapter has presented a simple test procedure for assessing the probability that a random sample could have come from a Pareto type I distribution. The procedure uses the log transformation to convert the data to an exponential distribution with an origin of zero. A modification of a test for the exponential proposed by Brain and Shapiro was used to assess this hypothesis where the test statistic has a chi-squared two degrees of freedom distribution for sample sizes of 10 or over. The p-value for a test can be obtained from tables of this distribution or simply by using an exponential with a mean of 2.0. Monte Carlo results showed that this approximation was close to a two degree of freedom chi-square distribution and the type I errors were very close to the nominal values. A Monte Carlo study indicated that the procedure had a high power against almost all distributions included in the study.

The estimation of the parameters for the type II test procedure is more complex because the maximum likelihood equations may not always converge. An alternative procedure to handle these cases, the use of probability weighted moments, was given. Once the estimates were obtained the same Brain and Shapiro technique was used to test for exponentiality. The resulting null distribution could be approximated by chi-squared one degree of freedom or the square of a standard normal random variable distribution. Simulations results indicated that the approximation could be used to represent the test statistic for samples of 30 or higher.

Thus both procedures have the advantage that no special tables are needed to compute the test statistic or find the p-values.

Acknowledgements

The authors are grateful to Dr. Scott Grimshaw for supplying a copy of the macro of the procedure to find the maximum likelihood estimators for the type II Pareto distribution.

References

1. Arnold, B. C. (1983). Pareto distributions, In *Statistical Distributions in Scientific Work Series*, Vol. 5, International Co-operative Publication House, Burtonsville, Maryland.

2. Arnold, B. C. and Laguna, L. (1977). On generalized Pareto distributions with applications to income data, In *International Studies in Economics*,

Monograph #10, Department of Economics, Iowa State University, Ames, Iowa.

3. Baxter, M. A. (1980). Minimum variance unbiased estimators of the parameters of the Pareto distribution, *Metrika*, **27**, 133–138.

4. Beirlant, J., de Wet, T., and Goegebeur, Y. (2006). A goodness-of-fit statistic for Pareto-type behaviour, *Journal of Computational and Applied Mathematics*, **186**, 99–116.

5. Brain, C. W. and Shapiro, S. S. (1983). A regression test for exponentiality: Censored and complete samples, *Technometrics*, **25**, 69–76.

6. Chernoff, H. and Lehmann, E. L. (1954). The use of maximum likelihood estimates in χ^2 tests for goodness of fit, *The Annals of Mathematical Statistics*, **25**, 579–586.

7. Choulakian, V. and Stephens, M. A. (2001). Goodness-of-fit tests for the generalized Pareto distribution, *Technometrics*, **43**, 478–484.

8. Cook, W. L. and Mumme, D. C. (1981). Estimation of Pareto parameters by numerical methods, In *Statistical Distributions in Scientific Work* (Eds., C. Taillie, G. P. Patil, and B. Baldessari), **5**, pp. 127–132, Reidel, Dordecht-Holland.

9. Cox, D. R. and Lewis, P. A. (1966). *The Statistical Analysis of a Series of Events*, Methune, London.

10. Davison, A. C. (1984). Modeling excesses over high thresholds, with an application, In *Statistical Extremes and Applications*, (Ed., J. Tiago de Oliveira), pp. 461–482, D. Reidel, Dordrecht.

11. Greenwood, P. S. and Nikulin, M. S. (1996). *A Guide to Chi-Squared Testing*, John Wiley & Sons, New York.

12. Grimshaw, S. D. (1993). Computing maximum likelihood estimates for the generalized Pareto distribution, *Technometrics*, **35**, 185–191.

13. Harris, C. M. (1968). The Pareto distribution as a queue service discipline, *Operations Research*, **16**, 307–313.

14. Hosking, J. R. M. and Wallis, J. R. (1987). Parameter and quantile estimation for the generalized Pareto distribution, *Technometrics*, **29**, 339–349.

15. Jackson, O. A. Y. (1967). An analysis of departures from the exponential distribution, *Journal of the Royal Society Statistical Society, Series B*, **29**, 540–549.

16. Klugman, S. A., Panjer, H. H., and Wilmot, G. E. (1998). *Loss Models: From Data to Decisions*, John Wiley & Sons, New York.

17. Malik, H. J. (1970). Estimation of the parameters of the Pareto distribution, *Metrika*, **15**, 126–132.

18. Pareto, V. (1897). *Cours d'economie Politique*, Vol. II, F. Rouge, Lausanne.

19. Saksena, S. K. (1978). Estimation of parameters in a Pareto distribution and simultaneous comparison of estimators, *Ph.D. Thesis*, Louisiana Tech University, Ruston.

20. Voinov, V. G. and Nikulin, M. S. (1993). *Unbiased Estimators and their Applications, Vol. I*, Kluwer, Boston.

Application of Inverse Problems in Epidemiology and Biodemography

A. Michalski

Institute of Control Sciences, Moscow, Russia

Abstract: Inverse problems play an important role in science and engineering. Estimation of boundary conditions on the temperature distribution inside a metallurgical furnace and reconstruction of tissue density inside a body on plane projections obtained with x-rays are some examples. Different problems in epidemiology, demography, and biodemography can be considered as solutions of inverse problems as well: when using observed data one estimates the process that generated the data. Examples are estimation of infection rate on dynamics of the disease, estimation of mortality rate on the sample of survival times, and estimation of survival in the wild on survival in the laboratory. A specific property of the inverse problem—the instability of a solution—is discussed and a procedure for the solution stabilization is presented. Examples of morbidity estimation on incomplete data, HIV infection rate estimation on dynamics of AIDS cases, and estimation of the survival function in a wild population on survival of captured animals are presented.

Keywords and Phrases: Inverse problem, epidemiology, biodemography, incomplete follow-up, HIV infection rate, AIDS, survival in wild

20.1   Introduction

Interpretation of observations in different disciplines of life science and engineering can be considered as estimation of a process using observations from another process related to the one estimated. Depending on the problem setting the objective can be estimation of a signal in the presence of noise, numerical calculation of derivatives, calculation of boundary conditions on the values of temperature distribution inside a metallurgical furnace, and reconstruction of tissue density inside a body on plane projections obtained with x-rays. Similar problems arise in epidemiology, when a disease prevalence (proportion of sick people in different age groups) can be obtained but incidence rate (probability of a healthy person to become sick during say, one year) is to be estimated. In demography and biodemography calculation of mortality rates form similar problems. The proportion of survived people is observed but the chance of dying during one year is of primary interest. These chances influence the numbers of survivors and are used in the calculation and projection of the life expectancy and the population age structure.

In all these examples the value of the "effect" can be estimated on population observations whereas the direct estimation of the "cause" is impossible or expensive. On the other hand information about the cause often is important for better understanding of the phenomenon investigated and mathematical methods for estimation of cause on effect data are needed. All these problems form a class of mathematical problems called *inverse problems* contrary to *forward problems* when the estimation process follows the cause–effect line. Many inverse problems important for practice have a solution which is very sensitive to disturbances in the data. In epidemiology, demography, and biodemography variations in data arise because of the probabilistic nature of the process and the limited number of observed subjects. As a result one has extremely large changes in the estimates even when the amount of data increases.

The inverse problems are presented in statistical analysis as well. Estimation of the probability density function on the independent sample is an inverse problem with an unstable solution. One has to apply additional constraints on the estimate to guarantee the convergence of the estimate to the real probability density function when the amount of data increases. In a histogram estimate the restriction can be applied in the form of dependence between the number of cells and the number of elements in the sample. In the kernel estimates the restriction is applied in the form of dependence between the kernel width and the sample size. The introduction of parametric estimation can be considered as a way to stabilize an unstable estimate as well.

Formal consideration of inverse problems, statistical consideration, and procedures for solution stabilization are presented in the next section. Three examples with the results of calculations are presented in the other sections. They are: estimation of morbidity on the results of incomplete follow-up, estimation of HIV infection rate on the dynamics of AIDS cases, and estimation of survival in a wild population on survival of the captured animals in the laboratory.

20.2 Definition and Solution of Inverse Problem

In formal terms the inverse problem is a problem of the solution of an operator equation

$$Ax = y, \tag{20.1}$$

where A is a bounded linear operator between infinite-dimensional functional Hilbert spaces X and Y; x and y are elements from these spaces. Function y plays the role of observations or effect; function x plays the role of cause-produced observed effect. It is supposed that operator A makes one-to-one mapping between spaces X and Y. The solution of Equation (20.1) is a function, defined as

$$x = A^{-1}y,$$

where A^{-1} is the inverse operator of A which is linear as well. It is proved that if the range $R(A)$ for A is nonclosed, then operator A^{-1} is unbounded [Tikhonov and Arsenin (1977) and Engl *et al.* (1996)]. The latter means that if one substitutes a "disturbed" function $y^\delta \in Y$ such that $\|y - y^\delta\| \le \delta$ in (20.1) then the disturbance in the corresponding solution $A^{-1}y^\delta$ may be infinite. Here $\|y\|$ denotes the norm of y. More precisely: for any small value δ and any large value Δ there exists a function $y_\Delta^\delta \in Y$ such that $\|y - y_\Delta^\delta\| \le \delta$ and $\|A^{-1}y - A^{-1}y_\Delta^\delta\| > \Delta$. The unboundedness of the inverse operator makes it impossible to guarantee that the solution found on the perturbed data will be close to the solution, corresponding to the unperturbed data.

The general approach to the solution of equations with an unbounded inverse operator, called ill-posed equations, was formulated in Tikhonov and Arsenin (1977) as the minimization of a regularized functional $J_\alpha(x) = \|Ax - y^\delta\|^2 + \alpha\|Bx\|^2$, where $\alpha > 0$ is a regularization parameter, and B is an unbounded operator defined at functional set $D(B) \subseteq X$ such that $Bx \subseteq X$. Minimization is to be done in $D(B)$, the region of definition of the operator B. The problem of proper selection of the regularization parameter value is widely discussed in the literature. For special case $B = D^s$, where D is a differential operator and s is some nonnegative real number, Natterer (1984) has shown that under the assumptions $\|D^p A^{-1}y\| \le E$ and $m\|D^{-\alpha}x\| \le \|Ax\| \le M\|D^{-\alpha}x\|$ with some constants E, m, and M, regularized solution x_α provides approximation of the real solution with bound $\|x_\alpha - A^{-1}y\| = O\left(\delta^{p/(\alpha+p)}\right)$ for $s \ge (p - \alpha)/2$ if α is chosen prior as $\alpha = c\delta^{2(\alpha+s)/(\alpha+p)}$ with some constant c. Posterior selection of a regularization parameter can be done using Morozov's discrepancy principle [Morozov (1993)] which prescribes selecting parameter α as the solution of the equation $\|Ax_\alpha - y^\delta\| = C\delta$, where $C \ge 1$ is a constant. The efficiency of this approach has been proved in many applications [Nair *et al.* (2003, 2005)]. Procedures of regularization parameter selection in the case of stochastic disturbances in y^δ are considered in Lukas (1998), and Engl *et al.* (2005).

The statistical estimation as an inverse problem was considered in Vapnik (1982), O'Sullivan (1986), and Evans and Stark (2002). The statistical estimation procedure can be considered as the minimization of an averaged risk functional on the empirical data. In nonparametric estimation the dimension of the estimate is infinite and the result is unstable just as in the case of solution of the ill-posed problem. The method of sieves [Geman and Hwang (1982) and Shen (1997)], spline and ridge regressions, and penalized likelihood are regularization methods for minimizing the empirical risk functional. The form of the averaged risk functional depends on the problem under consideration. For regression estimation the averaged risk functional is

$$J\left(x\right) = \int \left(y - x\left(t\right)\right)^2 dP\left(t, y\right),$$

where t and y are random variables with joint distribution function $P\left(t, y\right)$, and $x\left(t\right)$ is a function from a functional class F. The averaged risk value can be estimated using random sample $T = \{t_1, y_1, \dots, t_m, y_m\}$ of independent realizations of t and y by the empirical risk functional

$$J^e\left(x\right) = \frac{1}{m} \sum_{i=1}^{m} \left(y_i - x\left(t_i\right)\right)^2.$$

Minimization of the empirical risk in F is the classical *least square procedure* and can be used without supposition about conditional normality of the random variable y. If the class F is restricted by the smoothed functions, then the minimizer of $J^e\left(x\right)$ is the spline; the class F of polynomials corresponds to estimation of the polynomial regression.

The other form for the averaged risk functional is the Kullback–Leibler entropy

$$J\left(x\right) = - \int \ln p_x\left(t, y\right) dP\left(t, y\right),$$

where $p_x\left(t, y\right)$ is the probability density function for distribution of the random pair (t, y), which corresponds to the function $x\left(t\right)$. The empirical risk functional is proportional to the log-likelihood functional, obtained from the independent sample T,

$$J^e\left(x\right) = \frac{-1}{m} \sum_{i=1}^{m} \ln p_x\left(t_i, y_i\right),$$

minimization of which is the *method of maximal likelihood*. The constrained maximization of the log-likelihood functional leads to the *method of penalized likelihood maximization*.

Many procedures are used for selection of the smoothing parameter value which stands for the regularization parameter. The cross-validation technique and Bayesian approach are among them. Different approaches and methods are presented in Evans and Stark (2002). Vapnik (1982) described for this purpose the method of structural risk minimization. The method operates by an estimate for the uniform in subclass $F_c \subset F$ deviation between the empirical risk and the averaged risk, which can be obtained from the inequality

$$P\left\{\sup_{x \in F_c} |J(x) - J^e(x)| \geq \varepsilon\right\} \leq \eta,$$

which allows us to say that with probability not less than $1 - \eta$ it holds

$$\min_{x \in F_c} J(x) < \min_{x \in F_c} J^e(x) + \varepsilon(F_c, \eta).$$

The right part of the last inequality can be used to build the procedure for data-driven selection of the proper subclass F_c, which is equivalent to selection of the regularized parameter value. The details can be found in Vapnik (1982, 1998) and Chapelle *et al.* (2002).

A simple procedure for regularization parameter selection using a finite sample of observations was described in Mikhal'skii (1987). Suppose that in the sample $T = \{t_1, y_1, \ldots, t_m, y_m\}$ the elements t_j are fixed and the elements y_j are random, $y = \mathbf{A}x_0 + \xi$, y is a vector with coordinates y_i, x_0 is a vector with n coordinates presenting the real solution for the undisturbed equation, $\mathbf{A}$ is an $m \times n$ matrix, ξ is a random vector with m coordinates ξ_i such that $E(\xi_i) = 0$, and $var(\xi_i) = \sigma^2$, $cov(\xi_i, \xi_j) = 0$, and $i, j = 1, \ldots, m$. Denote x_α the regularized solution obtained by minimization of the functional $\|u - \mathbf{A}x\|^2 + \alpha\|\mathbf{B}x\|^2$ and $\mathbf{A}_\alpha = \mathbf{A}(\mathbf{A}^T\mathbf{A} + \alpha\mathbf{B}^T\mathbf{B})^{-1}\mathbf{A}^T$. For α such that m $> 2Tr\mathbf{A}_\alpha$, with probability no less than $1 - \eta$ the inequality is valid [Mikhal'skii (1987)],

$$E_{u,y}\|y - \mathbf{A}x_\alpha\|^2 \leq \frac{\|u - \mathbf{A}x_\alpha\|^2}{1 - 2Tr\mathbf{A}_\alpha/m} + \sigma^2 + \sqrt{r/\eta}. \tag{20.2}$$

The constant r is defined by eigenvalues of matrices $\mathbf{A}$ and $\mathbf{B}$, by the square norm of vector x_0, and by the second and the fourth moments of the random values ξ_i. The left side of (20.2) is the mean value of disagreement between the possible vectors of experimental and predicted data. The expectation is taken over y and u. To reduce this value one can use parameter α, which minimizes a criterion

$$I_\alpha = \|u - \mathbf{A}x_\alpha\|^2 / (1 - 2Tr\mathbf{A}_\alpha/m). \tag{20.3}$$

The quantity $\|u - \mathbf{A}x_\alpha\|^2$ is the square residual for empirical data.

The criterion I_α shows a resemblance to the cross-validation criterion $I_\alpha^{cv} = \|u - \mathbf{A}x_\alpha\|^2 / \left(1 - Tr\mathbf{A}_\alpha/m\right)^2$ [Stone (1974)]. For the large values of m these two criteria are equivalent because $\left(1 - Tr\mathbf{A}_\alpha/m\right)^2 = 1 - 2Tr\mathbf{A}_\alpha/m + o\left(1/m\right)$. For small values of m the criterion I_α produces better results than criterion I_α^{cv} [Mikhal'skii (1987)].

20.3   Estimation on Incomplete Follow-Up

In longitudinal studies a problem of incomplete response rate exists. This means that not all members of the investigated cohort participate in surveys, conducted in different years. In this case estimates should be corrected to avoid a possible bias. Let λ_i be a probability to diagnose the disease of interest, n_j is the number of examined people who were healthy before the ith survey, and d_i is the number of diagnosed cases in the ith survey. If all n_i people were diagnosed as being healthy in the $(i-1)$th survey then the relationship is valid,

$$E\left(d_i\right) = \lambda_i n_i.$$

If n_{i1} persons among n_i were not observed in the $(i-1)$th survey and were diagnosed as being healthy in the $(i-2)$th survey then the above relationship takes the form

$$
\begin{aligned}
E\left(d_i\right) &= \lambda_i \left(n_i - n_{i1}\right) + \left(\lambda_i + \lambda_{i-1}\right) n_{i1} + \mathrm{O}\left(\lambda_i \lambda_{i-1}\right) \\
&= \lambda_i n_i + \lambda_{i-1} n_{i1} + \mathrm{O}\left(\lambda_i \lambda_{i-1}\right).
\end{aligned}
$$

In the same way one can obtain the presentation

$$E\left(d_i\right) \approx \sum_{j=1}^{i} \lambda_j n_{ij},$$

where n_{ij} is the number of persons investigated in the ith survey, which participated last time in the jth survey and were diagnosed as being healthy, $n_{ii} = n_i$. In this consideration we assume that nonresponses at different years are independent events with constant probability and that there is no cure from the disease. The last assumption corresponds to the case of incurable disease and to the investigation of the first occurrence of the disease. Estimation for the disease incidences in different years obtain from the relationships

$$\frac{d_i}{n_{ii}} \approx \sum_{j=1}^{i} \frac{n_{ij}}{n_{ii}} \lambda_j, \qquad i = 1, \ldots,$$

which leads to the solution of a matrix equation

$$u = \mathbf{A}\lambda$$

with u denoting the vector of the proportion of diagnosed cases among observed people by years of investigation, and λ is a vector of probabilities for a healthy person to become sick during one year by years. $\mathbf{A}$ is a triangular matrix with 1 at the main diagonal and below the diagonal elements equal to the proportion of people, examined in the year i and healthy before, among those who skipped the examination in the year j after the last examination. In the case of a complete follow-up when all people participate in all surveys the matrix $\mathbf{A}$ is the identity matrix and the morbidity estimates for different years are just the ratio between the numbers of cases and the numbers of healthy people examined in the same year. Stabilization of the matrix equation was made by minimization of the functional

$$\|u - \mathbf{A}\lambda\|^2 + \alpha\Omega(\lambda)$$

with regularization functional $\Omega(\lambda) = \|\mathbf{B}\lambda\|^2 = \lambda^T\mathbf{B}^T\mathbf{B}\lambda$, $\mathbf{B}$ is a matrix with two nonzero diagonals. It holds -1 at the main diagonal and 1 at the second. This structure of the regularization functional reflects the hypothesis that the morbidity does not demonstrate sharp changes in subsequent years.

The described approach was applied for estimation of malignant neoplasm (ICD9 140-208) morbidity among participants in the clean-up operations after the accident at the Chernobyl Nuclear Power Station in 1986 [Michalski *et al.* (1996)]. The results of the annual health examinations of the clean-up workers were extracted from the database of the Russian National Medical-Dosimetric Registry, which at the end of 1993 contained information about 159,319 clean-up workers [Morgenstern *et al.* (1995)]. Each year in the period 1987–1993 about 70% of the registered people participated in the health examinations. Some people skipped one, two, or more examinations and then participated again. No correlation between nonparticipation in the health examination and the health status or any other factors were observed. In addition every year new people, who started work in the rectification zone, were registered and joined the annual health examinations. It was supposed that at the beginning of registration all people were healthy. The observed morbidity of malignant neoplasms demonstrated the rapid growth from 0 in 1986 up to 326 per 100,000 in 1993. This growth can be attributed to the effect of radiation, absorbed during work in the radiation-contaminated area, to other risk factors for health and to the gaps between the health examinations. In the last case the event of the disease is attributed to the year of the health examination even if it took place before but was missed because of missing the health examination in the proper year. The adjustment of the morbidity estimates to such follow-up incompleteness allows us to reduce the deformations and clarify the role of radiation and other risk factors in the morbidity dynamics.

Table 20.1. Number of examined people, number of diagnosed malignant neo-plasm cases, incidence estimates per 100,000 without and with adjustment for missing observations

Year of Survey	1987	1988	1989	1990	1991	1992	1993
Examined people	2955	6343	6472	7100	7061	7512	7367
Diagnosed cases	1	3	5	6	11	14	24
Incidence estimate (without adjustment)	34	47	77	84	156	186	326
Incidence estimate (with adjustment)	24	40	62	85	119	150	184

Table 20.1 presents the results of estimation using a random sample of records of 11,043 clean-up workers, registered in the Russian National Medical-Dosimetric Registry up to 1993. The table includes the number of people examined in different years, number of diagnosed cases, and two estimates for malignant neoplasm incidence, without adjustment for missing observations and with it. The value for the parameter α was selected using the criterion (20.3). Estimates show that adjustment for the missing observations reduces the rate of the malignant neoplasm morbidity growth in time. The effect of "morbid-ity accumulation" is to be adjusted in estimations of the health effects on the results of incomplete follow-up studies.

20.4   Estimation of HIV Infection Rate on the Dynamics of AIDS Cases

HIV infection is a "cause" for development of the AIDS syndrome. Monitoring of the HIV infection process is essential for control of HIV spread in different risk groups, for elaboration of HIV spread protection measures, and for projection of future development of an HIV/AIDS epidemic. One important characteristic of the epidemic is the current number of HIV-infected people in the population. Assessment of this number is difficult, needs big funds, and estimates made by independent experts can be very different.

One of the possible approaches to estimation of the number of HIV-infected people in a population or in a risk group is estimation of the HIV infection rate using the dynamics of AIDS case diagnoses. This approach is known as the backcalculation method and is widely applied in the statistical analysis of the HIV/AIDS epidemic [Brookmeyer and Gail (1988), Bacchetti et al. (1993),

Bellocco and Pagano (2001), and Sweeting *et al.* (2006)]. The main idea of the approach is to use the epidemiological data on AIDS to find a solution for the convolution equation, which describes the AIDS epidemic given HIV infection process. Different authors use different assumptions to produce the solution for the problem. Becker *et al.* (1991) considered HIV incidence at different years as Poisson distributed random values from which the likelihood for the observed AIDS counts was constructed and a smoothed EM algorithm was applied to make the nonparametric estimate for HIV incidence. Tan and Ye (2000) applied the Kalman filter approach for estimation of the HIV infection process by consideration of submodels: the stochastic model of the system, the model of the HIV epidemic, and the observation model for available AIDS data. Aalen *et al.* (1997) composed a discrete Markov chain model for HIV incidence estimation which incorporated information about time of HIV diagnosis and treatment. Sweeting *et al.* (2006) formulated the backcalculation method in a multistate formulation using a Bayesian framework. Many authors use the penalized likelihood maximization approach for construction of HIV-related estimates [Liao and Brookmeyer (1995) and Joly and Commenges (1999)].

In this section the method of estimating the HIV infection rate is constructed as a method for the regularized solution of an ill-posed integral equation. Application of the criterion (20.3) for regularization of the HIV infection rate estimate when the number of observations is small is demonstrated by the results of a simulation experiment. The number of people infected by HIV in year t at age x $\Psi(t, x)$ is related to the number of AIDS diagnoses in year t at age x $U(t, x)$ by an integral equation [Michalski (2005)]:

$$U(t, x) = \int_0^x L(x, s) \exp\left(-\int_s^x \mu_c(t - x + \tau, \tau)\, d\tau\right) \Psi(t - x + s, s)\, ds, \quad (20.4)$$

where $\mu_c(t, x)$ is mortality in year t at age x and $L(x, s)$ is the probability density function for distribution of AIDS diagnoses at age x if at age s a person was infected with HIV. This function includes a time period for AIDS development, time for AIDS "recognition" by the health care system, and probability to miss the case as well. Age-specific mortality is supposed to be known, function $L(x, s)$ can be estimated from the clinical data, and data about AIDS cases among patients who were infected with HIV during blood transfusion, from different specialized studies. Construction of a proper distribution function $L(x, s)$ is a complex task. It should reflect the manner of infection, effect of possible retroviral prevention, and lengthening of incubation period with time [Bacchetti *et al.* (1993), Deuffic and Costagliola (1999), and Tan and Ye (2000)]. In this chpater we do not consider all these problems and suppose the probability density function $L(x, s)$ to be given.

Write Equation (20.4) in matrix form

$$U = \mathbf{A}\Psi,$$

where U and Ψ are vectors composed of values of functions $U(.)$ and $\Psi(.)$ for corresponding birth cohorts, $\mathbf{A}$ is a block-diagonal matrix composed of triangular matrices with elements for the kth cohort,

$$a_{ij}^k = \begin{cases} 0 & s_j > x_i^k \\ L(x_i^k, s_j)\exp\left(-\int_{s_j}^{x_i^k} \mu_c\,(d_k + \tau, \tau)\,d\tau\right) & s_j \leq x_i^k \end{cases}.$$

The stabilized solution for (20.4) can be found by minimization of the functional

$$\|y - \mathbf{A}\Psi\|^2 + \alpha\Omega\,(\Psi),$$

and y is a vector composed of numbers of AIDS diagnoses in different years,

$$\Omega\,(\Psi) = \sum_k \frac{1}{m_k} \sum_{j=2}^{m_k} \left(\Psi_j^k - \Psi_{j-1}^k\right)^2.$$

The stabilized solution takes the form

$$\Psi_\alpha = \left(\mathbf{A}^T\mathbf{A} + \alpha\mathbf{D}\right)^{-1} \mathbf{A}^T y,$$

and matrix $\mathbf{D}$ is a block-diagonal matrix composed of tridiagonal matrices. For the kth cohort the matrix holds $2/m_k$ at the main diagonal, $-1/m_k$ at the other two diagonals, and $1/m_k$ as the first and the last elements in the matrix.

Results of HIV infection rate estimation from AIDS diagnoses dynamics were investigated using simulated data [Michalski (2005)]. In the simulations the number of new HIV-infected people in year t at age x was given by a hypothetical unimodal function

$$\Psi\,(t, x) = \begin{cases} 0 & x < 19 \\ 10^{-2}\exp\left(-\frac{(x-35)^2}{100}\right) & 19 \leq x \leq 45 \end{cases},$$

which supposes that there are no infection events at age younger than 19 years. The probability density function for the incubation period was used in form

$$L\,(x, s) = 0.1\exp\left(\frac{x - s}{10}\right),$$

which corresponds to 100% detection of the AIDS cases, constant intensity of the AIDS case development for HIV-infected person, and mean duration of incubation period equal to 10 years. The total mortality rate for ages 19–45 years was supposed to be 1% and independent of time and age. The role of HIV infection in the total mortality was not included in the present model because of its small effect on mortality for the countries with low prevalence of

Table 20.2. Simulated number of HIV-infected people by age (per 100,000) and its unstabilized and stabilized estimates

Age (Years)	31	32	33	34	35	36	37
Infected	852.1	913.9	960.7	990.0	1000.0	990.0	960.7
Not stabilized (estimates)	873.8	955.3	962.9	958.4	1118.0	1039.3	862.6
Stabilized (estimates)	939.5	953.2	972.6	989.8	995.6	976.1	935.0
Age (Years)	38	39	40	41	42	43	44
Infected	913.9	852.1	778.8	697.6	612.6	527.2	444.8
Not stabilized (estimates)	700.1	122.16	724.3	326.6	674.5	788.8	76.4
Stabilized (estimates)	885.2	828.8	740.3	652.0	593.9	548.2	508.9

HIV [United Nations (2003)]. The annual numbers of AIDS cases in ages 31–44 years was calculated by Equation (20.4). The calculated values were disturbed by 5% random uniformly distributed noise with zero mean to simulate the possible false-positive and false-negative AIDS diagnoses. All the parameters and functions are presented here for illustrative purpose.

Table 20.2 presents results of the investigation. The stabilization parameter value was selected using described criterion I_α (20.3). Comparison of the estimates shows that the stabilized estimate is closer to the given annual numbers of HIV-infected persons than the not stabilized. Application of the cross-validation criterion [Stone (1974)] for the regularization parameter value selection led to the solution which is close to the not stabilized one. This is a result of the small number of observations for the annual numbers of AIDS cases which was equal to 14.

20.5 Estimation of Survival in the Wild

Biodemography studies the effects of environmental and genetic factors on aging, disability, and mortality in animals [Carey and Vaupel (2005)]. The most informative results are obtained in the laboratory under controlled conditions and known date of the animal's birth. The last is extremely important in studies of aging. Investigation of aging and survival in the wild is of great interest as well because the organisms are observed in their natural surroundings which can be rather different from the artificial laboratory conditions [Finch and Austad (2001)]. Such investigations need a method to determine the age of capture in the wild animal. The capture–recapture method can give information about residual after capture survival but not about survival starting at birth. Muller et al. (2004) proposed to apply a mathematical technique for estimation survival in the wild population from the residual survival in the laboratory. Muller et al. (2004) supposed that the animals are randomly captured in a stable, stationary, and closed population. The probability to be captured does not depend on the individual age. These assumptions are artificial but they can be realistic under some conditions. The real population can be considered as stable, stationary, and closed for the capturing period which is shorter than the period of significant changes of population in number and in the age structure. In this case we are investigating the survival which is specific to the population at that very period. The assumption about equal probability for the animal to be captured at different ages looks reasonable if capture is made with a trap as was done in the investigation of Mediterranean fruit flies [Muller et al. (2004)].

Under the hypotheses of stationarity of wild population probability $P_c(x)$ to survive x days in the laboratory after capture is

$$P_c(x) = E_a\left(P\{X > x|a\}\right) = \int_0^\omega \frac{S_{lab}(a+x)}{S_{lab}(a)} p_w(a)\, da,$$

where $S_{lab}(a)$ is a probability to survive in the laboratory till the age at capture a, $p_w(a)$ is the probability density function of age at capture in the wild population, and ω is the maximal life span. In the stable wild population $p_w(a) = 1/e_0\, S_w(a)$ and

$$P_c(x) = \frac{1}{e_0} \int_0^\omega \frac{S_{lab}(a+x)}{S_{lab}(a)} S_w(a)\, da,$$

where e_0 is the life expectancy at birth in the wild. Probability to survive in the laboratory till the age a can be estimated from the reference cohort which, in the case of fruit flies, can be reared in the laboratory from the fruit collected in the same region where the flies were captured [Muller et al. (2004)]. The last equation can be simplified under a hypothesis that mortality in the laboratory does not differ from mortality in the wild, which does not look realistic but can be used as a starting point if the reference cohort is not available. The resulting equation is

$$P_c(x) = \frac{1}{e_0} \int_0^\omega S_w(x+a)da = \frac{1}{e_0} \int_x^\omega S_w(a)da. \qquad (20.5)$$

It is easy to obtain an analytical solution for this equation in the form

$$S_w(x) = \frac{d}{dx}P_c(x) \Big/ \frac{d}{dx}P_c(0).$$

This formula leads to the necessity to estimate the derivative from the probability to survive in the laboratory in captured animals $P_c(x)$, which is unstable. Muller *et al.* (2004) used the nonparametric kernel density estimate

$$\frac{d}{dx}P_c(x) = \frac{-1}{nh(n)}\sum_{i=1}^{n} K\left(\frac{x - x_i^*}{h(n)}\right),$$

where $x_1^*, \ldots, x_n^*$ is a sample of observed lifespans after capture; $h(n)$ is a sequence of proper selected values for bandwidth. The kernel functions were defined as $K(x) = 0.75\left(1 - x^2\right)$, at $[-1,1]$ in the derivative estimation and $K_0(x) = 12(x+1)(x+0.5)$ at $[-1,0]$ in estimation of the derivative value at $x = 0$.

The alternative way of estimation survival in the wild is the numerical solution of Equation (20.5) which leads to a matrix equation

$$P_c = \mathbf{A}S_w \qquad (20.6)$$

with triangular matrix

$$\mathbf{A} = \begin{pmatrix} 1/e_0 & 1/e_0 & \ldots & 1/e_0 \\ 0 & 1/e_0 & \ldots & 1/e_0 \\ 0 & 0 & \ldots & 1/e_0 \\ 0 & 0 & \ldots & 1/e_0 \end{pmatrix}.$$

The diagonal and subdiagonal elements of the matrix $\mathbf{A}$ are the inverse of the life expectancy e_0, which can be estimated from the reference cohort survival. The structure of matrix $\mathbf{A}$ is obtained from Equation (20.5) by a change from integration to summation with a unit step.

Solution of Equation (20.6) was investigated by simulation. The "survival in the wild" was modeled by the survival in the reference cohort of Mediterranean fruit flies reared in the laboratory (J. Carey's data, personal communication). This survival is presented in Figure 20.1 by empty circles. The vector of survival in the reference cohort was multiplied by the matrix $\mathbf{A}$ to model the residual laboratory survival for randomly captured flies. Small random disturbances were added to the residual survival to simulate an effect of estimation using a small number of captured animals. The resulting survival curve is presented in Figure 20.1 by crosses.

Figure 20.1 presents the results of the solution of Equation (20.6) by regularized functional minimization

$$J_\alpha(S) = \|P_c - \mathbf{A}S\|^2 + \alpha\|\mathbf{B}S\|^2$$

where matrix $\mathbf{B}$ holds -1 at the main diagonal and 1 at the second diagonal. The dashed line in Figure 20.1 presents the solution obtained for $a = 0.001$. One can see instability in the solution. The solid line in Figure 20.1 presents the solution obtained for α, which was selected by minimization on α of the criterion (20.3).

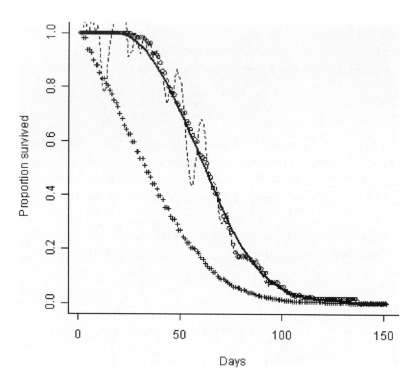

Figure 20.1. Survival in the wild (open circuits), calculated and randomly disturbed survival among captured flies (crosses), estimate for survival in the wild corresponding to small value (dashed line) and selected value for regularization parameter (solid line).

References

1. Aalen, O. O., Farewell, V. T., de Angelis, D., Day, N. E., and Gill, O. N. (1997). A Markov model for HIV disease progression including the effect of HIV diagnosis and treatment: Application to AIDS prediction in England and Wales, *Statistics in Medicine*, **16**, 2191–2210.

2. Bacchetti, P., Segal, M. R., and Jewell, N. P. (1993). Backcalculation of HIV infection rates, *Stat. Sci.*, **8**, 82–101.

3. Becker, N. G., Watson, L. F., and Carlin, J. B. (1991). A method of non-parametric back-projection and its application to AIDS data, *Statistics in Medicine*, **10**, 1527–1542.

4. Bellocco, R. and Pagano, M. (2001). Multinomial analysis of smoothed HIV back-calculation models incorporating uncertainty in the AIDS incidence, *Statistics in Medicine*, **20**, 2017–2033.

5. Brookmeyer, R. and Gail, M. H. (1988). A method for obtaining short-term projections and lower bounds on the size of the AIDS epidemic, *Journal of the American Statistical Society*, **83,** 301–308.

6. Carey, J. R. and Vaupel, J. W. (2005). Biodemography, In *Handbook of Population* (Eds., D. L. Poston, and M. Mickin), pp. 625–658, Springer-Verlag, Heidelberg.

7. Chapelle, O., Vapnik, V., and Bengio, Y. (2002). Model selection for small sample regression, *Machine Learning*, **48,** 9–23.

8. Deuffic, S. and Costagliola, D. (1999). Is the AIDS incubation time changing? A back-calculation approach, *Statistics in Medicine*, **18,** 1031–1047.

9. Engl, H. W., Hanke, M., and Neubauer, A. (1996). *Regularization of Inverse Problems*, Kluwer, Dordrecht.

10. Engl, H. W., Hofinger, A., and Kinderann, S. (2005). Convergence rates in the Prokhorov metric for assessing uncertainty in ill-posed problems, *Inverse Problems*, **21,** 399–412.

11. Evans, S. N. and Stark, P. N. (2002). Inverse problems as statistics, *Inverse Problems*, **18,** R55-R97.

12. Finch, C. E. and Austad, S. N. (2001). History and prospects: Symposium on organisms with slow aging, *Exp. Gerontol.* **36,** 593–597.

13. Geman, S. and Hwang, C-R. (1982). Nonparametric maximum likelihood estimation by the method of sieves, *Annals of Statistics*, **10,** 401–414.

14. Joly, P. and Commenges, D. (1999). A penalized likelihood approach for a progressive three-state model with censored and truncated data: application to AIDS, *Biometrics*, **55,** 887–890.

15. Liao, J. and Brookmeyer, R. (1995). An empirical Bayes approach to smoothing in backcalculation of HIV infection rates, *Biometrics*, **51,** 579–588.

16. Lukas, M. A. (1998). Comparison of parameter choice methods for regularization with discrete noisy data, *Inverse Problems*, **14,** 161–184.

17. Michalski, A. I. (2005). Estimation of HIV infected number in population on the dynamics of observed AIDS cases, In *Demography of HIV, Population and Crisises, 11* (Ed., B. P. Denisov), pp. 75–99, MSU, Moscow (*in Russian*).

18. Michalski, A. I., Morgenstern, W., Ivanov, V. K., and Maksyitov, M.A. (1996). Estimation of morbidity dynamics from incomplete follow-up studies, *Journal Epidemiology and Biostatistics*, **1,** 151–157.

19. Mikhal'skii, A. I. (1987). Choosing an algorithm of estimation based on samples of limited size, *Automatization and Remote Control*, **48**, 909–918.

20. Morgenstern, W., Ivanov, V. K., Michalski, A. I., Tsyb, A. F., and Schettler, G. (1995). *Mathematical Modelling with Chernobyl registry data*, Springer-Verlag, Berlin.

21. Morozov, V. A. (1993). *Regularization Methods for Ill-Posed Problems*, CRC Press, Boca Raton, FL.

22. Muller, H.-G., Wang, J.-L., Carey, J. R., Caswell-Chen, E. P., Chen, C., Papadopoulos, N., and Yao, F. (2004). Demographic window to aging in the wild: Constructing life tables and estimating survival functions from marked individuals of unknown age, *Aging Cell*, **3**, 125–131.

23. Nair, M. T., Pereverzev, S. V., and Tautenhahn, U. (2005). Regularization in Hilbert scales under general smoothing conditions, *Inverse Problems*, **21**, 1851–1869.

24. Nair, M. T., Schock, E., and Tautenhahn, U. (2003). Morozov's discrepancy principle under general source conditions, *Journal for Analysis and its Applications*, **22**, 199–214.

25. Natterer, F. (1984). Error bounds for Tikhonov regularization in Hilbert scales, *Applied Analysis*, **18**, 9–37.

26. O'Sullivan, F. (1986). A statistical perspective on ill-posed inverse problems, *Statistical Science*, **1**, 502–518.

27. Shen, X. (1997). On methods of sieves and penalization, *Annals of Statistics*, **25**, 2555–2591.

28. Stone, M. (1974). Cross-validation choice and assessment of statistical prediction, *Journal of the Royal Statistical Society, Series B*, **36**, 111–133.

29. Sweeting, M. J., de Angelis, D., and Aalen O. O. (2006). Bayesian back-calculation using a multi-state model with application to HIV, *Statistics in Medicine*, **24**, 3991–4007.

30. Tan, W.-Y., and Ye, Z. (2000). Estimation of HIV infection and incubation via state space models, *Mathematical Biosciences*, **167**, 31–50.

31. Tikhonov, A. N., and Arsenin, V. Y. (1977). *Solutions of Ill-Posed Problems*, John Wiley & Sons, New York.

32. United Nations (2003). The impact of HIV/AIDS on mortality, In *Workshop on HIV/AIDS and Adult Mortality in Developing Countries*, New York.

33. Vapnik, V. (1982). *Estimation of Dependencies Based on Empirical Data*, Springer-Verlag, Berlin.

34. Vapnik, V. (1998). *Statistical Learning Theory*, John Wiley & Sons, New York.

PART IV
Analysis of Censored Data

21

A Sampling-Based Chi-Squared Test for Interval-Censored Data

M. L. Calle[1] **and G. Gómez**[2]

[1] *Systems Biology Department, Universitat de Vic, Vic, Spain*
[2] *Statistics and Operational Research Department, Universitat Politècnica de Catalunya, Barcelona, Spain*

Abstract: The analysis of censored data has been mainly approached through nonparametric or semiparametric methods. One of the reasons for the wide use of these methods, as opposed to classical parametric approaches, lies in the difficulty of checking the validity of a parametric model when data are censored. In this work we propose a sampling-based chi-squared test of goodness-of-fit for censored data. The proposed algorithm is an extension of the Bayesian quantile chi-squared test proposed by Johnson (2004) for complete data.

Keywords and Phrases: Chi-squared test, goodness-of-fit test, interval censoring, survival analysis

21.1 Introduction

Although the use of parametric models, both in a frequentist or in a Bayesian framework, can be advisable in some situations, most applied methods in survival analysis are either non- or semiparametric. One of the reasons for the wide use of these methods, as opposed to classical parametric approaches, lies in the difficulty of checking the validity of a parametric model when data are censored. This is especially cumbersome under interval-censoring, which is a general censoring scheme that includes the usual right-censoring and left-censoring as special cases. Interval-censoring occurs when the exact survival time of each individual cannot be observed and its value is only known to lie within a certain random interval. This kind of censoring often occurs in longitudinal studies where patients are monitored periodically and the event of interest, for instance, the recurrence of a tumor, is only detectable at specific times of observation such as at the time of a medical examination.

The problem considered in this chapter is to test the composite null hypothesis that the survival time distribution belongs to a specific parametric family of distributions based on interval-censored data. We propose a sampling-based goodness-of-fit test based on a chi-squared statistic. Pearson's chi-squared test is one of the most classical tests of goodness-of-fit. As is well known, the application of this test stands on a finite partition of the sample space in r classes and in the discrepancy between the observed and the expected frequencies on each member of the partition under the null hypothesis. There are two problems when trying to apply this statistic to our censoring situation. The first one is that this statistic cannot be computed because the number of survival times in each class is not observable if data are interval-censored. To avoid this difficulty we propose the data-augmentation method for interval censoring proposed in Calle (2003) based on sampling iteratively from the posterior distribution of the parameter. The second problem that arises when trying to apply Pearson's statistic to a censoring situation relies on its asymptotic properties. Although the asymptotic distribution of Pearson's statistic under the simple null hypothesis is χ^2 with $r - 1$ degrees of freedom, when the parameter is unknown (composite hypothesis) and has to be estimated, its asymptotic distribution depends on the estimation method. In particular, if the parameter is estimated by maximum likelihood from the complete data the limit distribution of the statistic is no longer χ^2. For this reason some modifications of the classical Pearson's test have been proposed [see Greenwood and Nikulin (1996) for a detailed review of chi-squared testing methods]. In this work we base our approach on a different version of the chi-squared test, the so-called quantile chi-squared statistic which is more suitable for deriving asymptotical properties in our interval-censoring situation than the classical one.

The goodness-of-fit test for interval-censored data proposed in this chapter is an extension of the Bayesian quantile chi-squared test proposed by Johnson (2004) for complete data, described in Section 21.2. In Section 21.3 we propose a sampling-based goodness-of-fit test based on a quantile chi-squared statistic for interval-censored survival data. The results of a small simulation study to investigate the power of our test are presented in Section 21.4. A discussion concludes the chapter.

21.2   Johnson's Bayesian Chi-Squared Statistic

Let $X_1, \ldots, X_n$ be a random sample from a random variable X with cumulative distribution F_X. We wish to test the hypothesis H_0 that $F_X \in \mathcal{C}$ versus the alternative hypothesis that $F_X \notin \mathcal{C}$, where $\mathcal{C} = \{F_0(\cdot, \theta), \theta \in \Theta\}$ is a specific parametric family of distributions.

Johnson's quantile test fixes a vector $(p_1, \ldots, p_r)$ of probabilities such that $\sum_{j=1}^{r} p_j = 1$ and $r > s+1$ instead of considering a finite partition of the sample space. Define $u_i = p_1 + \cdots + p_j$ for $j = 1, \ldots, r-1 > s$. For each value u_i compute the inverse distribution function $F_0^{-1}(u_j; \theta)$ which defines a partition of the sample space: $A_1 = (-\infty, F_0^{-1}(u_1; \theta)], A_2 = (F_0^{-1}(u_1; \theta), F_0^{-1}(u_2; \theta)], \ldots, A_r = (F_0^{-1}(u_{r-1}; \theta), +\infty)$.

The goodness-of-fit quantile statistic is given by

$$X_n^2(\theta) = \sum_{j=1}^{r} \frac{(m_j(\theta) - np_j)^2}{np_j}, \tag{21.1}$$

where the count $m_j(\theta)$ is the random number of observations that fall into the jth class, A_j.

Note that the computation of $X_n^2(\theta)$ requires the value of the unknown parameter θ, which has to be somehow estimated. One of the good asymptotic properties of the statistic $X_n^2(\theta)$ given in (21.1) is that the value of θ can be replaced by its maximum likelihood estimate and $X_n^2(\theta)$ still behaves as a χ^2 distribution with $r - 1$ degrees of freedom, independently of the dimension of the parameter.

An alternative to maximum likelihood estimation would be to use, instead, the posterior distribution of θ in a Bayesian parametric framework. Specifically, Johnson (2004) proposed the following Bayesian quantile statistic,

$$X_n^2(\tilde{\theta}) = \sum_{j=1}^{r} \frac{(m_j(\tilde{\theta}) - np_j)^2}{np_j}, \tag{21.2}$$

which corresponds to the statistic $X_n^2(\theta)$ defined in (21.1) evaluated at a value $\tilde{\theta}$ of the posterior distribution

$$p(\theta|X_1, \ldots, X_n) = \prod_{i=1}^{n} f_0(X_i; \theta) \cdot \pi(\theta), \tag{21.3}$$

where $X_1, \ldots, X_n$ is a random sample from $F_0(\cdot; \theta)$, $f_0(X_i; \theta)$ denotes the corresponding density function, and $\pi(\theta)$ is the prior distribution of θ.

Using results on large sample properties of posterior distributions given in Chen (1985), Johnson (2004) proves that under the null hypothesis, the asymptotic distribution of $X_n^2(\tilde{\theta})$ is a χ^2 distribution independent of the dimension of the underlying parameter vector as we state next.

Proposition 21.2.1 *Under the null hypothesis, $H_0\colon F_X \in \mathcal{C} = \{F_0(\cdot, \theta), \theta \in \Theta\}$, the asymptotic distribution of the Bayesian quantile statistic $X_n^2(\tilde{\theta})$ is a χ^2 distribution with $r - 1$ degrees of freedom, independent of the dimension of the underlying parameter vector.*

Using Proposition (21.2.1), Johnson proposes the following algorithm to test H_0. Obtain a sample $\tilde{\theta}_1, \ldots, \tilde{\theta}_M$ from the posterior distribution of θ (21.3). For each of the sampled parameter values compute the corresponding quantile statistic and reject the null hypothesis H_0 whenever the obtained sample of quantiles, $X_n^2(\tilde{\theta}_1), \ldots, X_n^2(\tilde{\theta}_M)$, is not compatible with a chi-square distribution with $r - 1$ degrees of freedom. Johnson discusses several decision criteria, which we extend in Section 21.3.3, such as to use a random selected value from the posterior or to report the proportion of cases that exceed the critical value of the χ^2 test.

21.3   Sampling-Based Chi-Squared Test for Interval-Censored Data

In an interval-censoring problem the values of the random sample $X_1, \ldots, X_n$ are not observed and hence Johnson's test $X_n^2(\tilde{\theta})$ cannot be directly applied. The test we propose in this section, denoted by $Y_n^2(\tilde{\theta})$, is a sampling-based procedure which iteratively replaces $X_1, \ldots, X_n$ by imputed values $T_1, \ldots, T_n$ derived from the observed censoring intervals $[L_1, R_1], \ldots, [L_n, R_n]$ and applies Johnson's test (21.2) to $T_1, \ldots, T_n$. In what follows, we state formally the interval-censoring scheme, establishing the notation as well as the required assumptions and develop the sampling-based chi-squared test for this situation.

We assume that X is a positive random variable representing the time until the occurrence of a certain event with unknown distribution function F_X. Under interval-censoring the potential survival times of n individuals, namely, $X_1, \ldots, X_n$, cannot be observed and, instead, we observe intervals that contain them. Let $\mathcal{D} = \{[L_i, R_i], \quad 1 \leq i \leq n\}$ denote the observed censoring intervals.

This kind of censoring mechanism usually arises as a consequence of an intermittent inspection of each individual, for instance, from a sequence of examination times in a medical longitudinal study. In this situation, R_i indicates the time of the first visit where the event has been observed and L_i is the time of the previous visit.

We assume that the support of the inspection times is the positive real line and that the random inspection censoring process occurs noninformatively in the sense described in Gómez et al. (2004) and Oller et al. (2004). These assumptions are necessary for the consistent estimation of the whole time distribution F_X [Gentleman and Geyer (1994)].

To test the null hypothesis, H_0: $F_X \in \mathcal{C}$, where $\mathcal{C} = \{F_0(\cdot, \theta), \theta \in \Theta\}$, we propose the following sampling-based chi-squared test based on the data augmentation algorithm given in Calle (2003) to obtain a sample from the posterior distribution of the parameter of interest followed by Johnson's test.

A survival time is sampled for each individual under the null distribution with the restriction that the event occurred between L_i and R_i and the parameter θ is updated based on these complete imputed samples. Then, the proposed Bayesian quantile statistic given by (21.2) is computed based on the imputed sample. We denote this statistic by $Y_n^2(\tilde{\theta})$ in order to distinguish it from $X_n^2(\tilde{\theta})$ which would be computed from the real survival times, $X_1, \ldots, X_n$. This procedure can be formalized in the following three-step algorithm.

21.3.1 Iterative algorithm

1. For every $i = 1, \ldots, n$, impute a value T_i sampled from $F_0(x; \theta)$ truncated in the interval $[L_i, R_i]$; that is, the conditional density of T given the random interval $[L, R]$ is given, under the null hypothesis, by

$$f_{T|L,R}(t|l,r) = \frac{f_0(t; \theta)}{F_0(r; \theta) - F_0(l; \theta)} \mathbf{1}_{\{t:\ t \in [l,r]\}}(t). \qquad (21.4)$$

   We obtain an imputed sample $T_1, \ldots, T_n$.

2. Sample a new value $\tilde{\theta}$ of θ from its full conditional distribution given the complete imputed sample $T_1, \ldots, T_n$:

$$p(\theta|T_1, \ldots, T_n) = \prod_{i=1}^{n} f_0(T_i; \theta) \cdot \pi(\theta), \qquad (21.5)$$

   where $\pi(\theta)$ is the prior distribution for θ.

3. Given the imputed sample, compute the statistic

$$Y_n^2(\tilde{\theta}) = \sum_{j=1}^{r} \frac{(\tilde{m}_j(\tilde{\theta}) - np_j)^2}{np_j}, \qquad (21.6)$$

   where $\tilde{\theta}$ is the sampled value of θ obtained in Step 2 and $\tilde{m}_j$ is the number of imputed values $T_1, \ldots, T_n$ that fall into the jth class.

After iteratively performing the above algorithm and after a burn-in process of discarding the first sampled values one obtains a sample $Y_{1n}^2(\tilde{\theta}_1), \ldots, Y_{Kn}^2(\tilde{\theta}_K)$ of the statistic $Y_n^2(\tilde{\theta})$ which is the base for testing the null hypothesis as it is described in Section 21.3.3.

21.3.2 Asymptotic properties

The following propositions justify the use of the statistic $Y_n^2(\tilde{\theta})$ as a goodness-of-fit test for the distribution of X and give its asymptotic distribution.

Proposition 21.3.1 *At each iteration j of the proposed algorithm, for j sufficiently large, the marginal distribution of an imputed value, T_i^j, $i \in \{1, \ldots, n\}$, is*

$$F_T(t) = F_0(t; \tilde{\theta}_j) \iint_{\{(l,r):\, t \in [l,r]\}} \frac{F_X(r) - F_X(l)}{F_0(r; \tilde{\theta}_j) - F_0(l; \tilde{\theta}_j)} \, f_{L,R|X}(l, r|t) \, dlr,$$

where F_X is the true distribution of X and $\tilde{\theta}_j$ is a value from the posterior distribution of θ under the null distribution F_0 given $\mathcal{D}$.

PROOF. For ease of notation, we only specify the parameter vector of the null distribution. The marginal distribution of an imputed value, T_i^j, $i \in \{1, \ldots, n\}$, in Step j of the algorithm is

$$\begin{aligned}
f_T(t) &= \int_0^{+\infty} \int_0^{+\infty} f_{T|L,R}(t|l,r) f_{L,R}(l,r) \, dlr \\
&= \int_0^{+\infty} \int_0^{+\infty} f_{T|L,R}(t|l,r) \int_l^r f_{L,R|X}(l,r|x) f_X(x) dx \, dlr. \quad (21.7)
\end{aligned}$$

As detailed in Gómez *et al.* (2004) and in Oller *et al.* (2004), the noninformative censoring condition implies that the conditional distribution of L and R given X satisfies

$$f_{L,R|X}(l,r|x_1) = f_{L,R|X}(l,r|x_2), \quad \text{for any } x_1, x_2 \in [l,r]. \quad (21.8)$$

Therefore, the term $f_{L,R|X}(l,r|x)$ in the right-hand side of (21.7) can be factored out of the integral and $f_T(t)$ becomes:

$$\begin{aligned}
f_T(t) &= \int_0^{+\infty} \int_0^{+\infty} f_{T|L,R}(t|l,r) f_{L,R|X}(l,r|x) \int_l^r f_X(x) dx \, dlr \\
&= \int_0^{+\infty} \int_0^{+\infty} f_{T|L,R}(t|l,r) f_{L,R|X}(l,r|x)(F_X(r) - F_X(l)) \, dlr.
\end{aligned}$$

By construction in the proposed iterative algorithm (see Section 21.3.1), the conditional density of T given L and R is the truncated null distribution (21.4) and $f_T(t)$ can be written as

$$\begin{aligned}
f_T(t) &= \int_0^{+\infty} \int_0^{+\infty} f_{T|L,R}(t|l,r) f_{L,R|X}(l,r|x)(F_X(r) - F_X(l)) \, dlr \\
&= \int_0^{+\infty} \int_0^{+\infty} \frac{f_0(t; \tilde{\theta}_j) \cdot \mathbf{1}_{\{t:\, t \in [l,r]\}}(t)}{F_0(r; \tilde{\theta}_j) - F_0(l; \tilde{\theta}_j)} (F_X(r) - F_X(l)) f_{L,R|X}(l,r|x) \, dlr \\
&= f_0(t; \tilde{\theta}_j) \iint_{\{(l,r):\, t \in [l,r]\}} \frac{F_X(r) - F_X(l)}{F_0(r; \tilde{\theta}_j) - F_0(l; \tilde{\theta}_j)} f_{L,R|X}(l,r|x) \, dlr. \quad (21.9)
\end{aligned}$$

Using again the noninformative censoring condition (21.8), $f_{L,R|X}(l,r|x)$ can be substituted by $f_{L,R|X}(l,r|t)$ in expression (21.9) which proves the proposition. ∎

Proposition 21.3.2 *If the support of the inspection times process is* $[0, \infty)$ *the posterior distribution of* θ *is consistent.*

PROOF. We assume that the parameter of interest θ can be expressed as a functional of F_0; that is, there is a functional ψ such that $\theta = \psi(F_0)$. Because the support of the inspection times process is equal to $[0, \infty)$, it is guaranteed that Turnbull's nonparametric estimator $\hat{F}_n$ consistently estimates the distribution function F_X, or F_0 under H_0. Then we can define the plug-in estimator $\hat{\theta}_n = \psi(\hat{F}_n)$ which will converge in probability to $\theta = \psi(F_0)$.

On the other hand, as stated in Schervish (1995, see Theorem 7.78), the existence of a consistent estimate of θ implies the consistency of the posterior distribution of θ in the following sense: the posterior probability measure associated with $p(\theta|\mathcal{D})$ converges almost surely, as n tends to ∞, to the measure that concentrates all the mass in the true value θ_0 of θ. ∎

Proposition 21.3.3 *If the null hypothesis* $H_0 : F_X \in \mathcal{C}$ *is correct, that is, if the true distribution function of* X *is* $F_X = F_0(\cdot \; ; \theta_0) \in \mathcal{C}$, *the statistic* $Y_n^2(\tilde{\theta})$ *follows a chi-square distribution with* $r - 1$ *degrees of freedom as* $n \to \infty$.

PROOF. If the true distribution function of X is $F_X = F_0(\cdot \; ; \theta_0) \in \mathcal{C}$ it follows from Proposition 21.3.1 that the marginal distribution of the imputed values, T_i^j, $i \in \{1, \ldots, n\}$, is

$$F_T(t) = F_0(t; \tilde{\theta}_j) \iint_{\{(l,r): \; t \in [l,r]\}} \frac{F_0(r; \theta_0) - F_0(l; \theta_0)}{F_0(r; \tilde{\theta}_j) - F_0(l; \tilde{\theta}_j)} \; f_{L,R|X}(l, r|t) \; dl dr. \quad (21.10)$$

From Proposition 21.3.2, $F_0(r; \tilde{\theta}_j)$ converges in probability to $F_0(r; \theta_0)$ as j tends to infinity, and hence

$$\frac{F_0(r; \theta_0) - F_0(l; \theta_0)}{F_0(r; \tilde{\theta}_j) - F_0(l; \tilde{\theta}_j)} \quad (21.11)$$

converges to 1 in probability as j tends to infinity.

On the other hand, $f_{L,R|X}(l, r|x)$ is a density function in the support $\{(l, r) : x \in [l, r]\}$ and thus, the integral in (21.10) tends to 1, as j tends to infinity.

Thus the asymptotic distribution of the posterior $p(\theta|T_1, \ldots, T_n)$ (21.5), used in the computation of $Y_n^2(\tilde{\theta})$, is the same as the asymptotic distribution of $p(\theta|X_1, \ldots, X_n)$ (21.3), used in the computation of Johnson's statistic, $X_n^2(\tilde{\theta})$ (21.2). Therefore, under the null hypothesis the statistic $Y_n^2(\tilde{\theta})$ has the same asymptotic distribution as $X_n^2(\tilde{\theta})$, which is a χ^2 distribution with $r - 1$ degrees of freedom (Proposition 21.2.1). ∎

Proposition 21.3.4 *If the null hypothesis is false because the true distribution function of X is in fact given by $F_X = F_1(\cdot\,;\gamma) \notin \mathcal{C}$, then the marginal distribution of the imputed values T_i is*

$$F_T(t) = F_0(t;\theta) \iint_{\{(l,r):\ t\in[l,r]\}} \frac{F_1(r;\gamma) - F_1(l;\gamma)}{F_0(r;\theta) - F_0(l;\theta)}\ f_{L,R|X}(l,r|t)\ dlr.$$

Note that the integral represents the discrepancy between F_0 and F_1 that we are able to detect using this approach. Thus, the power of the test depends on one hand on the similarity between F_0 and F_1 and on the masses given by F_0 and F_1 to the censoring intervals.

21.3.3 Decision criteria

Once we have derived a sample $Y^2_{1n}(\tilde\theta_1),\ldots,Y^2_{Kn}(\tilde\theta_K)$ from $Y^2_n(\tilde\theta)$ [see (21.6)], and keeping in mind that the statistic $Y^2_n(\tilde\theta)$ follows a χ^2 distribution with $r-1$ degrees of freedom if the null hypothesis is correct, we need a decision criterion to calibrate the degree of similarity or dissimilarity of the sample's distribution with respect to a χ^2_{r-1} distribution.

Following Johnson (2004), the decision on whether to reject H_0 is to be based necessarily on the posterior distribution. Two different approaches are possible.

1. Sample a random value $Y^2_j = Y^2_{jn}(\tilde\theta_j)$ of the posterior distribution of $Y^2_n(\tilde\theta)$ and reject H_0 whenever $Y^2_j > \chi^2_\alpha(r-1)$ where $\chi^2_\alpha(r-1)$ denotes the $100(1-\alpha)$ percentile of a χ^2 distribution with $r-1$ degrees of freedom. Proposition 21.3.3 implies that such a test is an asymptotic α-level test for H_0 versus H_1. The performance of the proposed approach has been investigated through a simulation study where the null hypothesis of an exponential distribution was tested for different underlying distributions and different censoring levels (Section 21.4).

2. Alternatively to the above criteria we could base the decision on the proportion π of values Y^2_js, drawn from the posterior that exceed a specified critical value, say $\chi^2_{0.95}(r-1)$, from the $\chi^2(r-1)$ distribution and reject the null hypothesis if π is larger than a certain threshold, say 10%. Any excess in this proportion can be attributed either to the dependency between the sampled values of the posterior or to lack of fit. The problem with this approach is that so far there is no theoretical result on which to base the choice of the appropriate threshold for a given level α.

21.4 Simulation Study

We performed a small simulation study to analyze the power of the goodness-of-fit test of an exponential null distribution; that is, $H_0 : F_X \sim \exp(\theta)$, with unknown mean θ.

We considered three different alternative distributions:

1. Weibull (Weib(α, β)) with $\alpha = 3$ and $\beta = 1, 1.5, 2, 2.5$
2. Gamma (Gam(α, β)) with $\alpha = 3$ and $\beta = 1, 1.8, 2.4, 3$
3. Log-normal (Lnorm(μ, σ)) with $\mu = 0.5, 1, 1.5, 2$ and $\sigma = 0.7$

We choose the parameters of the alternative distributions in such a way that different degrees of similarity between the null and alternative distributions are taken into account. When $\beta = 1$ both the Weibull and the gamma distributions become the exponential distribution and as β increases they gradually drift away from the null distribution. Something similar happens with the log-normal distribution when $\sigma = 0.7$; for $\mu = 0.5$ the log-normal and the exponential distributions are relatively alike, however, their similarity decreases as the mean μ increases.

We simulated 200 samples of size 100 from each alternative distribution. The censoring process was generated independently of the lifetime process by sampling a Poisson process of visits for each individual where the times between consecutive visits followed an exponential distribution of mean parameter λ. Three different levels of censoring—low, moderate, and high—were generated according to $\lambda = 1$, $\lambda = 1.5$, and $\lambda = 2$, respectively. Note that the smaller the value of λ, the more frequent visits and the shorter the censoring intervals.

For each of these scenarios we performed the proposed chi-squared statistic [given in (21.6)] and rejected the null hypothesis following the first decision criterion described in Section 21.3.3. The power of the test is given in Table 21.1. Actually, for the Weibull and gamma distributions, the first column of the table corresponds to the significance level of the test. In addition, the results for the Weibull distribution are depicted in Figure 21.1.

This small simulation study shows that the power of the sampling-based goodness-of-fit test described in Section 21.3

1. Increases as the shape of the alternative distribution moves away from the shape of an exponential distribution. In particular, we can see in Figure 21.1 that the power to distinguish a Weibull distribution from an exponential distribution increases as the shape parameter β moves far from 1.

2. For low and moderate censoring the test performs very well, but for high censoring it is much more difficult to reject the null hypothesis.

Table 21.1. Power to reject the null hypothesis $H_0 : X \sim \exp(\theta = 3)$

$H_1 : \text{Weib}(\alpha = 3, \beta)$

Censoring level	$\beta = 1$	$\beta = 1.5$	$\beta = 2$	$\beta = 2.5$
Low: $\lambda = 1$	0.05	0.52	1	1
Moderate: $\lambda = 1.5$	0.03	0.47	0.94	1
High: $\lambda = 2$	0.05	0.41	0.80	0.97

$H_1 : \text{Gam}(\alpha = 3, \beta)$

Censoring level	$\beta = 1$	$\beta = 1.8$	$\beta = 2.4$	$\beta = 3$
Low: $\lambda = 1$	0.06	0.45	0.74	0.76
Moderate: $\lambda = 1.5$	0.07	0.37	0.68	0.85
High: $\lambda = 2$	0.05	0.3	0.53	0.69

$H_1 : \text{Lognorm}(\mu, \sigma = 0.7)$

Censoring level	$\mu = 0.5$	$\mu = 1$	$\mu = 1.5$	$\mu = 2$
Low: $\lambda = 1$	0.40	0.72	0.91	0.87
Moderate: $\lambda = 1.5$	0.39	0.66	0.77	0.85
High: $\lambda = 2$	0.24	0.41	0.66	0.72

3. In the case of heavy censoring it would be more appropriate to base the inferences on a nonparametric approach.

21.5   Discussion

This work presents a Bayesian method to test the fit of a given parametric distribution based on a sample of interval-censored observations. The methodology proposed is based on the posterior distribution and one of its main advantages is the ease of implementation. A second, and relevant, advantage is that the distribution of the statistic, under the null, follows a χ^2 distribution with $k - 1$ degrees of freedom independently of the dimension of the parameter space.

The simulation study to evaluate the power of the proposed statistic is so far restricted to one null hypothesis, three alternatives, and three degrees of censoring. This study should be extended by considering other null distributions, other alternative families, and different choices of both the dimension and the values of the vector of probabilities $(p_1, \ldots, p_r)$. A second interesting issue would be to study both theoretically and by simulation the properties of

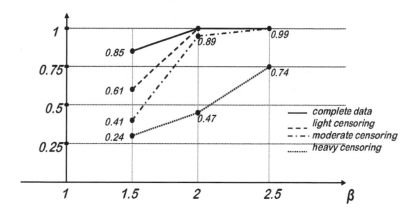

Figure 21.1. Power of the proposed quantile chi-squared test for interval-censoring.

the test based on the second decision criterion, that is, of the test based on the proportion of Ys above a certain value.

The assumption that the support of the inspection times process is $[0, \infty)$ is obviously necessary for consistent estimation of the whole failure time distribution F_0. One cannot estimate $F_0(t)$ at times where no individuals are inspected. If the inspection times are not dense, then the MLE consistently estimates only the restriction of F_0 to the support of the inspection time process.

The procedure is developed for all models in which observations are continuous and conditionally independent given the value of finite-dimensional parameter space, however, as discussed by Johnson (2004), the method could be extended to discrete random variables.

References

1. Calle, M. L. (2003). Parametric Bayesian analysis of interval-censored and doubly-censored survival data, *Journal of Probability and Statistical Science*, **1**, 103–118.

2. Chen, C. F. (1985). On asymptotic normality of limiting density functions with Bayesian implications, *Journal of the Royal Statistical Society, Series B*, **47**, 540–546.

3. Gentleman, R. and Geyer, C. J. (1994). Maximum likelihood for interval-censored data: Consistency and computation, *Biometrika*, **81**, 618–623.

4. Gómez, G., Calle, M. L., and Oller, R. (2004). Frequentist and Bayesian approaches for interval-censored data, *Statistical Papers*, **45**, 139–173.

5. Greenwood, P. E. and Nikulin, M. S. (1996). *A Guide to Chi-Squared Testing*, John Wiley & Sons, New York.

6. Johnson, V. E. (2004). A Bayesian chi-squared test for goodness-of-fit, *The Annals of Statistics*, **32**, 2361–2384.

7. Oller, R., Gómez, G., and Calle, M. L. (2004). Interval censoring: Model characterizations for the validity of the simplified likelihood, *The Canadian Journal of Statistics*, **32**, 315–325.

8. Schervish, M. J. (1995). *Theory of Statistics*, Springer-Verlag, New York.

22

Semiparametric Regression Models for Interval-Censored Survival Data, With and Without Frailty Effects

Philip Hougaard

Biostatistics Department, H. Lundbeck A/S, Valby, Denmark

Abstract: Interval-censored survival data occur when the time to an event is assessed by means of blood samples, urine samples, X-ray, or other screening methods that cannot tell the exact time of change for the disease, but only that the change has happened since the last examination. This is in contrast to the standard (naive) thinking that assumes that the change happens at the time of the first positive examination. Even though this screening setup is very common and methods to handle such data nonparametrically in the one-sample case have been suggested more than 30 years ago, it is still not a standard method. However, interval-censored methods are needed in order to consider onset and diagnosis as two different things, such as when we consider screening in order to diagnose a disease earlier. The reason for the low use of interval-censored methods is that in the nonparametric case, analysis is technically more complicated than standard survival methods based on exact or right-censored times. The same applies to proportional hazards models. This chapter covers semiparametric regression models, both of the proportional hazards type and of the corresponding frailty models, with proportional hazards conditional on a gamma-distributed frailty. With today's computing power, it is possible to handle these models and we should consider using interval-censoring methods in that case.

The whole approach can also be extended to handle truncation, differential mortality with and without the disease, multivariate data, and time-dependent covariates. However, various complexities appear in these models.

Keywords and Phrases: Frailty, interval-censoring, nonparametric estimation

22.1   Introduction

Interval-censored survival data refer to survival data where the times of events
are not known precisely; they are only known to lie in given intervals. This is
in contrast to the standard survival data setup, which assumes that all event
times are either known precisely, or they happen after the end of observation
(i.e., right-censored data).

For each subject one or more examinations are made over time to find out
if or when the subject gets the disease. It turns out that it is sufficient to know
that the event time is in an interval of the form $(L_i, R_i]$, where the left endpoint
is the time last seen without the disease, and the right endpoint is the first time
seen with the disease. Subjects with the disease at the first examination have
$L_i = 0$ and subjects that are never found to have the disease have $R_i = \infty$, that
is, are right-censored. For many diseases (e.g., diabetes type II), the natural
time scale is age, whereas for other cases (e.g., HIV infection), the natural time
scale is calendar time, in order to follow the spread of the infection.

If all subjects are studied at the same times, the data are grouped and can
easily be analysed. Here, we consider the more general case of individual inspection times. The inspection times are supposed to be generated independently
of the response process and not informative of the parameters governing the
response process. The likelihood then has the following form,

$$\prod_i \{S_i(L_i) - S_i(R_i)\}. \tag{22.1}$$

Strictly speaking, this likelihood is applicable when the inspection times are
fixed beforehand. If, instead, the inspection times are chosen randomly, the
density of this distribution enters as a factor. However, as this factor does not
influence the maximization, we may omit that term.

In the past, such data have often been analysed by various approximations.
Probably the most common approximation is to use the right endpoint for subjects with the disease; that is, we naively consider the onset of disease equal
to the diagnosis of disease. This is obviously biased and may lead to faulty
conclusions in, for example, screening studies, because the screening leads to a
smaller delay from onset to diagnosis, which has been interpreted as a higher
incidence; and the automatically longer survival time with the disease has been
interpreted as a true improvement of survival, although it could partly, or completely, be a consequence of the shifting of the time of diagnosis. With methods
for interval-censored data, we can correct for these problems and make a more
valid evaluation of the effect of screening. A second approximation is to use the
midpoint in the interval for subjects that are observed with the disease. This is
clearly better than the right endpoint, but may still not be optimal, in particular when times between inspections are long, or the inspection frequency varies

in the population. Rather than using an approximate method that requires justification in each case, it makes sense to consider and implement methods that account for the way that the data are collected.

22.2   Parametric Models

In the parametric case, the expression (22.1) can be directly optimized; all that is needed is to insert the relevant expressions for $S_i(t)$. As in other cases, the likelihood function is maximized by differentiating the expression with respect to the parameters, and then setting these derivatives to 0.

Standard asymptotic results apply and the estimate is normally distributed around the true value and with a variance that can be estimated by minus the inverse of the second derivative of the log-likelihood (the so-called observed information), similar in idea to what we get with right-censored data. We need to have some assumptions on the inspection times to make sure that all parameters can be identified. For example, if, in the one-sample case, all subjects are examined at the same time, say t_0, we can only estimate $S(t_0)$ and that only allows for identifying a single parameter.

It is easy to estimate in these models with standard software. For example, in SAS, there is proc lifereg, which is set up to fit Weibull, log-normal, log-logistic, and generalized gamma distributions. Other distributions can be handled by proc nlmixed, which is not dedicated to handle interval-censored data, but we only need to code the survivor function for the observations and this is easy in many models.

Overall, the parametric case is so simple that there are no excuses for not accounting for interval-censoring in a valid way. Indeed, it may in many cases be preferable to use parametric models. This chapter also explores the nonparametric case in order to evaluate precisely how far we can come in practice without a parametric assumption.

22.3   Nonparametric Models

By the nonparametric case, we refer to the one-sample case; that is, all times to disease are assumed to follow the same distribution, or in formulas $S_i(t) = S(t)$. It becomes much more complicated than the parametric case; and also more complicated than the nonparametric case for right-censored data. First, it is impossible to estimate the survivor function at all time points in a nonparametric way. This corresponds to the problem that the Kaplan–Meier estimate cannot determine the tail of the distribution, when the largest time value corresponds to a censoring. For interval-censored data, this problem can occur at any time point. We can only determine the values of the survivor function at the interval endpoints, that is, the collection of L_i and R_is, which we together call x-values. In many cases, several consecutive x-values will show identical survivor function values, and thus the survivor function between them is given as the common value. When two consecutive values do not agree, we have an interval with positive estimated probability and we cannot determine where in the interval the probability mass lies. That is, we can only determine the total probability of that interval. This was already realized by Peto (1973), who also describes a procedure to select a subset of the intervals, which will contain all the probability mass. It is those intervals between the x-values, which have a lower endpoint among the L-observations and an upper endpoint among the R-observations. To emphasize that these make up only a subset of the intervals, they are denoted as intervals $(P_j, Q_j]$, $j = 1, \ldots, k$. Typically, the number of intervals is much lower than the number of observations.

The likelihood is formally the same as described in Equation (22.1). When the $(P, Q]$-intervals have been determined, the likelihood can be reformulated as a function of the probabilities $p_1, \ldots, p_k$. Estimation consists of optimising the likelihood subject to the probabilities of these intervals being greater than or equal to 0 and, of course, with the condition that $\sum_{j=1}^{k} p_j = 1$. It is often the case that some of these intervals have zero estimated probability. It is popular to use the EM-algorithm to calculate the estimates as suggested by Turnbull (1976), but an alternative is a modified Newton–Raphson approach suggested by Peto (1973).

Regarding software, there is a SAS macro (called ice) and also Splus/R has facilities to calculate this estimate. This implies that it is no longer a problem to calculate the estimate.

During the last 15 years, a number of asymptotic results have become available, although mainly for current status data (only one inspection for each subject). If the inspection times are chosen among a finite set of potential inspection times, all we can estimate is the survivor function at these time points. These values follow standard asymptotics, that is, converge by order $\sqrt{n}$, and the variance can be estimated as minus the inverse of the observed information.

If the inspection times are chosen according to a continuous distribution, we can asymptotically determine $S(t)$ in all points, where the inspection time density is positive. However, asymptotic results are no longer standard. Convergence of the survivor function only follows an asymptotic order of $n^{1/3}$. For the case of current status data, this problem was considered by Groeneboom and Wellner (1992). To be precise, let the survivor function of T be $S(t)$, with density $f(t)$ and let the inspection time distribution have density $g(t)$. The sample consists of n independent identically distributed inspection times U_i, and for each subject the indicator $D_i = 1\{T_i \leq U_i\}$ is observed. The relation to the $(L, R]$-intervals is that if $D_i = 1$, the subject has the disease and thus $(L_i, R_i] = (0, U_i]$, and when $D_i = 0$, the subject is healthy at time U_i and thus $(L_i, R_i] = (U_i, \infty]$. Conditions needed for the asymptotic results are that $0 < S(t) < 1$, $f(t) > 0$, and $g(t) > 0$. It is then shown that as $n \to \infty$,

$$n^{1/3}\{\hat{S}_n(t) - S(t)\}/[\frac{1}{2}S(t)\{1 - S(t)\}f(t)/g(t)]^{1/3}$$

converges in distribution to $2Q$, where Q is the time point displaying the maximum value of the stochastic process $W(q) - q^2, q \in \Re$, where $W(q)$ is a standard two-sided Brownian motion, with $W(0) = 0$. This is a symmetric distribution. Keiding *et al.* (1996) have simulated this distribution and tabulated a number of quantiles. In particular for a 95% symmetric confidence interval, the relevant quantiles are ± 2.018. The asymptotic order is still $n^{1/3}$, when there is more than one inspection for each subject, under the additional assumption that these inspections cannot be closer in time than some $\epsilon > 0$. If the inspections are allowed to happen closer in time, the results are more complicated, but Groeneboom and Wellner (1992) have an example where they find an asymptotic order of $(n \log n)^{1/3}$.

Despite the slow convergence of the survivor function, it has been shown that the mean as well as other smooth functionals can be estimated under the standard order of $\sqrt{n}$. This needs additional assumptions of the distribution being concentrated on a finite interval $(0, \tau]$ and $g(t) > 0$ almost everywhere.

22.4   Proportional Hazards Models

The nonparametric model can be extended to the semiparametric proportional hazards model, defined as the hazard being of the form

$$\lambda(t; z) = \lambda_0(t) \exp(\beta' z), \tag{22.2}$$

where z is a vector of covariates with corresponding regression coefficients β and $\lambda_0(t)$ an arbitrary function describing the hazard as a function of time. The regression parameter β is the interesting parameter, whereas the hazard function is a nuisance parameter. This extends the proportional hazards model of Cox (1972) to interval-censored data, but the nice estimation methods of that paper cannot be used. This was already realized by Finkelstein (1986). Instead, the estimates can be found by generalizing the procedure from the nonparametric case. To do so, we need to express the model by means of the survivor function, for example, as

$$S(t; z) = \exp\{-\Lambda_0(t) \exp(\beta' z)\}, \tag{22.3}$$

where $\Lambda_0(t) = \int_0^t \lambda_0(u)du$ is the integrated hazard function. This is then inserted in Equation (22.1). The argument for selecting a subset of the intervals carries over without modification, because the argument does not request that the distributions be equal. This was noticed by Hougaard *et al.* (1994). Thus the mass is concentrated on the $(P, Q]$-intervals. Instead of using the probability parameters corresponding to each interval ($p_1, \ldots, p_k$ above), we may use the contributions to the integrated hazards for each interval, say $\theta_j = \Lambda_0(Q_j) - \Lambda_0(P_j)$, $j = 1, \ldots, k$. All of these need to be positive or zero. The condition that the probabilities sum to 1, is here substituted with $\hat{\theta}_k = \infty$.

Although dedicated software is not available for this model, it is possible to maximize the likelihood by extension of the methods for nonparametric models, either as a modified Newton–Raphson approach or by an EM algorithm.

Regarding asymptotics, Huang (1996) found the interesting result that the regression coefficients β could be estimated according to the standard asymptotic order of $\sqrt{n}$, whereas the integrated hazard $\Lambda_0(t)$ only can be estimated with an asymptotic order of $n^{1/3}$. This was done for current status data, but can probably be extended to general interval-censored data.

22.5 Conditional Proportional Hazards (Frailty Model)

The proportional hazards model described above is very useful for finding the effect of covariates as well as for testing their significance. However, it may still be relevant to extend the model, first of all, in its own right to obtain a more flexible model, when we think that the assumption of proportional hazards is not fulfilled and second as a means of goodness-of-fit checking the assumption of proportional hazards. A third purpose could be to perform a robustness check for a proportional hazards analysis, seeing that it is the same covariates that are influential in another regression model.

One choice is the gamma frailty model, which specifies that conditional on the individual unobserved frailty, say Y, the hazard has the form

$$\mu(t; z) = \mu_0(t)Y \exp(\beta' z). \tag{22.4}$$

This gives an interpretation of the population as consisting of subjects with different risks. This heterogeneity is modelled by the random variable Y. For our purpose here (for univariate data), this interpretation is not the key issue. Instead, it is seen as a tool to generate nonproportional hazards. As Y is unobserved, we have to assign a distribution to it and integrate it out, to obtain the marginal distribution. Here we use the gamma distribution with density

$$f(y) = \delta^\delta y^{\delta-1} \exp(-\delta y)/\Gamma(\delta), \tag{22.5}$$

which is formulated to have a mean of 1. After integration, we obtain the expression

$$S(t; z) = \{1 + \exp(\beta' z) M_0(t)/\delta\}^{-\delta}, \tag{22.6}$$

where $M_0(t) = \int_0^t \mu_0(u) du$. This is then inserted into Equation (22.1). This model will show converging hazards when Y has been integrated out. In that sense it is an extension of the proportional hazards in only one direction. Specifically, the hazard is

$$\mu_0(t) \exp(\beta' z)/\{1 + M_0(t) \exp(\beta' z)/\delta\}. \tag{22.7}$$

The ratio of this hazard between two subjects with covariates z_1, respectively, z_2 is $\exp\{\beta'(z_1 - z_2)\}$, when t is small and 1, when t is large. The special case $\delta = 1$ gives the proportional odds model. More details on the frailty model are described in Hougaard (2000).

The probability mass will be concentrated on the same $(P, Q]$-intervals as in nonparametric and proportional hazards cases, and again only the probabilities of these intervals can be determined. This model can be optimised in the same way as for the proportional hazards model; there is just an additional parameter δ. This model can be compared to the proportional hazards model by the likelihood ratio test, whereas the Wald test does not make sense as the hypothesis of proportional hazards is on the boundary corresponding to $\delta = \infty$.

Detailed asymptotic theory is not yet available, but it seems natural to have results similar to those of the proportional hazards model. Compared to that case, we do, however, need an extra assumption, namely that $\beta \neq 0$, in order to be able to identify δ.

22.6 Extensions

The above sections describe the simplest cases, but indeed there are many natural extensions that are important for practical applications. In most cases, parametric models can be handled without complications compared to the right-censored case. Therefore, the following comments are directed at the non- and semiparametric cases.

Accelerated failure times make an alternative regression model, which is easy to handle for parametric models. As expected from right-censored data, nonparametric models become technically more complicated than the hazard-based models, and therefore need a completely different set of methods. One such approach is described by Rabinowitz *et al.* (1995).

Left truncation means that observation starts conditional on the subject not having had the event before some time $V_i \geq 0$. For example, a dataset could consist of the subjects having some disease at a given time point, and who are then followed over time. The disease duration (time since diagnosis) may be more interesting than time since study start, but to handle the time scale of duration, we obtain truncated data. Turnbull (1976) mentions the possibility of truncation, but the suggested algorithm for finding intervals with positive mass is not correct. Actually, the procedure to find intervals with positive mass becomes more complex, and involves the truncation times as noted by Frydman (1994). More precisely, we can apply the Peto procedure, but combining the truncation times with the right-interval endpoints. Furthermore, it is possible that there is a positive mass in the interval from 0 to $V_{\min} = \min\{V_1, \ldots, V_n\}$. Outside these intervals, the maximum likelihood method does not assign probability and within these intervals we cannot identify where the mass lies. However, where the case without truncation leads to the likelihood being continuously defined on a closed parameter set and the interval probabilities being identifiable, this is no longer the case.

With truncation, we may experience first that the set where the likelihood is defined is not closed, which may imply that the supremum is not obtainable. Second, it is possible that the interval probabilities are not identifiable. A typical example of the first problem is that the first interval has a probability, say p_1, with a near-maximum likelihood estimate arbitrarily close to 1 and the contribution from the later intervals being maximized relatively independent of p_1. More precisely $1 - p_1$ cancels out from the likelihood terms, but we can only do that cancelling out when $p_1 < 1$. To take a specific example, suppose that one subject is truncated at time 0 and $(L, R]$ is $(0, 1]$ and that another subject is truncated at time 2 and has an event in the interval $(3, 6]$. The intervals with potential mass are then $(0, 1]$ and $(3, 6]$. The likelihood becomes $p_1 p_2 / p_2$, which only makes sense if $p_2 > 0$ (i.e., $p_1 < 1$). The supremum of the likelihood is 1, but this is only obtained under a limit of $p_1 \to 1$. The second problem implies that in some cases, only the sum of probabilities for two intervals can be determined, but not the individual interval probabilities. Hudgens (2005) describes specific conditions for existence and uniqueness of the maximum likelihood estimate. Asymptotic calculations are not much more complicated than without truncation if $V_{\min} = 0$. However, if $V_{\min}$ is positive, some models (such as the proportional hazards models) will not depend on the probability of the interval $(0, V_{\min}]$ and thus this probability cannot be identified, whereas other models (such as the frailty model with covariates) will require determination of a parameter for that interval.

General truncation, where the event is known to have happened within a union of intervals and truncation to be within another (larger) union of intervals is in many ways similar, although more complicated; and in particular there can be more than one set outside the union of all truncation sets. For more details, see Huber-Carol and Vonta (2004).

Mortality is often neglected, even though many of the events considered by means of interval-censored data reflect the presence of diseases or complications that may influence the risk of death. If the mortality is nondifferential (i.e., the same with the disease as without the disease) the standard theory is applicable, although we cannot talk about the probability (or survivor function) for the disease, but have to consider the hazard or integrated hazard of disease instead. Typically, we will expect a differential mortality in the direction so that patients with the disease have higher mortality than subjects without disease. This implies a risk of missing disease cases, because they have died without being diagnosed with the disease. To handle this case, we need to describe the life course as a multistate model of the illness–death type, and make a full estimation of all the potential transition hazards.

Multivariate data can either be family data, or multivariate data for a single subject. A common example of the second type is the age at eruption of teeth. All teeth are then checked at visits to a dentist at one or more times. Such data will also for the nonparametric estimation lead to a more complex interval-finding procedure and it is still not possible to identify the interval probabilities in all cases. As with truncated data, there are circumstances where only the sum of probabilities from several intervals can be determined in the maximum likelihood estimate. As for right-censored data, it can be difficult to illustrate the survivor function estimate graphically and difficult to determine measures of dependence, such as Spearman's ρ. It may therefore be sensible to simplify to a semiparametric model, such as describing the dependence by means of a frailty model, and letting the nonparametric component describe only the univariate distributions. In practice, this means that the frailty Y as defined above is shared between the family members, respectively, the teeth of an individual. Advantages of this approach are that the interval-finding procedure is reduced to that of Peto described above and that Spearman's ρ can be estimated, being a function of the frailty distribution. This will also simplify the model in the case of including covariates in a regression model.

Time-dependent covariates will spoil the interval-finding procedure if the covariate can change within an observation interval. A further problem with time-dependent covariates is that they can change in the period from the event happening until it is observed to have happened. Thus it is unclear whether a change in a covariate is a cause for the disease or a response to the disease under study.

22.7   Conclusion

The proportional hazards model has been suggested earlier for interval-censored data, but many researchers have found it too complicated to calculate the estimates and therefore, this has not yet become a standard model. However, with modern computing facilities, estimation is not that difficult, so it is possible to apply this model. Indeed, it is not difficult to extend to the gamma frailty model, which is useful for setting the proportional hazards model in perspective. So, we are now at a stage where the interval-censored data should be analysed as such, rather than by means of some approximation such as assuming that the disease started at the time of diagnosis.

Actually, the theory can be extended to many more interesting cases, both in the parametric and non-/semiparametric case. This includes accounting for truncation, differential mortality with and without the disease, multivariate data, and time-dependent covariates.

Overall, the parametric models are quite tractable, whereas the non-/semiparametric methods are more complicated than those used to form right-censored data.

References

1. Cox, D. R. (1972). Regression models and life tables (with discussion), *Journal of the Royal Statistical Society, Series B*, **34**, 187–220.

2. Finkelstein, D. M. (1986). A proportional hazards model for interval-censored failure time data, *Biometrics*, **42**, 845–854.

3. Frydman, H. (1994). A note on nonparametric estimation of the distribution function from interval-censored and truncated observations, *Journal of the Royal Statistical Society, Series B*, **56**, 71–74.

4. Groeneboom, P. and Wellner, J. A. (1992). *Information Bounds and Nonparametric Maximum Likelihood Estimation*, Birkhäuser, New York.

5. Hougaard, P. (2000). *Analysis of Multivariate Survival Data*, Springer-Verlag, New York.

6. Hougaard, P., Myglegaard, P., and Borch-Johnsen, K. (1994). Heterogeneity models of disease susceptibility, with application to diabetic nephropathy, *Biometrics*, **50**, 1178–1188.

7. Huang, J. (1996). Efficient estimation for the proportional hazards model with interval censoring, *Annals of Statistics,* **24**, 540–568.

8. Huber-Carol, C. and Vonta, I. (2004). Frailty models for arbitrarily censored and truncated data, *Lifetime Data Analysis,* **10**, 369–388.

9. Hudgens, M. G. (2005). On nonparametric maximum likelihood estimation with interval censoring and left truncation, *Journal of the Royal Statistical Society, Series B,* **67**, 573–587.

10. Keiding, N., Begtrup, K., Scheike, T. H., and Hasibeder, G. (1996). Estimation from current-status data in continuous time, *Lifetime Data Analysis,* **2**, 119–129.

11. Peto, R. (1973). Experimental survival curves for interval-censored data, *Applied Statistics,* **22**, 86–91.

12. Rabinowitz, D., Tsiatis, A., and Aragon, J. (1995). Regression with interval-censored data, *Biometrika,* **82**, 501–513.

13. Turnbull, B. W. (1976). The empirical distribution function with arbitrarily grouped, censored and truncated data, *Journal of the Royal Statistical Society, Series B,* **38**, 290–295.

23

Exact Likelihood Inference for an Exponential Parameter Under Progressive Hybrid Censoring Schemes

A. Childs,[1] **B. Chandrasekar,**[2] **and N. Balakrishnan**[1]

[1]*Department of Mathematics and Statistics, McMaster University, Hamilton, Ontario, Canada*
[2]*Department of Statistics, Loyola College, Chennai, India*

Abstract: The purpose of this chapter is to propose two types of progressive hybrid censoring schemes in life-testing experiments and develop exact inference for the mean of the exponential distribution. The exact distribution of the maximum likelihood estimator and an exact lower confidence bound for the mean lifetime are obtained under both types of progressive hybrid censoring schemes. Illustrative examples are finally presented.

Keywords and Phrases: Progressive censoring, hybrid censoring, life-testing, exponential distribution, maximum likelihood estimator, conditional moment-generating function, exact inference, lower confidence bound, truncated gamma density

23.1 Introduction

Epstein (1954) considered a hybrid censoring scheme in the context of life-testing experiments in which the experiment is terminated at time $T_1^* = \min\{X_{m:n}, T\}$, where $T \in (0, \infty)$ and $1 \leq m \leq n$ are fixed in advance, and $X_{m:n}$ denotes the mth failure time when n units are put on a life-test. By assuming exponential lifetimes for the units, Chen and Bhattacharyya (1988) derived the distribution of the maximum likelihood estimator (MLE) of the mean lifetime and also obtained an exact lower confidence bound for the mean lifetime. Because the termination time is at most T, as in a conventional Type-I censoring scheme, we refer to the above-mentioned scheme as a *Type-I hybrid censoring scheme (Type-I HCS)*. Basic details on some of these developments can be found in the book by Balakrishnan and Basu (1995).

Recently, Childs *et al.* (2003) obtained a simplified form for the exact distribution of the maximum likelihood estimator of the mean of an exponential distribution based on a Type-I HCS. These authors also proposed a new hybrid censoring scheme, called a *Type-II hybrid censoring scheme (Type-II HCS)*, in which the stopping time is $T_2^* = \max\{X_{m:n}, T\}$. They also derived some exact inference results for this new hybrid censoring scheme. In this chapter, we generalize the above-mentioned hybrid censoring schemes to the case when the observed sample is progressively censored. In Section 23.2, we consider a *Type-I progressive hybrid censoring scheme (Type-I PHCS)*, in which n items are put on test with censoring scheme $(R_1, R_2, \ldots, R_m)$ and stopping time $T_1^* = \min\{X_{m:m:n}, T\}$, where $X_{1:m:n} \leq X_{2:m:n} \leq \cdots \leq X_{m:m:n}$ are the ordered failure times resulting from the progressively censored experiment; see Balakrishnan and Aggarwala (2000). We then extend the results of Chen and Bhattacharyya (1988) and Childs *et al.* (2003) to this more general situation. In Section 23.3, we similarly generalize the results for the Type-II HCS by using the stopping time $T_2^* = \max\{X_{m:m:n}, T\}$, where again T and m are fixed in advance. This new progressive hybrid censoring scheme, which we call a *Type-II progressive hybrid censoring scheme (Type-II PHCS)* guarantees that at least m failure times will be observed. Some illustrative examples are presented finally in Section 23.4.

We should mention here that both Type-II PHCS and Type-I PHCS have some advantages and disadvantages. In the case of Type-I PHCS, the termination time is fixed by the experimenter which is a clear advantage. However, if θ (the unknown mean lifetime) is not small compared to T (the pre-fixed termination time), then with a high probability the experimentation would terminate at T. In addition, there is a disadvantage that far fewer than m failures may be observed which may have an adverse effect on the efficiency of the inferential procedure based on Type-I PHCS. In the case of Type-II PHCS, the termination time is unknown to the experimenter which is a disadvantage. In the case when θ is not small compared to T, with a high probability the experimentation would terminate at $X_{m:m:n}$ thus resulting in a longer life-test. However, there is a clear advantage that more than m failures may be observed which will result in efficient inferential procedures based on Type-II PHCS.

23.2 Results for Type-I Progressive Hybrid Censoring

Consider the following progressive Type-II censoring scheme. Experimentation begins at time 0 with n units placed on a life-test. Immediately following the first observed failure, R_1 surviving items are removed from the test at random. Similarly, following the second observed failure, R_2 surviving items are removed from the test at random. This process continues until, immediately following the mth observed failure, all the remaining $R_m = n - R_1 - \cdots - R_{m-1} - m$ items are removed from the experiment. In this experiment, the progressive censoring scheme $\boldsymbol{R} = (R_1, R_2, \ldots, R_m)$ is pre-fixed. The resulting m ordered failure times, which we denote by $X_{1:m:n}, X_{2:m:n}, \ldots, X_{m:m:n}$, are referred to as progressive Type-II right-censored order statistics. The special case of $R_1 = R_2 = \cdots = R_{m-1} = 0$ (so that $R_m = n - m$) is the case of conventional Type-II right-censored sampling. The joint probability density function of $(X_{1:m:n}, X_{2:m:n}, \ldots, X_{i:m:n})$, $i = 1, 2, \ldots, m$, is given by [Balakrishnan and Aggarwala (2000)]

$$f(x_1, x_2, \ldots, x_i) = \left\{ \prod_{j=1}^{i} \sum_{k=j}^{m} (R_k + 1) \right\} \prod_{j=1}^{i-1} f(x_j)\{1 - F(x_j)\}^{R_j}$$
$$\times \ f(x_i)\{1 - F(x_i)\}^{R_i^* - 1},$$
$$-\infty < x_1 < x_2 < \cdots < x_i < \infty, \qquad (23.1)$$

where $R_i^* = \sum_{k=i}^{m}(R_k + 1)$.

Suppose that the lifetimes of the n units put on test are independent and identically distributed as exponential random variables with pdf

$$f(x; \theta) = \frac{1}{\theta} e^{-x/\theta}, \qquad x > 0, \qquad \theta > 0.$$

Also suppose that the experiment is terminated at a random time $T_1^* = \min\{X_{m:m:n}, T\}$. Let D^* denote the number of observed failures up to time T_1^*. Then the likelihood function is given by

$$L(\theta) \propto \frac{1}{\theta^{D^*}} e^{-\frac{1}{\theta}\left[\sum_{i=1}^{D^*}(R_i+1)x_{i:m:n} + R_{D^*+1}^* T_1^*\right]},$$

and so the MLE is given by

$$\widehat{\theta} = \frac{1}{D^*} \left\{ \sum_{i=1}^{D^*}(R_i + 1)X_{i:m:n} + R_{D^*+1}^* T_1^* \right\}, \qquad D^* \geq 1.$$

Note that the MLE does not exist when $D^* = 0$. Let D denote the number of failures up to time T. Then,

$$\widehat{\theta} = \begin{cases} \frac{1}{D}\left\{ \sum_{i=1}^{D}(R_i + 1)X_{i:m:n} + R_{D+1}^* T \right\} & \text{if } D = 1, 2, \ldots, m - 1 \\ \frac{1}{m}\left\{ \sum_{i=1}^{m}(R_i + 1)X_{i:m:n} \right\} & \text{if } D = m. \end{cases}$$

In order to derive the moment-generating function of the above MLE $\widehat{\theta}$, we first present two lemmas. The proof of Lemma 23.2.1 can be found in Balakrishnan *et al.* (2002).

Lemma 23.2.1 *Let $f(x)$ and $F(x)$ denote the pdf and cdf of an absolutely continuous random variable X, and let $a_j > 0$ for $j = 1, 2, \ldots, r$. Then for $r \geq 1$, we have*

$$\int_{-\infty}^{x_{r+1}} \cdots \int_{-\infty}^{x_3} \int_{-\infty}^{x_2} \prod_{j=1}^{r} f(x_j)\{1 - F(x_j)\}^{a_j-1} dx_1 dx_2 \cdots dx_r$$

$$= \sum_{i=0}^{r} c_{i,r}(\boldsymbol{a}_r)\{1 - F(x_{r+1})\}^{b_{i,r}(\boldsymbol{a}_r)},$$

where $\boldsymbol{a}_r = (a_1, a_2, \ldots, a_r)$;

$$c_{i,r}(\boldsymbol{a}_r) = \frac{(-1)^i}{\left\{\prod_{j=1}^{i} \sum_{k=r-i+1}^{r-i+j} a_k\right\} \left\{\prod_{j=1}^{r-i} \sum_{k=j}^{r-i} a_k\right\}}, \qquad b_{i,r}(\boldsymbol{a}_r) = \sum_{j=r-i+1}^{r} a_j,$$

with the usual conventions that $\prod_{j=1}^{0} d_j \equiv 1$ and $\sum_{j=i}^{i-1} d_j \equiv 0$.

Lemma 23.2.2 *(a) For $d = 1, \ldots, m-1$, the conditional joint density of $X_{1:m:n}, X_{2:m:n}, \ldots, X_{d:m:n}$, given $D = d$, is*

$$f(x_1, x_2, \ldots, x_d | D = d)$$

$$= \frac{c'(n, d)\{1 - F(T)\}^{R_{d+1}^*}}{P(D = d)} \prod_{j=1}^{d} f(x_j)\{1 - F(x_j)\}^{R_j},$$

$$-\infty < x_1 < x_2 < \cdots < x_d < T,$$

where $c'(n, d) = \prod_{j=1}^{d} \sum_{k=j}^{m} (R_k + 1)$ for $d = 1, 2, \ldots, m$.
(b) The conditional joint density of $X_{1:m:n}, X_{2:m:n}, \ldots, X_{m:m:n}$, given $D = m$, is

$$f(x_1, x_2, \ldots, x_m | D = m) = \frac{c'(n, m)}{P(D = m)} \prod_{j=1}^{m} f(x_j)\{1 - F(x_j)\}^{R_j},$$

$$-\infty < x_1 < x_2 < \cdots < x_d < T.$$

PROOF. Part (a) is obtained by writing the event $\{D = d\}$ as $\{X_{d:m:n} \leq T, X_{d+1:m:n} > T\}$ and integrating with respect to x_{d+1} (from T to ∞) in the joint density function of $X_{1:m:n}, X_{2:m:n}, \ldots, X_{d+1:m:n}$ obtained from (23.1). Part (b) is straightforward, in view of (23.1). Hence, the lemma. ∎

Theorem 23.2.1 *The conditional moment-generating function of $\hat{\theta}$, given $D^* \geq 1$, is given by*

$$\phi_{\hat{\theta}}(w)$$

$$= (1 - q^n)^{-1} \sum_{d=1}^{m} \frac{c'(n, d)}{(1 - w\theta/d)^d} \sum_{i=0}^{d} c_{i,d}(R_1 + 1, \ldots, R_d + 1) q^{R_{d-i+1}^*(1 - w\theta/d)},$$

where $q = e^{-T/\theta}$.

PROOF. We first note that, conditional on $D \geq 1$, we can write

$$E(e^{w\widehat{\theta}}) = (1 - q^n)^{-1}$$

$$\times \left\{ \sum_{d=1}^{m-1} E(e^{w\widehat{\theta}}|D = d)P(D = d) + E(e^{w\widehat{\theta}}|D = m)P(D = m) \right\}.$$

$$(23.2)$$

From Part (a) of Lemma 23.2.2, we have for $d = 1, 2, \ldots, m - 1$,

$$E(e^{w\widehat{\theta}}|D = d)P(D = d) = c'(n, d)q^{R^*_{d+1}(1-w\theta/d)}$$

$$\times \int_0^T \cdots \int_0^{x_3} \int_0^{x_2} \prod_{j=1}^d f(x_j)\{1 - F(x_j)\}^{(R_j+1)(1-w\theta/d)-1}dx_1 dx_2 \cdots dx_d.$$

We now apply Lemma 23.2.1 with $a_j = (R_j + 1)(1 - w\theta/d)$ and then factor $(1 - w\theta/d)$ out of all of the a_js in order to obtain

$$E(e^{w\widehat{\theta}}|D = d)P(D = d)$$

$$= \frac{c'(n, d)}{(1 - \theta w/d)^d} \sum_{i=0}^d c_{i,d}(R_1 + 1, \ldots, R_d + 1)q^{(1-\theta w/d)R^*_{d-i+1}}. \quad (23.3)$$

Similarly, when $D = m$, we obtain

$$E(e^{w\widehat{\theta}}|D = m)P(D = m)$$

$$= c'(n, m) \int_0^T \cdots \int_0^{x_3} \int_0^{x_2} \prod_{j=1}^m f(x_j)$$

$$\times \{1 - F(x_j)\}^{(R_j+1)(1-w\theta/m)-1}dx_1 dx_2 \cdots dx_m$$

$$= \frac{c'(n, m)}{(1 - \theta w/m)^m} \sum_{i=0}^m c_{i,m}(R_1 + 1, \ldots, R_m + 1)q^{(1-\theta w/m)R^*_{m-i+1}},$$

$$(23.4)$$

where the first equality follows from Part (b) of Lemma 23.2.2 and the second equality follows from Lemma 23.2.1. The theorem then follows readily upon substituting (23.3) and (23.4) into (23.2). ∎

Remark 23.2.1 If we set $R_j = 0$ for $j = 1, 2, \ldots, m - 1$ so that $R_m = n - m$, then the Type-I progressive hybrid censoring scheme reduces to the classical Type-I hybrid censoring scheme discussed earlier by Chen and Bhattacharyya (1988). Hence, the above result is an extension of the results obtained by these authors, and gives a more elegant and compact representation of the moment-generating function of the MLE. Indeed, Theorem 23.2.1 reduces in this case to the one presented by Childs *et al.* (2003). In fact, in this case,

$$
\phi_{\widehat{\theta}}(w) = (1 - q^n)^{-1} \Bigg[\sum_{d=1}^{m-1} \binom{n}{d} \frac{q^{(n-d)(1-\theta w/d)}}{(1 - w\theta/d)^d} \left(1 - q^{(1-\theta w/d)}\right)^d
$$

$$
+ (1 - \theta w/m)^{-m} + m\binom{n}{m}(1 - \theta w/m)^{-m}
$$

$$
\times \sum_{k=1}^{m} \frac{(-1)^k}{n - m + k}\binom{m-1}{k-1} q^{(1-\theta w/m)(n-m+k)} \Bigg].
$$

Theorem 23.2.2 *The conditional pdf of $\widehat{\theta}$, given $D \geq 1$, is given by*

$$
f_{\widehat{\theta}}(x) = (1 - q^n)^{-1} \sum_{d=1}^{m} c'(n, d)
$$

$$
\times \sum_{i=0}^{d} c_{i,d}(R_1 + 1, \ldots, R_d + 1) q^{R^*_{d-i+1}} \gamma_d(x, R^*_{d-i+1}T/d),
$$

$$(23.5)$$

where

$$
\gamma_k(x, a) = \frac{(k/\theta)^k}{(k-1)!}\langle x - a\rangle^{k-1} e^{-\frac{k}{\theta}(x-a)},
$$

is the translated gamma density function and $\langle a\rangle = \max(a, 0)$.

PROOF. Consider the moment-generating function of $\widehat{\theta}$, given by

$$
M_{\widehat{\theta}}(w) = (1 - q^n)^{-1} \sum_{d=1}^{m}\sum_{i=0}^{d} c'(n, d)c_{i,d}(R_1 + 1, \ldots, R_d + 1) q^{R^*_{d-i+1}}
$$

$$
\times e^{wTR^*_{d-i+1}/d}(1 - \theta w/d)^{-d}.
$$

Because $e^{wTR^*_{d-i+1}/d}(1 - \theta w/d)^{-d}$ is the moment-generating function of $Y + TR^*_{d-i+1}/d$ at w, where Y is a gamma random variable with pdf $\gamma_d(x, 0)$, the theorem readily follows. ∎

Remark 23.2.2 Separating out the term corresponding to $d = m$ and $i = 0$ in the density function in (23.5), we can write

$$f_{\widehat{\theta}}(x)$$

$$= (1 - q^n)^{-1} \Bigg[\gamma_m(x, 0)$$

$$+ \sum_{d=1}^{m-1} c'(n, d) \sum_{i=0}^{d} c_{i,d}(R_1 + 1, \ldots, R_d + 1) q^{R^*_{d-i+1}} \gamma_d(x, R^*_{d-i+1} T/d)$$

$$+ c'(n, m) \sum_{i=1}^{m} c_{i,m}(R_1 + 1, \ldots, R_m + 1) q^{R^*_{m-i+1}} \gamma_m(x, R^*_{m-i+1} T/m) \Bigg].$$

Note that as $T \to \infty$, the above Type-I PHCS reduces to the usual progressive censoring scheme. In this case, the above-conditional pdf of $\widehat{\theta}$ simply becomes $\gamma_m(x, 0)$. Therefore, the above result generalizes the result of Viveros and Balakrishnan (1994) that $(2m\widehat{\theta})/\theta$ has a chi-square distribution with $2m$ degrees of freedom when the sample is progressively censored.

Corollary 23.2.1 *The mean and mean squared error of $\widehat{\theta}$ are given by*

(i) $E_\theta(\widehat{\theta}) = \theta + \frac{T}{(1-q^n)} \sum_{d=1}^{m} \frac{c'(n,d)}{d} \sum_{i=0}^{d} c_{i,d}(R_1 + 1, \ldots, R_d + 1)$
$$\times R^*_{d-i+1} q^{R^*_{d-i+1}}$$

and

(ii) $MSE(\widehat{\theta}) = (1 - q^n)^{-1} \sum_{d=1}^{m} \frac{c'(n,d)}{d} \sum_{i=0}^{d} c_{i,d}(R_1 + 1, \ldots, R_d + 1)$
$$\times q^{R^*_{d-i+1}} \{ \theta^2 + T^2 \left(R^*_{d-i+1} \right)^2 / d \}.$$

In order to derive a lower confidence bound for θ, we need the expression for $P(\widehat{\theta} > t)$ which is presented in the following theorem.

Theorem 23.2.3 *Given that $D^* \geq 1$,*

$$P(\widehat{\theta} > t) = (1 - q^n)^{-1} \sum_{d=1}^{m} \frac{c'(n, d)}{(d-1)!}$$

$$\times \sum_{i=0}^{d} c_{i,d}(R_1 + 1, \ldots, R_d + 1) q^{R^*_{d-i+1}} \Gamma(d, A_d(R^*_{d-i+1} T/d)),$$

where $\Gamma(a, z) = \int_z^\infty t^{a-1} e^{-t} dt$ *is the incomplete gamma function and* $A_k(a) = (k/\theta)\langle t - a \rangle$.

PROOF. Let

$$g_k(x, a) = \frac{(k/\theta)^k}{(k-1)!} (x - a)^{k-1} e^{-\frac{k}{\theta}(x-a)}.$$

Then,

$$
\int_t^\infty \gamma_k(x, a)dx
$$

$$
= \int_{\max(t,a)}^\infty g_k(x, a)dx
$$

$$
= \int_{\frac{k}{\theta}<t-a>}^\infty \frac{y^{k-1}}{(k-1)!}e^{-y}dy
$$

$$
\text{(upon making the substitution } y = (k/\theta)(x-a))
$$

$$
= \frac{\Gamma(k, A_k(a))}{(k-1)!}.
$$

■

23.3 Results for Type-II Progressive Hybrid Censoring

In the Type-II progressive hybrid censoring situation, the experiment is terminated at the random time $T^* = \max(X_{m:m:n}, T)$. Let D denote the number of failures that occur up to time T. If $X_{m:m:n} > T$, then the experiment is terminated at the mth failure with the withdrawals occurring after each failure according to the prespecified progressive censoring scheme $\boldsymbol{R} = (R_1, R_2, \ldots, R_m)$. However, if $X_{m:m:n} < T$, then instead of terminating the experiment by removing the remaining R_m units after the mth failure, we continue to observe failures (without any further withdrawals) up to time T. Therefore, $R_m = R_{m+1} = \cdots = R_d = 0$, where d is the observed value of D. In this case, we denote the resulting failure times by $X_{1:m:n}, X_{2:m:n}, \ldots, X_{m:m:n}, X_{m+1:n}, \ldots, X_{d:n}$.

The MLE of θ in this case is given by

$$
\widehat{\theta} = \begin{cases} \frac{1}{m}\sum_{i=1}^m (R_i + 1)X_{i:m:n} & \text{if } D = 0, 1, \ldots, m-1 \\ \frac{1}{D}\left[\sum_{j=1}^m (R_j + 1)X_{j:m:n} \right. \\ \quad \left. + \sum_{j=m+1}^D X_{j:n} + R'_D T\right] & \text{if } D = m, \ldots, n - \sum_{i=1}^{m-1} R_i, \end{cases}
$$

where $R'_D = n - D - R_1 - \cdots - R_{m-1}$, and $R_m = 0$ if $D \geq m$.

The proofs of the following lemma and theorems, which give the moment-generating function and pdf of $\widehat{\theta}$, as well as the corresponding expression for $P(\widehat{\theta} > t)$, are similar to those presented in the last section, and hence are omitted for brevity.

Lemma 23.3.1 *(a) For $d = 1, \ldots, m - 1$, the conditional joint density of $X_{1:m:n}, X_{2:m:n}, \ldots, X_{m:m:n}$, given $D = d$, is*

$$f(x_1, x_2, \ldots, x_m | D = d) = \frac{c'(n, m)}{P(D = d)} \prod_{j=1}^{m} f(x_j)\{1 - F(x_j)\}^{R_j},$$

$$-\infty < x_1 < \cdots < x_d < T < x_{d+1} < \cdots < x_m < \infty.$$

(b) For $d = m, m + 1, \ldots, n - R_1 - \cdots - R_{m-1}$, the conditional joint density of $X_{1:m:n}, X_{2:m:n}, \ldots, X_{m:m:n}, X_{m+1:n}, \ldots, X_{d:n}$, given $D = d$, is

$$f(x_1, \ldots, x_d | D = d) = \frac{c'(n, d)q^{R'_d}}{P(D = d)} \prod_{j=1}^{d} f(x_j)\{1 - F(x_j)\}^{R_j},$$

$$-\infty < x_1 < \cdots < x_d < T,$$

where $R_m = R_{m+1} = \cdots = R_d = 0$ and $R'_d = n - d - R_1 - \cdots - R_{m-1}$.

Theorem 23.3.1 *The moment-generating function of $\widehat{\theta}$ is given by*

$$
\begin{aligned}
\phi_{\widehat{\theta}}(w) &= E(e^{w\widehat{\theta}}) \\
&= \sum_{d=0}^{m-1} \frac{c'(n, d)}{(1 - w\theta/m)^m} \sum_{i=0}^{d} c_{i,d}(R_1 + 1, \ldots, R_d + 1)q^{R^*_{d-i+1}(1 - w\theta/m)} \\
&\quad + \sum_{d=m}^{n - R_1 - \cdots - R_{m-1}} \frac{c'(n, d)}{(1 - w\theta/d)^d} \\
&\quad \times \sum_{i=0}^{d} c_{i,d}(R_1 + 1, \ldots, R_d + 1)q^{[R'_d + b_{i,d}(R_1 + 1, \ldots, R_d + 1)](1 - w\theta/d)},
\end{aligned}
$$

where $b_{i,r}$ is as defined in Lemma 23.2.1.

Theorem 23.3.2 *The pdf of $\widehat{\theta}$ is given by*

$$
\begin{aligned}
f_{\widehat{\theta}}(x) &\\
&= \sum_{d=0}^{m-1} \sum_{i=0}^{d} c'(n, d)q^{R^*_{d-i+1}} c_{i,d}(R_1 + 1, \ldots, R_d + 1)\gamma_m(x, R^*_{d-i+1}T/m) \\
&\quad + \sum_{d=m}^{n - R_1 - \cdots - R_{m-1}} c'(n, d) \sum_{i=0}^{d} c_{i,d}(R_1 + 1, \ldots, R_d + 1) \\
&\quad \times q^{R'_d + b_{i,d}(R_1 + 1, \ldots, R_d + 1)}\gamma_d\left(x, [R'_d + b_{i,d}(R_1 + 1, \ldots, R_d + 1)]T/d\right),
\end{aligned}
$$

where, as in the last section, $\gamma_k(x, a)$ is the translated gamma density function.

Corollary 23.3.1 *The mean and mean squared error of $\widehat{\theta}$ are given by*

$$(i)\ E_\theta(\widehat{\theta})\ =\ \theta + \frac{T}{m}\sum_{d=0}^{m-1}\sum_{i=0}^{d}c'(n,d)R^*_{d-i+1}q^{R^*_{d-i+1}}c_{i,d}(R_1+1,\ldots,R_d+1)$$

$$+T\sum_{d=m}^{n-R_1-\cdots-R_{m-1}}\frac{c'(n,d)}{d}\sum_{i=0}^{d}c_{i,d}(R_1+1,\ldots,R_d+1)$$

$$\times[R'_d + b_{i,d}(R_1+1,\ldots,R_d+1)]q^{R'_d+b_{i,d}(R_1+1,\ldots,R_d+1)}$$

and

$$(ii)\ MSE(\widehat{\theta})$$

$$=\ \frac{1}{m}\sum_{d=0}^{m-1}c'(n,d)\sum_{i=0}^{d}q^{R^*_{d-i+1}}c_{i,d}(R_1+1,\ldots,R_d+1)$$

$$\times[\theta^2 + T^2(R^*_{d-i+1})^2/m]$$

$$+\sum_{d=m}^{n-R_1-\cdots-R_{m-1}}\frac{c'(n,d)}{d}\sum_{i=0}^{d}c_{i,d}(R_1+1,\ldots,R_d+1)$$

$$\times q^{R'_d+b_{i,d}(R_1+1,\ldots,R_d+1)}\left\{\theta^2 + T^2[R'_d+b_{i,d}(R_1+1,\ldots,R_d+1)]^2/d\right\}.$$

Theorem 23.3.3 *We have*

$$P(\widehat{\theta} > t)$$

$$=\ \sum_{d=0}^{m-1}\frac{c'(n,d)}{(m-1)!}\sum_{i=0}^{d}q^{R^*_{d-i+1}}c_{i,d}(R_1+1,\ldots,R_d+1)$$

$$\times\Gamma\left(m, A_m(R^*_{d-i+1}T/m)\right)$$

$$+\sum_{d=m}^{n-R_1-\cdots-R_{m-1}}\frac{c'(n,d)}{(d-1)!}\sum_{i=0}^{d}c_{i,d}(R_1+1,\ldots,R_d+1)$$

$$\times q^{R'_d+b_{i,d}(R_1+1,\ldots,R_d+1)}\Gamma\left(d, A_d([R'_d+b_{i,d}(R_1+1,\ldots,R_d+1)]T/d)\right),$$

where, as in the last section, $\Gamma(a,z)$ denotes the incomplete gamma function. It needs to be mentioned here that in the second sum of all the above results, we have $R_m = R_{m+1} = \cdots = R_d = 0$.

23.4   Examples

Assuming that $P_\theta(\widehat{\theta} > b)$ is a monotone increasing function of θ, a $100(1-\alpha)\%$ lower confidence bound for θ is obtained by solving the equation $\alpha = P_{\theta_L}(\widehat{\theta} > \widehat{\theta}_{\text{obs}})$ for θ_L. To illustrate this method, as well as the corresponding method for confidence intervals, we consider the data reported by Nelson (1982, p. 228) on times to breakdown of an insulating fluid in an accelerated test conducted at various voltages. Viveros and Balakrishnan (1994) generated the following Type-II progressively censored sample from these data.

i	1	2	3	4	5	6	7	8
$x_{i:8:19}$	0.19	0.78	0.96	1.31	2.78	4.85	6.50	7.35
R_i	0	0	3	0	3	0	0	5

In order to illustrate both cases of Type-I and Type-II progressive hybrid censoring schemes, we take $T = 6.0$. Table 23.1 presents the lower confidence bounds and $100(1-\alpha)\%$ confidence intervals for θ with $\alpha = 0.05, 0.1$ for values of m selected so as to illustrate both cases of progressive hybrid censoring schemes. We have also included the mean square error and standard error calculated from Corollaries 23.2.1 and 23.3.1. Note that when $m = 6$, we take $R_m = 7$ in the case of Type-I progressive hybrid censoring, and $R_m = 0$ in the case of Type-II progressive hybrid censoring (as described in Section 23.3).

Table 23.1. Inference for θ

				Type-I PHCS			
				LCB for θ		CI for θ	
m	$\widehat{\theta}_{\text{obs}}$	MSE	s.e.	$\alpha = .05$	$\alpha = .1$	$\alpha = .05$	$\alpha = .1$
6	9.3400	23.032	4.786	5.330	6.042	(4.802, 25.519)	(5.330, 21.472)
8	10.6817	35.100	5.833	6.004	6.766	(5.434, 26.093)	(6.004, 22.212)
				Type-II PHCS			
6	10.6817	16.600	4.045	6.019	6.781	(5.448, 26.084)	(6.019, 22.232)
8	9.0863	9.493	3.078	5.513	6.157	(5.027, 20.935)	(5.513, 18.167)

In Table 23.1, we see that the MLE for $m = 8$ in the case of Type-I PHCS is the same as for the Type-II PHCS when $m = 6$. The reason for this is that, in both these cases, the experiment is terminated at time $T = 6$ after observing the first 6 failures.

Acknowledgements

The first and third authors thank the Natural Sciences and Engineering Research Council of Canada for funding this research. This work was conducted during a summer visit of Professor B. Chandrasekar to McMaster University, Hamilton, Canada.

References

1. Balakrishnan, N. and Aggarwala, R. (2000). *Progressive Censoring: Theory, Methods, and Applications*, Birkhäuser, Boston.

2. Balakrishnan, N. and Basu, A. P. (Eds.) (1995). *The Exponential Distribution: Theory, Methods and Applications*, Gordon and Breach Science, Newark, N.J.

3. Balakrishnan, N., Childs, A., and Chandrasekar, B (2002). An efficient computational method for moments of order statistics under progressive censoring, *Statistics & Probability Letters*, **60**, 359–365.

4. Chen, S. and Bhattacharyya, G. K. (1988). Exact confidence bounds for an exponential parameter under hybrid censoring, *Communications in Statistics—Theory and Methods*, **17**, 1857–1870.

5. Childs, A., Chandrasekar, B., Balakrishnan, N., and Kundu, D. (2003). Exact likelihood inference based on Type-I and Type-II hybrid censored samples from the exponential distribution, *Annals of the Institute of Statistical Mathematics*, **55**, 319–330.

6. Epstein, B. (1954). Truncated life tests in the exponential case, *Annals of Mathematical Statistics*, **25**, 555–564.

7. Nelson, W. (1982). *Applied Life Data Analysis*, John Wiley & Sons, New York.

8. Viveros, R. and Balakrishnan, N. (1994). Interval estimation of parameters of life from progressively censored data, *Technometrics*, **36**, 84–91.

PART V
QUALITY OF LIFE

24

Sequential Analysis of Quality-of-Life Measurements Using Mixed Rasch Models

Véronique Sébille,[1] **Jean-Benoit Hardouin,**[1] **and Mounir Mesbah**[2]

[1]*Laboratoire de Biostatistique, Université de Nantes, Nantes, France*
[2]*Laboratoire de Statistique Théorique et Appliquée, Université Pierre et Marie Curie, Paris, France*

Abstract: Early stopping of clinical trials in the case of either beneficial or deleterious effect of a treatment on quality of life (QoL) is an important issue. QoL is usually evaluated using self-assessment questionnaires and responses to the items are usually combined into QoL scores assumed to be normally distributed. However, these QoL scores are rarely normally distributed and usually do not satisfy a number of basic measurement properties. An alternative is to use item response theory (IRT) models such as the Rasch model for binary items which takes into account the categorical nature of the items. In this framework, the probability of response of a patient on an item depends upon different kinds of parameters: the "ability level" of the person (which reflects his or her current QoL) and a set of parameters characterizing each item.

Sequential analysis and mixed Rasch models were combined in the context of phase II or III comparative clinical trials. The statistical properties of the triangular test (TT) were compared using mixed Rasch models and the traditional method based on QoL scores by means of simulations.

The type I error of the TT was correctly maintained for the methods based on QoL scores and the Rasch model assuming known item parameter values, but was higher than expected when item parameters were assumed to be unknown. The power of the TT was satisfactorily maintained when Rasch models were used but the test was underpowered with the QoL scores method. All methods allowed substantial reductions in average sample numbers as compared with fixed sample designs, especially the method based on Rasch models. The use of IRT models in sequential analysis of QoL endpoints seems to provide a more powerful method to detect therapeutic effects than the traditional QoL scores method and to allow for reaching a conclusion with fewer patients.

Keywords and Phrases: Quality of life, item response theory, Rasch models, triangular test, clinical trials, mixed models

24.1 Introduction

Many clinical trials attempt to measure health-related Quality of Life (QoL) which refers to "the extent to which one's usual or expected physical, emotional and social well-being are affected by a medical condition or its treatment" [Cella and Bonomi (1995), and Fairclough (2002)]. Early stopping of clinical trials either in the case of beneficial or deleterious effect of treatment on QoL is an important issue. However, each domain of health can have several components (e.g., symptoms, ability to function, disability) and translating these various domains of health into quantitative values to measure quality of life is a complex task, drawing from the field of psychometrics, biostatistics, and clinical decision theory. In clinical trials in which specific therapeutic interventions are being studied, a patient's QoL is usually evaluated using self-assessment questionnaires which consist of a set of questions called items (which can be dichotomous or polytomous) that are frequently combined to give scores. The common practice is to work on average scores which are generally assumed to be normally distributed. However, these average scores are rarely normally distributed and usually do not satisfy a number of basic measurement properties including sufficiency, unidimensionality, or reliability. An alternative is to use item response theory (IRT) models [Fischer and Molenaar (1995)], such as the Rasch model for binary items, which takes into account the categorical nature of the items by introducing an underlying response model relating those items to a latent parameter interpreted as the true individual QoL.

Early stopping of a trial can occur either for efficacy, safety, or futility reasons. Several early termination procedures have been developed to allow for repeated statistical analyses on accumulating data and for stopping a trial as soon as the information is sufficient to conclude. Among the sequential methods that have been developed over the last few decades [Pocock (1977), O'Brien and Fleming (1979), and Lan and De Mets (1983)], the sequential probability ratio test (SPRT) and the triangular test (TT), which were initially developed by Wald (1947) and Anderson (1960) and later extended by Whitehead to allow for sequential analyses on groups of patients [Whitehead and Jones (1979), and Whitehead and Stratton (1983)] have some of the interesting following features. They allow for: (i) early stopping under H_0 or under H_1; (ii) the analysis of quantitative, qualitative, or censored endpoints; (iii) type I and II errors to be correctly maintained at their desired planning phase values; and (iv) substantial sample size reductions as compared with the single-stage design (SSD).

Although sequential methodology is often used in clinical trials, IRT modelling, as a tool for scientific measurement, is not quite well established in the clinical trial framework despite a number of advantages offered by IRT to analyze clinical trial data [Holman et al. (2003a)]. Moreover, it has been suggested that IRT modelling offers a more accurate measurement of health status and thus should be more powerful to detect treatment effects [McHorney *et al.* (1997), Kosinski *et al.* (2003)]. The benefit of combining sequential analysis and IRT methodologies using mixed Rasch models for binary items has already been studied in the context of noncomparative phase II trials and seems promising [Sébille and Mesbah (2005)]. The joint use of IRT modelling and sequential analysis is extended to comparative phase II and phase III trials using the TT. The test statistics (score statistics and Fisher information for the parameter of interest) used for sequential monitoring of QoL endpoints are derived and studied through simulations.

24.2   IRT Models

Item response theory or more precisely parametric IRT, which was first mostly developed in educational testing, takes into account the multiplicity and categorical nature of the items by introducing an underlying response model [Fischer and Molenaar (1995)] relating those items to a latent parameter interpreted as the true individual QoL. In this framework, the probability of response of a patient on an item depends upon two different kinds of parameters: the "ability level" of the person (which reflects his or her current QoL) and a set of parameters characterizing each item. The basic assumption for IRT models is the unidimensionality property stating that the responses to the items of a questionnaire are influenced by one underlying concept (e.g., QoL) often called the latent trait and noted θ. In other words, the person's ability or the person's QoL should be the only variable affecting individual item response. Another important assumption of IRT models, which is closely related to the former, is the concept of local independence, meaning that items should be conditionally independent given the latent trait θ. Hence, the joint probability of a response pattern given the latent trait θ can be written as a product of marginal probabilities. Let X_{ij} be the answer for subject i to item j and let θ_i be the unobserved latent variable for subject i $(i = 1, \ldots, N; j = 1, \ldots, J)$:

$$P(X_{i1} = x_{i1}, \ldots, X_{iJ} = x_{iJ}/\theta_i) = \prod_{j=1}^{J} P(X_{ij} = x_{ij}/\theta_i). \qquad (24.1)$$

A last assumption for IRT models is the monotonicity assumption stating that the item response function $P(X_{ij} > k/\theta_i)$ is a nondecreasing function of θ_i, for all j and all k.

24.2.1 The Rasch model

For binary items, one of the most commonly used IRT models is the Rasch model, sometimes called the one-parameter logistic model [Rasch (1980)]. The Rasch model specifies the conditional probability of a patient's response X_{ij} given the latent variable θ_i and the item parameters β_j:

$$P(X_{ij} = x_{ij}/\theta_i, \beta_j) = f(x_{ij}/\theta_i, \beta_j) = \frac{e^{x_{ij}(\theta_i - \beta_j)}}{e^{\theta_i - \beta_j}}, \qquad (24.2)$$

where β_j is often called the difficulty parameter for item j ($j = 1, ..., J$). Contrasting with other IRT models, in the Rasch model, a patient's total score, $S_i = \sum_{j=1}^{J}$ is a sufficient statistic for a specific latent trait θ_i.

24.2.2 Estimation of the parameters

Several methods are available for estimating the parameters (the θs and βs) in the Rasch model [Fischer and Molenaar (1995)] including: joint maximum likelihood (JML), conditional maximum likelihood (CML), and marginal maximum likelihood (MML). JML is used when person and item parameters are considered as unknown fixed parameters. However, this method gives asymptotically biased and inconsistent estimates [Haberman (1977)]. The second method, CML, consists in maximizing the conditional likelihood given the total score in order to obtain the item parameter estimates. The person parameters are then estimated by maximizing the likelihood using the previous item parameter estimates. This method has been shown to give consistent and asymptotically normally distributed estimates of item parameters [Andersen (1970)]. The last method, MML, is used when the Rasch model is interpreted as a mixed model with θ as a random effect having distribution $h(\theta/\xi)$ with unknown parameters ξ. The distribution $h(.)$ is often assumed to belong to some family distribution (often Gaussian) and its parameters are jointly estimated with the item parameters. As with the CML method, the MML estimators for the item parameters are asymptotically efficient [Thissen (1982)]. Furthermore, because MML does not presume existence of a sufficient statistic (unlike CML), it is applicable to virtually any type of IRT model.

24.3 Sequential Analysis

24.3.1 Traditional sequential analysis

Let us assume a two-group parallel design with two treatment groups ($g = 1$ for the control group and $g = 2$ for the experimental treatment group) and that the primary endpoint is QoL at the end of the treatment period which is measured using a QoL questionnaire with J dichotomous items. In the traditional framework of sequential analysis [Wald (1947), Whitehead (1997), Jennison and Turnbull (1999)], QoL is assumed to be observed (not to be a latent variable) in each treatment group and the QoL score S_{ig} is used in place of the true latent trait θ_{ig} ($g = 1, 2$) at each sequential analysis. In that setting, the observed scores in each group ($s_{11}, s_{12}, \ldots$) and ($s_{21}, s_{22}, \ldots$) are assumed to follow some distribution often assumed to be Gaussian with unknown parameters μ_g ($g = 1, 2$) and common σ_S. Suppose we are testing the null hypothesis $H_0 : \mu_1 = \mu_2 = \mu$ against the one-sided alternative $H_1 : \mu_2 > \mu_1$. The following parameterization is often used for the measure of treatment difference (parameter of interest) $\phi_S = (\mu_2 - \mu_1)/\sigma_S$. The log-likelihood, which can be expressed according to both independent samples, and its derivatives can be used to derive the test statistics $Z(S)$ and $V(S)$, both evaluated under the null hypothesis. The test statistic $Z(S)$ is the efficient score for ϕ depending on the observed scores S, and the test statistic $V(S)$ is Fisher's information for ϕ.

More precisely, the test statistics $Z(S)$ and $V(S)$ are given by:

$$Z(S) = \frac{n_1 n_2}{(n_1 + n_2)D}(\bar{s}_2 - \bar{s}_1) \tag{24.3}$$

and

$$V(S) = \frac{n_1 n_2}{(n_1 + n_2)} - \frac{Z^2(S)}{2(n_1 + n_2)} \tag{24.4}$$

in which:

- n_g is the cumulated number of patients (since the beginning of the trial) in group g ($g = 1, 2$).

- $\bar{s}_g = (\sum_{j=1}^{n_g} s_{gj})/n_g$ where s_{gj} denotes the observed scores of patient j in group g.

- D is the maximum likelihood estimate of σ_S under the null hypothesis

$$D = \sqrt{\frac{Q}{n_1 + n_2} - \left(\frac{R}{n_1 + n_2}\right)^2}$$

with $Q = \sum_{j=1}^{n_1} s_{1j}^2 + \sum_{j=1}^{n_2} s_{2j}^2$ and $R = \sum_{j=1}^{n_1} s_{1j} + \sum_{j=1}^{n_2} s_{2j}$.

Details of the computations are described at length by Whitehead (1997).

24.3.2 Sequential analysis based on Rasch models

We are now interested in the latent case, that is, the case where θ_{ig} ($g = 1, 2$) is unobserved in each treatment group. Let us assume that the latent traits

θ_1 and θ_2 are random variables that follow normal distributions $N(\psi_1, \sigma_\theta^2)$ and $N(\psi_2, \sigma_\theta^2)$, respectively, and that we are testing $H_0 : \psi_1 = \psi_2 = \psi$ against $H_1 : \psi_1 < \psi_2$. A reparameterization can be performed so that $\varphi = (\psi_2 - \psi_1)/2$ is the parameter of interest and the nuisance parameter is made up of $\phi = (\psi_1 + \psi_2)/2$ and $\eta = (\sigma, \beta_1, \ldots, \beta_J)$ such that $\varphi = 0$ under H_0, $\psi_1 = \phi - \varphi$, and $\psi_2 = \varphi + \phi$. Assuming that $n_1 + n_2 = N$ data have been gathered so far in the two treatment groups, the log-likelihood of φ, ϕ, and η can be written as $l(\varphi, \phi, \eta) = l^{(1)}(\psi_1, \sigma_\theta, \beta_1, \ldots, \beta_J) + l^{(2)}(\psi_2, \sigma_\theta, \beta_1, \ldots, \beta_J)$. Assuming a Rasch model for patient's items responses, we can write:

$$l^{(g)}(\psi_g, \sigma_\theta, \beta_1, \ldots, \beta_J)$$

$$= \sum_{i=1}^{N} \log \left\{ \frac{1}{\sigma_\theta \sqrt{2\pi}} \int_{-\infty}^{+\infty} e^{-\frac{(\theta - \psi_g)^2}{2\sigma_\theta^2}} \prod_{j=1}^{J} \frac{e^{x_{ijg}(\theta - \beta_j)}}{1 + e^{\theta - \beta_j}} d\theta \right\}, \qquad g = 1, 2. \quad (24.5)$$

Let ϕ^* and $\eta^* = (\sigma_\theta^*, \beta_1^*, \ldots, \beta_J^*)$ be the estimates of ϕ and $\eta = (\sigma_\theta, \beta_1, \ldots, \beta_J)$ under the assumption that both series of data are drawn from the same distribution. There is no analytical solution for ϕ^* and η^* and numerical integration methods have to be used to estimate these parameters. The identifiability constraint $\sum_{j=1}^{J} \beta_j = 0$ is used.

The test statistics $Z(X)$ and $V(X)$, which were previously noted as $Z(S)$ and $V(S)$, are depending this time directly on X, the responses to the items. They can be derived in the following way.

$$Z(X) = \frac{\partial l(0, \phi^*, \sigma_\theta^*, \beta_1^*, \ldots, \beta_j^*)}{\partial \varphi}$$

$$= \frac{\partial l^{(2)}(\phi^*, \sigma_\theta^*, \beta_1^*, \ldots, \beta_j^*)}{\partial \psi_2} - \frac{\partial l^{(1)}(\phi^*, \sigma_\theta^*, \beta_1^*, \ldots, \beta_j^*)}{\partial \psi_1}. \quad (24.6)$$

That is, we need to evaluate

$$\sum_{i=1}^{N} \frac{\partial}{\partial \psi_g} \left[\log \left(\int_{-\infty}^{+\infty} h_{\psi_g, \sigma_\theta}(\theta) \prod_{j=1}^{J} f(x_{ijg}/\theta; \beta_j) d\theta \right) \right] \quad (24.7)$$

at $(\phi^*, \sigma_\theta^*, \beta_1^*, \ldots, \beta_J^*)$ for $g = 1, 2$ where $h_{\psi_g, \sigma_\theta}$ is the density of the normal distribution.

The test statistic $V(X)$ can sometimes be approximated under H_0 by

$$V(X) = -\frac{\partial^2 l(0, \phi^*, \sigma_\theta^*, \beta_1^*, \ldots, \beta_J^*)}{\partial \varphi^2}$$

$$= -\frac{\partial^2 l^{(2)}(\phi^*, \sigma_\theta^*, \beta_1^*, \ldots, \beta_J^*)}{\partial \psi_2^2} - \frac{\partial^2 l^{(1)}(\phi^*, \sigma_\theta^*, \beta_1^*, \ldots, \beta_J^*)}{\partial \psi_1^2} \quad (24.8)$$

when the two samples are large, of about the same size, and when φ is small.

Estimation of the statistics $Z(X)$ and $V(X)$ is done by maximising the marginal likelihood, obtained from integrating out the random effects. Quasi-Newton procedures can be used, for instance, to maximise the likelihood and adaptive Gaussian quadrature can be used to integrate out the random effects [Pinheiro and Bates (1995)].

24.3.3 The triangular test

For ease of general presentation of the sequential test we use the conventional notations Z and V. The TT uses a sequential plan defined by two perpendicular axes: the horizontal axis corresponds to Fisher's information V, and the vertical axis corresponds to the efficient score Z which represents the benefit as compared with H_0. For a one-sided test, the boundaries of the test delineate a continuation region (situated between these lines), from the regions of nonrejection of H_0 (situated beneath the bottom line) and of rejection of H_0 (situated above the top line). The boundaries depend on the statistical hypotheses (values of the expected treatment benefit, α, and β) and on the number of subjects included between two analyses. They can be adapted at each analysis when this number varies from one analysis to the other, using the "Christmas tree" correction [Siegmund (1979)]. The expressions of the boundaries for a one-sided test are well known [Sébille and Bellissant (2001)]. At each analysis, the values of the two statistics Z and V are computed and Z is plotted against V, thus forming a sample path as the trial goes on. The trial is continued as long as the sample path remains in the continuation region. A conclusion is reached as soon as the sample path crosses one of the boundaries of the test: nonrejection of H_0 if the sample path crosses the lower boundary, and rejection of H_0 if it crosses the upper boundary. This test and other types of group sequential tests are implemented in the computer program PEST 4 [MPS Research Unit (2000)] that can be used for the planning, monitoring, and analysis of comparative clinical trials.

24.4 Simulations

24.4.1 Simulation design

The statistical properties of the TT were evaluated with simulated data. We studied the type I error (α), the power $(1 - \beta)$, and the average sample number (ASN) of patients required to reach a conclusion. A thousand comparative clinical trials were simulated. The latent trait in the control group θ_{i1} was assumed to follow a normal distribution with mean λ_1 and variance $\sigma^2 = 1$ and the latent trait in the experimental group θ_{i2} was assumed to follow a normal distribution with mean $\lambda_2 = \lambda_1 + d$ and the same variance. The trial involved the comparison of the two hypotheses: $H_0 : d = 0$ against $H_1 : d > 0$.

We first assumed that the items under consideration formed part of a calibrated item bank, meaning that item parameters were assumed to be known [Holman *et al.* (2003b)]. We also investigated the more extreme case where all item parameters were assumed to be totally unknown and had therefore to be estimated at each sequential analysis. For both cases, the item parameters were uniformly distributed in the interval $[-2, 2]$ with $\sum_{j=1}^{J} \beta_j = 0$.

The traditional method consisted in using the observed QoL scores S, given by the sum of the responses to the items, which were assumed to follow a normal distribution. The $Z(S)$ and $V(S)$ statistics were computed within the well-known framework of normally distributed endpoints [Sébille and Bellissant (2001)].

We compared the use of Rasch modelling methods with QoL scores methods. To evaluate the effect of the number of items used for measuring QoL, we investigated QoL questionnaires with five or ten items. Moreover, different expected effect sizes (noted ES equal to $(\lambda_2 - \lambda_1)/\sigma = d$) ranging from small (0.4) to large (0.8) were investigated. The sequential analyses were performed every 40 included patients and $\alpha = \beta = 0.05$ for all simulations.

The simulations were performed using a C++ program, and the data analysed with the SAS software [Hardouin and Mesbah (2007)].

24.4.2   Results

Table 24.1. Type I error and power for the triangular test (TT) using the method based on QoL scores or the Rasch model for different values of the effect size and of the number of items (nominal $\alpha = \beta = 0.05$, 1000 simulations)

Effect Size	Number of Items	Type I Error			Power		
		QoL Scores	Rasch Model		QoL Scores	Rasch Model	
			β Known	β Unknown		β Known	β Unknown
0.4	5	0.027	0.039	0.058	0.758	0.951	0.926
0.4	10	0.045	0.044	0.082	0.852	0.952	0.926
0.5	5	0.039	0.048	0.077	0.736	0.944	0.908
0.5	10	0.057	0.064	0.088	0.838	0.951	0.931
0.6	5	0.045	0.056	0.072	0.736	0.934	0.907
0.6	10	0.052	0.057	0.083	0.846	0.952	0.934
0.7	5	0.044	0.046	0.076	0.743	0.938	0.912
0.7	10	0.054	0.049	0.079	0.844	0.947	0.932
0.8	5	0.049	0.041	0.069	0.741	0.943	0.924
0.8	10	0.055	0.049	0.080	0.836	0.949	0.941

Table 24.1 shows the type I error and power for the TT for different values of the effect size and of the number of items using the method based on QoL scores or the Rasch modelling method assuming either known or unknown item

parameter values. The significance level was usually close to the target value of 0.05 for the QoL scores method and the Rasch modelling method assuming known item parameter values. However, the significance level was always higher than the target value of 0.05 for the Rasch modelling method assuming unknown item parameter values for all effect sizes and number of items considered. The TT was quite close to the nominal power of 0.95 when the Rasch modelling method assuming known item parameter values was used, and a little lower than expected when unknown item parameter values were assumed. However, the TT was notably underpowered when the QoL scores method was used. Indeed, for the QoL scores method, as compared with the target power value of 0.95, there were decreases in power of approximately 22% and 11% with five and ten items, respectively. By contrast, for the Rasch modelling method assuming unknown item parameter values, the decrease in power was of about only 4% and 2% with five and ten items, respectively.

Table 24.2. Sample size for the single-stage design (SSD) and average sample number (ASN) required to reach a conclusion under H_0 and H_1 for the triangular test (TT) using the method based on QoL scores or the Rasch model for different values of the effect size and of the number of items (nominal $\alpha = \beta = 0.05$, 1000 simulations)

Effect Size	Number of Items	SSD	TT* H_0/H_1	QoL Scores H_0/H_1	Rasch Model	
					β Known H_0/H_1	β Unknown H_0/H_1
0.4	5	271	155/155	140/178	140/148	135/145
0.4	10	271	155/155	141/167	117/122	114/119
0.5	5	174	103/103	104/128	102/103	102/92
0.5	10	174	103/103	103/121	84/85	83/84
0.6	5	121	74/74	76/95	77/76	77/77
0.6	10	121	74/74	76/91	62/63	64/63
0.7	5	89	57/57	60/72	61/60	63/60
0.7	10	89	57/57	60/70	51/51	53/52
0.8	5	68	46/46	50/58	51/51	52/52
0.8	10	68	46/46	50/56	45/45	47/45

*Approximate ASN for the TT for a normally distributed endpoint.

Table 24.2 shows the ASN of the number of patients required to reach a conclusion under H_0 and H_1 for the TT for different values of the effect size and of the number of items using the method based on QoL scores or the Rasch modelling method assuming either known or unknown item parameter values. We also computed for comparison purposes the number of patients required by the single-stage design (SSD) and the approximate ASN for the TT computed with

PEST 4 when a normally distributed endpoint was assumed when planning the trial. As expected, the ASNs all decreased as the expected effect sizes increased whatever the method used. The ASNs under H_0 and H_1 were always smaller for all sequential procedures based either on QoL scores or Rasch modelling methods than the sample size required by the SSD for whatever values of effect size or number of items considered. The decreases in the ASNs under H_0 and H_1 were usually more marked when the Rasch modelling methods were used, assuming either known or unknown item parameter values, as compared with the methods based on QoL scores. Indeed, under H_0 (H_1) as compared with the SSD, there were decreases of approximately 37% (25%) and 41% (42%) in sample sizes for the QoL scores method and the Rasch modelling methods, respectively.

24.5   Discussion—Conclusion

We evaluated the benefit of combining sequential analysis and IRT methodologies in the context of phase II or phase III comparative clinical trials using QoL endpoints. We studied and compared the statistical properties of a group sequential method, the TT, using either mixed Rasch models assuming either known or unknown item parameter values or the traditional method based on QoL scores. Simulation studies showed that: (i) the type I error α was correctly maintained for the QoL scores method and the Rasch modelling method assuming known item parameter values but was always higher than expected for the Rasch modelling method assuming unknown item parameter values; (ii) the power of the TT was correctly maintained for the Rasch modelling method assuming known item parameter values and a little lower than expected when item parameters were assumed to be unknown, but the TT was particularly underpowered for the QoL scores method; and (iii) as expected, using group sequential analysis all methods allowed substantial reductions in ASNs as compared with the SSD, the largest reduction being observed with the Rasch modelling methods.

The different results that were obtained using the mixed Rasch models assuming either known or unknown item parameter values or the method based on QoL scores might be partly explained by looking at the distributions of the test statistics $Z(S)$, $V(S)$, $Z(X)$, and $V(X)$. According to asymptotic distributional results, we might expect the sequences of test statistics $(Z_1(S), Z_2(S), \ldots, Z_K(S))$ and $(Z_1(X), Z_2(X), \ldots, Z_K(X))$ to be multivariate normal with: $Z_k(S) \sim N(ES * V_k(S), V_k(S))$ and $Z_k(X) \sim N(ES * V_k(X), V_k(X))$, respectively, where ES denotes the effect size, for $k = 1, 2, \ldots, K$ analyses [Whitehead (1997), and Jennison and Turnbull (1999)]. Table 24.3 shows the distribution of the standardized test statistics under H_0 and H_1 (effect size equal to 0.5) that were estimated using the method based on QoL scores or the Rasch models assuming either known or unknown item parameter values. The estimation of the test statistics was performed at the second sequential analysis corresponding to a sample size of 80 patients. The normality assumption was not rejected using a Kolmogorov–Smirnov test, whatever the method used. Under H_0 or H_1, the null hypothesis of unit standard deviation (SD) was rejected when the estimation was performed with the mixed Rasch model assuming unknown item parameter values, the estimated SD being larger than expected. This feature might be to some extent responsible for the inflation of the type I error α under H_0 and might also partly explain the bit of underpowering of the TT that was observed under most H_1 hypotheses. Under H_1, the null hypothesis of 0 mean was rejected when the estimation was performed with the QoL scores method, the estimated mean value being lower than expected. This might explain why the TT was notably underpowered using the QoL scores method.

Table 24.3. Distribution of the standardized test statistics estimated using the method based on QoL scores or the Rasch model for different values of the number of items and for an effect size equal to 0.5, assuming that the vector of item parameter values β is either known or unknown (nominal $\alpha = \beta = 0.05$, 1000 simulations)

Number	H_0			H_1		
of	QoL Scores	Rasch Model		QoL Scores	Rasch Model	
Items		β Known	β Unknown		β Known	β Unknown
	Z′(S)	Z′(X)	Z′(X)	Z′(S)	Z′(X)	Z′(X)
5	−0.034	−0.005	−0.028	−0.654*	−0.009	−0.006
	(0.995)	(0.972)	(1.090)**	(1.014)	(0.978)	(1.086)**
10	−0.037	−0.003	−0.016	−0.423*	0.007	0.029
	(0.995)	(1.017)	(1.143)**	(1.009)	(0.996)	(1.131)**

Z′(S) and Z′(X) are the standardized test statistics for the method based on QoL scores and the Rasch model, respectively:

$$Z'(S) = \frac{Z(S) - ES.V}{\sqrt{V}} \quad \text{and} \quad Z'(X) = \frac{Z(X) - ES.V}{\sqrt{V}},$$

where ES is the effect size. Data are means (SD).
*$p < 0.001$ for testing the mean equal to 0.
**$p < 0.05$ for testing the standard deviation equal to 1.

Another important aspect is also to be noted for the mixed Rasch model assuming unknown item parameter values. The use of this model corresponds to a rather extreme case where no information is assumed to be known about the item parameters. This can be the case if no data have ever been collected using the corresponding QoL questionnaire, which is rarely the case. Otherwise, one could use data from another study using that specific QoL questionnaire to estimate the item parameters and then use these estimates in the Rasch model, because the item parameters are assumed to be parameters related only to the questionnaire and are therefore supposed to be invariant from one study to another (using the same QoL questionnaire). In our simulation study and in the example using the data from the phase III oncology trial, the item parameters were estimated at each sequential analysis, that is on 40, 80, 120,... patients because the group sequential analyses were performed every 40 patients. It is very likely that the amount of available data at each sequential analysis might be quite insufficient to satisfactorily estimate the item difficulty parameters, especially when estimating five or ten items with only 40 patients. The simulations were also performed using 80 patients for the first sequential analysis to estimate the item parameters and 40 more patients at each subsequent sequential analysis and this resulted in a type I error closer to the target value of 0.05 and higher power (data not shown). However, it has to be mentioned that such a feature might not be interesting for larger effect sizes (over 0.6) because the benefit in terms of ASNs offered by sequential analyses might then be overwhelmed by the fact that it will not be possible to stop the study before 80 patients have been included.

Other types of investigations on incorporating IRT methodologies in sequential clinical trials could also be interesting to perform such as: evaluating the impact on the statistical properties of the sequential tests of the amount of missing data (often encountered in practice and not investigated in our study) and missing data mechanisms (missing completely at random, missing at random, nonignorable missing data). In addition, other group sequential methods could also be investigated such as spending functions [Lan and De Mets (1983)] and Bayesian sequential methods [Grossman et al. (1994)], for instance. Finally, we only worked on binary items and polytomous items more frequently appear in health-related QoL questionnaires used in clinical trial practice. Other IRT models such as the partial credit model or the rating scale model [Fischer and Molenaar (1995)] would certainly be more appropriate in this context.

Item response theory usually provides more accurate assessment of health status as compared with the QoL scores method [McHorney et al. (1997), and Kosinski et al. (2003)]. The use of IRT methods in the context of sequential analysis of QoL endpoints provides a more powerful method to detect therapeutic effects than the traditional method based on QoL scores. Finally, there are a number of challenges for medical statisticians using IRT that may be worth mentioning. IRT was originally developed in educational research using samples of thousands or even ten thousands. Such large sample sizes are very rarely (almost never) attained in medical research where medical interventions are often assessed using less than 200 patients. The problem is even more crucial in the sequential analysis framework where the first interim analysis is often performed on fewer patients. Moreover, IRT and associated estimation procedures are conceptually more difficult than the QoL scores method often used in medical research. Perhaps one of the biggest challenges for medical statisticians will be to explain these methods well enough so that clinical researchers will accept them and use them. As in all clinical research but maybe even more in this context, there is a real need for good communication and collaboration between clinicians and statisticians.

References

1. Andersen, E. B. (1970). Asymptotic properties of conditional maximum likelihood estimators, *Journal of the Royal Statistical Society, Series B*, **32**, 283–301.

2. Anderson, T. W. (1960). A modification of the sequential probability ratio test to reduce the sample size, *Annals of Mathematical Statistics*, **31**, 165–197.

3. Cella, D. F. and Bonomi, A. E. (1995). Measuring quality of life: 1995 update, *Oncology*, **9**, 47–60.

4. Fairclough, D. L. (2002). *Design and Analysis of Quality of Life Studies in Clinical Trials*, Chapman & Hall/CRC, Boca Raton.

5. Fischer, G. H. and Molenaar, I. W. (1995). *Rasch Models, Foundations, Recent Developments, and Applications*, Springer-Verlag, New York.

6. Grossman, J., Parmar, M. K., Spiegelhalter, D. J., and Freedman, L. S. (1994). A unified method for monitoring and analysing controlled trials, *Statistics in Medicine*, **13**, 1815–1826.

7. Haberman, S. J. (1977). Maximum likelihood estimates in exponential response models, *Annals of Statistics*, **5**, 815–841.

8. Hardouin, J. B. and Mesbah M. (2007). The SAS macro-program %AnaQol to estimate the parameters of item response theory models, *Communications in Statistics—Simulation and Computation*, **36**, in press.

9. Holman, R., Glas, C. A. W., and de Haan, R. J. (2003a). Power analysis in randomized clinical trials based on item response theory, *Controlled Clinical Trials*, **24**, 390–410.

10. Holman, R., Lindeboom, R., Glas, C. A. W., Vermeulen, M., and de Haan, R. J. (2003b). Constructing an item bank using item response theory: The AMC linear disability score project, *Health Services and Outcomes Research Methodology*, **4**, 19–33.

11. Jennison, C., and Turnbull, B. W. (1999). *Group Sequential Methods with Applications to Clinical Trials*, Chapman & Hall/CRC, Boca Raton, FL.

12. Kosinski, M., Bjorner, J. B., Ware, J. E., Jr., Batenhorst, A., and Cady, R. K. (2003). The responsiveness of headache impact scales scored using 'classical' and 'modern' psychometric methods: A re-analysis of three clinical trials, *Quality of Life Research*, **12**, 903–912.

13. Lan, K. K. G. and De Mets, D. L. (1983). Discrete sequential boundaries for clinical trials, *Biometrika*, **70**, 659–663.

14. McHorney, C. A., Haley, S. M., and Ware, J. E. Jr. (1997). Evaluation of the MOS SF-36 physical functioning scale (PF-10): II. Comparison of relative precision using Likert and Rasch scoring methods, *Journal of Clinical Epidemiology*, **50**, 451–461.

15. MPS Research Unit. (2000). *PEST 4: Operating Manual*, The University of Reading, Reading, UK.

16. O'Brien, P. C. and Fleming, T. R. (1979). A multiple testing procedure for clinical trials, *Biometrics*, **35**, 549–556.

17. Pinheiro, J. C. and Bates, D. M. (1995). Approximations to the log-likelihood function in the nonlinear mixed-effects model, *Journal of Computational and Graphical Statistics*, **4**, 12–35.

18. Pocock, S. J. (1977). Group sequential methods in the design and analysis of clinical trials, *Biometrika*, **64**, 191–199.

19. Rasch, G. (1980). *Probabilistic Models for some Intelligence and Attainment Tests*. The University of Chicago Press, Chicago, IL.

20. Sébille, V. and Bellissant E. (2001). Comparison of the two-sided single triangular test to the double triangular test, *Controlled Clinical Trials*, **22**, 503–514.

21. Sébille, V. and Mesbah, M. (2005). Sequential analysis of quality of life Rasch measurements, In *Probability, Statistics and Modelling in Public Health* (Eds., M. Nikulin, D. Commenges, and C. Huber), Springer-Verlag, New York.

22. Siegmund, D. (1979). Corrected diffusion approximations in certain random walk problems, *Advances in Applied Probability*, **11**, 701–719.

23. Thissen, D. (1982). Marginal maximum likelihood estimation for the one-parameter logistic model, *Psychometrika*, **47**, 175–186.

24. Wald, A. (1947). *Sequential Analysis*, John Wiley and Sons, New York.

25. Whitehead, J. and Jones, D. R. (1979). The analysis of sequential clinical trials, *Biometrika*, **66**, 443–452.

26. Whitehead, J. and Stratton, I. (1983). Group sequential clinical trials with triangular continuation regions, *Biometrics*, **39**, 227–236.

27. Whitehead, J. (1997). *The Design and Analysis of Sequential Clinical Trials*, revised 2nd edition, John Wiley and Sons, Chichester.

25

Measuring Degradation of Quality-of-Life Related to Pollution in the SEQAP Study

S. Deguen,[1] **C. Segala,**[2] **and M. Mesbah**[3]

[1]*LAPSS, Ecole Nationale de Sante Publique, Rennes, France*
[2]*LSTA, Université Pierre et Marie Curie, Paris, France*
[3]*SEPIA-Santé, Melrand, France*

Abstract: Development of an instrument to measure subjective concepts is a long process involving only marginally effective participation of statisticians. Most of the time, the main work is done by sociologist, psychologist, or health policy decision makers even if statistical methodology is always the main scientific foundation. In this chapter, using the opportunity of a real epidemiological and environmental study, we mainly present the methodology used of construction of a quality of life instrument specific to air pollution disturbance with a large emphasis on its statistical part. These methods are based on classical and modern psychometrical measurement models chosen in order to select questions measuring a few clear unidimensional latent traits (subjective concepts).

Keywords and Phrases: Air quality, annoyances, perception quality of life, psychometrical models, pluridiciplinarity

25.1   Introduction

Air pollution may cause cardiorespiratory diseases, and more often annoyance reactions. Despite the large populations exposed to air pollution in our cities and numerous epidemiological studies demonstrating relationships between air pollution and health, few studies have been published on the quantitative relations between the exposure to pollution and the public perception of air quality. The SEQAP epidemiological study has for its main objective the measurement of the relationships between adults' perception of air pollution and air pollutant concentrations measured by monitoring networks in several French towns. Around 3000 subjects will be randomly selected from adults living in seven cities having different levels of air pollutant exposure. From each city, 450 subjects adults (age >18) will be chosen. Interviews will be conducted by phone, including questions on sociodemographic characteristics, occupation, smoking habits, household members, access to a car, health, plus a specific quality of life scale taking into account air pollution annoyance.

In this chapter, using the opportunity of a real ongoing epidemiological study, we mainly present the methodology of construction of a quality-of-life instrument specific to air pollution disturbance.

25.2   Material and Methods

25.2.1   Finding questions, using previous knowledge, and focus groups

During a preliminary step, the main goal was to answer the question: what do we want to measure? We found only few bibliographical references on the subject. Unlike most of the studies on perception of air pollution mainly based on assessment of satisfaction about air quality, we focused on assessment of degradation of quality of life explained by air pollution. The first step was to identify questions (qualitative items) related to that subjective concept. These questions (items) were chosen using a preliminary deep bibliographical research and four focus group meetings. Two different focus groups involved students in environmental health, another one included teachers known as experts on health environment and the last one included general people without any a priori knowledge of environmental science.

After this preliminary step, we created a form containing questions on annoyance reactions for different fields: health, daily life, local environment, and quality of life. The set of items (questions) analyzed here is presented in Appendix Table 25A.1.

25.2.2   Selecting questions, using a real sample, and psychometric methods

The second step consisted of testing this questionnaire on a small group of 83 subjects. All interviews were done by telephone. In order to get a preliminary sample including people living in places with contrasting levels of air pollution three different cities were chosen. Twenty-six interviews were obtained from people living in Le Havre, 16 inhabitants of Lyon, and 41 from people living in Rennes. We present in this chapter preliminary results of the analysis of the obtained data. The main interest of this preliminary study is to test the acceptability of the questionnaire and to eliminate very bad questions. The final validation study, and the selection of items will be based on the data of the large main survey, available later.

25.2.3 From principal component analysis to Cronbach alpha curves

Statistical validation of questionnaire methods are generally based on factorial models such as principal component analysis, that we do not explain in detail here (a lot of good books are easily available) and more recently on use of specific unidimensional psychometric measurement models. The most famous are classical parallel models or modern item response theory models. Without a clear a priori knowledge of the structure of the concepts that we want to measure, principal component analysis followed by a varimax is very helpful as an exploratory analysis. It allows us to find a subset of unidimensional items, that is, a set of observed items measuring the same latent unobserved "construct." Statistical validation of a questionnaire is generally based on an **internal** validation (based only on the information given by observed items data) and an **external** validation (based on joint information given by the observed items and other variables known as highly related to the measured construct).

The parallel model describing the unidimensionality of a set of variables

Let $X_1, X_2, \ldots, X_k$ be a set of observed quantitative variables measuring the same underlying unidimensional latent (unobserved) variable. We define X_{ij} as the measurement of subject i, $i = 1, \ldots, n$, given by a variable j, where $j = 1, \ldots, k$. The model underlying Cronbach's alpha is just a mixed one-way ANOVA model: $X_{ij} = \mu_j + \alpha_i + \varepsilon_{ij}$, where μ_j is a varying fixed (nonrandom) effect and α_i is a random effect with zero mean and standard error σ_α corresponding to subject variability. It produces the variance of the true latent measure ($\tau_{ij} = \mu_j + \alpha_i$). ε_{ij} is a random effect with zero mean and standard error σ corresponding to the additional measurement error. The true measure and the error are uncorrelated: $\text{cov}(\alpha_i, \varepsilon_{ij}) = 0$. This model is called a parallel model, because the regression lines relating any observed item X_j, $j = 1, \ldots, k$ and the true unique latent measure τ_j are parallel.

These assumptions are classical in experimental design. This model defines relationships among different kinds of variables: the observed score X_{ij}, the true score τ_{ij}, and the error ε_{ij}. It is interesting to make some remarks about assumptions underlying this model. The random part of the true measure of individual i is the same whatever variable j might be. α_i does not depend on j. The model is unidimensional. One can assume that, in their random part, all variables measure the same thing (α_i).

Reliability of an instrument

A measurement instrument gives us values that we call the observed measure. The reliability ρ of an instrument is defined as the ratio of the variance of the true over the variance of the observed measure. Under the parallel model, one can show that the reliability of any variable X_j (as an instrument to measure the true value) is given by:

$$\rho = \frac{\sigma_\alpha^2}{\sigma_\alpha^2 + \sigma^2},$$

which is also the constant correlation between any two variables. This coefficient is also known as the intraclass coefficient. The reliability coefficient ρ can be easily interpreted as a correlation coefficient between the true and the observed measure.

When the parallel model is assumed, the reliability of the sum of k variables equals:

$$\tilde{\rho} = \frac{k\rho}{k\rho + (1 - \rho)}.$$

This formula is known as the Spearman–Brown formula. Its maximum likelihood estimator, under the assumption of a normal distribution of the error and the parallel model, is known as Cronbach's alpha coefficient (CAC) [Cronbach (1951)]:

$$\alpha = \frac{k}{k-1}\left(1 - \frac{\sum\limits_{j=1}^{k} S_j^2}{S_{tot}^2}\right),$$

where

$$S_j^2 = \frac{1}{n-1}\sum_{i=1}^{n}(X_{ij} - \overline{X_j})^2 \quad \text{and} \quad S_{tot}^2 = \frac{1}{nk-1}\sum_{i=1}^{n}\sum_{j=1}^{k}(X_{ij} - \overline{X})^2.$$

Backward Cronbach alpha curve

The Spearman–Brown formula indicates a simple relationship between CAC and the number of variables. It is easy to show that the CAC is an increasing function of the number of variables. This formula is obtained under the parallel model.

A step-by-step curve of CAC can be built to assess the unidimensionality of a set of variables. The first step uses all variables to compute CAC. Then, at every successive step, one variable is removed from the scale. The removed variable is that one which leaves the scale with its maximum CAC value. This procedure is repeated until only two variables remain. If the parallel model is true, increasing the number of variables increases the reliability of the total score which is estimated by Cronbach's alpha. **Thus, a nondecrease of such**

curves after adding a variable would cause us to suspect strongly that the added variable did not constitute a unidimensional set with the other variables.

25.2.4 Modern measurement models and graphical modeling

Modern ideas about measurement models are more general. Instead of arbitrarily defining the relationship between observed and truth as an additive function (of the true and the error), they just focus on the joint distribution of the observed and the true variables $f(X, g\theta)$. We do not need to specify any kind of distance between X and θ. The residual error E and its relation to X and θ could be anything! E is not equal to $X - g\theta$. E could be any kind of **distance between the distributions** of X and θ.

This leads us naturally to graphical modeling. Graphical modeling [Lauritzen and Wermuth, (1989), and Whittaker (1990)] aims to represent the multidimensional joint distribution of a set of variables by a graph. We focus on conditional independence graphs. The interpretation of an independence graph is easy. Each multivariate distribution is represented by a graphic, which is built up by nodes and edges between nodes. Nodes represent one-dimensional random variables (observed or latent, i.e., nonobserved) whereas a missing edge between two variables means that those two variables are independent conditionally on the rest (all other variables in the multidimensional distribution). Such graphical modeling is also known as a Bayesian network, where, instead of latent variables, unknown parameters with a priori distribution are represented in the graphic.

The Rasch model [Fischer and Molenaar (1995)] in the psychometric context is probably the most popular of modern measurement models. It is defined for the outcome X taking two values (coded for instance 0 or 1):

$$P(X_{ij} = 1/\theta_i, \beta_j) = \frac{\exp(\theta_i - \beta_j)}{1 + \exp(\theta_i - \beta_j)}.$$

θ_i is the person parameter; it measures the ability of an individual i on the latent trait. It is the true latent variable in a continuous scale. It is the true score that we want to obtain, after the reduction of the k items to 1 *dimension*. β_j is the item parameter. It characterizes the level of difficulty of the item (the question). The Rasch model is a member of the item response models. The partial credit model [Fischer and Molenaar (1995), Andrich, et al. (1997), and Dorange *et al.* (2003)] is another member of the family of item response models; it is the equivalent of the Rasch model for ordinal categorical responses. Let

$P_{ijx} = P(X_{ij} = x)$; then

$$P_{ijx} = \frac{\exp\left(x\theta_i - \sum_{l=1}^{x} \beta_{jl}\right)}{\sum_{h=0}^{m_j} \exp\left(h\theta_i - \sum_{l=1}^{h} \beta_{jl}\right)},$$

for $x = 1.2, \ldots, m_j$ (m_j is the number of levels of item j); $i = 1, \ldots, N$ (number of subjects); $j = 1, \ldots, k$ (number of items). Under these models a reliability coefficient such as the Cronbach alpha can be derived [Hamon and Mesbah (2002)] and used in the same way as in parallel models, and a backward Cronbach alpha curve can be used as a first step followed by a goodness-of-fit test of the Rasch model. The Rasch model can be easily interpreted as a graphical model (see Figure 25.1) with observed items conditionally independent of the unobserved latent and any other external covariate. Moreover, another nice measurement property can be read from the graphics: with a good instrument (questionnaire) there is **no differential item functioning**. All external covariates must be conditionally independent with the observed items of the latent, and so, there are no edges between items and external covariates.

25.3   Results

Fifty-four ordinal items were used in the original form to measure the annoyance of air pollution. Four response levels were used for each item: "pas du tout" (never), "parfois" (sometimes), "souvent" (often), and "toujours" (always). Nine items (Seqap_18 to Seqap_26, adapted from the famous generic quality of life instrument $SF36$, were excluded from the current analysis. This set of items forms a clear separate dimension (psychological well-being, quality of life) already validated in various studies. Moreover, the original set of nine items was also used in a different place (end) of the questionnaire (Seqap_59 to Seqap_67). The only difference between the two formulations was the beginning of each question. In the new formulation, all questions (Seqap_18 to Seqap_26, started by, "Cette dernière semaine á cause de la pollution de l'air, avez-vous été," ("Last week, because of air pollution, have you been,") instead of the old formulation, "Au cours de ces 4 dernières semaines, y a-t-il eu des moments où vous vous êtes senti(e)" "In the course of the last four weeks have there been times when you felt."

At the first step, eight items with ceiling effects (more than 90% of persons answering "never") were excluded from the analysis. The descriptive analysis of the remaining items was carefully examined. For example, about 66% of questioned persons declared they noticed that the windows of their home were

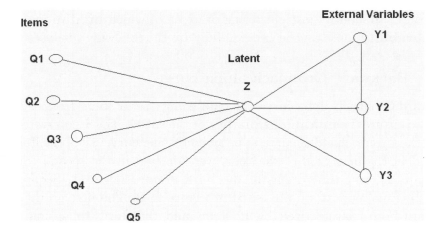

Figure 25.1. Graphical interpretation of the Rasch model.

dirty due to air pollution. It is interesting to underline that about a half of the sample of questioned persons declared having paid attention to air quality information. Then all remaining items were recoded in binary code: "never" versus all the other levels of possible response; the responses "sometimes", "often," and "always" were grouped together because of too small numbers of response per level. The list of items is presented in Appendix Table 25A.1.

25.3.1   Rotated principal component analysis

On this set of items, a principal component analysis was performed. The percentage of variance corresponding to the first latent root is 24%. The second latent root equals 7.6% and the third 6.4% of variance. Eleven latent roots were higher than one. A forced (limited to three factors) factorial analysis followed by a varimax rotation allowed us to identify three different groups of items. The number of factors was chosen coherently with the a priori chosen structure of the questionnaire (i.e., the number of constructs that one need to measure). More precisely, this part of the questionnaire was built in three sections each including questions about three separate concepts: air pollution annoyances (*i*) on own health, (*ii*) on own daily activities, or (*iii*) on own environment. Results are presented in Appendix Table 25A.2. For each item, only the maximum correlation between that item and the three factors is shown. So, a simple fast clustering of the items into factors can be derived by defining a cluster of items attached to any factor as those items with nondeleted correlation (see Appendix Table 25A.2). This fast clustering needs to be confirmed using the notion of **unidimensionality** and **separability** as below. Other, more sophisticated, methods related to Rasch models [Hardouin and Mesbah (2004)] could be used. So, this notion of **unidimensionality** of a set of items is the core of our methods. Rotated principal analysis is just an exploratory and preliminary analysis used in order to identify fast clustering of items of which **unidimensionality** and **separability** must be checked carefully by the following analyses.

25.3.2   Backward Cronbach alpha curve

A backward Cronbach alpha curve was built using a set of items from each group in order to ensure the **unidimensionality** of the subset. Few items were deleted to allow the Cronbach alpha curve to be an increasing curve: all of the items were conserved in the first group, two items were deleted in the second (Seqap_28 and Seqap_51), and three items in the third group (Seqap_11, Seqap_31 and Seqap_32). Final curves are presented in Figure 25.2. The first group and the second are both characterized by 12 items and the third dimension by only 7 items. The Cronbach α coefficients, higher than the reference value 0.70, indicate a good reliability in each group. The Cronbach α coefficient is lower in group 3 than in other groups because of fewer items in this group. The SAS® macro ANAQOL [Hardouin and Mesbah (2007)] was used to perform the backward Cronbach alpha curves.

25.3.3   Scoring procedure

A score has been estimated in each group: Score1, Score2, and Score3 for the first, second, and third group of items. For each group, and for each individual, a score is just the sum of item responses divided by the maximum total number of the same observed items. So, missing items are partly treated as missing at random. When the number of items is larger than the half number of the items in the groups, the score is considered as missing. A high score means many annoyances due to air pollution perceived by an individual (many items are coded "one" meaning "sometimes," "often," or "always"). A low score means few annoyances due to air pollution (many items are coded zero meaning "never").

25.3.4   Correlation items to scores

Correlations among each item and the three scores are shown in Appendix Table 25A.3. This can be considered as part of the internal validation done to ensure the **separability** of the subsets. We much check that for any item:

1. There is a strong correlation between that item and its own score.

2. Item correlations between that item and its own score are higher than the correlation between the same item and other scores.

   The first property is another view of the internal consistency condition of the subscale. The Cronbach alpha coefficient and intraclass coefficients are indicated

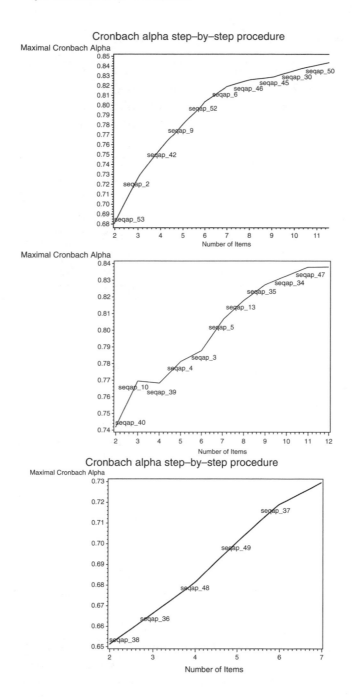

Figure 25.2. Cronbach alpha curves for the three final groups.

Table 25.1. Rasch item parameter estimates for group 1

Item	Location	SE	Residual	DF	Chisq	DF	Prob
Seqap_1	0.218	0.282	−2.590	65.89	7.294	2	0.026
Seqap_2	−0.209	0.278	−0.698	65.89	4.636	2	0.098
Seqap_6	0.278	0.283	0.414	65.89	1.444	2	0.486
Seqap_9	0.978	0.304	−1.085	65.89	1.725	2	0.422
Seqap_27	1.281	0.318	−0.849	65.89	2.045	2	0.360
Seqap_30	−0.679	0.279	1.606	65.89	0.093	2	0.955
Seqap_42	−1.240	0.289	0.012	64.98	0.269	2	0.874
Seqap_45	−1.626	0.300	0.255	64.98	0.643	2	0.725
Seqap_46	0.286	0.290	0.072	63.18	2.721	2	0.257
Seqap_50	0.089	0.289	1.167	61.37	5.288	2	0.071
Seqap_52	−1.044	0.285	−0.473	64.98	5.921	2	0.052
Seqap_53	1.668	0.354	−0.539	63.18	0.733	2	0.693

for each subscale in Appendix Table 25A.3. A deeper rigorous analysis involves use of adequate tests and methods, taking into account the multiplicity of those tests (FDR or Bonferoni). This is certainly an improvement that must be done. Anyway, the rule in the scientific area is to consider this step of the analysis as an exploratory step, which needs to be confirmed in a second step. So, we focus more on the strength of the associations than on the significance of the tests.

25.3.5   Rasch model

In our study, the item responses are categorical (ordinal), so unidimensionality must be better assessed using Rasch models. Original item response levels in our data were ordinal. So, the partial credit model must be used. Nevertheless, because we decided to dichotomize the item coding, only a simple Rasch model was used in this work. Results of Rasch analysis are partly shown in Table 25.1 and Figure 25.3. One can see that item Seqap_1 has an extreme fit residual value which indicates, that regarding Rasch model measurement that item is questionable. One can also see that items Seqap_45 and Seqap_53 are the most extremal in terms of difficulty in the first latent trait.

All groups were deeply analyzed with the Rasch model, but only a few results of group 1 are presented here. RUMM (Rasch unidimensional measurement models) software was used to perform the Rasch analysis and to produce the Table 25.1 and Figure 25.3.

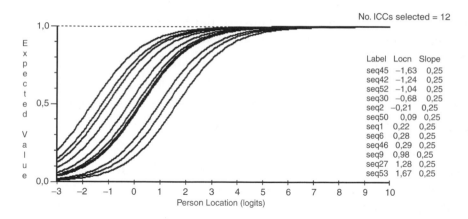

Figure 25.3. Item characteristic curves for the group 1.

25.3.6 External validation

Four external validations using available covariates in the questionnaire were also performed. Results of ANOVAs are in Appendix Table 25A.4. We can see that the individual's perception of air quality is strongly associated with the built degradation scores. There is a clear trend between degradation of the quality of life as described by the scores and their own perception of the air quality in general, or comparing (i) to the past, (ii) other areas, or (iii) other cities. More precisely, we can note that:

- About 40% of individuals think that the air quality they breathe is good; only 3.7% think that the air quality is excellent. We observed an increasing of the means score in the three groups with the increasing of air quality degradation perceived. This increase is statistically significant for the first two groups only ($p < 0.0001$ for group 1 and $p < 0.008$ for group 2).

- About 43% think that the air quality stays the same or becomes better. All three scores are higher when one thinks that the air quality become worse.

- 38% think that the air quality in their city is better than in other cities. All three scores are higher when one thinks that the air quality of his own city is worse.

- 41% think that the air quality of their area is better than in other areas of their cities. All three scores are higher when one thinks that the air quality of her own area is worse.

These results confirm those of the internal validation part and the preliminary work done by the team, including the focus groups. The built scores integrate the individual perception of the quality of the air. Scores 2 and 3 are significantly negatively correlated with the quality-of-life score based on items from the SF36 instrument, but no significant correlation appeared with the prognostic of depression in this study.

25.4 Discussion

Development of a quality-of-life questionnaire is a long and hard process. We need more than a single study to evaluate the quality of the instrument. We also need more than one simple statistical analysis to confirm the good reliability of such instrument. This is only the beginning.

In fact, the validation results in Appendix Table 25A.4 suggest that the three scales corresponding to these three components all behave in more or less the same way. Perhaps a single scale would have been enough? We decided to postpone the answer to this question. The previous results were based on a small pilot study. The big problem is that multivariate analysis of data was based on only 83 subjects. A subject-to-variable ratio of about 2 : 1 is surely insufficient for reliable multivariate analysis. So results are only useful to exclude "very bad" items to get a smaller questionnaire (items with low acceptability by people or low variability in the responses) and to reformulate some questions. The three identified dimensions here need to be confirmed by the final study based on the planned large study with a first part conducted between June and August 2006 to characterize summer pollution and a second part that will begin in November 2006 and finish in January 2007 to take into account winter pollution.

After the pilot study, it was easy to understand that some questions were very poor in their linguistic formulation: sometimes interviewers or, even, interviewees were very helpful in finding the obvious, that no one from the development team saw previously during the long phase of preparation!

So a long and careful preparation in the development of a questionnaire is very important. It must include exhaustive documentary research, planning and management of focus groups (often necessary), and organization of an unavoidable pilot study.

The goal of this chapter is to present the statistical part of the methodology of construction of a quality-of-life questionnaire specific to air pollution disturbance.

It is clear that building such a questionnaire in a field where no such questionnaire is available is not easy. Generally, when we want to develop a new instrument to measure some psychological dimension, we choose items (questions) from different available similar questionnaires.

So, the preliminary exhaustive documentary research is very important and very useful. Unfortunately, in this field, which is very new as a scientific research field, it is very difficult to find helpful material to build an instrument.

Most of the publications including key words "Air Pollution" and "Perception" are publications about people's satisfaction on "the Quality of Air." They include a lot of "public policy" researchers mainly interested in immediate people satisfaction. Our current work is in the intersection of epidemiology and sociology. So we focused on measurement of the individual perception of air pollution and its effect on individual quality of life.

The new list of questions on perception of air pollution is in Appendix Table 25A.5. It was used in the new large study. The statistical analysis, including the validation of the new version of the instrument, is in progress. Final results will be available elsewhere soon.

Acknowledgements

This work is funded by ADEME in the framework of Primequal-Predit. SEQAP is (Socio Epidémiologie Qualité de l'Air et Perception); LAPSS is (Laboratoire D'Analyses des Politiques Sociales et Sanitaires); SEPIA-santé is (Société d'études épidémiologiques et Analyses statistiques); LSTA is (Laboratoire de Statistique Théorique et Appliquée); ADEME is (Agence De l'Environnement et de la maîtrise de l'Energie); PRIMEQUAL is (Programme de Recherche Inter Organisme pour une meilleure Qualité de l'Air à l'Echelle Locale).

Appendix

Table 25A.1. Original item list with French labels: 37 items

Cette dernière semaine, avez vous:	
seqap_1	Été inquiet pour votre santé ACPA
seqap_2	Été inquiet pour la santé de vos proches ACPA
seqap_3	Eu les yeux qui piquent ACPA
seqap_4	Eu les yeux rouges ACPA
seqap_5	Eu le nez qui pique ACPA
seqap_6	Éternué ACPA
seqap_7	Ressenti des picotements dans la gorge ACPA

(continued)

(continued)

seqap_8	Eu la gorge sèche ACPA
seqap_9	Toussé ACPA
seqap_10	Eu du mal à respirer ACPA
seqap_11	Eu la peau sèche ACPA
seqap_13	Eu des maux de tête ACPA
seqap_17	Eu autres problèmes ACPA

Cette dernière semaine, ACPA:

seqap_27	Avez-vous changé certaines de vos habitudes?
seqap_28	Avez-vous modifié vos moyens de transports?
seqap_30	Avez vous été attentif aux informations sur la qualité de l'air?
seqap_31	Avez vous promené avec des enfants à l'extérieur?
seqap_32	Avez-vous pratiqué un sport à extérieur?
seqap_33	Êtes vous resté dans votre logement?
seqap_34	Avez vous aéré votre logement?
seqap_35	Avez-vous fermé les volets de votre logement?
seqap_36	Avez-vous parfumé l'intérieur de votre logement?
seqap_37	Avez-vous mis en marche la ventilation de votre logement?
seqap_38	Avez-vous évité d'ouvrir les fenêtres?
seqap_39	Avez-vous éprouve le besoin de vous laver plus fréquemment?
seqap_40	Avez-vous bu plus que d'habitude?
seqap_42	Avez-vous senti de mauvaises odeurs à l'extérieur de votre logement?
seqap_43	Avez-vous senti de mauvaises odeurs à l'intérieur de votre logement?
seqap_45	Avez-vous constaté que les fenêtres étaient sales?
seqap_46	Avez-vous constaté que vos rideaux sont sales?
seqap_47	votre maison était-elle pleine de poussière?
seqap_48	Avez-vous vu de la poussière en suspension dans l'air à l'extérieur?
seqap_49	Avez-vous vu de la poussière en suspension dans l'air à l'intérieur?
seqap_50	Le ciel a-t'il été gris?
seqap_51	Y a-t-il eu du brouillard?
seqap_52	Avez vous pensé que votre qualité de vie est dégradée par pollution?

Cette dernière question, ne concerne pas la dernière semaine, ACPA:

seqap_53	Avez-vous envisagé de déménager?

ACPA = à cause de la pollution de l'air.

Table 25A.2. Rotated factors pattern

Items	Factor1	Factor2	Factor3
seqap_1	0.75744		
seqap_2	0.66529		
seqap_3		0.51318	
seqap_4		0.69372	
seqap_5		0.48161	
seqap_6	0.47825		
seqap_7		0.44177	
seqap_8		0.45219	
seqap_9	0.54641		
seqap_10		0.51783	
seqap_11			0.29986
seqap_13		0.51745	
seqap_17			
seqap_27	0.70434		
seqap_28		0.38806	
seqap_30	0.60029		
seqap_31			−0.35862
seqap_32			−0.47117
seqap_33			0.79712
seqap_34		0.64588	
seqap_35		0.67352	
seqap_36			0.48367
seqap_37			0.47392
seqap_38			0.57005
seqap_39		0.42328	
seqap_40		0.55086	
seqap_42	0.56447		
seqap_43			0.58047
seqap_45	0.47847		
seqap_46	0.47497		
seqap_47		0.34992	
seqap_48			0.47846
seqap_49			0.50076
seqap_50	0.38471		
seqap_51		0.30685	
seqap_52	0.53886		
seqap_53	0.57123		
Variance	8.930	2.817	2.381

Table 25A.3. Pearson correlation coefficient among items and scores

Group	Item	SCORE		
		Score 1	Score 2	Score 3
	seqap_1	0.770	0.495	0.262
	seqap_2	0.679	0.346	0.314
	seqap_6	0.562	0.502	0.289
	seqap_9	0.661	0.667	0.458
	seqap_27	0.622	0.261	0.440
	seqap_30	0.526	0.146	0.077
Group 1: $\alpha = 0.84$; $\rho = 0.30$	seqap_42	0.626	0.341	0.204
	seqap_45	0.576	0.352	0.284
	seqap_46	0.553	0.322	0.352
	seqap_50	0.521	0.350	0.194
	seqap_52	0.634	0.366	0.362
	seqap_53	0.542	0.344	0.200
	seqap_3	0.391	0.632	0.227
	seqap_4	0.231	0.685	0.232
	seqap_5	0.400	0.522	0.262
	seqap_7	0.519	0.602	0.389
	seqap_8	0.514	0.693	0.512
	seqap_10	0.432	0.625	0.342
Group 2: $\alpha = 0.83$; $\rho = 0.29$	seqap_13	0.301	0.574	0.355
	seqap_34	0.082	0.435	0.145
	seqap_35	0.225	0.537	0.360
	seqap_39	0.451	0.598	0.450
	seqap_40	0.347	0.636	0.414
	seqap_47	0.356	0.494	0.250
	seqap_33	0.294	0.402	0.696
	seqap_36	0.203	0.280	0.579
	seqap_37	0.075	0.302	0.505
Group 3: $\alpha = 0.72$; $\rho = 0.28$	seqap_38	0.534	0.349	0.714
	seqap_43	0.373	0.364	0.596
	seqap_48	0.249	0.416	0.624
	seqap_49	0.232	0.328	0.582

Table 25A.4. External validation

Response level	Frequency	Score 1		Score 2		Score 3	
		Mean[a]	(sd)	Mean	(sd)	Mean	(sd)
The quality of the air that you inhale is:							
Excellent	3	2.78	(4.8)	0.00	(0)	4.76	(8.2)
Very good	4	2.08	(4.2)	2.08	(4.2)	0.00	(0.0)
Good	33	29.78	(22.5)	17.17	(20.2)	16.45	(21.7)
Poor	30	53.67	(27.7)	23.81	(23.6)	20.47	(24.5)
Bad	11	62.72	(21.3)	39.39	(27.7)	25.11	(28.7)
Do you think that the quality of the air:							
Became better	9	33.33	(25.0)	12.04	(13.2)	6.88	(11.7)
Stayed the same	25	27.54	(23.2)	9.81	(12.6)	16.00	(24.1)
Became worse	45	51.16	(29.1)	30.23	(23.4)	21.59	(24.5)
Compared to the other cities, the quality of the air of your city is:							
Better	29	28.18	(24.1)	16.09	(21.7)	15.76	(22.4)
Similar	17	35.34	(28.6)	21.07	(25.5)	18.49	(24.6)
Worse	30	54.64	(28.7)	24.44	(25.1)	19.20	(25.1)
Compared to the other districts of your city, the quality of the air of your district is:							
Better	33	31.19	(24.1)	15.19	(16.6)	16.45	(24.7)
Similar	32	39.94	(28.6)	21.35	(25.7)	16.22	(20.9)
Worse	15	94.00	(28.7)	29.29	(25.7)	23.81	(25.1)
Quality of Life Score is:							
Less than 75	40	34.75	(29.6)	25.69	(21.6)	24.00	(27.5)
More than 75	43	27.68	(23.6)	11.31	(13.7)	10.34	(19.3)
SALSA Prognostic of Depression is:							
Negative	60	27.68	(26.3)	16.69	(18.5)	14.43	(22.7)
Positive	17	32.87	(22.5)	18.46	(17.6)	23.33	(28.2)

[a] Mean (standard deviation) of the scores by level response.

Table 25A.5. New list of questions produced after the analysis: 32 items

Cette dernière semaine, avez-vous

Seqap_1	Été inquiét pour votre santé ACPA?[a]
Seqap_2	Été inquiét pour la santé de vos proches ACPA?
Seqap_3	Eu les yeux qui piquent (ou qui pleurent) ACPA?
Seqap_4	Eu les yeux rouges ACPA?
Seqap_5	Eu le nez qui pique ACPA?
Seqap_6	Éternuez ACPA?
Seqap_7	Ressenti des picotements dans la gorge ACPA?
Seqap_8	Eu la gorge sèche ACPA?
Seqap_9	Toussé ACPA?
Seqap_10	eu du mal à respirer ACPA?
Seqap_11	Eu des problèmes de peau (sècheresse, rougeurs ACPA?
Seqap_13	Eu des maux de tête ACPA?
Seqap_16	Eu des allergies déclenchées par la pollution de l'air?
Seqap_30	Été attentif aux informations sur la qualité de l'air?
Seqap_28	Modifié vos moyens de transports ACPA?
Seqap_27	Changé vos habitudes de loisirs ACPA
Seqap_33	Cette dernière semaine, êtes-vous resté dans votre logement ACPA?
Seqap_34	Aéré ou ventillé votre logement ACPA?
Seqap_35	Fermé les volets de votre logement ACPA?
Seqap_36	Parfumé l'intérieur de votre logement ACPA?
Seqap_38	Évité d'ouvrir les fénêtres ACPA?
Seqap_40	bu Plus que d'habitude ACPA?
Seqap_39	éprouvé le besoin de vous laver plus fréquemment (mains, visage)
Seqap_42	Senti de mauvaises odeurs à l'extérieur de votre logement ACPA?
Seqap_43	Senti de mauvaises odeurs à l'intérieur de votre Logement ACPA?
Seqap_45	constaté que les fenêtres de votre logement étaient sales ACPA?
Seqap_46	Constaté que vos rideaux étaient sales ACPA?
Seqap_55	Vu de la poussière noire à l'intérieur de votre logement ACPA?
Seqap_56	Vu de la poussière noire à l'extérieur de votre logement ACPA?
Seqap_50	Constaté que le ciel était gris ACPA?
Seqap_52	Pensé que votre qualité de vie était dégradée par la pollution de l'air?
Seqap_53	Envisagé de déménager ACPA?

[a] ACPA = À cause de la pollution de l'air.

References

1. Andrich, D., de Jong, J. H. A. L., and Sheridan, B. E. (1997). Diagnostic opportunities with the Rasch model for ordered response categories, In *Applications of Latent Trait and Latent Class Models in the Social Sciences* (Eds., J. Rost and R. Langeheine), pp. 59–70, Waxmann, Munster.

2. Cronbach, L. J. (1951). Coefficient alpha and the internal structure of tests, *Psychometrika*, **16**, 297–334.

3. Fischer, G. H. and Molenaar, I. W. (1995). *Rasch Models, Foundations, Recent Developments and Applications*, Springer-Verlag, New York.

4. Dorange, C., Chwalow, J., and Mesbah, M. (2003). Analysing quality of life data with the ordinal Rasch model and NLMixed SAS procedure, In *Proceedings of the International Conference on Advance in Statistical Inferential Methods "ASIM2003"* (Ed., KIMEP Ed, Almaty), pp. 41–73.

5. Hamon, A. and Mesbah, M. (2002). Questionnaire reliability under the Rasch model, In *Statistical Methods for Quality of Life Studies: Design, Measurement and Analysis* (Eds., M. Mesbah, B. F. Cole, and M. L. T. Lee), pp. 155–168, Kluwer Academic, Boston.

6. Hardouin, J. B. and Mesbah, M. (2004). Clustering binary variables in subscales using an extended Rasch model and Akaike information criterion, *Communication in Statistics—Theory and Methods*, **33**, 1277–1294.

7. Hardouin, J.-B. and Mesbah, M. (2007). The SAS macro-program ANAQOL to estimate the parameters of item responses theory models, *Communication in Statistics—Simulation and Computation*, **36**, 437–455.

8. Lauritzen, S. L. and Wermuth, N. (1989). Graphical models for association between variables, some of which are qualitative and some quantitative, *Annals of Statistics*, **17**, 31–57.

9. Whittaker, J. (1990). *Graphical Models in Applied Multivariate Statistics*, First Edition, John Wiley & Sons, New York.

26

A Bayesian Ponders "The Quality of Life"

Mounir Mesbah[1] and Nozer D. Singpurwalla[2]

[1]*Laboratoire de Statistique Théorique et Appliquée, Université Paris 6, Paris, France*
[2]*Department of Statistics, The George Washington University, Washington, DC, USA*

Abstract: The notion of quality of life (QoL) has recently received a high profile in the biomedical, the bioeconomic, and the biostatistical literature. This is despite the fact that the notion lacks a formal definition. The literature on QoL is fragmented and diverse because each of its constituents emphasizes its own point of view. Discussions have centered around ways of defining QoL, ways of making it operational, and ways of making it relevant to medical decision making. An integrated picture showing how all of the above can be brought together is desirable. The purpose of this chapter is to propose a framework that does the above. This we do via a Bayesian hierarchical model. Our framework includes linkages with item response theory, survival analysis, and accelerated testing. More important, it paves the way for proposing a definition of QoL.

This is an expository chapter. Our aim is to provide an architecture for conceptualizing the notion of QoL and its role in health care planning. Our approach could be of relevance to other scenarios such as educational, psychometric, and sociometric testing, marketing, sports science, and quality assessment.

Keywords and Phrases: Health care planning, hierarchical modeling, information integration, survival analysis, quality control, utility theory

26.1   Introduction and Overview

A general perspective on the various aspects of the QoL problem can be gained from the three-part paper of Fitzpatrick *et al.* (1992). For an appreciation of the statistical issues underlying QoL, the recent book by Mesbah, *et al.* (2002) is a good starting point. In the same vein is the paper of Cox *et al.* (1992) with the striking title, "Quality of Life Assessment: Can We Keep It Simple?" Reviewing the above and other related references on this topic, it is our position that QoL assessment can possibly be kept simple, but not too simple! To get a sense as to why we come upon this view, we start by selectively quoting phrases from

the writings of several prominent workers in the field. These quotes give a feel
for the diverse issues that the topic of this chapter spawns, and this in turn
helps us conceptualize what the notion of QoL could be. The quotes also set
the stage for developing a foundation for the Bayesian framework we propose.
Our sense is that Bayesian involvement in this arena is practically nonexistent
[cf. Mesbah *et al.* (2002)]. Yet, as we hope to show here, it is only a Bayesian
framework that is able to:

(*i*) Pull together the several apparently conflicting issues that the QoL problem raises.

(*ii*) Provide a foundation for defining QoL.

(*iii*) Formally place the notion of QoL in the context of medical decision
making.

Quotations (*a*) through (*d*) below pertain to a characterization of QoL,
whereas quotes (*e*) through (*j*) pertain to the properties that a metric for QoL
should possess; quotes (*k*) through (*l*) pertain to the uses of QoL. The emphases
(in italics) are ours.

26.1.1   Selective quotations on QoL

(*a*) "QoL can be considered as a *global holistic judgment*," Cox *et al.* (1992).

(*b*) "The term QoL misleadingly suggests an *abstract and philosophical approach*," Fitzpatrick *et al.* (1992).

(*c*) "QoL is defined as an individual's perception of their position in life in the
context of the culture and the value system in which they live in relation
to their goals, standards, and concerns," WHOQoL Group (1994).

(*d*) "We need to look at the QoL measure from individual as well as population
perspectives," Sen (2002).

(*e*) "Patients' judgments of QoL differ substantially from clinicians," Fitzpatrick *et al.* (1992).

(*f*) "Who Should Measure QoL, Doctor or Patient?" Slevin *et al.* (1988).

(*g*) "Although the concept of QoL is *inherently subjective* and definitions vary,
the content of the various instruments shows similarities," Fitzpatrick
et al. (1992).

(*h*) "... process may be enhanced by including people with a wide range
of backgrounds in the assessment process; for example, doctors, nurses,
patients, etc.," Fitzpatrick *et al.* (1992).

(i) "Many instruments reflect the multidimensionality of QoL," Fitzpatrick *et al.* (1992).

(j) "Summing disparate dimensions is not recommended, because contrary trends for different aspects of QoL are missed," Fitzpatrick *et al.* (1992).

(k) "In health economics QoL measures have ... more controversially (become) the means of prioritizing funding," Fitzpatrick *et al.* (1992).

(l) "The best understood application of QoL measures is in clinical trials, where they provide evidence of the effects of interventions," Fitzpatrick *et al.* (1992).

There is a variant of the notion of QoL, namely, the quality adjusted life (QAL). This variant is designed to incorporate the QoL notion into an analysis of survival data and history. A motivation for introducing QAL has been the often expressed view that medical interventions may prolong life, but that the discomfort that these may cause could offset any increase in longevity. The following four quotes provide some sense of the meaning of QAL.

(m) "QAL is an index combining survival and QoL...," Fitzpatrick *et al.* (1992).

(n) "QAL is a measure of the medical and psychological adjustments needed to induce an affordable QoL for patients undergoing problems," Sen (2002).

(o) "QAL is a patients' survival time weighted by QoL experience where the weights are based on utility values – measured on the unit interval," Cole and Kilbridge (2002).

(p) "QAL has emerged as an important yardstick in many clinical studies; this typically involves the lifetime as the primary endpoint with the incorporation of QAL or QoL measures through appropriate utility scores that are obtained through appropriate item analysis schemes," cf. Zhao and Tsiatis (2000).

26.1.2   Overview of this chapter

The above quotes encapsulate the essence of the QoL and its variant, the QAL. They indicate the diverse constituencies that are attracted to a QoL metric and the controversies that each constituency raises. For our objectives, the quotes provide ingredients for proposing a definition of QoL and developing a metric for measuring it. As a first step, it appears to us that any satisfactory discourse on QoL should encompass the involvement of three interest groups, the clinicians, the patients (or their advocates), and an economic entity, such as managers of health care programs. How do these three parties interact with one another? Are they adversarial, or do clinicians and patients engage in a co-operative game against a health care provider? The Bayesian paradigm is able to provide a general framework for articulating the above decision-making/game-theoretic scenario with linkages to statistical inference, life-data analysis, and information integration. The three-party framework, perhaps the first of its kind in the literature on QoL, is a central aspect of this chapter. Its architecture is discussed in Section 26.2, with Figure 26.1 providing an overall perspective. Sections 26.3 and 26.4 pertain to a treatment of a QoL-related questionnaire and bear relationship to the work on statistical aspects of item response theory [cf. Johnson and Albert (1999)]. What is special here is a strategy for integrating information from the clinician and the patient. The architecture of Section 26.2, and the material of Sections 26.3 and 26.4 open the door for proposing a definition of QoL, and a metric for assessing it. Our proposed metric is *probability*, and this may be seen as a key contribution of this chapter; it is discussed in Section 26.5. Section 26.6 concludes the chapter by summarizing its key contributions; the chapter ends with a few words about our choice of its title.

In proposing a unique probability-based approach for defining QoL, we recognize that some may prefer to define QoL in different ways, each definition relevant to a specific context. The WHO interpretation comes closest to ours in the sense that it is a composite, context-independent definition, such as the one we are proposing here.

26.2   The Three-Party Architecture

To facilitate a *normative* discourse on the topic of QoL and QAL, we need to introduce a three-party setup involving a decision-maker $\mathcal{D}$, a patient $\mathcal{P}$, and a clinician $\mathcal{C}$. We see $\mathcal{D}$ as a health management organization, or some economic entity. In principle $\mathcal{P}$ could also serve as a decision maker, but undesirable as it may sound, this these days is not the case. Health care decisions tend to be made by others, albeit in consultation with clinicians and patients. Inputs to $\mathcal{D}$ are provided by $\mathcal{P}$ via a set of responses to QoL questionnaires, and also by $\mathcal{C}$ via clinical and psychological assessments. The responses of $\mathcal{P}$ and $\mathcal{C}$ could also be interpreted as their decisions, but in the architecture we propose, it is $\mathcal{D}$'s *actions* that we are aiming to prescribe. Thus even though our setup entails three parties (each of whom can be seen as a decision maker), it is the decisions of $\mathcal{D}$ that we strive to consider. In order that $\mathcal{D}$'s actions be coherent, $\mathcal{D}$ needs to integrate (or fuse) the inputs of $\mathcal{C}$ and $\mathcal{P}$, and a strategy for facilitating this integration is another key element of this chapter; see Section 26.4. The interplay among $\mathcal{P}$, $\mathcal{C}$, and $\mathcal{D}$, described above, is illustrated by the decision tree of Figure 26.1.

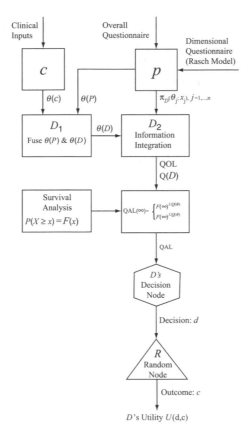

Figure 26.1. $\mathcal{D}$'s decision tree using QAL consideration (the unifying perspective of QAL).

The quantities $\theta(\mathcal{P})$, $\theta(\mathcal{C})$, and $\theta(\mathcal{D})$ are explained later in Sections 26.3 through 26.5. The hexagon denotes $\mathcal{D}$'s decision node and the triangle is a random node $\mathcal{R}$. At the decision node $\mathcal{D}$ takes one of several possible actions available to $\mathcal{D}$; let these actions be denoted by a generic d. At $\mathcal{R}$, we would see the possible outcomes of decision d. The quantity $U(d, c)$ at the terminus of the tree represents to $\mathcal{D}$ the utility of a decision d when the outcome is c. With medical decisions it is often the case that d influences c.

The quantity $Q(\mathcal{D})$ is $\mathcal{P}$'s QoL assessed by $\mathcal{D}$ subsequent to fusing the inputs of $\mathcal{P}$ and $\mathcal{C}$; $Q(\mathcal{D}) \in [0, 1]$. Let $P(X \geq x)$ denote $\mathcal{P}$'s *survival function*; this is assessed via survival data history on individuals judged exchangeable with $\mathcal{P}$, plus other covariate information that is specific to $\mathcal{P}$. Together with $P(X \geq x)$ and $\theta(\mathcal{D})$, $\mathcal{D}$ is able to assess $\mathcal{P}$'s QAL. There are two strategies for doing this. One is through the accelerated life model whereby $\mathrm{QAL}(x) = P(XQ(\mathcal{D}) \geq x)$. The other is via a proportional life model whereby $\mathrm{QAL}(x) = (P(X \geq x))^{1/Q(\mathcal{D})}$. Note that the QAL metric is, like the survival function, indexed by x. The effect of both of the above is to dampen the survival function of the life-time X towards degeneracy at 0. If $Q(\mathcal{D}) = 1$, then $\mathcal{D}$ uses $P(X \geq x)$ as is, without making adjustments to it. We see in the above a linkage with survival analysis and accelerated testing for developing the QAL metric. The remainder of this chapter is devoted to $\mathcal{D}$'s assessment of $Q(\mathcal{D})$ and a definition of QoL.

26.3   The Rasch Model for $\mathcal{P}$s Input to QoL

An approach for eliciting $\mathcal{P}$'s inputs to his or her QoL assessment is via the Rasch model of item response theory; see, for example, Fischer and Molenaar (1995). In stating the above we have put the cart before the horse, because QoL has not as yet been formally defined. However, as we show, the Rasch model can help us define QoL. Specifically, $\mathcal{P}$ is asked for binary (yes/no) responses to a battery of k questions pertaining to a certain dimension, say mobility, of $\mathcal{P}$'s life. Let $X_{ij} = 1(0)$ if $\mathcal{P}$ responds in the affirmative (negative) to the ith question, $i = 1, \ldots, k$ of the jth dimension, $j = 1, \ldots, m$. Then according to the Rasch model

$$P(X_{ij} = x_{ij}|\theta_j, \beta_{ij}) = \frac{e^{x_{ij}(\theta_j - \beta_{ij})}}{1 + e^{\theta_j - \beta_{ij}}},$$

where the parameter θ_j encapsulates $\mathcal{P}$'s ability to undertake the dimension of interest (such as mobility), and β_{ij} is a nuisance parameter that reflects, in some sense, the intensity of the ith question. For example, with mobility as a dimension, the first question may pertain to walking and the second to climbing a flight of stairs. The second is more intense than the first. Accordingly, we assume that the β_{ij}s are ordered and take values in $\mathbb{R}$, so that $-\infty < \beta_{1j} < \beta_{2j} < \cdots < \beta_{kj} < \infty$. In the standard Rasch model $\theta_j \in \mathbb{R}$, but for reasons that become clear later, we modify the model and require that $\theta_j \in [0, 1]$. Letting

$$P(X_{ij} = 1|\theta_j, \beta_{ij}) \stackrel{\text{def}}{=} p(\theta_j, \beta_{ij}),$$

we see that the said restriction on θ_j forces $p(\theta_j, \beta_{ij})$ to lie in the envelope shown by the shaded region of Figure 26.2.

The S-shapedness of the envelope is merely illustrative. But the point we wish to make here is that because θ_j encapsulates $\mathcal{P}$'s ability regarding a particular dimension, θ_j must clearly be an ingredient of $\mathcal{P}$'s QoL, loosely interpreted; it is therefore a key parameter that is of interest to us. In what follows, our focus is on θ_j.

Whereas the discussion so far has focused on questions to $\mathcal{P}$ regarding m specific dimensions, the QoL questionnaire also includes a question that is all-encompassing such as, "How would you rate your overall quality of life?" or a question such as, "How would you rate your overall condition?" Generally

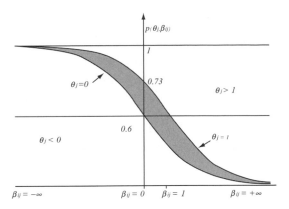

Figure 26.2. Envelope showing the range of values for $p(\theta_j, \beta_{ij})$.

such omnibus questions generate a response on a multinomial scale, but here we assume that $\mathcal{P}$'s response takes values in the continuum $[0, 1]$, with 1 denoting excellent. Let $\theta(\mathcal{P})$ denote $\mathcal{P}$'s response to an omnibus question.

26.3.1   The case of a single dimension: $\mathcal{D}$'s assessment of θ_j

Given the responses $x_j = (x_{1j}, \ldots, x_{kj})$ to a set of k questions pertaining to dimension j, the likelihood of θ_j and $\beta_j = (\beta_{1j}, \ldots, \beta_{kj})$ under the Rasch model is

$$\mathcal{L}(\theta_j, \beta_j; x_j) = \prod_{i=1}^{k} \frac{e^{x_{ij}(\theta_j - \beta_{ij})}}{1 + e^{\theta_j - \beta_{ij}}}, \tag{26.1}$$

for $\theta_j \in [0, 1]$ and $-\infty < \beta_{1j} < \cdots < \beta_{kj} < +\infty$.

If we suppose, as is reasonable to do so, that θ_j and β_j are a priori independent with $\pi(\theta_j)$ and $\pi(\beta_j)$ denoting their respective prior densities, then by treating β_j as a nuisance parameter and integrating it out, the posterior distribution of θ_j is

$$\pi(\theta_j; x_j) \propto \int_{\beta_j} \mathcal{L}(\theta_j, \beta_j; x_j) \pi(\theta_j) \pi(\beta_j) d\beta_j. \tag{26.2}$$

The question now arises as to what should $\pi(\theta_j)$ and $\pi(\beta_j)$ be? In order to answer this question we first need to ask who specifies these priors, $\mathcal{P}$, $\mathcal{C}$, or $\mathcal{D}$? The answer has to be either $\mathcal{C}$ or $\mathcal{D}$, because $\mathcal{P}$ cannot satisfy a prior and then respond to a questionnaire. Furthermore, in principle, these priors have to be $\mathcal{D}$'s priors because it is $\mathcal{D}$'s decision process that we are describing. Thus, the posterior of Equation (26.2) pertains to $\mathcal{D}$, and to underscore this feature we denote the left-hand side of Equation (26.2) by $\pi_{\mathcal{D}}(\theta_j; \underset{\sim}{x}_j)$, and also index the two priors in question by the subscript $\mathcal{D}$. Because $\mathcal{D}$'s conduct has to be altruistic, $\pi_{\mathcal{D}}(\theta_j)$ has to reflect neutrality, and following standard convention we take $\pi_{\mathcal{D}}(\theta_j)$ to be uniform over $[0, 1]$. $\mathcal{D}$'s choice of $\pi_{\mathcal{D}}(\underset{\sim}{\beta}_j)$ is more involved because $\underset{\sim}{\beta}_j$ is a constrained set. One possibility is that $\pi_{\mathcal{D}}(\underset{\sim}{\beta}_j)$ is an *Ordered Dirichlet*; the specifics remain to be explored. We suggest here mere possibilities.

26.4   The Case of Multiple Dimensions: Fusing Information

Based on $\mathcal{P}$'s responses to the QoL questionnaire covering the m dimensions of interest, $\mathcal{D}$ has at hand the m posterior distributions $\pi_{\mathcal{D}}(\theta_j; \underset{\sim}{x}_j)$, $j = 1, \ldots, m$, and also $\theta(P)$.

Because each θ_j encapsulates $\mathcal{P}$'s ability with respect to dimension j, it makes sense to suppose that the θ_js are positively dependent. One way to conceptualize this positive dependence is that each θ_j bears a relationship to some parameter, say $\theta(\mathcal{D})$, where $\theta(\mathcal{D})$ encapsulates the overall quality of life, as perceived by $\mathcal{D}$. Because all the θ_js are related to the same $\theta(\mathcal{D})$, they are positively dependent. The two questions that now arise are: how should $\mathcal{D}$ assess $\theta(\mathcal{D})$, and how should $\mathcal{D}$ encode the positive dependence between the θ_js. The first question is addressed below in Section 26.4.1; the second in Section 26.4.2.

26.4.1 $\mathcal{D}$'s assessment of $\theta(\mathcal{D})$

We have mentioned, in Section 26.3, that the QoL questionnaire to $\mathcal{P}$ encompasses an overall quality of life question, and that $\mathcal{P}$'s response to this question is a number $\theta(\mathcal{P})$, where $0 \leq \theta(\mathcal{P}) \leq 1$. The role of the clinician $\mathcal{C}$ has yet to enter our discussion. Accordingly, $\mathcal{D}$ also elicits from $\mathcal{C}$ an assessment of $\mathcal{P}$'s overall quality of life via a number $\theta(\mathcal{C})$, where as with $\theta(\mathcal{P})$, the values taken by $\theta(\mathcal{C})$ are in the continuum $[0, 1]$. The number $\theta(\mathcal{C})$ declared by $\mathcal{C}$ is based on clinical and psychological assessments conducted by $\mathcal{C}$ on $\mathcal{P}$. In order to avoid $\mathcal{C}$ being biased by $\mathcal{P}$'s responses, $\mathcal{D}$ must ensure that $\mathcal{C}$ does not have access to $\theta(\mathcal{P})$ and also the $\underset{\sim}{x}_j$s, $j = 1, \ldots, m$. With $\theta(\mathcal{P})$ and $\theta(\mathcal{C})$ at hand, $\mathcal{D}$ is now able to fuse these two quantities via Bayes' law to obtain an assessment of $\theta(\mathcal{D})$ as follows.

$$P_{\mathcal{D}}\left((\theta(\mathcal{D}); \theta(\mathcal{P}), \theta(\mathcal{C}))\right) \overset{\text{def}}{=} \hat{\pi}_{\mathcal{D}}(\theta(\mathcal{D}))$$

$$\propto \mathcal{L}(\theta(\mathcal{D}); \theta(\mathcal{P}), \theta(\mathcal{C}))\pi_{\mathcal{D}}(\theta(\mathcal{D})). \tag{26.3}$$

The quantity $\mathcal{L}(\theta(\mathcal{D}); \theta(\mathcal{P}), \theta(\mathcal{C}))$ denotes $\mathcal{D}$'s likelihood that $\mathcal{P}$ will declare a $\theta(\mathcal{P})$, and $\mathcal{C}$ will declare a $\theta(\mathcal{C})$, were $\theta(\mathcal{D})$ to be a measure of $\mathcal{P}$'s overall quality of life. This likelihood will encapsulate any biases that $\mathcal{P}$ and $\mathcal{C}$ may have in declaring their $\theta(\mathcal{P})$ and $\theta(\mathcal{C})$, respectively, as perceived by $\mathcal{D}$, and also any correlations between the declared values by $\mathcal{P}$ and $\mathcal{C}$. The nature of this likelihood remains to be investigated. The quantity $\pi_{\mathcal{D}}(\theta(\mathcal{D}))$ is $\mathcal{D}$'s prior for $\theta(\mathcal{D})$, and following our previous convention, we assume that it is uniform on $[0, 1]$. This completes our discussion on $\mathcal{D}$'s assessment of $\theta(\mathcal{D})$. It involves a $\theta(\mathcal{P})$, $\theta(\mathcal{C})$ and connotes information integration by $\mathcal{D}$ at one level.

26.4.2 Encoding the positive dependence between the θ_js

One way to capture the positive dependence between the θ_js is through mixtures of independent sequences. Specifically, we suppose, as if is reasonable to do so, that given $\theta(\mathcal{D})$ the θ_js are independent, with θ_j having a probability density function of the form $f_{\mathcal{D}}(\theta_j | \theta(\mathcal{D}))$, $j = 1, \ldots, m$. The subscript $\mathcal{D}$ associated with f denotes the fact that the probability density in question is that of $\mathcal{D}$. A strategy for obtaining $f_{\mathcal{D}}(\theta_j | \theta(\mathcal{D}))$ is described later, subsequent to Equation (26.5).

With $\pi_{\mathcal{D}}(\theta_j; \underset{\sim}{x}_j)$, $j = 1, \ldots, m$, and $\widehat{\pi}_{\mathcal{D}}(\theta(\mathcal{D}))$ at hand, $\mathcal{D}$ may extend the conversation to $\theta(\mathcal{D})$ and obtain the joint distribution of $\theta_1, \ldots, \theta_m$ as

$$P_{\mathcal{D}}(\theta_1, \ldots, \theta_m; \underset{\sim}{x}_{j1}, \ldots, \underset{\sim}{x}_{jm}, \theta(\mathcal{P}), \theta(\mathcal{C}))$$

$$= \int_{\theta(\mathcal{D})} P(\theta_1, \ldots, \theta_m | \theta(\mathcal{D}); \underset{\sim}{x}_1, \ldots, \underset{\sim}{x}_m) \widehat{\pi}_{\mathcal{D}}(\theta(\mathcal{D})) d\theta(\mathcal{D}); \qquad (26.4)$$

in writing out the above, we have assumed that the $\underset{\sim}{x}_j$s, $j = 1, \ldots, m$, have no bearing on $\theta(\mathcal{D})$, once $\theta(\mathcal{P})$ and $\theta(\mathcal{C})$ have been declared by $\mathcal{P}$ and $\mathcal{C}$, respectively. Applying the multiplication rule, and supposing that the $\underset{\sim}{x}_i$s, $i \neq j$ have no bearing on θ_j, $j = 1, \ldots, m$, the right-hand side of the above equation becomes

$$\int_{\theta(\mathcal{D})} \prod_{j=1}^{m} f_{\mathcal{D}}(\theta_j | \theta(\mathcal{D}); \underset{\sim}{x}_j) \widehat{\pi}_{\mathcal{D}}(\theta(\mathcal{D})) d\theta(\mathcal{D}). \qquad (26.5)$$

We now invoke Bayes' law to write

$$f_{\mathcal{D}}(\theta_j | \theta(\mathcal{D}); \underset{\sim}{x}_j) \propto f_{\mathcal{D}}(\theta(\mathcal{D}) | \theta_j; \underset{\sim}{x}_j) \pi_{\mathcal{D}}(\theta_j; \underset{\sim}{x}_j),$$

where $f_{\mathcal{D}}(\theta(\mathcal{D}) | \theta_j; \underset{\sim}{x}_j)$ is $\mathcal{D}$'s probability density of $\theta(\mathcal{D})$ were $\mathcal{D}$ to know θ_j, and in the light of $\underset{\sim}{x}_j$. A strategy for specifying this probability density is to suppose that $\theta(\mathcal{D})$ is uniform and symmetric around θ_j, with endpoints $\theta_j \pm \epsilon$, for some $\epsilon > 0$; furthermore with θ_j assumed known, $\underset{\sim}{x_j}$ has no role to play. The quantity $\pi_{\mathcal{D}}(\theta_j; \underset{\sim}{x_j})$ has been obtained in Section 26.3.1. With the above in place, we may now write Equation (26.4) as

$$P_{\mathcal{D}}(\theta_1, \ldots, \theta_m; \underset{\sim}{x_1}, \ldots, \underset{\sim}{x_m}, \theta(\mathcal{P}), \theta(\mathcal{C}))$$

$$\propto \int_0^1 \prod_{j=1}^m f_{\mathcal{D}}(\theta(\mathcal{D})|\theta_j)\pi_{\mathcal{D}}(\theta_j; \underset{\sim}{x_j})\hat{\pi}_{\mathcal{D}}(\theta(\mathcal{D}))d\theta(\mathcal{D}). \qquad (26.6)$$

This expression entails the impact of responses of all questions in the QoL questionnaire, dimension-specific and overall, and also $\mathcal{C}$'s assessment of $\mathcal{P}$'s overall quality of life. Furthermore, it entails $\mathcal{D}$'s uniform priors on θ_j, $j = 1, \ldots, m$, and $\theta(\mathcal{D})$. We have therefore provided here a hierarchical Bayesian mechanism that fuses all sources of information available to $\mathcal{D}$, from both the patient and the clinician. The architecture is quite general in the sense that if besides the clinician, inputs of others — such as the clergy, the nurses, and the sociologists — are desired by $\mathcal{D}$, then these too can be incorporated. All $\mathcal{D}$ needs to do here is prescribe a likelihood of the form given by Equation (26.3). The main issues that remain to be addressed, but only from a technical point of view, are the specification of a prior for the ordered β_is, and a model for $\underset{\sim}{\theta}$'s likelihood for $\theta(\mathcal{D})$, with $\theta(\mathcal{P})$ and $\theta(\mathcal{C})$ fixed. The conceptual setup poses no obstacles.

26.5   Defining the Quality of Life

Once $\mathcal{D}$ is able to obtain $P_{\mathcal{D}}(\theta_1 x_1, \ldots, \underset{\sim}{x_m}, \theta(\mathcal{P}), \theta(\mathcal{C}))$ via Equation (1.4), a definition of QoL emerges naturally. Specifically, for some given constants a_i, $a_i \in [0, 1]$, $i = 1, \ldots, m$, the QoL as assessed by $\mathcal{C}$, is defined as

$$Q(\mathcal{D}) = P_{\mathcal{D}}(\theta_1 \geq a_1, \ldots, \theta_m \geq a_m; \underset{\sim}{x_1}, \ldots, \underset{\sim}{x_m}, \theta(\mathcal{P}), \theta(\mathcal{C})). \qquad (26.7)$$

Thus $Q(\mathcal{D})$, the QoL is a probability. It is specific to $\mathcal{D}$ (but based on inputs from $\mathcal{P}$ and $\mathcal{C}$), and is indexed by constants a_i, $i = 1, \ldots, m$.

There is a precedence for our definition, in the sense that reliability is also defined as a probability, and it is indexed by a mission time. The definition (26.7) can be invoked in other contexts as well; the one that comes to mind immediately is in quality control, wherein one needs to define quality in terms of multiple attributes. The metric for QoL is therefore a number between zero and one, the number being deduced via definition (26.7), and as such, it is unique. The expression for $Q(\mathcal{D})$ is attractive because it incorporates inputs from $\mathcal{P}$ and $\mathcal{C}$, and this it does coherently via the calculus of probability.

There could be other possible ways for defining QoL. A few of these would be to consider $\min_j(\theta_j)$, $\max_j(\theta_j)$, or $mean_j(\theta_j)$, and to let QoL be a quantity such as

$$\text{QoL} = \mathcal{P}_{\mathcal{D}}(\min_j(\theta_j) \geq a)$$

for some $a \in [0, 1]$. Whereas the proposed definition(s) are appropriate in all situations, it is not clear whether a unique definition of QoL is palatable to all constituents. We see some merits to having a unique yardstick.

26.6 Summary and Conclusions

In this chapter we have proposed an approach for addressing a contemporary problem that can arise in many scenarios, the one of interest to us coming from the health sciences vis-a-vis the notion of "quality of life." What seems to be common to these scenarios is information from diverse sources that needs to be integrated, considerations of multidimensionality, and the need to make decisions whose consequences are of concern. Previous work on problems of this type has been piecemeal with statisticians mainly focusing on the frequentist aspects of item response models. Whereas such approaches have the advantages of "objectivity", they do not pave the path of integrating information from multiple sources. The approach of this chapter is based on a hierarchical Bayesian architecture. In principle, our architecture is able to do much, if not all, that is required by the users of QoL indices. The architecture also leads to a strategy by which QoL can be defined and measured in a formal manner. The current literature on this topic does not address the matter of definition. This chapter is expository in the sense that it outlines an encompassing and unifying approach for addressing the QoL and QAL problem. The normative development of this chapter has the advantage of coherence. However, this coherence is gained at the cost of simplicity. Some multidimensional priors with a restricted sample space are involved, and these remain to be articulated. So do some likelihoods. Finally, there is the matter of computations. However, all these limitations are only of a technical nature and these can eventually be addressed. We are continuing our work on such matters, including an application involving real data and real scenarios. The purpose of this chapter was to show how a Bayesian approach can address a contemporary problem, and the overall strategy that can be used to develop such an approach. The novel aspects of this chapter are: the conceptualization of the QoL problem as a scenario involving three groups of individuals, a structure whereby information from several sources can be integrated, and a definition of the notion of QoL.

Finally, there is the matter of our choice of a title for this chapter. As remarked by a colleague, our choice of the singular for the title of a chapter with two co-authors seems intriguing. A few words about this would be a nice way to close this chapter. The first co-author (MM) has been deeply involved in the QoL problem for a long time, and has contributed much to its (non-Bayesian) literature; the references attest to this fact. The second co-author (NS) with much guidance from the first about the state of the art of the work in this field, has brought in the Bayesian perspective, more as a matter of curiosity than a challenge. The title reflects the disposition of the second co-author.

Acknowledgements

The comments of a meticulous referee, whose inputs have helped develop a more balanced document, are gratefully acknowledged. N. D. Singpurwalla's work has been supported in part by The Office of Naval Research Grant N00014-06-1-0037 with The George Washington University.

References

1. Cole, B. F. and Kilbridge, K. L. (2002). Quality-adjusted survival analysis, In *Statistical Methods for Quality of Life Studies* (Eds., M. Mesbah, B. Cole, and M. T. Lee), pp. 267–277, Kluwer, Boston.

2. Cox, D. R., Fitzpatrick, R., Fletcher, A. E., Gore, S. M., Spiegelhalter, D. J., and Jones, D. R. (1992). Quality-of-life assessment: Can we keep it simple?, *Journal of the Royal Statistical Society, Series A*, **155**, 353–393.

3. Fischer, G. H. and Molenaar, I. W., Eds. (1995). *Rasch Models: Foundations, Recent Developments, and Applications*, Papers from the workshop held in Vienna, February 25–27, 1993, Springer-Verlag, New York.

4. Fitzpatrick, R., Fletcher, A., Gore, S., Jones, D. Spiegelhalter, D., and Cox D. (1992). Quality of life measures in health care, Parts I, II, and III, *British Medical Journal* **305**, 1074–1077.

5. Johnson, V. E. and Albert, J. H. (1999). *Ordinal Data Modeling*, Springer-Verlag, New York.

6. Mesbah, M., Cole, B. F., and Lee, M. L. T. (Eds.) (2002). *Statistical Design, Measurements and Analysis of Health Related Quality of Life*, Kluwer, Amsterdam.

7. Sen, P. K. (2002). Measures of quality adjusted life and quality of life deficiency: Statistical perspectives, In *Statistical Methods for Quality of Life Studies* (Eds., M. Mesbah, B. Cole, and M. T. Lee), pp. 255–266, Kluwer, Boston.

8. Slevin, M., Plant H., Lynch D., Drinkwater I., and Gregory, W. M. (1988). Who should measure quality of life, the doctor or the patient?, *British Journal of Cancer*, **57**, 109–112.

9. WHOQoL Group (1994). The development of the World Health Organization quality of life assessment instrument, In *Quality of Life Assessment: International Perspectives* (Eds., J. Orley and W. Kuyken), Springer-Verlag, Heidelberg, Germany.

10. Zhao, H. and Tsiatis, A. A. (2000). Estimating mean quality of lifetime with censored data, *Sankhyā, Series B*, **62**, 175–188.

PART VI
INFERENCE FOR PROCESSES

27

On the Goodness-of-Fit Tests for Some Continuous Time Processes

Sergueï Dachian[1] **and Yury A. Kutoyants**[2]

[1]*Laboratoire de Mathématiques, Université Blaise Pascal, Aubière, France*
[2]*Laboratoire de Statistique et Processus, Université du Maine, Le Mans, France*

Abstract: We present a review of several results concerning the construction of the Cramér–von Mises and Kolmogorov–Smirnov type goodness-of-fit tests for continuous time processes. As the models we take a stochastic differential equation with small noise, ergodic diffusion process, Poisson process, and self-exciting point processes. For every model we propose the tests which provide the asymptotic size α and discuss the behaviour of the power function under local alternatives. The results of numerical simulations of the tests are presented.

Keywords and Phrases: Hypotheses testing, diffusion process, Poison process, self-exciting process, goodness-of-fit tests

27.1 Introduction

The goodness-of-fit tests play an important role in classical mathematical statistics. Particularly, the tests of Cramér–von Mises, Kolmogorov–Smirnov, and chi-squared are well studied and allow us to verify the correspondence of the mathematical models to the observed data [see, e.g., Durbin (1973) or Greenwood and Nikulin (1996)]. A similar problem, of course, exists for the continuous-time stochastic processes. The diffusion and Poisson processes are widely used as mathematical models of many evolution processes in biology, medicine, physics, financial mathematics, and in many other fields. For example, some theory can propose a diffusion process

$$\mathrm{d}X_t = S_* (X_t) \, \mathrm{d}t + \sigma \, \mathrm{d}W_t, \qquad X_0, \qquad 0 \leq t \leq T$$

as an appropriate model for description of the real data $\{X_t, 0 \leq t \leq T\}$ and we can try to construct an algorithm to verify if this model corresponds well to these data. The model here is totally defined by the trend coefficient $S_* (\cdot)$, which is supposed (if the theory is true) to be known. We do not discuss here the problem of verification if the process $\{W_t, 0 \leq t \leq T\}$ is Wiener. This problem is much more complicated and we suppose that the *noise is white Gaussian*. Therefore we have a basic hypothesis defined by the trend coefficient $S_*(\cdot)$ and we have to test this hypothesis against any other alternative. Any other means that the observations come from stochastic differential equation

$$\mathrm{d}X_t = S(X_t)\,\mathrm{d}t + \sigma\,\mathrm{d}W_t, \qquad X_0, \qquad 0 \leq t \leq T,$$

where $S(\cdot) \neq S_*(\cdot)$. We propose some tests which are in some sense similar to the Cramér–von Mises and Kolmogorov–Smirnov tests. The advantage of classical tests is that they are distribution-free; that is, the distribution of the underlying statistics does not depend on the basic model and this property allows us to choose the *universal thresholds* which can be used for all models.

For example, if we observe n independent identically distributed random variables $(X_1, \ldots, X_n) = X^n$ with distribution function $F(x)$ and the basic hypothesis is simple, $F(x) \equiv F_*(x)$, then the Cramér–von Mises W_n^2 and Kolmogorov–Smirnov D_n statistics are

$$W_n^2 = n \int_{-\infty}^{\infty} \left[\hat{F}_n(x) - F_*(x)\right]^2 \,\mathrm{d}F_*(x), \qquad D_n = \sup_x \left|\hat{F}_n(x) - F_*(x)\right|,$$

respectively. Here

$$\hat{F}_n(x) = \frac{1}{n} \sum_{j=1}^{n} 1_{\{X_j < x\}}$$

is the empirical distribution function. Let us denote by $\{W_0(s), 0 \leq s \leq 1\}$ a Brownian bridge, that is, a continuous Gaussian process with

$$\mathbf{E}W_0(s) = 0, \qquad \mathbf{E}W_0(s)W_0(t) = t \wedge s - st.$$

Then the limit behaviour of these statistics can be described with the help of this process as follows.

$$W_n^2 \Longrightarrow \int_0^1 W_0(s)^2 \,\mathrm{d}s, \qquad \sqrt{n}D_n \Longrightarrow \sup_{0 \leq s \leq 1} |W_0(s)|.$$

Hence the corresponding Cramér–von Mises and Kolmogorov–Smirnov tests

$$\psi_n(X^n) = 1_{\{W_n^2 > c_\alpha\}}, \qquad \phi_n(X^n) = 1_{\left\{\sqrt{n}D_n > d_\alpha\right\}}$$

with constants c_α, d_α defined by the equations

$$\mathbf{P}\left\{\int_0^1 W_0(s)^2 \,\mathrm{d}s > c_\alpha\right\} = \alpha, \qquad \mathbf{P}\left\{\sup_{0 \leq s \leq 1} |W_0(s)| > d_\alpha\right\} = \alpha$$

are of asymptotic size α. It is easy to see that these tests are distribution-free [the limit distributions do not depend of the function $F_* (\cdot)$] and are consistent against any fixed alternative [see, e.g., Durbin (1973)].

It is interesting to study these tests for a *nondegenerate set of alternatives*, that is, for alternatives with limit power function less than 1. It can be realized on the close nonparametric alternatives of the special form making this problem asymptotically equivalent to the *signal in Gaussian noise* problem. Let us put

$$F(x) = F_* (x) + \frac{1}{\sqrt{n}} \int_{-\infty}^{x} h\left(F_* (y)\right) \, dF_*(y),$$

where the function $h(\cdot)$ describes the alternatives. We suppose that

$$\int_0^1 h(s) \, ds = 0, \qquad \int_0^1 h(s)^2 \, ds < \infty.$$

Then we have the following convergence [under a fixed alternative, given by the function $h(\cdot)$],

$$W_n^2 \Longrightarrow \int_0^1 \left[\int_0^s h(v) \, dv + W_0(s) \right]^2 ds,$$

$$\sqrt{n} D_n \Longrightarrow \sup_{0 \leq s \leq 1} \left| \int_0^s h(v) \, dv + W_0(s) \right|.$$

We see that this problem is asymptotically equivalent to the following *signal in Gaussian noise* problem,

$$dY_s = h_* (s) \, ds + dW_0(s), \qquad 0 \leq s \leq 1. \tag{27.1}$$

Indeed, if we use the statistics

$$W^2 = \int_0^1 Y_s^2 \, ds, \qquad D = \sup_{0 \leq s \leq 1} |Y_s|$$

then under hypothesis $h(\cdot) \equiv 0$ and alternative $h(\cdot) \neq 0$ the distributions of these statistics coincide with the limit distributions of W_n^2 and $\sqrt{n} D_n$ under the hypothesis and alternative, respectively.

Our goal is to see how such kinds of tests can be constructed in the case of continuous-time models of observation and particularly in the cases of some diffusion and point processes. We consider the diffusion processes with small noise, ergodic diffusion processes, and Poisson processes with Poisson and self-exciting alternatives. For the first two classes we just show how Cramér–von Mises and Kolmogorov–Smirnov type tests can be realized using some known results and for the last models we discuss this problem in detail.

27.2   Diffusion Process with Small Noise

Suppose that the observed process is the solution of the stochastic differential equation

$$dX_t = S(X_t)\, dt + \varepsilon\, dW_t, \qquad X_0 = x_0, \qquad 0 \le t \le T, \qquad (27.2)$$

where $W_t, 0 \le t \le T$ is a Wiener process [see, e.g., Liptser and Shiryayev (2001)]. We assume that the function $S(x)$ is two times continuously differentiable with bounded derivatives. These are not the minimal conditions for the results presented below, but this assumption simplifies the exposition. We are interested in the statistical inference for this model in the asymptotics of small noise: $\varepsilon \to 0$. The statistical estimation theory (parametric and nonparametric) was developed in Kutoyants (1994).

Recall that the stochastic process $X^\varepsilon = \{X_t, 0 \le t \le T\}$ converges uniformly in $t \in [0, T]$ to the deterministic function $\{x_t, 0 \le t \le T\}$, which is a solution of the ordinary differential equation

$$\frac{dx_t}{dt} = S(x_t), \qquad x_0, \qquad 0 \le t \le T. \qquad (27.3)$$

Suppose that the function $S_*(x) > 0$ for $x \ge x_0$ and consider the following problem of hypotheses testing,

$$\mathcal{H}_0 : S(x) = S_*(x), \qquad x_0 \le x \le x_T^*$$
$$\mathcal{H}_1 : S(x) \ne S_*(x), \qquad x_0 \le x \le x_T^*,$$

where we denoted by x_t^* the solution of equation (27.3) under hypothesis $\mathcal{H}_0$:

$$x_t^* = x_0 + \int_0^t S_*(x_v^*)\, dv, \qquad 0 \le t \le T.$$

Hence, we have a simple hypothesis against the composite alternative.

The Cramér–von Mises (W_ε^2) and Kolmogorov–Smirnov (D_ε) type statistics for this model of observations can be

$$W_\varepsilon^2 = \left[\int_0^T \frac{dt}{S_*(x_t^*)^2} \right]^{-2} \int_0^T \left(\frac{X_t - x_t^*}{\varepsilon\, S_*(x_t^*)^2} \right)^2 dt,$$

$$D_\varepsilon = \left[\int_0^T \frac{dt}{S_*(x_t^*)^2} \right]^{-1/2} \sup_{0 \le t \le T} \left| \frac{X_t - x_t^*}{S_*(x_t^*)} \right|.$$

It can be shown that these two statistics converge (as $\varepsilon \to 0$) to the following functionals,

$$W_\varepsilon^2 \Longrightarrow \int_0^1 W(s)^2\, ds, \qquad \varepsilon^{-1} D_\varepsilon \Longrightarrow \sup_{0 \le s \le 1} |W(s)|,$$

where $\{W(s), 0 \le s \le 1\}$ is a Wiener process [see Kutoyants (1994)]. Hence the corresponding tests

$$\psi_\varepsilon(X^\varepsilon) = 1_{\{W_\varepsilon^2 > c_\alpha\}}, \qquad \phi_\varepsilon(X^\varepsilon) = 1_{\{\varepsilon^{-1} D_\varepsilon > d_\alpha\}}$$

with the constants c_α, d_α defined by the equations

$$\mathbf{P}\left\{\int_0^1 W(s)^2 \, \mathrm{d}s > c_\alpha\right\} = \alpha, \qquad \mathbf{P}\left\{\sup_{0 \le s \le 1} |W(s)| > d_\alpha\right\} = \alpha \qquad (27.4)$$

are of asymptotic size α. Note that the choice of the thresholds c_α and d_α does not depend on the hypothesis (distribution-free). This situation is quite close to the classical case mentioned above.

It is easy to see that if $S(x) \ne S_*(x)$, then $\sup_{0 \le t \le T} |x_t - x_t^*| > 0$ and $W_\varepsilon^2 \to \infty$, $\varepsilon^{-1} D_\varepsilon \to \infty$. Hence these tests are consistent against any fixed alternative. It is possible to study the power function of this test for local (contiguous) alternatives of the following form,

$$\mathrm{d}X_t = S_*(X_t) \, \mathrm{d}t + \varepsilon \, \frac{h(X_t)}{S_*(X_t)} \, \mathrm{d}t + \varepsilon \, \mathrm{d}W_t, \qquad 0 \le t \le T.$$

We describe the alternatives with the help of the (unknown) function $h(\cdot)$. The case $h(\cdot) \equiv 0$ corresponds to the hypothesis $\mathcal{H}_0$. One special class of such nonparametric alternatives for this model was studied in Iacus and Kutoyants (2001).

Let us introduce the composite (nonparametric) alternative

$$\mathcal{H}_1 : h(\cdot) \in \mathcal{H}_\rho,$$

where

$$\mathcal{H}_\rho = \left\{h(\cdot) : \int_{x_0}^{x_T} h(x)^2 \, \mu(\mathrm{d}x) \ge \rho\right\}.$$

To choose the alternative we have to make precise the "natural for this problem" distance described by the measure $\mu(\cdot)$ and the rate of $\rho = \rho_\varepsilon$. We show that the choice

$$\mu(\mathrm{d}x) = \frac{\mathrm{d}x}{S_*(x)^3}$$

provides for the test statistic the following limit,

$$W_\varepsilon^2 \longrightarrow \int_0^1 \left[\int_0^s h_*(v) \, \mathrm{d}v + W(s)\right]^2 \, \mathrm{d}s,$$

where we denoted

$$h_*(s) = u_T^{1/2} h(x_{u_T s}^*), \qquad u_T = \int_0^T \frac{\mathrm{d}s}{S_*(x_s^*)^2}.$$

We see that this problem is asymptotically equivalent to the *signal in white Gaussian noise* problem:

$$dY_s = h_* (s) \, ds + dW (s), \qquad 0 \leq s \leq 1, \tag{27.5}$$

with the Wiener process $W (\cdot)$. It is easy to see that even for fixed $\rho > 0$ without further restrictions on the smoothness of the function $h_* (\cdot)$, *uniformly good* testing is impossible. For example, if we put

$$h_n (x) = c \, S_* (x)^3 \cos [n (x - x_0)]$$

then for the power function of the test we have

$$\inf_{h(\cdot) \in \mathcal{H}_\rho} \beta (\psi_\varepsilon, h) \leq \beta (\psi_\varepsilon, h_n) \longrightarrow \alpha.$$

The details can be found in Kutoyants (2006). The construction of the uniformly consistent tests requires a different approach [see Ingster and Suslina (2003)].

Note as well that if the diffusion process is

$$dX_t = S (X_t) \, dt + \varepsilon \sigma (X_t) \, dW_t, \qquad X_0 = x_0, \qquad 0 \leq t \leq T,$$

then we can put

$$W_\varepsilon^2 = \left[\int_0^T \left(\frac{\sigma (x_t^*)}{S_* (x_t^*)} \right)^2 dt \right]^{-2} \int_0^T \left(\frac{X_t - x_t^*}{\varepsilon \, S_* (x_t^*)^2} \right)^2 dt$$

and have the same results as above [see Kutoyants (2006)].

27.3   Ergodic Diffusion Processes

Suppose that the observed process is the one-dimensional diffusion process

$$dX_t = S (X_t) \, dt + dW_t, \qquad X_0, \qquad 0 \leq t \leq T, \tag{27.6}$$

where the trend coefficient $S (x)$ satisfies the conditions of the existence and uniqueness of the solution of this equation and this solution has ergodic properties; that is, there exists an invariant probability distribution $F_S (x)$, and for any integrable w.r.t. this distribution function $g (x)$ the law of large numbers holds

$$\frac{1}{T} \int_0^T g (X_t) \, dt \longrightarrow \int_{-\infty}^\infty g (x) \, dF_S (x).$$

These conditions can be found, for example, in Kutoyants (2004).

Recall that the invariant density function $f_S(x)$ is defined by the equality

$$f_S(x) = G(S)^{-1} \exp\left\{2\int_0^x S(y) \, dy\right\},$$

where $G(S)$ is the normalising constant.

We consider two types of tests. The first one is a direct analogue of the classical Cramér–von Mises and Kolmogorov–Smirnov tests based on empirical distribution and density functions and the second follows the considered-above (small noise) construction of tests.

The invariant distribution function $F_S(x)$ and this density function can be estimated by the *empirical distribution function* $\hat{F}_T(x)$ and by the *local time type* estimator $\hat{f}_T(x)$ defined by the equalities

$$\hat{F}_T(x) = \frac{1}{T}\int_0^T 1_{\{X_t < x\}} \, dt, \qquad \hat{f}_T(x) = \frac{2}{T}\int_0^T 1_{\{X_t < x\}} \, dX_t,$$

respectively. Note that both of them are unbiased,

$$\mathbf{E}_S\hat{F}_T(x) = F_S(x), \qquad \mathbf{E}_S\hat{f}_T(x) = f_S(x),$$

admit the representations

$$\eta_T(x) = -\frac{2}{\sqrt{T}}\int_0^T \frac{F_S(X_t \wedge x) - F_S(X_t)F_S(x)}{f_S(X_t)} \, dW_t + o(1),$$

$$\zeta_T(x) = -\frac{2f_S(x)}{\sqrt{T}}\int_0^T \frac{1_{\{X_t > x\}} - F_S(X_t)}{f_S(X_t)} \, dW_t + o(1),$$

and are $\sqrt{T}$ asymptotically normal (as $T \to \infty$)

$$\eta_T(x) = \sqrt{T}\left(\hat{F}_T(x) - F_S(x)\right) \Longrightarrow \mathcal{N}\left(0, d_F(S,x)^2\right),$$

$$\zeta_T(x) = \sqrt{T}\left(\hat{f}_T(x) - f_S(x)\right) \Longrightarrow \mathcal{N}\left(0, d_f(S,x)^2\right).$$

Let us fix a simple (basic) hypothesis

$$\mathcal{H}_0 : S(x) \equiv S_*(x).$$

Then to test this hypothesis we can use these estimators for construction of the Cramér–von Mises and Kolmogorov–Smirnov type test statistics

$$W_T^2 = T\int_{-\infty}^{\infty} \left[\hat{F}_T(x) - F_{S_*}(x)\right]^2 \, dF_{S_*}(x),$$

$$D_T = \sup_x \left|\hat{F}_T(x) - F_{S_*}(x)\right|,$$

and

$$V_T^2 = T \int_{-\infty}^{\infty} \left[\hat{f}_T(x) - f_{S_*}(x)\right]^2 \, dF_{S_*}(x),$$

$$d_T = \sup_x \left|\hat{f}_T(x) - f_{S_*}(x)\right|,$$

respectively. Unfortunately, all these statistics are not distribution-free even asymptotically and the choice of the corresponding thresholds for the tests is much more complicated. Indeed, it was shown that the random functions $(\eta_T(x), x \in R)$ and $(\zeta_T(x), x \in R)$ converge in the space $(\mathcal{C}_0, \mathfrak{B})$ (of continuous functions decreasing to zero at infinity) to the zero mean Gaussian processes $(\eta(x), x \in R)$ and $(\zeta(x), x \in R)$, respectively, with the covariance functions [we omit the index S_* of functions $f_{S_*}(x)$ and $F_{S_*}(x)$ below]:

$$R_F(x, y) = \mathbf{E}_{S_*}[\eta(x)\eta(y)]$$

$$= 4\mathbf{E}_{S_*}\left(\frac{[F(\xi \wedge x) - F(\xi)F(x)][F(\xi \wedge y) - F(\xi)F(y)]}{f(\xi)^2}\right)$$

$$R_f(x, y) = \mathbf{E}_{S_*}[\zeta(x)\zeta(y)]$$

$$= 4f(x)f(y)\mathbf{E}_{S_*}\left(\frac{\left[1_{\{\xi > x\}} - F(\xi)\right]\left[1_{\{\xi > y\}} - F(\xi)\right]}{f(\xi)^2}\right).$$

Here ξ is a random variable with the distribution function $F_{S_*}(x)$. Of course,

$$d_F(S, x)^2 = \mathbf{E}_S\left[\eta(x)^2\right], \qquad d_f(S, x)^2 = \mathbf{E}_S\left[\zeta(x)^2\right].$$

Using this weak convergence it is shown that these statistics converge in distribution (under hypothesis) to the following limits (as $T \to \infty$),

$$W_T^2 \Longrightarrow \int_{-\infty}^{\infty} \eta(x)^2 \, dF_{S_*}(x), \qquad T^{1/2}D_T \Longrightarrow \sup_x |\eta(x)|,$$

$$V_T^2 \Longrightarrow \int_{-\infty}^{\infty} \zeta(x)^2 \, dF_{S_*}(x), \qquad T^{1/2}d_T \Longrightarrow \sup_x |\zeta(x)|.$$

The conditions and the proofs of all these properties can be found in Kutoyants (2004), where essentially different statistical problems were studied, but the calculus is quite close to what we need here.

Note that the Kolmogorov–Smirnov test for ergodic diffusion was studied in Fournie (1992) [see as well Fournie and Kutoyants (1993) for further details], and the weak convergence of the process $\eta_T(\cdot)$ was obtained in Negri (1998).

The Cramér–von Mises and Kolmogorov–Smirnov type tests based on these statistics are

$$\Psi_T(X^T) = 1_{\{W_T^2 > C_\alpha\}}, \qquad \Phi_T(X^T) = 1_{\{T^{1/2}D_T > D_\alpha\}},$$

$$\psi_T(X^T) = 1_{\{V_T^2 > c_\alpha\}}, \qquad \phi_T(X^T) = 1_{\{T^{1/2}d_T > d_\alpha\}}$$

with appropriate constants.

The contiguous alternatives can be introduced in the following way,

$$S(x) = S_*(x) + \frac{h(x)}{\sqrt{T}}.$$

Then we obtain for the Cramér–von Mises statistics the limits [see Kutoyants (2004)]:

$$W_T^2 \Longrightarrow \int_{-\infty}^{\infty} \left[2\mathbf{E}_{S_*} \left([1_{\{\xi < x\}} - F_{S_*}(x)] \int_0^\xi h(s)\,\mathrm{d}s \right) + \eta(x) \right]^2 \mathrm{d}F_{S_*}(x),$$

$$V_T^2 \Longrightarrow \int_{-\infty}^{\infty} \left[2f_{S_*}(x)\mathbf{E}_{S_*} \int_\xi^x h(s)\,\mathrm{d}s + \zeta(x) \right]^2 \mathrm{d}F_{S_*}(x).$$

Note that the transformation $Y_t = F_{S_*}(X_t)$ simplifies the writing, because the diffusion process Y_t satisfies the differential equation

$$\mathrm{d}Y_t = f_{S_*}(X_t) \left[2S_*(X_t)\,\mathrm{d}t + \mathrm{d}W_t \right], \qquad Y_0 = F_{S_*}(X_0)$$

with reflecting bounds in 0 and 1 and (under hypothesis) has uniform on $[0,1]$ invariant distribution. Therefore,

$$W_T^2 \Longrightarrow \int_0^1 V(s)^2\,\mathrm{d}s, \qquad T^{1/2}D_T \Longrightarrow \sup_{0 \le s \le 1} |V(s)|,$$

but the covariance structure of the Gaussian process $\{V(s), 0 \le s \le 1\}$ can be quite complicated.

To obtain an asymptotically distribution-free Cramér–von Mises type test we can use another statistic, which is similar to that of the preceding section. Let us introduce

$$\tilde{W}_T^2 = \frac{1}{T^2} \int_0^T \left[X_t - X_0 - \int_0^t S_*(X_v)\,\mathrm{d}v \right]^2 \mathrm{d}t.$$

Then we have immediately (under hypothesis)

$$\tilde{W}_T^2 = \frac{1}{T^2} \int_0^T W_t^2\,\mathrm{d}t = \int_0^1 W(s)^2\,\mathrm{d}s,$$

where we put $t = sT$ and $W(s) = T^{-1/2}W_{sT}$. Under the alternative we have

$$\tilde{W}_T^2 = \frac{1}{T^2} \int_0^T \left[W_t + \frac{1}{\sqrt{T}} \int_0^t h(X_v)\,\mathrm{d}v \right]^2 \mathrm{d}t$$

$$= \frac{1}{T} \int_0^T \left[\frac{W_t}{\sqrt{T}} + \frac{t}{T}\frac{1}{t} \int_0^t h(X_v)\,\mathrm{d}v \right]^2 \mathrm{d}t.$$

The stochastic process X_t is ergodic, hence

$$\frac{1}{t} \int_0^t h(X_v)\, dv \longrightarrow \mathbf{E}_{S_*} h(\xi) = \int_{-\infty}^{\infty} h(x) f_{S_*}(x)\, dx \equiv \rho_h$$

as $t \to \infty$. It can be shown [see Section 2.3 in Kutoyants (2004), where we have the similar calculus in another problem] that

$$\tilde{W}_T^2 \Longrightarrow \int_0^1 [\rho_h\, s + W(s)]^2\, ds.$$

Therefore the power function of the test $\psi(X^T) = 1_{\{\tilde{W}_T^2 > c_\alpha\}}$ converges to the function

$$\beta_\psi(\rho_h) = \mathbf{P}\left(\int_0^1 [\rho_h\, s + W(s)]^2\, ds > c_\alpha \right).$$

Using standard calculus we can show that for the corresponding Kolmogorov–Smirnov type test the limit will be

$$\beta_\phi(\rho_h) = \mathbf{P}\left(\sup_{0 \le s \le 1} |\rho_h\, s + W(s)| > c_\alpha \right).$$

These two limit power functions are the same as in the next section devoted to self-exciting alternatives of the Poisson process. We calculate these functions with the help of simulations in Section 27.5 below.

Note that if the diffusion process is

$$dX_t = S(X_t)\, dt + \sigma(X_t)\, dW_t, \qquad X_0, \qquad 0 \le t \le T,$$

but the functions $S(\cdot)$ and $\sigma(\cdot)$ are such that the process is ergodic then we introduce the statistics

$$\hat{W}_T^2 = \frac{1}{T^2\, \mathbf{E}_{S_*}\left[\sigma(\xi)^2\right]} \int_0^T \left[X_t - X_0 - \int_0^t S_*(X_v)\, dv \right]^2 dt.$$

Here ξ is a random variable with the invariant density function

$$f_{S_*}(x) = \frac{1}{G(S_*)\, \sigma(x)^2} \exp\left\{ 2 \int_0^x \frac{S_*(y)}{\sigma(y)^2}\, dy \right\}.$$

This statistic under hypothesis is equal to

$$\hat{W}_T^2 = \frac{1}{T^2\, \mathbf{E}_{S_*}\left[\sigma(\xi)^2\right]} \int_0^T \left[\int_0^t \sigma(X_v)\, dW_v \right]^2 dt$$

$$= \frac{1}{T\, \mathbf{E}_{S_*}\left[\sigma(\xi)^2\right]} \int_0^T \left[\frac{1}{\sqrt{T}} \int_0^t \sigma(X_v)\, dW_v \right]^2 dt.$$

The stochastic integral by the central limit theorem is asymptotically normal

$$\eta_t = \frac{1}{\sqrt{t \mathbf{E}_{S_*} \left[\sigma \left(\xi\right)^2\right]}} \int_0^t \sigma \left(X_v\right) \mathrm{d} W_v \implies \mathcal{N}\left(0, 1\right)$$

and moreover it can be shown that the vector of such integrals converges in distribution to the Wiener process

$$\left(\eta_{s_1 T}, \ldots, \eta_{s_k T}\right) \implies \left(W\left(s_1\right), \ldots, W\left(s_k\right)\right)$$

for any finite collection of $0 \le s_1 < s_2 < \cdots < s_k \le 1$. Therefore, under mild regularity conditions it can be proved that

$$\hat{W}_T^2 \implies \int_0^1 W\left(s\right)^2 \, \mathrm{d} s.$$

The power function has the same limit,

$$\beta_\psi \left(\rho_h\right) = \mathbf{P}\left(\int_0^1 \left[\rho_h \, s + W\left(s\right)\right]^2 \mathrm{d} s > c_\alpha\right).$$

but with

$$\rho_h = \frac{\mathbf{E}_{S_*} h \left(\xi\right)}{\sqrt{\mathbf{E}_{S_*} \left[\sigma \left(\xi\right)^2\right]}}.$$

Similar consideration can be done for the Kolmogorov–Smirnov type test too.

We see that both tests cannot distinguish the alternatives with $h\left(\cdot\right)$ such that $\mathbf{E}_{S_*} h\left(\xi\right) = 0$. Note that for ergodic processes usually we have $\mathbf{E}_S S\left(\xi\right) = 0$ and $\mathbf{E}_{S_* + h/\sqrt{T}} \left[S_*\left(\xi\right) + T^{-1/2} h\left(\xi\right)\right] = 0$ with corresponding random variables ξ, but this does not imply $\mathbf{E}_{S_*} h\left(\xi\right) = 0$.

27.4 Poisson and Self-Exciting Processes

The Poisson process is one of the simplest point processes and before taking any other model it is useful first of all to check the hypothesis that the observed sequence of events, say, $0 < t_1, \ldots, t_N < T$ corresponds to a Poisson process. It is natural in many problems to suppose that this Poisson process is periodic of known period, for example, many daily events, signal transmission in optical communication, season variations, and so on. Another model of point processes frequently used as well is the self-exciting stationary point process introduced in Hawkes (1972). As any stationary process it can also describe the periodic changes due to the particular form of its spectral density.

Recall that for the Poisson process $X_t, t \geq 0$ of intensity function $S(t), t \geq 0$ we have (X_t is the counting process)

$$\mathbf{P}\{X_t - X_s = k\} = (k!)^{-1} (\Lambda(t) - \Lambda(s))^k \exp\{\Lambda(s) - \Lambda(t)\},$$

where we suppose that $s < t$ and put

$$\Lambda(t) = \int_0^t S(v) \, \mathrm{d}v.$$

The self-exciting process $X_t, t \geq 0$ admits the representation

$$X_t = \int_0^t S(s, X) \, \mathrm{d}s + \pi_t,$$

where $\pi_t, t \geq 0$ is a local martingale and the intensity function

$$S(t, X) = S + \int_0^t g(t - s) \, \mathrm{d}X_s = S + \sum_{t_i < T} g(t - t_i).$$

It is supposed that

$$\rho = \int_0^\infty g(t) \, \mathrm{d}t < 1.$$

Under this condition the self-exciting process is a stationary point process with the rate

$$\mu = \frac{S}{1 - \rho}$$

and the spectral density

$$f(\lambda) = \frac{\mu}{2\pi |1 - G(\lambda)|^2}, \qquad G(\lambda) = \int_0^\infty e^{\mathrm{i}\lambda t} g(t) \, \mathrm{d}t$$

[see Hawkes (1972) or Daley and Vere-Jones (2003) for details].

We consider two problems: Poisson against another Poisson and Poisson against a close self-exciting point process. The first one is to test the simple (basic) hypothesis

$$\mathcal{H}_0 : S(t) \equiv S_*(t), \qquad t \geq 0$$

where $S_*(t)$ is a known periodic function of period τ, against the composite alternative

$$\mathcal{H}_1 : S(t) \neq S_*(t), \qquad t \geq 0,$$

but $S(t)$ is always τ-periodic.

Let us denote $X_j(t) = X_{\tau(j-1)+t} - X_{\tau(j-1)}$, $j = 1, \ldots, n$, suppose that $T = n\tau$, and put

$$\hat{\Lambda}_n(t) = \frac{1}{n} \sum_{j=1}^{n} X_j(t).$$

The corresponding goodness-of-fit tests of Cramér–von Mises and Kolmogorov–Smirnov type can be based on the statistics

$$W_n^2 = \Lambda_*(\tau)^{-2} n \int_0^\tau \left[\hat{\Lambda}_n(t) - \Lambda_*(t)\right]^2 d\Lambda_*(t),$$

$$D_n = \Lambda_*(\tau)^{-1/2} \sup_{0 \le t \le \tau} \left|\hat{\Lambda}_n(t) - \Lambda_*(t)\right|.$$

It can be shown that

$$W_n^2 \Longrightarrow \int_0^1 W(s)^2 \, ds, \qquad \sqrt{n}\, D_n \Longrightarrow \sup_{0 \le s \le 1} |W(s)|,$$

where $\{W(s), 0 \le s \le 1\}$ is a Wiener process [see Kutoyants (1998)]. Hence these statistics are asymptotically distribution-free and the tests

$$\psi_n(X^T) = 1_{\{W_n^2 > c_\alpha\}}, \qquad \phi_n(X^T) = 1_{\{\sqrt{n}D_n > d_\alpha\}}$$

with the constants c_α, d_α taken from Equations (27.4), are of asymptotic size α.

Let us describe the close contiguous alternatives which asymptotically reduce this problem to the *signal in the white Gaussian noise* model (27.5). We put

$$\Lambda(t) = \Lambda_*(t) + \frac{1}{\sqrt{n\Lambda_*(\tau)}} \int_0^t h(u(v)) \, d\Lambda_*(v), \qquad u(v) = \frac{\Lambda_*(v)}{\Lambda_*(\tau)}.$$

Here $h(\cdot)$ is an arbitrary function defining the alternative. Then if $\Lambda(t)$ satisfies this equality we have the convergence

$$W_n^2 \Longrightarrow \int_0^1 \left[\int_0^s h(v) \, dv + W(s)\right]^2 ds.$$

This convergence describes the power function of the Cramér–von Mises type test under these alternatives.

The second problem is to test the hypothesis

$$\mathcal{H}_0 : S(t) = S_*, \qquad t \ge 0$$

against nonparametric close (contiguous) alternative

$$\mathcal{H}_1 : S(t) = S_* + \frac{1}{\sqrt{T}} \int_0^t h(t-s) \, dX_t, \qquad t \ge 0.$$

We consider the alternatives with the functions $h\left(\cdot\right) \geq 0$ having compact support and bounded.

We have $\Lambda_*\left(t\right) = S_*\,t$ and for some fixed $\tau > 0$ we can construct the same statistics

$$W_n^2 = \frac{n}{S_*\tau^2} \int_0^\tau \left[\hat\Lambda_n\left(t\right) - S_*\,t\right]^2 \mathrm{d}t, \qquad D_n = \left(S_*\,\tau\right)^{-1/2} \sup_{0\leq t\leq\tau} \left|\hat\Lambda_n\left(t\right) - S_*\,t\right|.$$

Of course, they have the same limits under hypothesis

$$W_n^2 \Longrightarrow \int_0^1 W\left(s\right)^2 \mathrm{d}s, \qquad \sqrt{n}D_n \Longrightarrow \sup_{0\leq s\leq 1} \left|W\left(s\right)\right|.$$

To describe their behaviour under any fixed alternative $h\left(\cdot\right)$ we have to find the limit distribution of the vector

$$\mathbf{w}_n = \left(w_n\left(t_1\right), \ldots, w_n\left(t_k\right)\right), \qquad w_n\left(t_l\right) = \frac{1}{\sqrt{S_*\tau}\,n} \sum_{j=1}^n \left[X_j\left(t_l\right) - S_*t_l\right],$$

where $0 \leq t_l \leq \tau$. We know that this vector under hypothesis is asymptotically normal

$$\mathcal{L}_0\left\{\mathbf{w}_n\right\} \Longrightarrow \mathcal{N}\left(\mathbf{0}, \mathbf{R}\right)$$

with covariance matrix

$$\mathbf{R} = \left(R_{lm}\right)_{k\times k}, \qquad R_{lm} = \tau^{-1} \min\left(t_l, t_m\right).$$

Moreover, it was shown in Dachian and Kutoyants (2006) that for such alternatives the likelihood ratio is locally asymptotically normal; that is, the likelihood ratio admits the representation

$$Z_n\left(h\right) = \exp\left\{\Delta_n\left(h, X^n\right) - \frac{1}{2}\,\mathrm{I}\left(h\right) + r_n\left(h, X^n\right)\right\},$$

where

$$\Delta_n\left(h, X^n\right) = \frac{1}{S_*\sqrt{\tau n}} \int_0^{\tau n} \int_0^{t-} h\left(t - s\right) \mathrm{d}X_s \left[\mathrm{d}X_t - S_*\mathrm{d}t\right],$$

$$\mathrm{I}\left(h\right) = \int_0^\infty h\left(t\right)^2 \mathrm{d}t + S_* \left(\int_0^\infty h\left(t\right) \mathrm{d}t\right)^2$$

and

$$\Delta_n\left(h, X^n\right) \Longrightarrow \mathcal{N}\left(0, \mathrm{I}\left(h\right)\right), \qquad r_n\left(h, X^n\right) \to 0. \tag{27.7}$$

To use the third Le Cam's lemma we describe the limit behaviour of the vector $\left(\Delta_n\left(h, X^n\right), \mathbf{w}_n\right)$. For the covariance $\mathbf{Q} = \left(Q_{lm}\right), l, m = 0, 1, \ldots, k$ of this vector we have

$$\mathbf{E}_0\Delta_n\left(h, X^n\right) = 0, \qquad Q_{00} = \mathbf{E}_0\Delta_n\left(h, X^n\right)^2 = \mathrm{I}\left(h\right)\left(1 + o\left(1\right)\right).$$

Furthermore, let us denote $d\pi_t = dX_t - S_*dt$ and $H(t) = \int_0^{t^-} h(t-s) \, dX_s$; then we can write

$$Q_{0l} = \mathbf{E}_0 \left[\Delta_n (h, X^n) w_n (t_l) \right]$$

$$= \frac{1}{nS_*^{3/2}\tau} \mathbf{E}_0 \left(\sum_{j=1}^{n} \int_{\tau(j-1)}^{\tau j} H(t) \, d\pi_t \sum_{i=1}^{n} \int_{\tau(i-1)}^{\tau(i-1)+t_l} d\pi_t \right)$$

$$= \frac{1}{n\tau\sqrt{S_*}} \sum_{j=1}^{n} \int_{\tau(j-1)}^{\tau(j-1)+t_l} \mathbf{E}_0 H(t) \, dt = \frac{t_l}{\tau} \sqrt{S_*} \int_0^{\infty} h(t) \, dt \ (1 + o(1)),$$

because

$$\mathbf{E}_0 H(t) = S_* \int_0^{t^-} h(t-s) \, ds = S_* \int_0^{\infty} h(s) \, ds$$

for the large values of t [such that $[0, t]$ covers the support of $h(\cdot)$].

Therefore, if we denote

$$\bar{h} = \int_0^{\infty} h(s) \, ds$$

then

$$Q_{0l} = Q_{l0} = \frac{t_l}{\tau} \sqrt{S_*} \, \bar{h}.$$

The proof of Theorem 1 in Dachian and Kutoyants (2006) can be applied to the linear combination of $\Delta_n (h, X^n)$ and $w_n (t_1), \dots, w_n (t_k)$ and this yields the asymptotic normality

$$\mathcal{L}_0 \Big(\Delta_n (h, X^n), \mathbf{w}_n \Big) \Longrightarrow \mathcal{N}(\mathbf{0}, \mathbf{Q}).$$

Hence by the third lemma of Le Cam we obtain the asymptotic normality of the vector $\mathbf{w}_n$,

$$\mathcal{L}_h \Big(\mathbf{w}_n \Big) \Longrightarrow \mathcal{L} \left(W(s_1) + s_1 \sqrt{S_*} \, \bar{h}, \dots, W(s_k) + s_k \sqrt{S_*} \, \bar{h} \right),$$

where we put $t_l = \tau s_l$. This weak convergence together with the estimates such as

$$\mathbf{E}_h \left| w_n (t_1) - w_n (t_2) \right|^2 \le C \left| t_1 - t_2 \right|$$

provides the convergence (under alternative)

$$W_n^2 \Longrightarrow \int_0^1 \left[\sqrt{S_*} \, \bar{h} \, s + W(s) \right]^2 ds.$$

We see that the limit experiment is of the type

$$dY_s = \sqrt{S_*} \, \bar{h} \, ds + dW(s), \qquad Y_0 = 0, \qquad 0 \le s \le 1.$$

The power $\beta(\psi_n, h)$ of the Cramér–von Mises type test $\psi_n(X^n) = 1_{\{W_n^2 > c_\alpha\}}$ is a function of the real parameter $\rho_h = \sqrt{S_*}\, h$,

$$\beta(W_n, h) = \mathbf{P}\left(\int_0^1 [\rho_h\, s + W(s)]^2\, \mathrm{d}s > c_\alpha\right) + o(1) = \beta_\psi(\rho_h) + o(1).$$

Using the arguments of Lemma 6.2 in Kutoyants (1998) it can be shown that for the Kolmogorov–Smirnov type test we have the convergence

$$\sqrt{n}D_n \Longrightarrow \sup_{0 \le s \le 1} |\rho_h\, s + W(s)|.$$

The limit power function is

$$\beta_\phi(\rho_h) = \mathbf{P}\left(\sup_{0 \le s \le 1} |\rho_h\, s + W(s)| > d_\alpha\right).$$

These two limit power functions are obtained by simulation in the next section.

27.5   Simulation

First, we present the simulation of the thresholds c_α and d_α of our Cramér–von Mises and Kolmogorov–Smirnov type tests. Because these thresholds are given by the equations (27.4), we obtain them by simulating 10^7 trajectories of a Wiener process on [0,1] and calculating empirical $1 - \alpha$ quantiles of the statistics

$$W^2 = \int_0^1 W(s)^2\, \mathrm{d}s \quad \text{and} \quad D = \sup_{0 \le s \le 1} |W(s)|,$$

respectively. Note that the distribution of W^2 coincides with the distribution of the quadratic form

$$W^2 = \sum_{k=1}^\infty \frac{\zeta_k^2}{(\pi k)^2}, \qquad \zeta_k \text{ i.i.d. } \sim \mathcal{N}(0,1)$$

and both distributions are extensively studied [see (1.9.4(1)) and (1.15.4) in Borodin and Salmienen (2002)]. The analytical expressions are quite complicated and we would like to compare by simulation c_α and d_α with the real (finite time) thresholds giving the tests of exact size α, that is, c_α^T and d_α^T given by equations

$$\mathbf{P}\{W_n^2 > c_\alpha^T\} = \alpha \quad \text{and} \quad \mathbf{P}\{\sqrt{n}D_n > d_\alpha^T\} = \alpha,$$

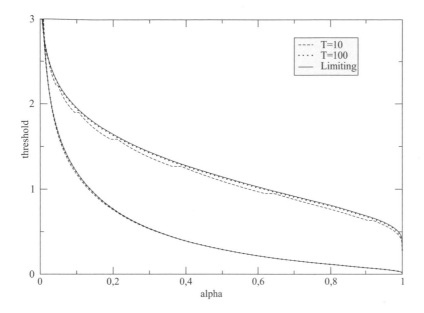

Figure 27.1. Threshold choice.

respectively. We choose $S^* = 1$ and obtain c_α^T and d_α^T by simulating 10^7 trajectories of a Poisson process of intensity 1 on $[0,T]$ and calculating empirical $1 - \alpha$ quantiles of the statistics W_n^2 and $\sqrt{n}D_n$. The thresholds simulated for $T = 10$, $T = 100$, and for the limiting case are presented in Figure 27.1. The lower curves correspond to the Cramér–von Mises type test, and the upper ones to the Kolmogorov–Smirnov type test. As we can see, for $T = 100$ the real thresholds are already indistinguishable from the limiting ones, especially in the case of the Cramér–von Mises type test.

It is interesting to compare the asymptotics of the Cramér–von Mises and Kolmogorov–Smirnov type tests with the locally asymptotically uniformly most powerful (LAUMP) test

$$\hat{\phi}_n(X^n) = 1_{\{\delta_T > z_\alpha\}}, \qquad \delta_T = \frac{X_{n\tau} - S_* n\tau}{\sqrt{S_* n\tau}}$$

proposed for this problem in Dachian and Kutoyants (2006). Here z_α is the $1 - \alpha$ quantile of the standard Gaussian law, $\mathbf{P}(\zeta > z_\alpha) = \alpha$, $\zeta \sim \mathcal{N}(0, 1)$. The limit power function of $\hat{\phi}_n$ is

$$\beta_{\hat{\phi}}(\rho_h) = \mathbf{P}(\rho_h + \zeta > z_\alpha).$$

In Figure 27.2 we compare the limit power functions $\beta_\psi(\rho)$, $\beta_\phi(\rho)$, and $\beta_{\hat{\phi}}(\rho)$. The last one can clearly be calculated directly, and the first two are obtained by

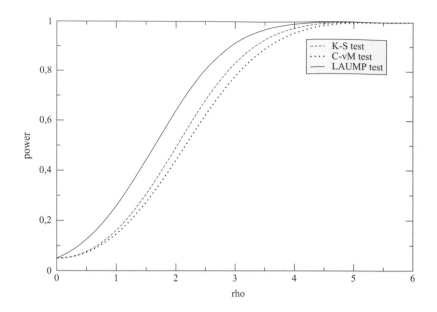

Figure 27.2. Limit power functions.

simulating 10^7 trajectories of a Wiener process on [0,1] and calculating empirical frequencies of the events

$$\left\{ \int_0^1 [\rho\, s + W(s)]^2 \, \mathrm{d}s > c_\alpha \right\} \quad \text{and} \quad \left\{ \sup_{0 \le s \le 1} |\rho\, s + W(s)| > d_\alpha \right\},$$

respectively.

The simulation shows the exact (quantitative) comparison of the limit power functions. We see that the power of the LAUMP test is higher than the two others and this is of course evident. We see also that the Kolmogorov–Smirnov type test is more powerful that the Cramér–von Mises type test.

References

1. Borodin, A. N. and Salmienen, R. (2002). *Handbook of Brownian Motion–Facts and Formulae, (2nd ed.)*, Birkhäuser, Basel.

2. Dachian, S. and Kutoyants, Yu. A. (2006). Hypotheses testing: Poisson versus self-exciting, *Scandinavian Journal of Statistics*, **33**, 391–408.

3. Daley, D. J. and Vere-Jones, D. (2003). *An Introduction to the Theory of Point Processes. vol. I. (2nd ed.)*, Springer-Verlag, New York.

4. Durbin, J. (1973). *Distribution Theory for Tests Based on the Sample Distribution Function*, SIAM, Philadelphia.

5. Fournie, E. (1992). Un test de type Kolmogorov-Smirnov pour processus de diffusions ergodic, *Rapport de Recherche*, **1696**, INRIA, Sophia-Antipolis.

6. Fournie, E. and Kutoyants, Yu. A. (1993). Estimateur de la distance minimale pour des processus de diffusion ergodiques, *Rapport de Recherche*, **1952**, INRIA, Sophia-Antipolis.

7. Greenwood, P. E. and Nikulin, M. (1996). *A Guide to Chi-Squared Testing*, John Wiley & Sons, New York.

8. Hawkes, A. G. (1972). Spectra for some mutually exciting point processes with associated variable, In *Stochastic Point Processes*, (Ed., P. A. W. Lewis), John Wiley & Sons, New York.

9. Iacus, S. and Kutoyants, Yu. A. (2001). Semiparametric hypotheses testing for dynamical systems with small noise, *Mathematical Methods of Statistics*, **10**, 105–120.

10. Ingster, Yu. I. and Suslina, I. A. (2003). *Nonparametric Goodness-of-Fit Testing Under Gaussian Models*, Springer-Verlag, New York.

11. Kutoyants, Yu. A. (1994). *Identification of Dynamical Systems with Small Noise*, Kluwer, Dordrecht.

12. Kutoyants, Yu. A. (1998). Statistical inference for spatial Poisson processes, In *Lecture Notes in Statistics*, **134**, Springer-Verlag, New York.

13. Kutoyants, Yu. A. (2004). *Statistical Inference for Ergodic Diffusion Processes*, Springer-Verlag, London.

14. Kutoyants, Yu. A. (2006). Goodness-of-fit tests for perturbed dynamical systems, in preparation.

15. Liptser, R. S. and Shiryayev, A. N. (2001). *Statistics of Random Processes. II. Applications,* (2nd ed.) Springer-Verlag, New York.

16. Negri, I. (1998). Stationary distribution function estimation for ergodic diffusion process, *Statistical Inference for Stochastic Processes*, **1**, 1, 61–84.

28

Nonparametric Estimation of Integral Functionals for Semi-Markov Processes with Application in Reliability

Nikolaos Limnios[1] and Brahim Ouhbi[2]

[1]*Université de Technologie de Compiègne, Laboratoire de Mathématiques Appliquées, Compiègne, France*
[2]*Ecole Nationale Supérieure d'Arts et Métiers, Meknès, Maroc*

Abstract: This chapter is concerned with moment calculus and estimation of integral functionals of semi-Markov processes. We prove that the nth moment performance function verifies the Markov renewal equation and we derive a simple formula for the first two moments of the integral functional in the finite-state semi-Markov case. We propose an estimator for each one of the two quantities. Then we prove their asymptotic properties. We end this chapter by proposing the confidence intervals for the first moment. As an illustration example, we give a numerical application.

Keywords and Phrases: Integral functional, semi-Markov process, nonparametric estimation, hitting time moments, consistency, asymptotic normality, confidence interval, reliability, performability

28.1 Introduction

Integral functionals are very important in stochastic theory and applications. They are used as compensators in martingale theory [see, e.g., Koroliuk and Limnios (2005)]. In particular, in some applications they are very useful, for example, in statistics as empirical estimators for stationary distributions in semi-Markov processes [Limnios (2006)], in some reliability studies including availability, in performance evaluation of computer systems [Ciardo *et al.* (1990), Csenki (1995), and Limnios and Oprişan (2001)], in performability analysis [Meyer (1981)], in storage processes [Prabhu (1980)], in economics/rewards [Papadopoulou (2004)], in survival analysis [Heutte and Huber (2002)], and so on.

Let us consider a stochastic process $Z_t, t \geq 0$, with state space a set E. Define a real-valued measurable function v defined on E. Define the following process

$$\Phi(t) := \int_0^t v(Z_s)ds, \qquad t \geq 0.$$

In this chapter we give estimation results concerning the process $\Phi(t), t \geq 0$. In particular we give explicit formulas for all moments and estimation of the first two.

The chapter is organized as follows. Section 28.2 presents a short background on semi-Markov processes needed in the sequel of the chapter. Section 28.3 gives the derivation of all moments of the functional Φ. Section 28.4 gives estimation results of the first two moments of the functional Φ, and Section 28.5 gives confidence interval results for these moments. Finally, Section 28.6, presents a numerical example of a three-state semi-Markov process.

28.2   The Semi-Markov Setting

Let us give in this section the essential background on semi-Markov processes, needed in the next sections for integral functional estimation of semi-Markov processes. Here we follow closely Limnios and Oprişan (2001).

Consider a finite set, say E, and an E-valued stochastic process $Z = (Z_t)_{t \in \mathbf{R}_+}$. Let $0 = S_0 < S_1 < \cdots < S_n < S_{n+1} < \cdots$ be the jump times of Z, and $J_0, J_1, J_2, \ldots$ the successive visited states of Z. Note that S_0 may also take positive values.

If the stochastic process $(J_n, S_n)_{n \in \mathbf{N}}$ is a Markov renewal process (MRP), with state space E, that is, it verifies a.s. the following equality

$$\mathbb{P}(J_{n+1} = j, S_{n+1} - S_n \leq t \mid J_0, \ldots, J_n; S_1, \ldots, S_n)$$
$$= \mathbb{P}(J_{n+1} = j, S_{n+1} - S_n \leq t \mid J_n)$$

for any $j \in E$, $n \in \mathbf{N}$, and any $t \in \mathbf{R}_+$, then Z is called a semi-Markov process (SMP). Thus the process (J_n, S_n) is a Markov chain with state space $E \times \mathbf{R}_+$ and transition kernel $Q_{ij}(t) := \mathbb{P}(J_{n+1} = j, S_{n+1} - S_n \leq t \mid J_n = i)$ called the semi-Markov kernel. Let α be the initial distribution row vector of Z; that is, $\alpha(i) = \mathbb{P}(Z_0 = i)$, $i \in E$. The process (J_n) is the embedded Markov chain (EMC) of Z with state space E and transition probabilities $P(i, j) := Q_{ij}(\infty) = \mathbb{P}(J_{n+1} = j \mid J_n = i)$.

The semi-Markov process Z is connected to the MRP (J_n, S_n) through

$$Z_t = J_n, \quad \text{if} \quad S_n \leq t < S_{n+1}, \qquad t \geq 0, \quad \text{and} \quad J_n = Z_{S_n}, \qquad n \geq 0.$$

For example, a Markov process with state space $E = \mathbb{N}$ and Q-matrix $A = (a_{ij})_{i,j \in E}$ is a special semi-Markov process with semi-Markov kernel

$$Q_{ij}(t) = \frac{a_{ij}}{a_i}(1 - e^{-a_i t}),$$

where $a_i := -a_{ii}$, $i \in E$.

Define also $X_n := S_n - S_{n-1}$, $n \geq 1$, the interjump times, and the process $(N(t))_{t \in \mathbb{R}_+}$, which counts the number of jumps of Z in the time interval $(0, t]$. Let us also define the number $N_i(t)$ of visits of Z to state $i \in E$ up to time t. To be specific,

$$N(t) := \sup\{n \geq 0 : S_n \leq t\}, \qquad N_i(t) := \sum_{k=1}^{N(t)} \mathbf{1}_{\{J_k = i\}} = \sum_{k=1}^{\infty} \mathbf{1}_{\{J_k = i, S_n \leq t\}}.$$

If we consider the (possibly delayed) renewal process $(S_n^i)_{n \geq 0}$ of successive times of visits to state i, then $N_i(t)$ is the counting process of renewals. Denote by μ_{ii} the mean recurrence time of (S_n^i); that is, $\mu_{ii} = \mathbb{E}[S_2^i - S_1^i]$.

Let us denote by $Q(t) = (Q_{ij}(t), \ i, j \in E)$, $t \geq 0$, the semi-Markov kernel of Z. Then we can write:

$$Q_{ij}(t) := \mathbb{P}(J_{n+1} = j, X_{n+1} \leq t \mid J_n = i) \quad = \quad P(i,j)F_{ij}(t),$$
$$t \geq 0, i, j \in E, \quad (28.1)$$

where $P(i,j) := \mathbb{P}(J_{n+1} = j \mid J_n = i)$ is the transition kernel of the EMC (J_n), and $F_{ij}(t) := \mathbb{P}(X_{n+1} \leq t \mid J_n = i, J_{n+1} = j)$ is the conditional distribution function of the interjump times. Let us define also the distribution function $H_i(t) := \sum_{j \in E} Q_{ij}(t)$ and its mean value m_i, which is the mean sojourn time of Z in state i.

Generally H_i is a distribution function, hence Q_{ij} is a subdistribution; that is, $Q_{ij}(\infty) \leq 1$ and $H_i(\infty) = 1$, with $Q_{ij}(0-) = H_i(0-) = 0$. In the case where $F_{ij}(t)$ does not depend on the arrival state j, then we write $F_i(t)$, instead of $F_{ij}(t)$, and we have $F_i(t) = H_i(t)$.

Let us define, for any i and j in E, the instantaneous transition rate $\lambda_{ij}(t)$ of a semi-Markov kernel, under absolute continuity of $Q_{ij}(t)$, by:

$$\lambda_{ij}(t) = \begin{cases} \frac{q_{ij}(t)}{1 - H_i(t)} & \text{if } p_{ij} > 0 \text{ and } H_i(t) < 1 \\ 0 & \text{otherwise,} \end{cases}$$

where $q_{ij}(t)$ is the Radon–Nikodym derivative of $Q_{ij}(t)$, with respect to Lebesgue measure on $\mathbb{R}_+$. Let us set

$$\Lambda_{ij}(t) = \int_0^t \lambda_{ij}(u)du$$

and

$$\Lambda_i(t) = \Sigma_{j=1}^s \Lambda_{ij}(t),$$

the cumulative transition rates.

For every $i, j \in E$ and $t \in \overline{\mathbb{R}}_+$, we have:

$$Q_{ij}(t) := \int_0^t \exp(-\Lambda_i(u))\lambda_{ij}(u)du.$$

So, its derivative, with respect to t, is

$$Q'_{ij}(t) = p_{ij}f_{ij}(t) = \exp(-\Lambda_i(t))\lambda_{ij}(t).$$

Consider now the n-fold convolution of Q by itself. For any $i, j \in E$,

$$Q_{ij}^{(n)}(t) = \begin{cases} \sum_{k \in E} \int_0^t Q_{ik}(ds)Q_{kj}^{(n-1)}(t-s) & n \geq 2 \\ Q_{ij}(t) & n = 1 \\ \delta_{ij}\mathbf{1}_{\{t \geq 0\}} & n = 0. \end{cases}$$

It is easy to prove (e.g., by induction) that

$$Q_{ij}^{(n)}(t) = \mathbb{P}_i(J_n = j, S_n \leq t). \tag{28.2}$$

Let us define the Markov renewal function $\psi_{ij}(t)$, $i, j \in E, t \geq 0$, by

$$\psi_{ij}(t) := \mathbb{E}_i[N_j(t)] = \sum_{n=0}^\infty Q_{ij}^{(n)}(t) \quad =: \quad (I - Q(t))^{(-1)}(i,j). \tag{28.3}$$

Another important function is the semi-Markov transition function

$$P_{ij}(t) := \mathbb{P}(Z_t = j \mid Z_0 = i), \qquad i, j \in E, t \geq 0,$$

which is the conditional marginal distribution of the process. In matrix form, we have

$$P(t) = (I - Q(t))^{(-1)} * (I - H(t)), \tag{28.4}$$

where $H(t)$ is the diagonal matrix $diag(H_i(t), i = 1, \ldots, s)$ and $*$ stands for the Stieltjes convolution (here in matrix form).

In the sequel, we suppose that the state space $E = \{1, \ldots, s\}$ is a finite set and that the distribution functions H_i are not degenerated. Let us suppose also that the mean sojourn times are finite; that is, $m_i < \infty$ for any $i \in E$. Furthermore, let us suppose that the distribution functions G_{ii}, of the recurrence time in state i, $i \in E$, are not arithmetic, that is, not concentrated on $\{ka : k \in \mathbb{N}\}$, for some $a > 0$.

Let us define also the stationary distribution $\pi(i), i \in E$, of the semi-Markov process Z. We get from the Markov renewal theorem [see, e.g., Limnios and Oprişan (2001)]

$$P_{ij}(t) \longrightarrow \pi(j), \qquad t \to \infty, \qquad i, j \in E. \tag{28.5}$$

28.3   Integral Functionals

Let us consider a right-continuous semi-Markov process Z_t, $t \geq 0$, with state space E and a function $v : E \to \mathbf{R}$. Define the following integral functional

$$\Phi(t) = \int_0^t v(Z_s)ds, \qquad t \geq 0. \tag{28.6}$$

For a fixed time $t > 0$, define now the moments of this functional

$$\phi_n(i,t) = \mathbf{E}_i\Phi(t)^n, \qquad n = 1, 2, \ldots. \tag{28.7}$$

Then we have the following result.

Proposition 28.3.1 *The nth moment of the performance function verifies the Markov renewal equation*

$$\phi_n(i,t) - \sum_{i \in E} \int_0^t Q_{ij}(ds)\phi_n(j, t - s) = G_n(i,t), \tag{28.8}$$

where

$$G_n(i,t) := (v(i)t)^n \overline{F}_i(t) + \sum_{k=1}^n \binom{n}{k}(v(i))^k \sum_{i \in E} \int_0^t s^k \phi_{n-k}(j, t - s)Q_{ij}(ds).$$

PROOF. For fixed $i \in E$ and $t \geq 0$, let us define the characteristic function of $\Phi(t)$,

$$\varphi_\lambda(i,t) := \mathbb{E}_i[e^{\iota\lambda\Phi(t)}], \qquad (\iota = \sqrt{-1}). \tag{28.9}$$

So, we have

$$\phi_n(i,t) = (-\iota)^n \frac{\partial^n}{\partial\lambda^n}\varphi_\lambda(i,t)\Big|_{\lambda=0}. \tag{28.10}$$

By a renewal argument we get

$$\varphi_\lambda(i,t) = e^{\iota\lambda v(i)t}\overline{F}_i(t) + \sum_{i \in E} \int_0^t e^{\iota\lambda v(i)s}\varphi_\lambda(j, t - s)Q_{ij}(ds). \tag{28.11}$$

By differentiating n times the above equation, with respect to λ, and putting $\lambda = 0$, we get the claimed result. ∎

For a finite state space $E = \{1, 2, \ldots, s\}$ define the vector

$$\phi_n(t) = (\phi_n(1, t), \ldots, \phi_n(s, t)).$$

Then we have the following special result.

Corollary 28.3.1 *The first two moments of the integral functional are given by:*

$$\phi_n(t) = \alpha(I - Q)^{(-1)} * G_n(t), \qquad n = 1, 2,$$

where $G_n(t) = diag(g_n(1,t), \dots, g_n(s,t))$, $n = 1, 2$,

$$g_1(i,t) = v(i)[t\overline{F}_i(t) + \int_0^t uF_i(du)],$$

$$g_2(i,t) = (v(i)t)^2\overline{F}_i(t) + (v(i))^2 \int_0^t u^2 F_i(du)$$

$$+ 2v(i) \sum_{j \in E} \int_0^t u\phi_1(j, t-u)Q_{ij}(du).$$

PROOF. By solving the above Markov renewal equation (28.8), we get the desired result. ∎

28.4   Nonparametric Estimation of Moments

In this section we give estimators of the first two moments for the integral functional based on the explicit formulas given in Corollary 28.3.1 and derive their asymptotic properties, that is, consistency and asymptotic normality. Consider a censored MRP history at fixed time T, which is described by

$$\mathcal{H}(T) = (J_0, J_1, \dots, J_{N_T}, X_1, X_2, \dots, X_{N_T}).$$

The likelihood function associated with $\mathcal{H}(T)$ is

$$L = \alpha(J_0)(1 - K(U_T, J_{N_T})) \prod_{l=0}^{N_T-1} p(J_l, J_{l+1})f(J_l, J_{l+1}, X_{l+1}),$$

where

$$U_T = T - S_{N_T},$$
$$1 - K(x, j) = \mathbb{P}(X_{N_T+1} > x | J_{N_T} = j);$$

then

$$l_1(T) = \log L_1(T) = \sum_{k=0}^{N_T-1} \left[\log \lambda_{J_k, J_{k+1}}(X_{k+1}) - \Lambda_{J_k}(X_{k+1}) \right] - \Lambda_{J_{N_T}}(U_T).$$

Let $(v_k)_{0 \le k \le M}$ be a regular subdivision of $[0, T]$, with step $\Delta_T = T/M$ and $M = [T^{1+\epsilon}]$, $0 < \epsilon < 1$ and $[x]$ is the integer part of x. We approximate the transition rate $\lambda_{ij}(t)$ by

$$\lambda_{ij}^*(t) = \sum_{k=0}^{M-1} \lambda_{ijk} 1_{[v_k, v_{k+1}[}(t).$$

So, the log-likelihood is given by

$$l_1(T) = \sum_{i,j} \sum_{k=0}^{M-1} (d_{ijk} \log \lambda_{ijk} - \lambda_{ijk} \nu_{ik}),$$

where

$$\nu_{ik} = \sum_{l=0}^{N_T-1} (X_{k+1} \wedge v_{k+1} - v_k) 1_{\{J_l = i, X_{k+1} \ge v_k\}} + (U_T \wedge v_{k+1} - v_k) 1_{\{J_{N_T} = i, U_T \ge v_k\}}$$

and

$$d_{ijk} = \sum_{l=0}^{N_T-1} 1_{\{J_l = i, J_{l+1} = j, X_{l+1} \in I_k\}}.$$

Hence the MLE of λ_{ijk} is given by

$$\widehat{\lambda}_{ijk} = \begin{cases} d_{ijk}/\nu_{ik} & \text{if} \quad \nu_{ik} > 0 \\ 0 & \text{otherwise.} \end{cases}$$

We define the semi-Markov kernel estimator

$$\widehat{Q}_{ij}(t, T) = \int_0^t \exp(-\widehat{\Lambda}_i(u, T)) \widehat{\lambda}_{ij}(u, T) du.$$

Then the estimator of the Markov renewal matrix is given by

$$\widehat{\psi}(t, T) = \sum_{l=0}^{\infty} \widehat{Q}^{(l)}(t, T).$$

Define now the following estimators for the first two moments of the integral functional $\phi_n(t)$, $n = 1, 2$,

$$\widehat{\phi}_n(t, T) := \alpha \widehat{\psi} * \widehat{G}_n(t, T), \qquad n = 1, 2,$$

where

$$\widehat{\phi}_n(t, T) = (\widehat{\phi}_n(1, t, T), \dots, \widehat{\phi}_n(s, t, T))^\top$$

and

$$\widehat{G}_n(t, T) = \text{diag}(\widehat{g}_n(1, t, T), \dots, \widehat{g}_n(s, t, T)),$$

$n = 1, 2$, and

$$\widehat{g}_1(i, t, T) = v(i) \frac{1}{N_i(T)} \sum_{l=1}^{N_i(T)} (X_{il} \wedge t), \qquad (28.12)$$

with X_{il} the lth sojourn time in state i, and

$$\widehat{g}_2(i, t, T) = (v(i))^2 \frac{1}{N_i(T)} \sum_{l=1}^{N_i(T)} [X_{il} \wedge t]^2$$

$$+ 2v(i) \sum_{j \in E} \int_0^t u \widehat{\phi}_1(j, t - u, T) \widehat{Q}_{ij}(du, T). \qquad (28.13)$$

Theorem 28.4.1 (Consistency) *The estimators $\widehat{\phi}_n(t, T)$, $n = 1, 2$ of the first two moments of the integral functional are strongly uniformly consistent on $[0, L]$, for any $L > 0$; that is,*

$$\sup_{0 \le t \le L} \left\| \widehat{\phi}_n(t, T) - \phi_n(t) \right\| \xrightarrow{\mathbf{P}_i - a.s.} 0, \qquad T \to \infty, \qquad n = 1, 2,$$

where $\|\cdot\|$ is the Euclidean norm in $\mathbb{R}^s$.

PROOF. Let us prove that the first moment of the integral functional is strongly uniformly consistent. Firstly observe that

$$g_1(i, t) = v(i)[t\overline{F}_i(t) + \int_0^t uF_i(du)] = v(i)\mathbb{E}[t \wedge X_{il}].$$

We have that [see Theorem 3 in Ouhbi and Limnios (1999)],

$$\sup_{t \in [0, \infty)} \left| \overline{F}_i(t) - \widehat{\overline{F}}_i(t) \right|$$

converges to zero. Then

$$\sup_{t \in [0, L]} \left| v(i)[t\overline{F}_i(t) - t\widehat{\overline{F}}_i(t)] \right| + \sup_{t \in [0, L]} \left| \int_0^t u[F_i(du) - \widehat{F}_i(du)] \right| \xrightarrow{\mathbf{P}_i - a.s.} 0, \qquad T \to \infty.$$

$$(28.14)$$

On the other hand, from Theorem 5 in Ouhbi and Limnios (1999), we have that

$$\sup_{0 \le t \le T} \left| \widehat{\psi}_{ij}(t, T) - \psi_{ij}(t) \right| \xrightarrow{\mathbf{P}_i - a.s.} 0, \qquad T \to \infty. \qquad (28.15)$$

From (28.14) and (28.15) we get the desired result for the first moment.

For the second moment, observe that

$$
\begin{aligned}
g_2(i,t) &:= (v(i)t)^2 \overline{F}_i(t) + (v(i))^2 \int_0^t u^2 F_i(du) \\
&\quad + 2v(i) \sum_{j \in E} \int_0^t u\phi_1(j, t-u) Q_{ij}(du) \\
&= [v(i)]^2 \mathbb{E}[(X_{il} \wedge t)^2] + 2v(i) \sum_{j \in E} \int_0^t u\phi_1(j, t-u) Q_{ij}(du).
\end{aligned}
$$

So, estimator (28.13) of $g_2(i,t)$ can be written

$$
(v(i))^2 \frac{1}{N_i(T)} \sum_{l=1}^{N_i(T)} [X_{il} \wedge t]^2 + 2v(i) \sum_{j \in E} \int_0^t u\widehat{\phi}_1(j, t-u, T)\widehat{Q}_{ij}(du, T).
$$

In the same manner as in the first part of the proof we get the desired result. ∎

Theorem 28.4.2 (Normality) *For any fixed t, $t \in [0, \infty)$, $T^{1/2}(\widehat{\phi}_1(t, T) - \phi_1(t))$ converges in distribution to a centered normal random variable with variance*

$$
\begin{aligned}
\sigma^2(t) &= \sum_{i=1}^{s} \sum_{j=1}^{s} \mu_{ii}\{(W_{ij})^2 * Q_{ij} - (W_{ij} * Q_{ij})^2 \\
&\quad + \int_0^\infty [\int_0^\infty v(j)(x \wedge (t-u)) dA_i(u)]^2 dQ_{ij}(x) \\
&\quad - [\int_0^\infty \int_0^\infty v(j)(x \wedge (t-u)) dA_i(u) dQ_{ij}(x)]^2 \\
&\quad + 2\int_0^\infty W_{ij}(t-x) \int_0^\infty v(j)(x \wedge (t-u)) dA_i(u) dQ_{ij}(x) \\
&\quad - 2(W_{ij} * Q_{ij})(t)(A_i * (v(j)(x \wedge .)))(t)\},
\end{aligned}
$$

where for $t \in \mathbb{R}_+$:

$$
\begin{aligned}
A_i(t) &= \sum_{k=1}^{s} \alpha_k v(i) \psi_{ki}(t), \\
W_{kl}(t) &= \sum_{i=1}^{s} \sum_{j=1}^{s} \alpha_i v(i)(\psi_{ik} * \psi_{lj} * I_j)(t), \\
I_j(t) &= \int_0^t \overline{F}_j(u) du.
\end{aligned}
$$

PROOF. It is easy to see that

$$
\begin{aligned}
T^{1/2}&(\widehat{\phi}_1(t,T) - \phi_1(t)) \\
&= \sum_{i\in E}\sum_{j\in E}\alpha_i v(j)T^{1/2}[(\widehat{I}_j * \widehat{\psi}_{ij})(t) - (I_j * \psi_{ij})(t)] \\
&= \sum_{i\in E}\sum_{j\in E}\alpha_i v(j)T^{1/2}[(\widehat{I}_j - I_j) * (\widehat{\psi}_{ij} - \psi_{ij})(t) \\
&\quad + (\widehat{I}_j - I_j) * \psi_{ij}(t) + I_j * (\widehat{\psi}_{ij} - \psi_{ij})(t)].
\end{aligned}
\tag{28.16}
$$

The first term on the right-hand side of (28.16) converges to zero. Then $T^{1/2}(\widehat{\phi}_1(t) - \phi_1(t))$ has the same limit as the r.v.

$$
\sum_{i=1}^{s}\sum_{j\in U}\alpha_i v(j)T^{1/2}\left[\frac{1}{N_j(T)}\sum_{r=1}^{N_j(T)}((X_{jl}\wedge t) - I_j) * \psi_{ij}(t) \right. \\
\left. + \left(\sum_{k=1}^{s}\sum_{l=1}^{s}I_j * \psi_{ik} * \psi_{lj}\right) * (\widehat{Q}_{kl} - Q_{kl})(t)\right],
$$

which can be written as

$$
\sum_{k=1}^{s}\sum_{l=1}^{s}\frac{T^{1/2}}{N_k(T)}\sum_{r=1}^{N_k(T)}[1_{\{J_r=k,k\in U,J_{r+1}=l\}}(X_r\wedge t - I_k) * A_k(t) \\
+ (W_{kl} * (1_{\{J_{r+1}=l,X_r\leq.\}} - Q_{kl})(t))1_{\{J_r=k\}}].
$$

Because $T/N_k(T) \to \mu_{kk}$ (a.s.) (the mean recurrence time in state k), we get the desired result by the central limit theorem for semi-Markov process of Pyke and Schaufele (1964) applied to the function

$$
\begin{aligned}
f(J_r, J_{r+1}, X_n) &= \mu_{kk}A_k * ((X_n\wedge t) - I_k)1_{\{J_r=k,k\in U,J_{r+1}=l\}} \\
&\quad + \mu_{kk}W_{kl} * (1_{\{J_{r+1}=l,X_r\leq.\}} - Q_{kl})(t)1_{\{J_r=k\}}.
\end{aligned}
$$

■

28.5 Confidence Intervals for the Moments

An estimator of $\sigma^2(t)$, denoted $\widehat{\sigma}^2(t,T)$, is obtained by replacing Q and ψ by their estimators $\widehat{Q}$ and $\widehat{\psi}$, respectively, in the above expression. Then it is easy to prove the following theorem.

Theorem 28.5.1 *For any fixed* $t \geq 0$, *the estimator* $\widehat{\sigma}^2(t, T)$ *is uniformly strongly consistent in the sense that*

$$\sup_{t \in [0,L]} |\widehat{\sigma}^2(t, T) - \sigma^2(t)| \longrightarrow 0 \quad a.s., \quad as \quad T \to \infty,$$

for any fixed $L > 0$.

We can construct confidence intervals for the first moment of the integral functionals.

Theorem 28.5.2 *The r.v.* $(\sqrt{T}/\widehat{\sigma}(t, T))(\widehat{\phi}_1(t, T) - \phi_1(t))$ *converges in distribution to a standard normal random variable.*

Hence for $\alpha \in (0, 1)$, an approximate $100(1 - \alpha)\%$ confidence interval for $\phi_1(t))$ is

$$\widehat{\phi}_1(t, T) - z_{\frac{\alpha}{2}} \frac{\widehat{\sigma}(t, T)}{\sqrt{T}} \leq \phi_1(t, T) \leq \widehat{\phi}_1(t, T) + z_{\frac{\alpha}{2}} \frac{\widehat{\sigma}(t, T)}{\sqrt{T}},$$

where $z_{\alpha/2}$ is the upper $\alpha/2$ quantile of the standard normal distribution.

28.6   Numerical Application

Let us consider a three-state semi-Markov system as illustrated in Figure 28.1, where $F_{12}(x) = 1 - \exp(-\lambda_1 x)$, $F_{21}(x) = 1 - \exp[-(x/\alpha_1)^{\beta_1}]$, $F_{23}(x) = 1 - \exp[-(x/\alpha_2)^{\beta_2}]$, and $F_{31}(x) = 1 - \exp(-\lambda_2 x)$, for $x \geq 0$. $\lambda_1 = 0.1$, $\lambda_2 = 0.2$, $\alpha_1 = 0.3$, $\beta_1 = 2$, $\alpha_2 = 0.1$, and $\beta_2 = 2$.

The transition probability matrix of the embedded Markov chain (J_n) is:

$$P = \begin{pmatrix} 0 & 1 & 0 \\ p & 0 & 1-p \\ 1 & 0 & 0 \end{pmatrix},$$

where p is given by

$$p = \int_0^\infty [1 - F_{23}(x)] dF_{21}(x).$$

The function v is defined by $v(1) = 1.0$, $v(2) = 0.6$, and $v(3) = 0$.

If we simulate one trajectory for different censored times $T_1 < T_2 < \cdots < T_r$, we see that $\widehat{\phi}_1(i, t, T_k)$ converges to the true curve of $\phi_1(i, t)$ as k increases. See Figure 28.2.

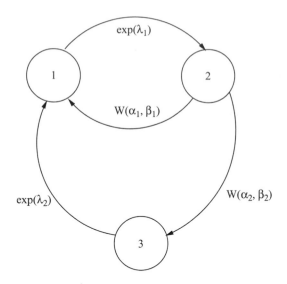

Figure 28.1. A three-state semi-Markov system.

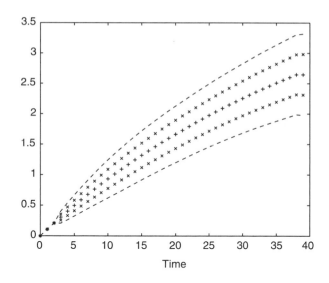

Figure 28.2. Mean value of the integral functional estimation of the three-state semi-Markov system and its 95% and 80% nonparametric interval confidence.

References

1. Asmussen, S. (1987). *Applied Probability and Queues*, John Wiley & Sons, New York.

2. Basawa, I. V. and Prakasa Rao, B. L. S. (1980). *Statistical Inference for Stochastic Processes*, Academic Press, London.

3. Ciardo, G., Marie, R. A., Sericola, B., and Trivedi, K. S. (1990). Performability analysis using semi-Markov reward processes, *IEEE Transactions on Computers*, **39**, 1251–1264.

4. Csenki, A. (1995). Dependability for systems with a partitioned state space, *Lecture Notes in Statistics*, Vol. 90, Springer-Verlag, Berlin.

5. Gihman, I. I. and Skorohod, A. V. (1974). *Theory of Stochastic Processes*, Vol. 2, Springer-Verlag, Berlin.

6. Heutte, N. and Huber, C. (2002). Semi-Markov models for quality of life data with censoring, In *Statistical Methods for Quality of Life Studies* (Eds., M. Mesbah, B. F. Cole, and M.L.-T. Lee), pp. 207–218, Kluwer, Dordrecht.

7. Janssen, J. and Limnios, N. (Eds.) (1999). *Semi-Markov Models and Applications*, Kluwer, Dordrecht.

8. Korolyuk, V. S. and Limnios, N. (2005). *Stochastic Systems in Merging Phase Space*, World Scientific, Singapore.

9. Limnios, N. (2006). Estimation of the stationary distribution of semi-Markov processes with Borel state space, *Statistics & Probability Letters*, **76**, 1536–1542.

10. Limnios, N. and Oprişan, G. (1999). A general framework for reliability and performability analysis of semi-Markov systems, *Applied Stochastic Models in Business and Industry*, **15**, 353–368.

11. Limnios, N. and Oprişan, G. (2001). *Semi–Markov Processes and Reliability*, Birkhäuser, Boston.

12. Limnios, N. and Ouhbi, B. (2003). Empirical estimators of reliability and related functions for semi-Markov systems, In *Mathematical and Statistical Methods in Reliability* (Eds., B. Lindqvist and K. Doksum), World Scientific, Singapore.

13. Meyer, J. (1980). On evaluating the performability of degradable computer systems, *IEEE Transactions on Computers*, **29**, 720–731.

14. Ouhbi, B. and Limnios, N. (1999). Non-parametric estimation for semi-Markov processes based on their hazard rate, *Statist. Infer. Stoch. Processes*, **2**, 151–173.

15. Ouhbi, B. and Limnios, N. (2003). Nonparametric reliability estimation of semi-Markov processes, *Journal of Statistical Planning and Inference*, **109**, 155–165.

16. Papadopoulou, A. (2004). Economic rewards in non-homogeneous semi-Markov systems, *Communications in Statistics—Theory and Methods*, **33**, 681–696.

17. Parzen, E. (1999). *Stochastic Processes*, SIAM Classics, Philadelphia.

18. Prabhu, N. U. (1980). *Stochastic Storage Processes*, Springer-Verlag, Berlin.

19. Pyke, R. and Schaufele, R. (1964). Limit theorems for Markov renewal processes, *Annals of Mathematical Statistics*, **35**, 1746–1764.

29

Estimators for Partially Observed Markov Chains

Ursula U. Müller,[1] **Anton Schick,**[2] **and Wolfgang Wefelmeyer**[3]

[1]*Department of Statistics, Texas A&M University, College Station, TX, USA*
[2]*Department of Mathematical Sciences, Binghamton University, Binghamton, NY, USA*
[3]*Mathematisches Institut, Universität zu Köln, Köln, Germany*

Abstract: Suppose we observe a discrete-time Markov chain only at certain periodic or random time points. Which observation patterns allow us to identify the transition distribution? In the case where we can identify it, how can we construct (good) estimators? We discuss these questions both for nonparametric models and for linear autoregression.

Keywords and Phrases: Markov chain, linear autoregression, partial observation, periodic skipping, random skipping, empirical estimator, deconvolution

---

29.1 Introduction

For Markov chains only observed at certain periodic or random time points we discuss when one can identify the underlying transition distribution, and how one can construct estimators of linear functionals of the stationary distribution in nonparametric models, and of the innovation density in linear autoregression. By Markov chain we mean a Markov process in discrete time, with arbitrary state space.

In Section 29.2 we consider nonparametric estimators of linear functionals of the form $E[h(X_0, X_1)]$ of a real-valued first-order stationary Markov chain. We introduce different periodic and random partial observation patterns. If nothing is known about the structure of the transition distribution, consistent estimation of $E[h(X_0, X_1)]$ is, in general, impossible unless one occasionally sees adjacent pairs (X_{j-1}, X_j). We can use these pairs to construct an empirical estimator of $E[h(X_0, X_1)]$. In the simplest such situation, with every third of the realizations of the chain unobserved, we show how to use the information across the gaps for improving the empirical estimator. The approach carries over to the other observation patterns, and to higher-order Markov chains. In Section 29.3 we assume that the Markov chain is a first-order linear autoregressive process. In this case we can even treat observation patterns in which we never see adjacent

419

pairs, assuming only that we know the sign of the autoregression parameter. In the simplest such situation, only every second realization of the process is observed. We construct deconvolution-type estimators for the innovation density in this case. Again the approach carries over to more complicated observation patterns, and to higher-order linear autoregressive processes.

29.2   Nonparametric Estimators

29.2.1   Full observations

Let $X_0, \ldots, X_n$ be observations of a real-valued stationary and uniformly ergodic first-order Markov chain with transition distribution $Q(x, dy)$. We can identify Q from the stationary distribution of an adjacent pair (X_0, X_1), which in turn is identified from sufficiently many linear functionals $E[h(X_0, X_1)]$, for example, from the distribution function $(s, t) \mapsto E[\mathbf{1}(X_0 \leq s, X_1 \leq t)]$ of (X_0, X_1). It suffices therefore to study estimation of such functionals. Let h be a bounded measurable function on $\mathbb{R}^2$. A natural estimator of $Eh = E[h(X_0, X_1)]$ is the empirical estimator

$$\mathbb{E}h = \frac{1}{n} \sum_{j=1}^{n} h(X_{j-1}, X_j).$$

It admits the martingale approximation

$$n^{1/2}(\mathbb{E}h - Eh) = n^{-1/2} \sum_{j=1}^{n} (Ah)(X_{j-1}, X_j) + o_p(1) \qquad (29.1)$$

with

$$(Ah)(x, y) = h(x, y) - Q_x h + \sum_{k=1}^{\infty} (Q_y^k h - Q_x^{k+1} h),$$

where $Q_x h = \int h(x, y) Q(x, dy)$ and $Q_x^k h = \int Q_y h Q^{k-1}(x, dy)$ for $k = 2, 3, \ldots$. Hence by the martingale central limit theorem, $n^{1/2}(\mathbb{E}h - Eh)$ is asymptotically normal with variance $E[(Ah)^2(X_0, X_1)]$. See Meyn and Tweedie (1993, Chapter 17), for these results and for generalizations. In nonparametric models, with nothing known about the structure of the transition distribution, $\mathbb{E}h$ is efficient in the sense of Hájek and LeCam; see Penev (1991), Bickel (1993), Greenwood and Wefelmeyer (1995), and Bickel and Kwon (2001) for different proofs.

29.2.2 Periodic skipping

Suppose now that we observe only some of the realizations, in a deterministic pattern that repeats itself periodically, say with period m. Specifically, in the first period we observe at k times $1 \leq i_1 < \cdots < i_k \leq m$ and then at times $m + i_1, \ldots, 2m + i_1, \ldots$, for $n + 1$ periods, say. Then we observe up to time $(n + 1)m$ and have $(n + 1)k$ observations. Here it is understood that we *know* how many realizations we skip. The *skip lengths* are

$$s_1 = i_2 - i_1, \ldots, \qquad s_{k-1} = i_k - i_{k-1}, \qquad s_k = m + i_1 - i_k.$$

1. In the simplest case, some of the skip lengths are 1. For example, let $m = 3$, $k = 2$, $i_1 = 1$, $i_2 = 2$. Then every third realization is missing. A simple estimator of $E[h(X_0, X_1)]$ is the empirical estimator based on observed pairs (X_{3j-2}, X_{3j-1}) of successive realizations of the chain. Such an estimator does not use the information in the nonadjacent pairs (X_{3j-1}, X_{3j+1}), and we should be able to find better estimators, in the sense of smaller asymptotic variance (unless the observations happen to be independent). In the next section we describe how one could use the information in the nonadjacent pairs to improve on the empirical estimator.

2. Suppose that none of the skip lengths is 1, but they have no common divisor. Then we can represent 1 as a linear combination of skip lengths. Suppose, for example, that $m = 5$, $k = 2$, $i_1 = 1$, $i_2 = 3$. Then the skip lengths are $s_1 = 2$, $s_2 = 3$, and, because $1 = 3 - 2$, we can write $Q = Q^{-2}Q^3$. We can therefore identify Q from Q^2 and Q^3, which in turn can be estimated from the pairs (X_{5j+1}, X_{5j+3}) and (X_{5j-2}, X_{5j+1}), respectively. To estimate the inverse of a transition distribution, decompose the state space into a finite number of sets and invert the corresponding empirical transition matrix.

3. If the skip lengths have a common divisor, Q is not identifiable. Suppose, for example, that $m = 2$, $k = 1$, $i_1 = 1$. Then we skip every second realization. The remaining observations allow us to estimate Q^2, but this does not identify the root Q uniquely. In certain parametric and semiparametric models we can, however, still (nearly) identify Q, for example, if the chain follows a first-order linear autoregressive model; see Section 29.3.

29.2.3 Observing two out of three

Suppose we observe (X_{3j-2}, X_{3j-1}) for $j = 1, \ldots, n$. A simple estimator for $E[h(X_0, X_1)]$ is the empirical estimator

$$\mathbb{E}h = \frac{1}{n} \sum_{j=1}^{n} h(X_{3j-2}, X_{3j-1}).$$

The information in the nonadjacent pairs (X_{3j-1}, X_{3j+1}) can be used as follows. Write (X, Y, Z) for $(X_{3j-1}, X_{3j}, X_{3j+1})$. We want to estimate $E[h(X,Y)]$. Introduce the conditional expectations

$$h_\ell(X, Z) = E(h(X,Y)|X, Z) \quad \text{and} \quad h_r(X, Z) = E(h(Y, Z)|X, Z).$$

We have

$$E[h_\ell(X, Z)] = E[h_r(X, Z)] = E[h(X, Y)].$$

If we knew h_ℓ and h_r, we could estimate $E[h(X,Y)]$ by empirical estimators

$$\frac{1}{n} \sum_{j=1}^{n} h_\ell(X_{3j-1}, X_{3j+1}) \quad \text{and} \quad \frac{1}{n} \sum_{j=1}^{n} h_r(X_{3j-1}, X_{3j+1})$$

or smoothed versions of these. We do not know h_ℓ and h_r and suggest replacing them by estimators as follows. Assume that the finite-dimensional stationary distributions of the chain have Lebesgue densities. Let p_1, p_2, p_3 denote the densities of X, (X, Y), (X, Y, Z), respectively. Write g for the density of (X, Z). Note that

$$g(x, z) = \int p_3(x, y, z)\, dy.$$

We have

$$h_\ell(x, z) = \frac{\int h(x, y) p_3(x, y, z)\, dy}{g(x, z)}.$$

Write

$$p_3(x, y, z) = \frac{p_2(x, y) p_2(y, z)}{p_1(y)}.$$

Estimate p_2 by a kernel estimator based on the adjacent pairs (X_{3j-2}, X_{3j-1}),

$$\hat{p}_2(x, y) = \frac{1}{n} \sum_{i=1}^{n} k_b(x - X_{3j-2}) k_b(y - X_{3j-1}),$$

where $k_b(x) = k(x/b)/b$ with k a kernel and b a bandwidth. Estimate p_1 by

$$\hat{p}_1(y) = \frac{1}{2} \left(\int \hat{p}_2(x, y)\, dx + \int \hat{p}_2(y, z)\, dz \right).$$

Then we can estimate p_3 by

$$\hat{p}_3(x, y, z) = \frac{\hat{p}_2(x, y) \hat{p}_2(y, z)}{\hat{p}_1(y)}$$

and g by

$$\bar{g}(x, z) = \int \hat{p}_3(x, y, z)\, dy.$$

We arrive at the following estimator for h_ℓ,

$$\hat{h}_\ell(x, z) = \frac{\int h(x, y)\hat{p}_3(x, y, z)\,dy}{\bar{g}(x, z)}.$$

Rather than looking at the empirical estimator $(1/n)\sum_{j=1}^n \hat{h}_\ell(X_{3j-1}, X_{3j+1})$, it is technically convenient to look at the smoothed version

$$\mathbb{E}_\ell h = \int \hat{h}_\ell(x, z)\hat{g}(x, z)\,dx\,dz,$$

where $\hat{g}$ is a kernel estimator of g based on nonadjacent pairs (X_{3j-1}, X_{3j+1}),

$$\hat{g}(x, z) = \frac{1}{n}\sum_{j=1}^n k_b(x - X_{3j-1})k_b(z - X_{3j+1}).$$

Similarly,

$$\hat{h}_r(x, z) = \frac{\int h(y, z)\hat{p}_3(x, y, z)\,dy}{\bar{g}(x, z)}$$

and

$$\mathbb{E}_r h = \int \hat{h}_r(x, z)\hat{g}(x, z)\,dx\,dz.$$

Under appropriate conditions, the three estimators $\mathbb{E}h$, $\mathbb{E}_\ell h$, and $\mathbb{E}_r h$ can be shown to be asymptotically normal. We can take linear combinations of them to obtain estimators with smaller asymptotic variance than the empirical estimator $\mathbb{E}h$. The best weights are expressed in terms of the variances and covariances of the three estimators. They depend on the unknown distribution but can be estimated empirically. Consider, for example, the empirical estimator $\mathbb{E}h = (1/n)\sum_{j=1}^n h(X_{3j-2}, X_{3j-1})$ based on the observations (X_{3j-2}, X_{3j-1}), $j = 1, \ldots, n$. The observations follow a Markov chain with transition distribution of (X_{3j+1}, X_{3j+2}) given $(X_{3j-2}, X_{3j-1}) = (v, w)$ not depending on v and defined by

$$R(w, dy, dz) = Q^2 \otimes Q(w, dy, dz) = Q^2(w, dy)Q(y, dz).$$

We can apply the martingale approximation (29.1) to obtain

$$n^{1/2}(\mathbb{E}h - Eh) = n^{-1/2}\sum_{j=1}^n (Bh)(X_{3j-1}, X_{3j+1}, X_{3j+2}) + o_p(1)$$

with

$$(Bh)(w, y, z) = h(y, z) - R_w h + \sum_{k=1}^\infty (R_z^k h - R_w^{k+1} h).$$

By the martingale central limit theorem, $\mathbb{E}h$ is asymptotically normal with variance $E[(Bh)^2(X_2, X_4, X_5)]$ of the form

$$Eh^2 - (Eh)^2 + 2\sum_{k=1}^{\infty} E[(h(X_1, X_2) - Eh)h(X_{3k+1}, X_{3k+2})].$$

This variance can be estimated empirically, by

$$\mathbb{E}h^2 - (\mathbb{E}h)^2 + 2\sum_{k=1}^{m(n)} \frac{1}{n-k} \sum_{j=1}^{n-k} (h(X_{3j-2}, X_{3j-1}) - \mathbb{E}h)h(X_{3(j+k)-2}, X_{3(j+k)-1})$$

with $m(n)$ slowly increasing to infinity. [Compare Müller *et al.* (2001).] Similar martingale approximations can be obtained for $\mathbb{E}h_\ell$ and $\mathbb{E}h_r$, and their variances and the covariances of the three estimators can be estimated similarly as the variance of $\mathbb{E}h$.

29.2.4   Random skipping

Suppose that, after an observation at time j, we make the next observation at time $j+s$ with probability a_s. Then the skip lengths are i.i.d. random variables S_i, $i = 0, 1, \ldots$, with values in $\mathbb{N}$ and distribution given by $A(\{s\}) = a_s$, $s \in \mathbb{N}$. Set $T_0 = 0$ and $T_j = \sum_{i=0}^{j-1} S_i$, and write $Y_j = X_{T_j}$. Suppose we observe the pairs (S_j, Y_j) for $j = 0, \ldots, n$, say. They form a Markov chain with transition distribution

$$R(x, ds, dy) = A(ds)Q^s(x, dy).$$

Let N_s denote the observed number of skip lengths $S_j = s$. We can estimate a_s by N_s/n. Estimation of $E[h(X_0, X_1)]$ is similar to the case of periodic skipping considered above. In particular, if a_1 is positive, a simple estimator of $E[h(X_0, X_1)]$ is the empirical estimator

$$\frac{1}{N_1} \sum_{S_j=1} h(Y_j, Y_{j+1}).$$

The information in the pairs (Y_j, Y_{j+1}) with skip lengths $S_j = 2, 3, \ldots$ can be exploited similarly as for periodic skipping.

29.2.5   Skipping at random

In the previous section we have assumed that the skip lengths are independent of the Markov chain. It is, however, conceivable that the skip lengths depend on the previous state. Let $A(x, ds)$ denote the skip length distribution out of state x. Then we observe pairs (S_j, Y_j) for $j = 0, \ldots, n$ with transition distribution

$$R(x, ds, dy) = A(x, ds)Q^s(x, dy).$$

This factorization is analogous to the factorization $Q(x, dy)A(x, y, ds)$ of the transition distribution of a Markov renewal process; for efficient estimation in semiparametric models of the corresponding semi-Markov process see Greenwood *et al.* (2004). The name "skipping at random" is chosen because of the similarity with responses "missing at random" in regression models; for efficient semiparametric estimation see Müller *et al.* (2006). Recent monographs treating missing data are Little and Rubin (2002), van der Laan and Robins (2003), and Tsiatis (2006). Random skipping as considered above, with A not depending on x, would correspond to "missing totally at random". We can estimate $a_s(x) = A(x, \{s\})$ by the kernel estimator

$$\hat{a}_s(x) = \frac{\sum_{i=1}^n k_b(x - Y_i)\mathbf{1}(S_i = s)}{\sum_{i=1}^n k_b(x - Y_i)},$$

where $k_b(x) = k(x/b)/b$ with k a kernel and b a bandwidth. Again, if $a_1(x) = A(x, \{1\})$ is positive with positive probability, a simple estimator of the expectation $E[h(X_0, X_1)]$ can be based on the observed pairs of successive observations:

$$\sum_{j=0}^{n-1} \frac{\mathbf{1}(S_j = 1)}{\hat{a}_1(Y_j)} h(Y_j, Y_{j+1}).$$

Again, the information in the pairs (Y_j, Y_{j+1}) with skip lengths $S_j = 2, 3, \ldots$ can be exploited similarly as for periodic skipping.

29.3 Linear Autoregression

29.3.1 Full observations

Let $X_0, \ldots, X_n$ be observations from a stationary first-order autoregressive linear model

$$X_j = \vartheta X_{j-1} + \varepsilon_j \tag{29.2}$$

with $|\vartheta| < 1$ and i.i.d. innovations ε_j that have mean zero, finite variance, and density f. This is a first-order Markov chain with transition distribution $Q(x, dy) = f(y - \vartheta x) \, dy$, parametrized by ϑ and f. A simple estimator for ϑ is the least squares estimator

$$\bar{\vartheta} = \frac{\sum_{j=1}^n X_{j-1} X_j}{\sum_{j=1}^n X_{j-1}^2}.$$

We can use it to estimate the innovation ε_j by the residual $\bar{\varepsilon}_j = X_j - \bar{\vartheta} X_{j-1}$. An estimator for the innovation density f is the residual-based kernel estimator

$$\hat{f}(x) = \frac{1}{n} \sum_{j=1}^n k_b(x - \bar{\varepsilon}_j),$$

where $k_b(x) = k(x/b)/b$ with k a kernel and b a bandwidth.

29.3.2 Observing one out of two

As mentioned in Section 29.2, the transition distribution of a Markov chain is not identifiable if observations are skipped periodically with skip lengths having a common divisor. In the simplest such case, only every second of the realizations of the chain is observed. The situation is much better for autoregression (29.2). Then the transition distribution is still identifiable, up to the sign of ϑ. To see this, suppose that we observe $X_0, X_2, \ldots, X_{2n}$ and write

$$X_{2j} = \vartheta^2 X_{2j-2} + \eta_{2j} \tag{29.3}$$

with

$$\eta_{2j} = \varepsilon_{2j} + \vartheta \varepsilon_{2j-1}. \tag{29.4}$$

The X_{2j} again follow a first-order linear autoregressive model, now with autoregression parameter $s = \vartheta^2$ and innovation η_{2j}. The nonuniqueness of the square root of the two-step transition distribution Q^2 reduces to the nonuniqueness of the square root of ϑ^2. Let us assume that we know the sign of ϑ; say ϑ is positive. This knowledge is realistic in many applications. We can estimate ϑ^2 by the least squares estimator

$$\hat{s} = \frac{\sum_{j=1}^{n} X_{2j-2} X_{2j}}{\sum_{j=1}^{n} X_{2j-2}^2}.$$

Then $\hat{\vartheta} = \hat{s}^{1/2}$ estimates ϑ.

It remains to estimate f. We introduce three different approaches. All are solutions of certain deconvolution problems. Write $\varphi_Y(t) = E[\exp(itY)]$ for the characteristic function of a random variable Y.

1. The most straightforward estimator for f uses only the autoregressive representation (29.2), which implies

$$\varphi_X(t) = \varphi_{\vartheta X}(t)\varphi_\varepsilon(t) = \varphi_X(\vartheta t)\varphi_\varepsilon(t).$$

Estimate φ_X by the empirical characteristic function

$$\hat{\varphi}_X(t) = \frac{1}{n}\sum_{j=1}^{n} \exp(itX_{2j}).$$

An estimator for φ_ε is then given by

$$\hat{\varphi}_{\varepsilon,1}(t) = \frac{\hat{\varphi}_X(t)}{\hat{\varphi}_X(\hat{\vartheta}t)}.$$

Let K be a kernel, φ_K its characteristic function, and b a bandwidth that tends to zero as n tends to infinity. By Fourier inversion we arrive at an estimator for f,

$$\hat{f}_1(x) = \frac{1}{2\pi}\int \exp(-itx)\varphi_K(bt)\hat{\varphi}_{\varepsilon,1}(t)\,dt.$$

2. Another estimator for f uses only the moving average representation (29.4) of the η_{2j}. It is based on the approach of Belomestny (2003); see also Belomestny and Prokhorov (2003) and Belomestny (2005). Belomestny considers i.i.d. random variables Y_1 and Y_2 and estimates their density on the basis of i.i.d. observations distributed as $\vartheta Y_1 + Y_2$. The moving average representation (29.4) is of this form, but we do not know ϑ and do not observe the η_{2j} and must replace them by an estimator $\hat{\vartheta}$ and residuals $\hat{\eta}_{2j} = X_{2j} - \hat{s} X_{2j-2}$. From (29.4) we obtain

$$\varphi_\eta(t) = \varphi_\varepsilon(t)\varphi_{\vartheta\varepsilon}(t) = \varphi_\varepsilon(t)\varphi_\varepsilon(\vartheta t).$$

Iteratively solving for φ_ε we arrive at the representation

$$\varphi_\varepsilon(t) = \frac{\varphi_\eta(t)}{\varphi_\varepsilon(\vartheta t)} = \prod_{r=0}^{\infty} \frac{\varphi_\eta(\vartheta^{2r}t)}{\varphi_\eta(\vartheta^{2r+1}t)}.$$

Estimate φ_η by the residual-based empirical characteristic function

$$\hat{\varphi}_\eta(t) = \frac{1}{n}\sum_{j=1}^{n} \exp(it\hat{\eta}_{2j}).$$

An estimator for φ_ε is then given by

$$\hat{\varphi}_{\varepsilon,2}(t) = \prod_{r=0}^{N} \frac{\hat{\varphi}_\eta(\hat{s}^r t)}{\hat{\varphi}_\eta(\hat{\vartheta}^{2r+1}t)}$$

with N tending to infinity. By Fourier inversion we arrive at a second estimator for f,

$$\hat{f}_2(x) = \frac{1}{2\pi}\int \exp(-itx)\varphi_K(bt)\hat{\varphi}_{\varepsilon,2}(t)\,dt.$$

3. A third estimator for f uses (29.2) together with the autoregression representation (29.3) of the observations X_{2j}. They give

$$\varphi_X(t) = \varphi_X(\vartheta t)\varphi_\varepsilon(t) \quad \text{and} \quad \varphi_X(t) = \varphi_X(\vartheta^2 t)\varphi_\eta(t)$$

and hence

$$\varphi_\varepsilon(t) = \frac{\varphi_X(\vartheta^2 t)\varphi_\eta(t)}{\varphi_X(\vartheta t)}.$$

An estimator for φ_ε is therefore given by

$$\hat{\varphi}_{\varepsilon,3}(x) = \frac{\hat{\varphi}_X(\hat{s}t)\hat{\varphi}_\eta(t)}{\hat{\varphi}_X(\hat{\vartheta}t)}.$$

By Fourier inversion we arrive at a third estimator for f,

$$\hat{f}_3(x) = \frac{1}{2\pi}\int \exp(-itx)\varphi_K(bt)\hat{\varphi}_{\varepsilon,3}(t)\,dt.$$

The estimator $\hat{f}_1$ is the easiest to calculate. However, the representation of φ_ε as a ratio $\varphi_X/\varphi_{\vartheta X}$ does not lead to a good estimator of φ_ε and f. It is comparable with the usual deconvolution estimators treated in the literature; see Fan (1991) for their convergence rates, which can be very slow. The estimators $\hat{f}_2$ and $\hat{f}_3$ do not have this disadvantage, at least not to the same extent. This is easier to explain for $\hat{f}_3$, which is based on the representation of φ_ε as $\varphi_{\vartheta^2 X}\varphi_\eta/\varphi_{\vartheta X}$ whose tail behavior is governed by the numerator. Of course, $\hat{\varphi}_{\varepsilon,3}$ and $\hat{f}_3$ are preferable because they are simpler than $\hat{\varphi}_{\varepsilon,2}$ and $\hat{f}_2$. Apart from this, $\hat{f}_2$ and $\hat{f}_3$ have similar convergence rates.

Let g denote the density of the innovation η_{2j}. Paradoxically, it can be estimated at a better rate than the density of the innovation ε_j of the fully observed time series. From (29.4) we have the representation

$$g(y) = \int f(y - \vartheta x)f(x)\,dx$$

and can estimate g by the plug-in estimator

$$\hat{g}(y) = \int \hat{f}(y - \hat{\vartheta}x)\hat{f}(x)\,dx,$$

where $\hat{f}$ is $\hat{f}_2$ or $\hat{f}_3$. The estimator $\hat{g}$ can be root-n consistent; compare Frees (1994), Schick and Wefelmeyer (2004a, 2007), and Giné and Mason (2007) for related results.

29.3.3 Higher lags

Versions of the three estimators $\hat{f}_1$, $\hat{f}_2$, $\hat{f}_3$ can also be constructed if we observe the AR(1) process each kth time only. We have seen that an AR(1) process, observed every second time, is again AR(1), with different innovation distribution and autoregression parameter. If we observe the process each kth time only, we also have an AR(1) process

$$X_{kj} = \vartheta^k X_{k(j-1)} + \eta_{kj} \tag{29.5}$$

with innovations

$$\eta_{kj} = \sum_{i=0}^{k-1} \vartheta^i \varepsilon_{kj-i}. \tag{29.6}$$

Suppose we observe $X_0, X_k, \ldots, X_{kn}$. Then ϑ^k can be estimated by the least squares estimator

$$\hat{s} = \frac{\sum_{j=1}^{n} X_{k(j-1)}X_{kj}}{\sum_{j=1}^{n} X_{k(j-1)}^2}.$$

If k is even, we cannot identify the sign of ϑ and will again assume that we know ϑ to be positive. Then $\hat{\vartheta} = \hat{s}^{1/k}$ estimates ϑ.

A version of $\hat{f}_1$ is obtained by using again the Fourier inverse of

$$\hat{\varphi}_{\varepsilon,1}(t) = \frac{\hat{\varphi}_X(t)}{\hat{\varphi}_X(\hat{\vartheta}t)},$$

now with the empirical characteristic function

$$\hat{\varphi}_X(t) = \frac{1}{n}\sum_{j=1}^{n}\exp(itX_{kj}).$$

In view of (29.5) and (29.6) we obtain

$$\varphi_X(t) = \varphi_\eta(t)\varphi_X(\vartheta^k t) \tag{29.7}$$

and then, by the representation (29.2),

$$\varphi_\varepsilon(t) = \frac{\varphi_X(t)}{\varphi_X(\vartheta t)} = \frac{\varphi_\eta(t)\varphi_X(\vartheta^k t)}{\varphi_X(\vartheta t)}. \tag{29.8}$$

A version of $\hat{\varphi}_{\varepsilon,3}$ is therefore

$$\hat{\varphi}_{\varepsilon,3}(t) = \frac{\hat{\varphi}_\eta(t)\hat{\varphi}_X(\hat{s}t)}{\hat{\varphi}_X(\hat{\vartheta}t)},$$

now with empirical characteristic function

$$\hat{\varphi}_\eta(t) = \frac{1}{n}\sum_{j=1}^{n}\exp(it\hat{\eta}_{kj})$$

based on residuals $\hat{\eta}_{kj} = X_{kj} - \hat{s}X_{k(j-1)}$. An estimator for f is now obtained by Fourier inversion of $\hat{\varphi}_{\varepsilon,3}$.

For a version of the second estimator, $\hat{f}_2$, we apply (29.7) repeatedly to (29.8) and obtain

$$\varphi_\varepsilon(t) = \frac{\varphi_\eta(t)\varphi_X(\vartheta^k t)}{\varphi_\eta(\vartheta t)\varphi_X(\vartheta^{k+1}t)} = \frac{\varphi_\eta(t)}{\varphi_\eta(\vartheta t)}\prod_{r=1}^{\infty}\frac{\varphi_\eta(\vartheta^{kr}t)}{\varphi_\eta(\vartheta^{kr+1}t)}.$$

From this we obtain a version of $\hat{\varphi}_{\varepsilon,2}$ and hence of $\hat{f}_2$.

29.3.4   Higher-order autoregression

Generalizations of our results to higher-order autoregression are not straightforward. In general we lose the Markov property. Consider an AR(2) process

$$X_j = \vartheta_1 X_{j-1} + \vartheta_2 X_{j-2} + \varepsilon_j,$$

with innovations ε_j as before. Assume that the polynomial $1 - \vartheta_1 z - \vartheta_2 z^2$ does not have zeroes on the closed complex unit disk. Suppose we observe the process at even times only. We have

$$X_{2j} = \vartheta_1 X_{2j-1} + \vartheta_2 X_{2j-2} + \varepsilon_{2j}.$$

Replacing X_{2j-1} by its AR(2) representation, we obtain

$$X_{2j} = (\vartheta_1^2 + \vartheta_2) X_{2j-2} + \vartheta_1 \vartheta_2 X_{2j-3} + \varepsilon_{2j} + \vartheta_1 \varepsilon_{2j-1}. \tag{29.9}$$

Iterating this for odd-numbered indices, we arrive at an ARMA(∞,∞) representation for X_{2j},

$$X_{2j} = (\vartheta_1^2 + \vartheta_2) X_{2j-2} + \sum_{i=1}^{\infty} \vartheta_1^2 \vartheta_2^i X_{2j-2i-2} + \varepsilon_{2j} + \vartheta_1 \varepsilon_{2j-1} + \sum_{i=1}^{\infty} \vartheta_1 \vartheta_2^i \varepsilon_{2j-2i-1}.$$

If we replace all X_{2j-i} by their AR(2) representations, we arrive at an AR(∞) representation for X_{2j}.

A simpler representation is obtained if we subtract

$$\vartheta_2 X_{2j-2} = \vartheta_2 (\vartheta_1 X_{2j-3} + \vartheta_2 X_{2j-4} + \varepsilon_{2j-2})$$

from (29.9). This gives the ARMA(2,2) representation

$$X_{2j} - (\vartheta_1^2 + 2\vartheta_2) X_{2j-2} + \vartheta_2^2 X_{2j-4} = \varepsilon_{2j} + \vartheta_1 \varepsilon_{2j-1} - \vartheta_2 \varepsilon_{2j-2}.$$

The parameters are identifiable if we know their signs.

Such a representation can be obtained for arbitrary ARMA(p,q) processes observed at even times. Introduce polynomials $\varrho(z) = 1 + \varrho_1 z + \cdots + \varrho_p z^p$ and $\varphi(z) = 1 + \varphi_1 z + \cdots + \varphi_q z^q$. Assume that ϱ does not vanish on the closed complex unit disk. Define the backshift operator by $BX_j = X_{j-1}$. Consider the ARMA(p,q) process

$$\varrho(B) X_j = \varphi(B) \varepsilon_j,$$

with ε_j as before. Let $\varrho_1^*, \ldots, \varrho_p^*$ denote the zeroes of ϱ. They lie outside the unit disk. Factor ϱ as

$$\varrho(z) = \prod_{i=1}^{p} (z - \varrho_i^*).$$

Introduce the polynomials

$$\varrho_2(z) = \prod_{i=1}^{p} (z - \varrho_i^{*2}), \qquad \varrho_+(z) = \prod_{i=1}^{p} (z + \varrho_i^*).$$

We can write

$$\varrho_2(z^2) = \prod_{i=1}^{p} (z^2 - \varrho_i^{*2}) = \prod_{i=1}^{p} (z + \varrho_i^*)(z - \varrho_i^*) = \varrho_+(z) \varrho(z)$$

and obtain an ARMA($p,p+q$) representation for the ARMA(p,q) process observed at even times only:

$$\varrho_2(B^2)X_{2j} = \varrho_+(B)\varphi(B)\varepsilon_{2j}.$$

We *retain* a Markovian representation if we have observations in blocks of length at least equal to the order of the process. For example, suppose we do not see every third observation of the AR(2) process, so our observations are (X_{3j-2}, X_{3j-1}) for $j = 1, \ldots, n$, say. Then we can write

$$X_{3j+1} = (\vartheta_1^2 + \vartheta_2)X_{3j-1} + \vartheta_1\vartheta_2 X_{3j-2} + \varepsilon_{3j+1} + \vartheta_1\varepsilon_{3j}$$

and

$$X_{3j+2} = \vartheta_1 X_{3j+1} + \vartheta_1\vartheta_2 X_{3j-1} + \vartheta_2^2 X_{3j-2} + \varepsilon_{3j+2} + \vartheta_2\varepsilon_{3j}.$$

This means that the observations (X_{3j-2}, X_{3j-1}) follow an alternating autoregressive process, with orders alternating between 2 and 3, and independent innovations $\eta_{3j+1} = \varepsilon_{3j+1} + \vartheta_1\varepsilon_{3j}$, $j = 1, \ldots, n$, and $\eta_{3j+2} = \varepsilon_{3j+2} + \vartheta_2\varepsilon_{3j}$, $j = 1, \ldots, n$, respectively. Note, however, that for fixed j the innovations η_{3j+1} and η_{3j+2} depend on each other. The observations (X_{3j-2}, X_{3j-1}) can also be viewed as a two-dimensional autoregressive process of order 3.

In both cases described above we have obtained ARMA(p,q) representations for the partially observed process. Such representations can again be used to construct estimators for the innovation density. Consider an ARMA(2,2) process of the form

$$X_j + aX_{j-1} + bX_{j-2} = \varepsilon_j + c\varepsilon_{j-1} + d\varepsilon_{j-2} = \eta_j.$$

To construct an estimator analogous to $\hat{f}_2$, write

$$\varphi_\varepsilon(t) = \frac{\varphi_\eta(t)}{\varphi_\varepsilon(ct)\varphi_\varepsilon(dt)},$$

replace $\varphi_\varepsilon(ct)$ and $\varphi_\varepsilon(dt)$ by such ratios to obtain

$$\varphi_\varepsilon(t) = \frac{\varphi_\eta(t)\varphi_\varepsilon(c^2t)\varphi_\varepsilon(d^2t)\varphi_\varepsilon^2(cdt)}{\varphi_\eta(ct)\varphi_\eta(dt)},$$

and iterate these steps to obtain an infinite product in terms of φ_η. An estimator for φ_η can be based on residuals $\hat{\eta}_j = X_j + \hat{a}X_{j-1} + \hat{b}X_{j-2}$.

Acknowledgements

Anton Schick was supported in part by NSF Grant DMS 0405791. We thank an editor and a referee for their suggestions.

References

1. Belomestny, D. (2003). Rates of convergence for constrained deconvolution problem, Technical Report, arXiv:math.ST/0306237.

2. Belomestny, D. (2005). Reconstruction of a general distribution from the distribution of some statistics, *Theory of Probability and Its Applications*, **49**, 1–15.

3. Belomestny, D. and Prokhorov, A. V. (2003). On the problem of reconstructing the general distribution from the distribution of a linear statistic, *Moscow University Mathematics Bulletin*, **58**, 1–6.

4. Bickel, P. J. (1993). Estimation in semiparametric models, In *Multivariate Analysis: Future Directions* (Ed., C. R. Rao), pp. 55–73, North-Holland, Amsterdam.

5. Bickel, P. J. and Kwon, J. (2001). Inference for semiparametric models: Some questions and an answer (with discussion), *Statistica Sinica*, **11**, 863–960.

6. Fan, J. (1991). On the optimal rates of convergence for nonparametric deconvolution problems, *Annals of Statistics*, **19**, 1257–1272.

7. Frees, E. W. (1994). Estimating densities of functions of observations, *Journal of the American Statistical Association*, **89**, 517–525.

8. Giné, E. and Mason, D. (2007). On local U-statistic processes and the estimation of densities of functions of several sample variables, *Annals of Statistics*, **35**(3), 1105–1145.

9. Greenwood, P. E. and Wefelmeyer, W. (1995). Efficiency of empirical estimators for Markov chains, *Annals of Statistics*, **23**, 132–143.

10. Greenwood, P. E., Müller, U. U., and Wefelmeyer, W. (2004). Efficient estimation for semiparametric semi-Markov processes, *Communications in Statistics Theory and Methods*, **33**, 419–435.

11. Little, R. J. A. and Rubin, D. B. (2002). *Statistical Analysis With Missing Data*, Second Edition, Wiley Series in Probability and Statistics, Wiley-Interscience, Hoboken, NJ.

12. Meyn, S. P. and Tweedie, R. L. (1993). *Markov Chains and Stochastic Stability*, Communications and Control Engineering Series, Springer-Verlag, London.

13. Müller, U. U., Schick, A., and Wefelmeyer, W. (2001). Improved estimators for constrained Markov chain models, *Statistics & Probability Letters*, **54**, 427–435.

14. Müller, U. U., Schick, A., and Wefelmeyer, W. (2006). Imputing responses that are not missing, In *Probability, Statistics and Modelling in Public Health* (Eds., N. Nikulin, D. Commenges, and C. Huber), pp. 350–363, Springer-Verlag, New York.

15. Penev, S. (1991). Efficient estimation of the stationary distribution for exponentially ergodic Markov chains, *Journal of Statistical Planning and Inference*, **27**, 105–123.

16. Schick, A. and Wefelmeyer, W. (2004a). Root n consistent and optimal density estimators for moving average processes, *Scandinavian Journal of Statistics*, **31**, 63–78.

17. Schick, A. and Wefelmeyer, W. (2004b). Functional convergence and optimality of plug-in estimators for stationary densities of moving average processes. *Bernoulli*, **10**, 889–917.

18. Schick, A. and Wefelmeyer, W. (2007). Root-n consistent density estimators of convolutions in weighted L_1-norms, *Journal of Statistical Planning and Inference*, **137**(6), 1765–1774.

19. Tsiatis, A. A. (2006). *Semiparametric Theory and Missing Data*, Springer Series in Statistics, Springer-Verlag, New York.

20. Van der Laan, M. J. and Robins, J. M. (2003). *Unified Methods for Censored Longitudinal Data and Causality*, Springer Series in Statistics, Springer-Verlag, New York.

30

On Solving Statistical Problems for the Stochastic Processes by the Sufficient Empirical Averaging Method

Alexander Andronov,[1] **Evgeniy Chepurin,**[2] **and Asaf Hajiyev**[3]

[1]*Faculty of Transport and Mechanical Engineering, Riga Technical University, Riga, Latvia*
[2]*Faculty of Mechanics and Mathematics, Moscow State University, Moscow, Russia*
[3]*Department of Probability and Statistics, Institute of Cybernetic, Baku, Azerbaijan*

Abstract: A problem of the statistical estimation of stochastic process functionals is considered. The sufficient empirical averaging method is used. The method requires the existence of the complete sufficient statistics for unknown parameters. Some examples are considered.

Keywords and Phrases: Stochastic process, functional, complete sufficient statistic

30.1 Introduction

The problems of the calculation of optimal point estimates for characteristics of random process functionals, characteristics of scattering of these estimates, and also estimates of observed significance levels for a criteria adequacy of model and experimental data occasionally can be successfully solved by using the *sufficient empirical averaging* (SEA) method that has been proposed by Chepurin (1994, 1995, 1999). The method of obtaining statistical results on the basis of the SEA method consists of the following steps. Let a statistical model $(Y, \mathcal{B}, \mathcal{P})$ generate sample data $y \in Y$ and admit a complete sufficient statistic $S(y)$. Here Y is a sampling space, $\mathcal{B} = \{A\}$ is a sigma-algebra on Y, $\mathcal{P} = \{P\{A; \theta\}, \theta \in \Theta\}$ is a family of probability measures, and Θ is the parametric space. It is proposed that y is generated by a probability measure with the unknown parameter θ_0, y is a trajectory of $Y(t)$, $0 \le t \le T$, and $Y(t)$ is a random process. Let us define the conditional distribution $Q(A; s_0) = P\{A|S(y) = s_0; \theta_0\}$. Note that $Q(\cdot; s_0)$ is free of $\theta_0 \in \Theta$. Suppose also that we can simulate a sequence of data variants $y_1^*, \ldots, y_B^*$, where i.i.d. random variables y_i^* are generated by $Q(\cdot; s_0)$. It is well known [Lehmann (1983)] that each data variant y_i^* is statistically equivalent to y.

Consider at first problems of unbiased point estimation of $g(\theta_0) = E\{G(T, Y(t)$ for $0 \le t \le T); \theta_0\}$, where $G(T, Y(t), \ 0 \le t \le T)$ is interesting for the functional of $Y(t)$. Let $z(y)$ be an easily calculated unbiased estimator for $g(\theta_0)$; that is, $E\{z(y); \theta_0\} = g(\theta_0)$. Then the SEA estimate of $g(\theta_0)$ is

$$\hat{g}_B(S) = B^{-1} \sum_{i=1}^{B} z(y_i^*). \qquad (30.1)$$

Let $\hat{g}^0(S) = E\{z(y)|S\}$. It is the uniformly minimum variance unbiased estimator of $g(\theta)$. If $V\{z(y); \theta_0\} < \infty$ then Equation (30.1) gives the consistent estimate of $\hat{g}^0(S)$ as $B \to \infty$, $E\{\hat{g}_B(S); \theta\} = g(\theta)$ and calculated by means of B data variance

$$V_B\{\hat{g}_B(S); \theta_0\} = V\{\hat{g}^0(S); \theta_0\} + \frac{1}{B}(V\{z(y); \theta_0\} - V\{\hat{g}^0(S); \theta_0\}). \qquad (30.2)$$

From Equation (30.2) it is easy to choose B for desired proximity of $\hat{g}_B(s)$ and $\hat{g}^0(s)$. Often one can also get an unbiased estimator for $V\{\hat{g}^0(s); \theta\}$ and other scattering characteristics of $\hat{g}^0(s)$. Notice that many of the unbiased estimation problems can be solved without difficult calculation of probability measures $Q(\cdot; s_0)$ and $E\{G(T, Y(t)$ for $0 \le t \le T); \theta_0\}$.

Furthermore, everywhere it is supposed that

$$z(y) = G(T, Y(t) \quad for \quad 0 \le t \le T).$$

The chapter is organized as follows. The next section contains a description of the base model. The further two sections are devoted to plans of observations. Procedures of data variant generation are considered in Section 30.5. Numerical examples are given in the last section.

30.2   Base Model

We consider the labelled random process $Y(t)$ that is determined by the sequence $\{\tau_n, \eta_n\}$, $n = 1, 2, \ldots$, where $\tau_n \in R_+^1$ is a moment of the process events (of the process jumps) and $\eta_n = (\eta_{n,1}, \eta_{n,2}, \ldots, \eta_{n,m})^T$ is the corresponding label $\eta_n \in R^m$. Note that a part of η_n can be integers. It is supposed that the sequences $\{\tau_n\}$ and $\{\eta_n\}$ are independent. Furthermore let $K(t) = max\{n : \tau_n \le t\}$ be a number of the process events on the interval $[0, t]$. It is known that the sample trajectory of the process $K(t)$ is statistically equivalent to an evolution of the sequence $\{\tau_n\}$, the jump moments of the process $K(t)$.

Many problems of queueing theory, reliability, insurance, inventory, and so on can be presented as search problems of the expectation for a functional $G(T, Y(t), 0 < t \leq T)$ where T is a fixed time moment. Let θ_0 be a generating parameter of the process $Y(t)$. If its value is unknown then there arises a search problem of the optimal unbiased estimate for $E\{G(T, Y(t), 0 < t \leq T); \theta_0\}$. Note that the corresponding unbiased estimate exists for special observation plans about the process $Y(t)$ only. Thus it exists for the following plans, for example.

- Plan of A-type: the process $Y(t)$ is observed in the interval $\{0, T\}$.
- Plan of B-type: a time moment of observation ending coincides with $\tau_{n(0)}$, where $n(0)$ is such that

$$P\{K(T) \leq n(0); \theta_0\} = 1. \tag{30.3}$$

Unfortunately for the substantial practical problems usually it is impossible to find an analytical expression for the optimal unbiased estimate. On the other hand it is often possible to find the unbiased estimate that is very close to the optimal one. These estimates can be obtained by using the *sufficient empirical averaging* method.

30.3 On a Class of Processes with the Complete Sufficient Statistics for the Plans of A-Type

In the current section it is supposed that $\theta_0 = (\theta_{0,1}, \theta_{0,2})$ where $\theta_{0,1}$ determines the distribution of the sequence $\{\tau_n\}$, $\theta_{0,2}$ determines the distribution of the label sequence $\{\eta_n\}$. We suppose that the statistical model generating the process $Y(t)$ admits a complete sufficient statistic $S_1 = K(T)$ for the sequence $\{\tau_1, \tau_2, \ldots, \tau_{K(T)}\}$. It means that joint probability density of the random sequence $\{\tau_1, \tau_2, \ldots, \tau_{K(T)}; K(T)\}$ can be represented in the following way,

$$Lc'(\tau_1, \tau_2, \ldots, \tau_{K(T)}; K(T)) = V(t_1, t_2, \ldots, t_k)exp\{-\theta_{0,1}k + a_1(\theta_{0,1}) + b_1(k)\},$$

where $V(t_1, t_2, \ldots, t_k)$ is an arbitrary joint probability density of the vector $\{\tau_1, \tau_2, \ldots, \tau_k\}$ on the set $0 < t_1 < t_2 < \cdots < t_k \leq T$.

Here and below $a_i(.)$ and $b_i(.)$ are components of density representation for the one-index exponential family.

Furthermore let S_2 be a restricted complete sufficient statistic for the family of the conditional random sequence of the labels $\{\eta_1, \eta_2, \ldots, \eta_{K(T)}|K(T) = k\}$. It is simple to show that $S = (S_1, S_2)$ is the complete sufficient statistic for $\theta_0 = (\theta_{0,1}, \theta_{0,2})$. As for a structure of $Y^*(t)$ (a date variant for the labelled random process), it is described in the following way. $Y^*(t)$ is determined uniquely by the sequence

$$(t_1^*, \eta_1^*), (t_2^*, \eta_2^*), \ldots, (t_k^*, \eta_k^*),$$

where $(t_1^*, t_2^*, \ldots, t_k^*)$ are generated by the probability density $V(.)$ and $(\eta_1^*, \eta_2^*, \ldots, \eta_k^*)$ are a date variant for the sequence of the labels $(\eta_1, \eta_2, \ldots, \eta_k)$ provided fixed values of the complete sufficient statistic S_2.

Let us consider an important particular example of the point process, for which $K(t)$ is the complete sufficient statistic.

Example. Mixed Poisson process. Let $K(t)$, $0 \le t \le T$, be the standard Poisson process with the parameter $\lambda > 0$, with λ a realization of the random variable Λ with the probability density from the one-index exponential family:

$$Lc'(\Lambda) = exp\{-\lambda/\sigma_0 + a_2(\lambda) + b_2(\sigma_0)\},$$

so $\theta_{0,1} = 1/\sigma_0$.

Let us show that $K(T)$ is the complete sufficient statistic and the conditional probability density $Lc'(\tau_1, \tau_2, \ldots, \tau_{K(T)} | K(T) = k)$ coincides with the probability density of the order statistic set for a sample from k independent but distributed on $[0, T]$ random variables. Actually (below $t_0 = 0$)

$$Lc'(\tau_1, \tau_2, \ldots, \tau_{K(T)}; K(T) = k) = \int_0^\infty \left(\prod_{i=1}^k \lambda e^{-\lambda(t_i - t_{i-1})} \right) \exp\{-\lambda (T - t_k)\}$$

$$\exp\left\{ -\frac{\lambda}{\sigma_0} + a_2(\lambda) + b_2(\sigma_0) \right\} d\lambda$$

$$= \frac{k!}{T^k} \int_0^\infty \frac{1}{k!} (\lambda T)^k e^{-\lambda T} \exp\left\{ -\frac{\lambda}{\sigma_0} + a_2(\lambda) + b_2(\sigma_0) \right\} d\lambda.$$

If we keep in mind that

$$Lc'(POIS(\Lambda T)) = \int_0^\infty \frac{1}{k!} (\lambda T)^k e^{-\lambda T} \exp\left\{ -\frac{\lambda}{\sigma_0} + a_2(\lambda) + b_2(\sigma_0) \right\} d\lambda$$

is the unconditional probability density of the random variable $K(T)$ then the above formulated statement about the structure of $Lc'(\tau_1, \tau_2, \ldots, \tau_{K(T)} | K(T) = k)$ becomes obvious.

Note that if we get

$$a_2(\lambda) = \ln \frac{\lambda^{a_0 - 1}}{\Gamma(a_0)}, \qquad b_2(\sigma_0) = -\ln \sigma_0^{a_0},$$

in other words if we assume Λ has gamma distribution with known form parameter a_0 and unknown scale parameter σ_0, then for the unconditional probability we have the negative binomial distribution:

$$P_S\{K(T) = k;\ \theta_{0,1}\} = \binom{a_0 + k - 1}{k} \left(\frac{1}{\sigma_0 T + 1}\right)^k \left(\frac{\sigma_0 T}{\sigma_0 T + 2}\right)^{a_0}.$$

Let us show the completeness of the unconditional distribution of $K(T)$. Actually let us have $E\{d_{K(T)};\ \theta_{0,1}\} \equiv 0$ for some sequence $\{d_0, d_1, \ldots\}$ and for all $\theta_{0,1} = \sigma_0$. Then

$$\sum_{k=0}^{\infty} d_k \int_0^{\infty} \frac{(\lambda T)^k}{k!} e^{-\lambda T} \exp\left\{-\frac{\lambda}{\sigma_0} + a_2(\lambda) + b_2(\sigma_0)\right\} d\lambda$$

$$= \int_0^{\infty} \left(\sum_{k=0}^{\infty} d_k \frac{(\lambda T)^k}{k!} e^{-\lambda T}\right) \exp\left\{-\frac{\lambda}{\sigma_0} + a_2(\lambda) + b_2(\sigma_0)\right\} d\lambda.$$

Now from the completeness of the distribution of the random variable Λ follows that

$$\sum_{k=0}^{\infty} d_k \frac{1}{k!} (\lambda T)^k e^{\lambda T} = 0 \ almost\ probably\ for\ all\ \lambda.$$

In turn, from the completeness of the Poisson distribution it follows that $d_k = 0$ for $k = 0, 1, \ldots$, so $K(T)$ is the complete sufficient statistic.

30.4 On Complete Sufficient Statistics for a Class of Labeled Processes with the Plans of B-Type

Let the sequence $\{\tau_n\}$ correspond to a recurrent flow for which sequential intervals $\varsigma_n = \tau_n - \tau_{n-1}$ are independent identically distributed random variables with the distribution density

$$Lc'(\varsigma_n) = \begin{cases} 0, & u \le \mu_0, \\ \sigma_0^{-1} \exp\{-(u - \mu_0)/\sigma_0\}, & u > \mu_0, \end{cases} \tag{30.4}$$

where $\sigma_0 > 0, \mu_0 > M$.

Here μ_0 and σ_0 are unknown parameters but M is a known value. We have a sample $\varsigma_1, \varsigma_2, \ldots, \varsigma_r$ of size r for corresponding random variables $\{\varsigma_n\}$, by that

$$r = n(0) \ge \left[\frac{T}{M}\right] + 1. \tag{30.5}$$

It is well known that the complete sufficient statistic for parameters μ_0 and σ_0 is the pair $S_1 = (\varsigma_{\min}, \Xi)$, where $\varsigma_{\min} = \min\{\varsigma_1, \varsigma_2, \ldots, \varsigma_r\}$,

$$\Xi = \sum_{i=1}^{r}(\varsigma_i - \varsigma_{\min}).$$

Furthermore let labels $\{\eta_n\}$ be a sequence of independent identically distributed random variables having complete sufficient statistics. Let S_2 be that value calculating the base of a sample of size at least $n(0)$. Obviously $S = (S_1, S_2)$ is the complete sufficient statistic for the considered random process.

Now we are able to generate the data variants of the described random process $Y^*(t)$ using statistics S_1 and S_2.

30.5   On Procedures of Data Variant Generation

The problem of a data variant generation is crucial for the possibility of realization of the considered method. To simulate the data variant it is necessary to know the conditional distribution of the data variant and to generate corresponding random variables. Usually it is very difficult to find an explicit form for the conditional distribution, because it is a distribution on the hypersurface in a space of high dimension [see Andronov *et al.* (2005)]. On the other hand, to generate corresponding random variables is a complicated problem too. Here two ways are possible. Firstly, often we can generate the random variables of interest directly, without knowledge of the corresponding distribution. Such examples were given by Chepurin (1995, 1999) and Engen and Lillegard (1997). Let us illustrate this approach.

We consider a procedure of data variant generation for distribution (30.4) on a base of the complete sufficient statistic $S_1 = (\varsigma_{\min}, \Xi)$, that has been calculated on a sample of size r. We want to show how it is possible to generate a typical data variant $\varsigma_1^*, \varsigma_2^*, \ldots, \varsigma_r^*$.

We generate a random integer number N that has the uniform distribution on set $\{1, 2, \ldots, r\}$ and set $\varsigma_N^* = \varsigma_{\min}$. Furthermore, $r - 1$ independent exponentially distributed with parameter 1 random variables $\vartheta_1, \vartheta_2, \ldots, \vartheta_{r-1}$ are generated and their sum $\tilde{\Xi} = \vartheta_1 + \vartheta_2 + \cdots + \vartheta_{r-1}$ is calculated. Finally we end the generation procedure setting

$$\varsigma_n^* = \begin{cases} \vartheta_n \Xi/\tilde{\Xi} + \varsigma_{\min}, & n < N, \\ \vartheta_{n-1}\Xi/\tilde{\Xi} + \varsigma_{\min}, & n > N. \end{cases}$$

Secondly, it is possible to apply *Gibbs sampling*; see Gentle (2002). This approach uses a decomposition of the multivariate probability density into a marginal and then a sequence of conditionals. We begin with the univariate marginal distribution (provided fixed value of the corresponding complete sufficient statistic) and generate the first random variable χ_n^*. Then we recount the value of the statistic and use one for the generation of the next random variable χ_{n-1}^* and so on.

We illustrate this approach for a sample $\chi_1, \chi_2, \ldots, \chi_n$ from the normal population $N(\mu, \sigma)$. In this case the complete sufficient statistic is $S = (\mu_n^*, \sigma_n^{2*})$,

$$\mu_n^* = \frac{1}{n}\sum_{i=1}^{n}\chi_i, \qquad \sigma_n^{2*} = \frac{1}{n-1}\sum_{i=1}^{n}(\chi_i - \mu_n^*)^2.$$

The conditional random variable χ_n^* by the condition $S = (\mu_n^*, \sigma_n^{2*})$ has the following probability density.

$$Lc'\left(\chi_n^* | \mu_n^*, \sigma_n^{2*}\right) = \frac{\sqrt{n}\,\Gamma\left(\frac{n-1}{2}\right)}{(n-1)\sqrt{\pi\sigma_n^{2*}}\,\Gamma\left(\frac{n-2}{2}\right)}\left(1 - \frac{n}{(n-1)^2\sigma_n^{2*}}(x - \mu_n^*)^2\right)^{\frac{n}{2}-2},$$

$$\mu_n^* - \frac{n-1}{\sqrt{n}}\sqrt{\sigma_n^{2*}} \le x \le \mu_n^* + \frac{n-1}{\sqrt{n}}\sqrt{\sigma_n^{2*}}.$$

Now we generate χ_n^* using, for example, *acceptance/rejection* or *inverse cumulative distribution function* methods. Furthermore, we recount the value of the statistic S by the formulas

$$\mu_{n-1}^* = \frac{1}{n-1}(n\mu_n^* - \chi_n^*), \qquad \sigma_{n-1}^{2*} = \frac{n-1}{n-2}\left(\sigma_n^{2*} - \frac{1}{n}(\chi_n^* - \mu_{n-1}^*)^2\right).$$

The consequent iterations give the sequence $\chi_n^*, \chi_{n-1}^*, \ldots, \chi_4^*, \chi_3^*$. Two last values are calculated by formulas

$$\chi_2^* = \mu_2^* + \sqrt{\frac{1}{2}\sigma_2^{2*}}, \qquad \chi_2^* = \mu_1^* - \sqrt{\frac{1}{2}\sigma_2^{2*}}.$$

30.6   Numerical Examples

Example 1 (Ruin problem) We consider the following modification of the classical model of an insurance risk business [Grandell (1991)]. An insurance company has initial capital of size u. The claims occur according to a mixed Poisson process as described in the third section. The costs of the claims are described by a sequence $\{\eta_1, \eta_2, \ldots\}$ of independent and identically distributed random variables, having normal distribution. The premium income of the company is defined by a positive real constant c.

Table 30.1. Estimates $\hat{\Psi}(u, 50)$ of ruin probability $\Psi(u, 50)$

u	100	110	120	130	140	150	160	170	180
$\hat{\Psi}(u, 50)$	0.996	0.988	0.966	0.927	0.844	0.812	0.727	0.643	0.529

u	190	200	210	220	230	240	250	260	270
$\hat{\Psi}(u, 50)$	0.445	0.327	0.263	0.195	0.135	0.111	0.070	0.051	0.026

The *risk process* Y is defined by

$$Y(t) = ct - \sum_{n=1}^{K(t)} \eta_n. \tag{30.6}$$

The *ruin probability till time moment* T for the company having initial capital u is defined by

$$\Psi(u, T) = P\{u + Y(t) < 0 \text{ for some moment } t \in (0, T)\}.$$

Constants T and c are known. Parameters of the mixed Poison process and the normal distribution are unknown, but complete sufficient statistics $K(T)$ and (μ_n^*, σ_n^{2*}) are given. Our aim is to estimate ruin probability $\Psi(u, T)$.

For that we apply the usual simulation. Necessary random variables are generated as described in Section 30.5.

The results we received are presented in Table 30.1. They correspond to the following values of the constants and statistics: $c = 0.01$, $T = 50$, $K(T) = 20$, $n = 20$, $\mu_{20}^* = 40$, and $\sigma_{20}^{2*} = 10$. Number B of the simulation runs equals 2000.

With respect to the above-considered statements, the presented values are close to minimum variance unbiased estimates of the ruin probabilities.

Example 2 (Queueing system) Let us consider a queueing system with two servers. Interarrival times of customers $\varsigma_1, \varsigma_2, \ldots$ are i.i.d. random variables, which have shifted exponential distribution (30.4).

The servers are different (nonhomogeneous). Service times are i.i.d. random variables having exponential distribution with various parameters $\sigma_0^{(1)}$ and $\sigma_0^{(2)}$ for the servers. These parameters are unknown. If both servers are busy when a customer arrives, then the customer must join a queue (i.e., wait in line). From the queue customers go to the server in accordance with their own arrival times. If both servers are empty when a customer arrives then the customer goes to a server that has been cleared earlier. Let's find the nonstationary distribution of the number $Y(t)$ of customers in the system at the time moment t, $0 < t < T$:

$$P_j(t) = P\{Y(t) = j\}, \qquad j = 0, 1, \ldots.$$

Table 30.2. Estimates for probabilities $\{P_j(t)\}$ of the number of customers in the system

t	0	1	2	3	4	5	6	7
$\hat{P}_0(t)$	1	0.556	0.348	0.247	0.219	0.198	0.186	0.178
$\hat{P}_1(t)$	0	0.444	0.478	0.466	0.412	0.409	0.402	0.370
$\hat{P}_2(t)$	0	0	0.163	0.229	0.266	0.263	0.261	0.272
$\hat{P}_3(t)$	0	0	0.011	0.053	0.084	0.096	0.105	0.123
$\hat{P}_4(t)$	0	0	0	0.005	0.018	0.030	0.037	0.042
$\hat{P}_{\geq 5}(t)$	0	0	0	0	0.001	0.004	0.009	0.015
t	8	9	10	11	12	13	14	15
$\hat{P}_0(t)$	0.170	0.158	0.156	0.157	0.155	0.157	0.154	0.159
$\hat{P}_1(t)$	0.365	0.366	0.356	0.367	0.355	0.340	0.353	0.341
$\hat{P}_2(t)$	0.266	0.272	0.265	0.259	0.265	0.264	0.257	0.265
$\hat{P}_3(t)$	0.127	0.125	0.136	0.127	0.131	0.139	0.135	0.134
$\hat{P}_4(t)$	0.050	0.054	0.058	0.060	0.064	0.062	0.061	0.060
$\hat{P}_{\geq 5}(t)$	0.022	0.026	0.028	0.031	0.032	0.038	0.040	0.041

We assume that originally the system was empty.

Let us remember that parameters μ_0 and σ_0 of distribution (30.4) and $\sigma_0^{(1)}$ and $\sigma_0^{(2)}$ are unknown but we have three samples of sizes r, n_1, n_2: interarrival times, and service times of the first and the second servers. Let $T < rM$, $r \leq n_1 \leq n_2$. The complete sufficient statistics for the interarrival time distribution (30.4) and data variant generation have been considered earlier. The complete sufficient statistics for parameters of exponential distribution of server times are the sums $S^{(1)}$ and $S^{(2)}$.

Our example corresponds to a general outline of Section 30.2. The random process $Y(t)$ is univariate and means the number of customers in the system at the time moment t. The probabilities of interest $\{P_j(t)\}$ are expectations of indicator functions $\{\chi_j(t)\}$ of events $\{Y(t) = j\} : \chi_j(t) = 1$ if event $\{Y(t) = j\}$ takes place and $\chi_j(t) = 0$ otherwise.

As usual these expectations are estimated by simulation of a corresponding queueing process. The received results are given in Table 30.2. They correspond to the following input data: $r = 30$, $n_1 = 22$, $n_2 = 22$, $\varsigma_{\min} = 0.5$, $\Xi = 20$, $S^{(1)} = 30$, $S^{(2)} = 40$, $T = 15$, $B = 1000$. According to the above, the presented values are close to minimum variance unbiased estimates of $\{P_j(t)\}$.

Finally it is possible to conclude that the supposed approach effectively applies to various models of queueing theory, reliability, inventory, insurance, and so on for practical problem solving [see, e.g., Kopytov and Zhukovskaya (2006)].

References

1. Andronov, A., Zhukovskaya, C., and Chepurin, E. (2005). On application of the sufficient empirical averaging method to systems simulation, In *Proceedings of the 12th International Conference on Analytical and Stochastic Modelling Technique and Applications*, pp. 144–150, Riga, Latvia.

2. Chepurin, E. V. (1994). The statistical methods in theory of reliability, *Obozrenije Prikladnoj i Promishlennoj Matematiki, Ser. Verojatnost i Statistika*, **1**, 279–330. (In Russian)

3. Chepurin, E. V. (1995). The statistical analysis of the Gauss data based on the sufficient empirical averaging method, In *Proceedings of the Russian University of People's Friendship. Series Applied Mathematics and Informatics*, pp. 112–125. (In Russian)

4. Chepurin, E. V. (1999). On analytic-computer methods of statistical inferences of small size data samples, In *Proceedings of the International Conference Probabilistic Analysis of Rare Events*, (Eds., V. V. Kalashnikov and A. M. Andronov), pp. 180–194, Riga Aviation University, Riga, Latvia.

5. Engen, S. and Lillegard, M. (1997). Stochastic simulations conditioned of sufficient statistics, *Biometrica*, **84**, 235–240.

6. Gentle, J. E. (2002). *Elements of Computational Statistics*, Springer-Verlag, New York.

7. Grandell, J. (1991). *Aspects of Risk Theory*, Springer-Verlag, New York.

8. Kopytov, E. and Zhukovskaya, C. (2006). Application of the sufficient empirical averaging method for inventory control problem solving, In *Proceeding of the International Conference Statistical Methods for Biomedical and Technical Systems* (Ed., F. Vonta), pp. 340–346, Limassol, Cyprus.

9. Lehmann, E. L. (1983). *Theory of Point Estimation*, John Wiley & Sons, New York.

PART VII
Designs

31

Adaptive Designs for Group Sequential Clinical Survival Experiments

Eric V. Slud

Statistics Program, University of Maryland, College Park, MD, USA

Abstract: Randomized two-group clinical survival experiments now commonly allow at least one interim look, enabling possible early stopping in order to meet ethical concerns. Various authors have also studied the possibility of interim design modifications to adapt to unexpected accrual or control-group mortality rates. This chapter formulates trial design as a decision-theoretic problem with a finite number of interim looks and a large class of loss functions, in the setting of a statistic with the asymptotic behavior of Brownian motion with drift, as in Leifer and Slud (2002). A more general action space can specify adaptive designs allowing the option of continued follow-up without new accrual past an interim look, as was introduced in Koutsoukos *et al.* (1998). An optimal two-look design is displayed in the first formulation, and a seven-look design in the second, and both types of adaptation are given a unified decision-theoretic motivation.

Keywords and Phrases: Accrual stopping, Bayesian decision theory, nonrandomized decision rule, loss function, nuisance parameter, stopping boundary

31.1 Introduction

Group sequential designs are designs in which experimental data on two-group treatment comparisons can be scrutinized at a finite number of interim look-times with the possibility of early termination of the experiment in such a way as to maintain a prescribed experimentwise significance level and power against a fixed alternative. Such designs first appeared for two-group randomized clinical trials with normally distributed quantitative responses in the mid-1960s. By the late 1970s, methods had appeared which took explicit account of the staggered entry, follow-up time, and delayed response of clinical trials with

survival-time endpoints. By the early 1980s, such methods were firmly established theoretically. Tsiatis (1982) showed that the repeatedly computed log-
rank–numerator statistic at a series of fixed scheduled interim look-times would
under standard conditions behave in large two-sample trials as a sequence of
independent-increment Gaussian variables, with mean 0 under the null hypothesis $\mathbf{H}_0$ of no treatment effect and with steady positive drift proportional to
variance under local proportional-hazard alternatives. As the theory developed,
look-times were allowed to be random (stopping-times for the observed information process), and additional classes of statistics including weighted log-rank
statistics (with weight functions also estimated from pooled two-group Kaplan–
Meier survival function estimators) were justified to be usable in the same way
as the log-rank, although the log-rank is the heavy practical favorite.

Slud and Wei (1982) showed how variance increments could be progressively
estimated while allowing early stopping by means of an α *-spending schedule*.
In a (one-sided) trial of sample size n, with the statistic $S_k/\sqrt{n}$ calculated at
the kth look-time t_k, a threshold or boundary b_k is used to stop the trial early
with rejection of $\mathbf{H}_0$ if $S_k/\sqrt{n} \geq b_k$, where b_k is found inductively, in terms of
the estimated large-sample variance V_k of $S_k/\sqrt{n}$, to satisfy

$$\alpha_k \approx \Pr(S_j/\sqrt{n} < b_j \quad \text{for} \quad 1 \leq j < k, \quad S_k/\sqrt{n} \geq b_k), \qquad (31.1)$$

where the values $\alpha_1, \ldots, \alpha_K$ are prescribed and sum to the experimentwise
significance level α. The times at which interim looks might be taken can be
allowed to be random stopping-times, for example, to be level-crossing times
for the proportional-hazard parameter's *information*, which is proportional to
the log-rank variance and thus also to the number of observed failure events.
Moreover, the choice of the specific value α_k need not be made until the $k - 1$th
look-time [Lan and DeMets (1983)]. The asymptotic theory underlying this
extension was given by Slud (1984) and other authors, establishing that under
local (contiguous) proportional-hazard alternatives the repeatedly computed
log-rank statistic considered as a stochastic process behaves asymptotically in
large samples as a time-changed Brownian motion with drift. The history of
these developments from the viewpoint of trial design, along with practical
recommendations on the choice among early-stopping designs as of 1984, can
be found in Fleming *et al.* (1984). The context of these results in the setting
of repeated significance testing within exponential families can be found in
Siegmund (1985).

Later progress on the specification of early-stopping boundaries included
generalizations beyond our scope here (more general statistics, adjustment for
covariates, modified formulations of repeated significance testing, etc.), but also
developed optimization methods. Tsiatis and co-authors restricted attention to
parametrically restricted families of boundaries and computed the ones that
minimized expected trial duration over boundaries with prescribed size and

average power against specified alternatives, whereas Jennison (1987) undertook a brute-force (grid-search) computation of optimal boundaries in the sense of minimizing a weighted linear combination of type-II error probabilities and expected sample sizes over specified alternatives, for given significance level.

Clinical investigators often find at the times of interim looks in clinical trials that planned accrual goals have not been met, or that due to noncompliance, lower than expected tolerated doses, or better survival than expected in the control group, power will be less than planned for against clinically meaningful alternatives. For this and other, ethical, reasons, there has been a perceived need for *adaptive* (group-) sequential trial designs accommodating flexibility in accrual rates through the spacing of look-times. However, the designs must explicitly take account of such flexibility: Proschan *et al.* (1992) nicely illustrate the adverse effects on the significance level of modifying look-time definitions and other trial assumptions in midtrial. Various authors [Bauer and Köhne (1994), Proschan and Hunsberger (1995), and others cited in Burman and Sonesson (2006)] have proposed methods of accommodating design changes (usually in sample size) after an interim look, resulting in procedures with valid experimentwise significance levels based on weighted combinations of statistic increments calculated up to and after the design changes. But there is active controversy [see Burman and Sonesson (2006), with discussion] concerning whether such adaptations are a good idea, or are even ethical, considering the loss of power they entail against the originally envisioned alternatives.

The accelerating pace of biomedical discovery due to the genomics revolution, discussed by Sen (2008) in this volume, highlights the dramatic opportunity costs from protracted clinical trials and from incorrect decisions based on them. A principled statistical response should take account of those costs, as well as the important ethical costs that arise from clinical trial errors. The approach followed in this chapter is decision-theoretic. We consider clinical trial designs which "adapt" to interim results subject to experimentwise type I and II error probability constraints, in such a way as to minimize the expected values of realistically structured loss functions.

This chapter has three objectives: first, in Section 31.2, to describe the Bayesian decision problem of Leifer and Slud (2002) incorporating multi-look trials with general loss components which penalize trial length and incorrect decisions as a function of the treatment-group difference parameter ϑ; second (Section 31.3), to describe how optimal decision procedures require later look-times and stopping-boundaries to depend on earlier observed statistic values, especially in the two-look case; and third, to describe a decision problem (in Section 31.2.2) motivating new design elements including those of Koutsoukos *et al.* (1998) described in Section 31.4, allowing group-sequential trials an option to stop accrual with or without early stopping, while maintaining experimentwise significance level.

31.2   Decision-Theoretic Formulation

Many theoretical results [Tsiatis (1982), Slud (1984), and Siegmund (1985)] justify that the sequence of two-sample (weighted-)log-rank statistics calculated at interim looks of a multi-look staggered-accrual clinical trial with survival endpoints under local proportional-hazard alternatives (and also more general classes of alternatives) is asymptotically equivalent in large datasets to sampled values of a Wiener process with drift, $X(t) = W(t) + \vartheta\, t$. Here ϑ is an unknown real parameter quantifying positive or negative relative prognosis for treatment-versus control-group patients in the trial. The natural timescale for estimation of the treatment difference parameter ϑ is *information time* [Siegmund (1985), and Andersen *et al.* (1993)], that is, the information about ϑ in the data up to time t. Increments of time are transformed by this statistical timescale, regarded as a function of nuisance parameters under near-null alternatives (i.e., those with $\vartheta \approx 0$). The nuisance parameters—all statistical parameters of the accrual, censoring, and survival mechanisms of the trial other than ϑ—are assumed to be consistently estimated at times of interim analysis of the data.

The objective of the trial is inference on ϑ to distinguish the null hypothesis $\vartheta \leq 0$ against alternatives with $\vartheta > 0$: process data $X(\tau_j)$ may be observed (only) at an increasing sequence of discrete times τ_j, $1 \leq j \leq K$, with τ_j allowed to be determined from $(\tau_i, X(\tau_i), i < j)$ (and, possibly, auxiliary randomizations independent of the data). The upper-bound K on the number of look-times is generally nonrandom and fixed, and the trial ends at the first time τ_ν for which either $\nu = K$ or $\tau_{\nu+1} = \tau_\nu$, at which time a binary decision $\chi \in \{0,1\}$ is made as a function of all observable data $(\tau_i,\ X(\tau_i),\ i \leq \nu)$. When actions $(\tau_i,\ 1 \leq i \leq \nu)$ and χ have been taken, losses are measured in terms of $\tau_\nu = t$ and $\chi = z \in \{0,1\}$, when ϑ is the correct alternative (drift) parameter assumed distributed according to a prior distribution π on **R**, by

$$L(t,z,\vartheta) \;=\; \begin{cases} c_1(t,\vartheta) + z\, c_2(\vartheta) + (1-z)\, c_3(t,\vartheta), & \text{if } \vartheta \leq 0, \\[2mm] c_1(t,\vartheta) + (1-z)\, c_2(\vartheta) + z\, c_3(t,\vartheta), & \text{if } \vartheta > 0. \end{cases} \tag{31.2}$$

Here z denotes the indicator of rejection of the null hypothesis $\mathbf{H}_0 : \vartheta \leq 0$. The functions c_1, c_2, and c_3 represent, respectively, the costs of trial duration, of incorrect terminal decision, and of correct, but late, terminal decision. These costs are general enough to apply to realistic clinical trial scenarios, both from the point of view of public health and of the drug developer. The interim looks are not assigned direct costs, because data-monitoring committees do in any case monitor the interim results of clinical trials for treatment-safety issues and ethically driven early stopping.

The cost functions are assumed to be π-integrable for each (t, z), nondecreasing and piecewise smooth in t, and to satisfy for all (t, z, ϑ):

$$c_1(0, \vartheta) = c_3(0, \vartheta) = 0, \qquad c_3(t, \vartheta) < c_2(\vartheta) . \tag{31.3}$$

In addition, π is assumed to place positive mass in small neighborhoods of $\vartheta = 0$ and $\vartheta = \vartheta_1 > 0$, and $c_1(\cdot, \vartheta)$ is assumed to grow to ∞ for π-almost all ϑ.

In this setting, the decision problem is to choose decision rules

$$\delta = \left(\{\tau_j\}_{j=1}^K, \ \nu, \ \chi \right) \tag{31.4}$$

to minimize the expected loss or *risk function*

$$r(\delta) \ = \ \int E_\vartheta \big(L(\tau_\nu, \chi, \vartheta) \big) \, d\pi(\vartheta) \tag{31.5}$$

subject for fixed $\alpha, \ \beta > 0$ to the type I and II error probability constraints

$$E_{\vartheta=0}(\chi) \le \alpha, \qquad E_{\vartheta=\vartheta_1}(1 - \chi) \le \beta, \tag{31.6}$$

where $\vartheta_1 > 0$ is a fixed alternative deemed to be sufficiently distant from the null hypothesis value $\vartheta = 0$ to be a medically significant treatment difference.

This decision-theoretic problem is the one defined by Leifer and Slud (2002). It can be analyzed, standardly, in terms of Lagrange multipliers (Berger 1985) so that the constraints (31.6) are omitted and the loss-function is replaced [after a reduction showing there is no loss of generality in assuming $\pi_0 \equiv \pi(\{0\}) > 0$ and $\pi_1 \equiv \pi(\{\vartheta_1\}) > 0$] by

$$L_{\lambda_0, \lambda_1}(t, z, \vartheta) \ \equiv \ L(t, z, \vartheta) + \frac{\lambda_0}{\pi_0} I_{[\vartheta=0]} + \frac{\lambda_1}{\pi_1} I_{[\vartheta=\vartheta_1]}. \tag{31.7}$$

Up to this point, "adaptivity" of the clinical trial design is embodied in the flexibility of actions $(\{\tau_j\}_{j=1}^K, \chi)$: because data are re-examined at all of the look-times $\tau_1, \ldots, \tau_\nu$, especially good or bad performance of the treatment group can lead to early decision (rejection or acceptance of H_0 with $\nu < K$), and nuisance parameters such as accrual rates and control group survival distribution can be re-estimated. Flexibility of clinical trial design has two aspects: first, that action–space coordinates permit decision at many possible times, but second, that investigators' actions defining the times of later interim looks at the data may depend functionally on aspects of the nuisance parameters that do not directly appear in the reward or cost functions driving the trial, but which do affect expected costs.

Although the interim look-times $\{\tau_i, 1 \le i \le K\}$ that are designed into a clinical trial add logistical complexity, they can be justified not only because of the economy in expected sample size and other costs common to all sequential methods [Siegmund (1985)], but also because of the range of surprises—lower than expected accrual, or higher than expected treatment-group survival, reflected in a lower than expected rate of increase of statistical information about ϑ as a function of calendar time—under which the trial can still achieve desired experimentwise type I and type II error probabilities.

This last feature of group-sequential trials is underappreciated. In the starkest comparison, that between sequential and fixed-sample trials, the group-sequential trial is not only more economical on average under expected rates of accrual, but more robust in maintaining acceptable power under a variety of erratic accrual rates and other unexpected trial characteristics leading to slow increase of information with calendar time. We formulate the issue mathematically in the following brief section.

31.2.1 Inference in a random-information environment

Again let the action–space consist of elements $(\{\tau_j\}_{j=1}^K, \chi)$—stopping-times and final binary decision—based upon data available only at times τ_j from a Wiener process with drift $X(t) = W(A(t)) + \vartheta A(t)$, conditionally given the variance function $A(t)$. However, we now view $A(\cdot)$ itself as a smoothly increasing random function of time independent of $W(\cdot)$, with $A(t)$ observable at time t, and with a known or conjectured probability law μ_A but with the trajectory definitely *not* known in advance. Note that the conditional statistical information about ϑ given $A(t)$, based on any subset of the data history $(X(s), \ s \leq t)$ which includes the observation $X(t)$, coincides with $A(t)$. This is our idealized model of all of the surprises in a clinical trial which may have an impact on statistical information about ϑ. The observability of $A(t)$ at look-time t corresponds to the large-sample estimability of nuisance parameters.

Assume that the loss-function for the inference problem is exactly as given in (31.2)–(31.3) and either (31.6) or (31.7), but even a very simple cost structure such as $c_1(t, \vartheta) = t$, $c_2(\vartheta) = 0 = c_3(t, \vartheta)$ can be used to convey the main idea. The prior probability law $\pi(\cdot)$ for ϑ must now be coupled with a probability law μ_A for $A(\cdot)$ regarded as an independent "parameter" of the decision problem. Then risks (31.5) must be replaced by expectations taken jointly over $(\vartheta, A(\cdot))$ with respect to the product prior measure $\pi \times \mu_A$, in order to define the problem anew as a Bayesian decision problem, and again the constraints (31.6) are replaced by Lagrange multipliers when L in (31.5) is replaced by (31.7). A slightly different form of the decision-theoretic problem would average in Bayesian fashion over $d\pi(\vartheta)$ but treat unknown $A(\cdot)$ in minimax fashion, that is, would replace (31.5) by its maximum or supremum over functions $A(\cdot)$ in some class.

The point of this section is that an essentially nondeterministic and unknown $A(\cdot)$ makes even an otherwise "fixed-sample" procedure—one with $K = 1$ and τ_1 deterministic—depend on an uncertain amount of statistical information. Evidently a group-sequential procedure that makes use of one or more looks at the data to estimate features of a very uncertain $A(\cdot)$ can be found which will outperform such a fixed-sample procedure: the logistical costs of interim looks should be borne in order that adequate power be available under an ensemble of possible trajectories for $A(\cdot)$. The desirability of a multi-look procedure would derive from the requirement for robustness against alternative models $A(\cdot)$, even if we would have been satisfied, scientifically and ethically, with a fixed-sample one-look procedure under the common assumptions of uniform accrual and approximately constant withdrawal rates and control-group failure rate often used to derive the power of clinical trials.

Intuitively speaking, the observability of $(A(s),\ s \le t)$ at look-times t will force optimal Bayes decision procedures to allow more interim look-times than they would under the same cost structures with deterministic $A(\cdot)$. Finding simple examples in which this can be proved is an attractive current research problem. In any case, it is intuitively clear that in problems with random $A(\cdot)$, independent of ϑ and with histories observable at interim look-times, all optimal Bayes decisions must necessarily, under mild restrictions on μ_A, have number ν of interim looks equal to the upper bound K with positive probability. [If not, we could reason by contradiction and find a procedure that alters an existing decision rule δ by including an interim look before τ_1, thereby narrowing the class of possible $A(\cdot)$ trajectories, and later employs this information to improve on δ.]

31.2.2 Extended actions affecting information growth

We can imagine other sorts of violations of standard clinical trial assumptions that still other aspects of design flexibility might overcome. For example, there might be time trends in patient prognosis, occurring in random fashion but with overall effect estimable at interim look-times. This kind of violation of the usual *iid* assumptions about accrued patients will again have the effect of randomizing the information process $A(t)$: if these trends have no effect on treatment difference, then nothing new is needed beyond the formulation of the previous section. However, we can also imagine that at interim looks, a pattern of nonconstant treatment-to-control group hazard ratios might begin to emerge, such as an indication of treatment group differences occurring only at later times-on-test. In that case, a new degree of design freedom might be desirable: to prolong follow-up of already accrued patients without allowing any new patients to be accrued. Here again the motivation might be not primarily power under standard conditions but robustness of trial size and power characteristics under nonstandard ones.

One apparent obstacle to the exercise of this kind of design freedom is the need to show how a group-sequential design might allow an option to terminate accrual but extend follow-up, while maintaining a fixed experimentwise significance level. However, the design of Koutsoukos *et al.* (1998) described below in Section 31.4 does show this, and therefore serves as a "proof of concept."

31.3   Two-Look Optimal Decision Rules

Leifer and Slud (2002, revised 2007) show that optimal Bayesian decision rules for (31.7), in the standard setting of Section 31.2 without randomized information function or observable data other than X, have the following properties.

1. There is a finite, nonrandom constant $t_* > 0$, which may be made uniform with respect to compact sets of pairs $(\lambda_0, \lambda_1) \in \mathbf{R}_+^2$, such that $\tau_\nu \leq t_*$.

2. For each triple (α, β, r) lying on the (closed) lower boundary of the three-dimensional convex set of triples

$$\left(E_{\vartheta=0}(\chi), \ E_{\vartheta=\vartheta_1}(\chi), \ \int E_\vartheta(L(\tau_\nu, \chi, \vartheta)) \, \pi(d\vartheta) \right) \tag{31.8}$$

of randomized decision rules, there exists a possibly randomized decision rule for which (α, β, r) is exactly equal to the triple (31.8).

3. Every minimum risk, possibly randomized, decision rule for the decision problem with the loss-function (31.7) has a terminal decision χ which is a.s. equal to a nonrandom function of the form $\chi = I_{[X(\tau_\nu) \geq w(\tau_\nu)]}$, with $w(\cdot)$ uniquely defined implicitly through the equation

$$\int a_1(y, \lambda_0, \lambda_1, \vartheta) \, e^{\vartheta w(y) - \vartheta^2 y/2} \, \pi(d\vartheta) = 0,$$

where

$$a_1(t, \lambda_0, \lambda_1, \vartheta) = (c_2(\vartheta) - c_3(t, \vartheta)) (2I_{[\vartheta \leq 0]} - 1) + \frac{\lambda_0}{\pi_0} I_{[\vartheta=0]} - \frac{\lambda_1}{\pi_1} I_{[\vartheta=\vartheta_1]}.$$

4. Generically for the loss-function (31.7), that is, after a small random perturbation of the cost-function c_1 preserving the assumptions, for almost every pair (λ_0, λ_1), the optimal decision rule minimizing the Bayesian risk for loss function (31.7) is unique and nonrandomized and can be computed by backward induction.

We provide an example of such an optimized nonrandomized Bayes two-look decision rule, taken from Leifer and Slud (2002). Consider $\alpha = .025$, $\beta = .1$, and $\vartheta_1 = \log(1.5)$, with time scaled so that a fixed-sample ($K = 1$) trial with this size and type II error probability has duration $\tau_1 = 1$. We exhibit an optimal rule, with $K = 2$, for the discrete prior and loss-function defined (after taking $c_3(t, \vartheta) \equiv 0$) through the following table:

e^ϑ = Hazard Ratio	0.9	1.0	1.25	1.5	1.75
$1.51 \cdot \pi(\{\vartheta\})$	0.2	1.0	0.2	0.1	0.01
$c_1(t, \vartheta)$	t	t	t	t	t
$c_2(\vartheta)$	200	100	50	250	500

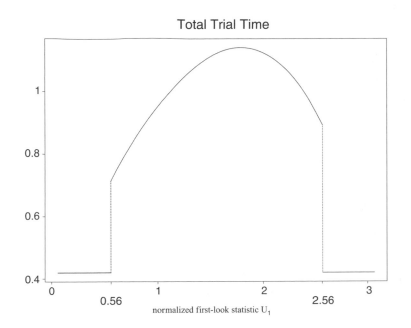

Figure 31.1. Second look-time τ_2 in example of Section 31.3, for fixed $\tau_1 = 0.42$, as a function of normalized statistic $U_1 = X(\tau_1)/\sqrt{\tau_1}$.

The optimized (nonrandomized) procedure has three elements: an initial look-time at $\tau_1 = .42$, a second look-time $\tau_2(U_1)$ defined as a function of $U_1 \equiv X(\tau_1)/\sqrt{\tau_1}$ and displayed in Figure 31.1, and a final rejection boundary $b(U_1)$ displayed in Figure 31.2 defining the rejection indicator as $\chi = I_{[X(\tau_2)/\sqrt{\tau_2} \geq b(U_1)]}$. These functions do completely describe the group-sequential procedure: the time-τ_1 rejection and acceptance boundaries are determined in Figure 31.1 through the observation that termination with $\nu = 1$ occurs whenever $\tau_2 = \tau_1$, that is, when $U_1 < 0.56$ or $U_1 > 2.56$, and the time-τ_1 decision (rejection-indicator) χ is 1 on $[U_1 > 2.56]$ and 0 on $[U_1 < 0.56]$.

31.4 Modified Trial Designs with Accrual-Stopping

We conclude by describing a clinical trial design of Koutsoukos *et al.* (1998) extending that of Section 31.2, which allows the flexibility of modifying accrual without stopping follow-up, effectively reducing, but not to 0, the rate at which information about the survival difference parameter ϑ unfolds. (As was mentioned in our motivating discussion in Section 31.2.2, the continuing increment of information relates primarily to large times on test, which may be particularly valuable information under some circumstances.) The notation concerning the

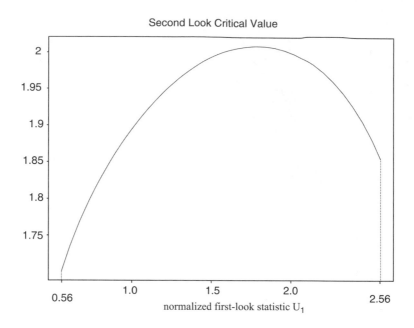

Figure 31.2. Rejection boundary at τ_2 as a function of $U_1 = X(\tau_1)/\sqrt{\tau_1}$ in the optimized two-look procedure of Section 31.3.

repeatedly calculated statistic $S_j/\sqrt{n}$ with (estimated) variance V_j is as in the introduction. In this design, the look-times $\tau_j = j$ are evenly spaced, because at most one time-unit of further follow-up is allowed when accrual is stopped, and at the end of such a follow-up period the trial is stopped. Immediate termination of the trial, respectively, with acceptance or rejection, is determined by extreme boundaries $C_{U,j}$ and $C_{L,j}$ of fixed shape (here, $C_{U,j} = C_U$ is constant and $C_{L,j}$ of the form $C_L + c_0 V_j$ for suitably chosen constants C_L, c_0); but accrual is also stopped when $S_j/\sqrt{n}$ crosses a less extreme boundary $C_{A,j} < C_U$ (or in any case, when $j = K - 1$), and rejection or acceptance is determined at the look-time following accrual-termination by a different boundary $C_{R,j}$.

> The trial is stopped outright at j, with rejection, if $S_j/\sqrt{n} \geq C_U$, and with acceptance of H_0, if $S_j/\sqrt{n} \leq C_{L,j}$.

> The accrual (i.e., entry) of new patients is disallowed at time j if $C_{A,j} \leq S_j/\sqrt{n} < C_U$, in which case the trial is stopped at time $j+1$, with final rejection if $S_{j+1}/\sqrt{n} \geq C_{R,j+1}$ and acceptance otherwise.

Boundaries of this type can be computed to have fixed size and power against a fixed alternative, and the free parameters in C_U, $C_{A,j}$, $C_{R,j+1}$ can be optimized with respect to a loss function containing costs for wrong decisions and trial durations under a range of alternatives weighted by a prior π. Details of calculation of such optimized boundaries can be found in Koutsoukos *et al.* (1998). An example of the resulting boundaries, in a trial with experimentwise significance level $\alpha = 0.025$ and power 0.8 against a hazard-ratio alternative of 1.4, is exhibited in Figures 31.3 and 31.4, which are taken from slides prepared by L. Rubinstein. In these figures, the boundaries plotted are those corresponding to the normalized statistics $S_j/\sqrt{nV_j}$, and the variances

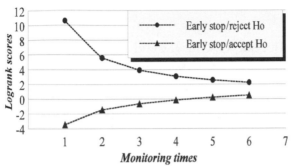

■ The upper bound is a standard O'Brien-Fleming upper bound for a 7 look design, with α=.025.

■ The lower bound is an asymmetric lower bound taken from an O'Brien-Fleming 6 look design, yielding .05 probability of crossing for Δ=1.4 (for which the trial has power 80%).

Figure 31.3. Immediate rejection and acceptance boundaries, respectively, $C_U/\sqrt{V_j}$ (plotted with filled dots) and $C_{L,j}/\sqrt{V_j}$ (filled triangles) for normalized log-rank statistics $S_j/\sqrt{nV_j}$ in a particular case of the Koutsoukos *et al.* (1998) boundaries described in Section 31.4.

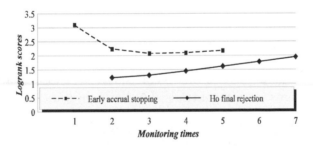

■ The H$_0$ final rejection (1-sided) bound is optimized with respect to power against a defined mix of alternative hypotheses.

■ The early accrual stopping bound and rejection bound, together, yield .05 conditional probability of failure to reject H$_0$ after stopping accrual at the boundary (assuming a defined mix of alternative hypotheses).

Figure 31.4. Accrual-stopping and final rejection boundaries, respectively, $C_{A,j}/\sqrt{V_j}$ (plotted with filled squares) and $C_{R,j}/\sqrt{V_j}$ (filled diamonds) for normalized log-rank statistics $S_j/\sqrt{nV_j}$ in the same example of the Koutsoukos *et al.* (1998) boundaries as in Figure 31.3.

V_j for log-rank statistics $S_j/\sqrt{n}$ were calculated under an assumption of constant failure rates for a two-armed clinical trial with patient arrivals following a homogeneous Poisson process.

References

1. Andersen, P., Borgan, O. Gill, R., and Keiding, N. (1993). *Statistical Methods Based on Counting Processes*, Springer-Verlag, New York.

2. Bauer, P. and Köhne, K. (1994). Evaluation of experiments with adaptive interim analyses, *Biometrics*, **50**, 1029–1041.

3. Berger, J. (1985). *Statistical Decision Theory and Bayesian Analysis*, Springer-Verlag, New York.

4. Burman, C.-F. and Sonesson, C. (2006). Are flexible designs sound?, *Biometrics*, **62**, 664–669, including discussion.

5. Fleming, T., Harrington, D., and O'Brien, P. (1984). Designs for group sequential tests, *Controlled Clinical Trials*, **5**, 348–361.

6. Hald, A. (1975). Optimum double sampling tests of given strength I: The normal distribution, *Journal of the American Statistical Association*, **70**, 451–456.

7. Jennison, C. (1987). Efficient group sequential tests with unpredictable group sizes, *Biometrika*, **77**, 577–513.

8. Koutsoukos, A., Rubinstein, L., and Slud, E. (1998). Early accrual-stopping sequential designs for clinical trials, *US National Cancer Institute*, preprint.

9. Lan, G. and DeMets, D. (1983). Discrete sequential boundaries for clinical trials, *Biometrika*, **70**, 659–663.

10. Leifer, E. and Slud, E. (2002, rev. 2007). Optimal time-adaptive repeated significance tests, preprint.

11. Liu, Q., Proschan, M., and Pledger, G. (2002). A unified theory of two-stage adaptive designs, *Journal of the American Statistical Association*, **97**, 1034–1041.

12. Proschan, M. and Hunsberger, S. (1995). Designed extension of studies based on conditional power, *Biometrics*, **51**, 1315–1324.

13. Proschan, M., Follmann, D., and Waclawiw, M. (1992). Effects of assumption violations on Type I error rate in group sequential monitoring, *Biometrics*, **48**, 1131–1144.

14. Sen, P. K. (2008). Clinical trials and the genomic evolution: some statistical perspectives. In *Statistical Models and Methods for Biomedical and Technical Systems*, F. Vonta, M. Nikulin, N. Limnios and C. Huber eds., 537–551, Birkhäuser, Boston.

15. Siegmund, D. (1985). *Sequential Analysis: Tests and Confidence Intervals*, Springer-Verlag, New York.

16. Slud, E. (1984). Sequential linear rank tests for two-sample censored survival data, *Annals of Statistics*, **12**, 551–571.

17. Slud, E. and Wei, L. J. (1982). Two-sample repeated significance tests based on the modified Wilcoxon statistic, *Journal of the American Statistical Association*, **77**, 862–868.

18. Tsiatis, A. (1982). Repeated significance testing for a general class of statistics used in censored survival analysis, *Journal of the American Statistical Association*, **77**, 855–861.

32

Optimal Two-Treatment Repeated Measurement Designs for Two Periods

Stratis Kounias and Miltiadis Chalikias

Department of Mathematics, University of Athens, Greece

Abstract: Repeated measurement designs, with $t = 2$ treatments, n (experimental) units, and $p = 2$ periods are examined. The parameters of interest are the difference of direct treatment effects and the difference of residual effects. Discrete optimal designs, that minimize the variance of the parameters of interest, are given for all values of n. D-optimal designs for the difference of direct as well as for the difference of residual effects are also given. The model examined is with uncorrelated observations following a continuous distribution with constant variance. Optimal designs are also derived when treatment-period interactions are included in the model.

Keywords and Phrases: Direct effects, residual effects, treatment-period interaction, projection matrix

32.1   Introduction

In repeated measurement or crossover or changeover designs, every unit is exposed, in every one of p consecutive periods, to one out of t treatments; we keep the term repeated measurement designs. Let $RMD(t, n, p)$ denote this class of repeated measurement designs. Here we restrict our attention to the case $t = 2$ and $p = 2$. Hedayat and Zhao (1990) examine optimal two-period, t-treatment designs and prove the existence of universal optimality of direct treatment effects. Mathews (1987, 1990) and Kushner (1997) investigate optimal two-treatment designs and give some optimal designs for three and four periods in the presence of autocorrelated errors. Carriere and Reinsel (1992, 1993) and Carriere and Huang (2000) study a nearly optimal four-sequence two-period design and investigate the effect of correlation between measurements within subjects. Many workers, for example, Grizzle (1965), focused on the AB, BA design in which patients effects are random. Hedayat and Yang (2003, 2004), Cheng and Wu (1980), Kunert (1983, 1984), Kunert and Stufken (2002), Laska and Meisner (1985), and Kushner (1997, 1998) have studied universally optimal designs. The review paper by Stufken (1996) and the revised edition of Jones and Kenward (2003) give valuable information and many references on the subject. For applications in clinical research see Senn (1993).

32.2 Sequence Enumeration and the Model

32.2.1 Enumeration of sequences

With two treatments A and B there are 2^p treatment sequences. A very convenient way of enumerating them is to use the binary system, setting 0 for A and 1 for B. Then the enumeration is $0, \ldots, 2^p - 1$. So in five periods to the sequence $BABBA$ corresponds the number 13 because $1 \cdot 2^0 + 0 \cdot 2^1 + 1 \cdot 2^2 + 1 \cdot 2^3 + 0 \cdot 2^4 = 13$. In two periods we have the one-to-one correspondence $AA \leftrightarrow 0, BA \leftrightarrow 1, AB \leftrightarrow 2, BB \leftrightarrow 3$. Let u_i, $i = 0, 1, \ldots, 2^p - 1$, denote the number of units allocated to the ith sequence. In this setting a design d is defined if the sequences contained in d and the number of units allocated to each sequence are given. Hence in four periods, the design d, that consists of the sequences: $12 \leftrightarrow AABB$ with five units and $10 \leftrightarrow ABAB$ with four units, is denoted by $d = \{u_{12} = 5, u_{10} = 4\}$.

32.2.2 The model

The model, without treatment-period interaction, is:

$$Y_{ijk} = \mu + \tau_{ij} + \pi_j + \delta_{i,j-1} + \gamma_{ik} + e_{ijk}, \qquad (32.1)$$

$i = 0, 1, \ldots, 2^p - 1$, $j = 1, 2, \ldots, p$, $k = 1, 2, \ldots, n_i$, $\delta_{i,0} = 0$ where i refers to the sequence employed, j to the period, and k to the unit within the ith sequence. $\tau_{ij} \in \{\tau_A, \tau_B\}$ is the direct effect of the treatment applied in the jth period of the ith sequence, $\delta_{i,j-1} \in \{\delta_A, \delta_B\}$ is the residual effect of the treatment applied in the $(j-1)$th period of the ith sequence, π_j is the jth period effect, and γ_{ik} is the effect of the kth unit of the ith sequence. The errors are independent within each sequence and among sequences and have 0 mean and constant variance σ^2; e_{ijk} has a continuous distribution. It does not make any difference, as regards the optimality of designs, if instead of γ_{ik} we set γ_i in the model as the effect of the ith sequence, which is proved in Theorem 32.2.2.

The model (32.1) in vector form is $Y = Xb + e$, where Y is $(pn) \times 1$, the design matrix X is $(pn) \times s$, b is $s \times 1$, e is the $(pn) \times 1$ vector, and s is the number of unknown parameters. From now on, for convenience, we use the same symbol for the parameter and the corresponding vector of the design matrix in (32.1); from the context it is clear what is meant each time.

Theorem 32.2.1 *In the model (32.1) the parameters $\tau_A, \tau_B, \delta_A, \delta_B$ are not estimable. Also the parameters $(\tau_A + \tau_B), (\delta_A + \delta_B)$ are not estimable.*

PROOF. It is known that if some vectors in the design matrix are linearly dependent, then the corresponding parameters are not estimable. Observe that the vectors $\pi_1, \delta_A, \delta_B$ are linearly dependent because $\pi_1 + \delta_A + \delta_B = \mu = 1_{pn}$, hence none of these parameters is estimable. Similarly $\tau_A + \tau_B = 1_{pn}$, so the parameters $\tau_A, \tau_B, (\tau_A + \tau_B)$ are not estimable. ∎

If we are interested in some and not in all the parameters, then we write the vector of parameters $b = (b_1', b_2')'$ where b_1 are the r parameters of interest and $X = (X_1 | X_2)$, then $Xb = X_1 b_1 + X_2 b_2$. The following relation gives the least squares estimate of the parameter vector b_1,

$$X_1'(I_{pn} - P(X_2))X_1 \hat{b_1} = X_1'(I_{pn} - P(X_2))Y, \qquad (32.2)$$

where X_1 is $(pn) \times r$, $P(X_2) = X_2(X_2'X_2)^- X_2'$ is the $(pn) \times (pn)$ projection matrix onto the linear space of the columns of X_2, and the variance matrix of the estimated parameters is

$$\mathrm{var}(\hat{b_1}) = \sigma^2 (X_1'(I_{pn} - P(X_2))X_1)^{-1} = \sigma^2 Q^{-1}, \qquad (32.3)$$

where $Q = X_1'(I_{pn} - P(X_2))X_1$. In the case of one parameter Q is the square of the distance of X_1 from the linear space $L(X_2)$ of the columns of X_2.

32.2.3 Calculation of Q

The difficulty in calculating Q is the computation of $P(X_2)$ and this is done in two steps. First reparameterise the model and second get rid of the nuisance parameters, that is, the sequence effects $\gamma_0, \gamma_1, \ldots, \gamma_m$, $m = 2^p - 1$.

Reparameterising we end up with the $p + 1$ parameters $(\tau_A - \tau_B), (\delta_A - \delta_B)/2, \tilde{\pi}_1, \ldots, \tilde{\pi}_{p-1}$ and the $2^p - 1 = m$ nuisance parameters $\tilde{\gamma}_0, \ldots, \tilde{\gamma}_m$, with corresponding vectors in the design matrix $(\tau_A, (\delta_A - \delta_B), \pi_1, \ldots, \pi_{p-1}, \gamma_0, \ldots, \gamma_m)$.

To get rid of the nuisance parameters $\tilde{\gamma}_0, \ldots, \tilde{\gamma}_m$ we write $X_2 = (Z|W)$, where X_1 contains r vectors, corresponding to the r parameters of interest, the $(np) \times m$ matrix Z contains the vectors $\gamma_0, \ldots, \gamma_m$ and W contains the remaining $p + 1 - r$ vectors. The $p + 1$ vectors are $(\tau_A, (\delta_A - \delta_B), \pi_1, \ldots, \pi_{p-1})$.

To calculate $P(X_2)$ use the form of the generalized inverse of a block matrix given in Searle (1971, p. 27). An equivalent form was given by Kunert (1984); that is,

$$P(X_2) = P(Z) + P((I - P(Z))W) \Leftrightarrow pr([Z|W]) = pr(Z) + pr(pr^\perp(Z)W). \qquad (32.4)$$

The $(np) \times r$ matrix X_1 is written $X'_1 = \{(1_{u_0} \otimes X_{10})' \cdots (1_{u_m} \otimes X_{1m})'\}$, where X_{1i} is $p \times r$ and $\otimes$ is the Kronecker product. The $(np) \times m$ matrix Z is written $Z' = \{(Z_1 \otimes (1_{u_0} \otimes 1_p))' \cdots (Z_{m+1} \otimes (1_{u_m} \otimes 1_p))'\}$, where $Z_1 = (1, 0, \ldots, 0), \ldots, Z_m = (0, \ldots, 0, 1)$ are $1 \times (m+1)$. The $(np) \times (p+1-r)$ matrix W is written $W' = \{(1_{u_0} \otimes W_{20})' \cdots (1_{u_m} \otimes W_{2m})'\}$, where W_{2i} is $p \times (p+1-r)$, $i = 0, 1, \ldots, m$.

Lemma 32.2.1 *If X_1, Z, W are as given above, then*

$$Q = X'_1(I_{pn} - P(X_2))X_1 = (R - q'M^-q)/p \qquad (32.5)$$

$$R = \sum_{i=0}^{m} u_i\{pX'_{1i}X_{1i} - (X'_{1i}1_p)(1'_pX_{1i})\} \qquad (32.6)$$

$$q' = \sum_{i=0}^{m} u_i\{pX'_{1i}W_{2i} - (X'_{1i}1_p)(1'_pW_{2i})\} \qquad (32.7)$$

$$M = \sum_{i=0}^{m} u_i\{pW'_{2i}W_{2i} - (W'_{2i}1_p)(1'_pW_{2i})\}. \qquad (32.8)$$

PROOF. $Q = (X_1)'(I_{pn} - P(X_2))X_1$ and $X_2 = (Z|W)$, where $Z = (np)x(m+1)$; then from (32.4) we have $P(X_2) = P(Z) + P((I_{pn} - P(Z))W)$ and then $Q = (X_1)'(I_{pn} - P(Z))X_1 - q'M^-q$. $P(Z)$ is easily computed,

$$R/p = (X_1)'(I_{pn} - P(Z))X_1, \qquad (X_1)'(I_{pn})X_1 = \sum_{i=0}^{m} u_i(X_{1i})'X_{1i},$$

$$(X_1)'P(Z)X_1 = \sum_{i=0}^{m} u_i((X_{1i})'1_p)((1_p)'X_{1i})/p,$$

$$q'/p = (X_1)'(I_{pn} - P(Z))W = \sum_{i=0}^{m} u_i\{p(X_{1i})'W_{2i} - ((X_{1i})'1_p)((1_p)'W_{2i})\}/p,$$

$$M/p = W'(I_{pn} - P(Z))W = \sum_{i=0}^{m} u_i\{p(W_{2i})'W_{2i} - ((W_{2i})'1_p)((1_p)'W_{2i})\}/p.$$

∎

Remark 32.2.1 (i) M is nonnegative definite as is clear from (32.4).

(ii) By taking the dual design (i.e., interchanging A and B in all the sequences of the design), the values of R, q, M remain invariant because $u_i \leftrightarrow u_{m-i}$, $X_{1i} \leftrightarrow X_{1,m-i}$, and $W_{2i} \leftrightarrow W_{2,m-i}$. Hence if a design is optimal so is its dual design.

Theorem 32.2.2 *If in the model (32.1) the unit effect γ_{ik} is replaced by the sequence effect γ_i, then the values of Q, R, q, M given in (32.5)–(32.8) remain invariant.*

PROOF. Replacing u_i, X_{1i}, W_{2i} in the relations (32.5)–(32.8), with $1, X_{1ik} = X_{1i}, W_{2ik} = W_{2i}$ and summing over k, we end up at the same results. ∎

32.3 Optimal Designs for Two Periods

Here $p = 2$ and there exist the following four treatment sequences in two periods, AA, BA, AB, BB. Let u_i, $i = 0, 1, 2, 3$ be the number of units allocated respectively to the four sequences. When $u_0 = u_3 = 0$, then $(\tau_A - \tau_B), (\delta_A - \delta_B)/2$ are not estimable because the vector $\tau_A + (\delta_A - \delta_B) + \gamma_2$ is a vector of 0s. If $u_1 = u_2 = 0$, then $\tau_A - \tau_B$ is not estimable because the vectors τ_A and γ_0 are identical. When $u_0 = u_2 = 0$ or $u_1 = u_3 = 0$, then $(\delta_A - \delta_B)/2$ is nonestimable, because the vectors $(\delta_A - \delta_B), \pi_1, \mu$ are linearly dependent, then M is singular and taking its generalized inverse we find $Q = u_1(n - u_1)/(2n)$, $Q = u_2(n - u_2)/(2n)$, respectively.

32.3.1 Optimal designs for direct effects

The $(2n) \times 1$ vector $X_1 = \tau_A$ corresponds to the parameter $\tau = (\tau_A - \tau_B)$ of the difference of direct effects, then $X_{10} = (1\ 1)'$, $X_{11} = (0\ 1)'$, $X_{12} = (1\ \ 0)'$, $X_{13} = (0\ 0)'$.

Also the $(2n) \times 2$ matrix W contains the vectors $\pi_1, (\delta_A - \delta_B)$ associated with the parameters $\pi_1, (\delta_A - \delta_B)/2$. The first column of W is the $(2n) \times 1$ vector $((1\ 0), (1\ 0), \ldots, (1\ 0))'$ and the second column corresponds to $(\delta_A - \delta_B)$. Hence $W_{20} = (0\ 1)'$, $W_{21} = (0\ -1)'$, $W_{22} = (0\ 1)'$, and $W_{23} = (0\ -1)'$.

From (32.6)–(32.8) we obtain $R = u_1 + u_2 = n - (u_0 + u_3)$, $q' = (q_1, q_2) = \{(u_1 - u_2), (u_1 + u_2)\}$, $M = m_{ij}$, $i, j = 1, 2$, $m_{11} = m_{22} = n$, $m_{12} = m_{21} = -(u_0 - u_1 + u_2 - u_3)$, and from (32.5) obtain

$$Q = \{(u_0 u_2)/(u_0 + u_2) + (u_1 u_3)/(u_1 + u_3)\}/2. \tag{32.9}$$

The maximum value of Q is denoted by Q^*.

Theorem 32.3.1 *The optimal design for estimating the difference of direct effects is:*
  (a) n even: $u_0 = u_2 = k, u_1 = u_3 = (n - 2k)/2$, $k = 0, 1, \ldots, n/2$ with

$$var(\hat{\tau_A} - \hat{\tau_B}) = \sigma^2 (Q^*)^{-1} = \sigma^2 (8/n).$$

(b) n odd: $|u_0 - u_2| = 1$, $u_0 + u_2 = n$, $u_1 = u_3 = 0$ or $|u_1 - u_3| = 1$, $u_1 + u_3 = n$, $u_0 = u_2 = 0$ with

$$var(\hat{\tau}_A - \hat{\tau}_B) = \sigma^2 (Q^*)^{-1} = \sigma^2 (8n)/(n^2 - 1).$$

PROOF. Because u_0, u_1, u_2, u_3 are nonnegative integers with $u_0 + u_1 + u_2 + u_3 = n$, then $(u_i u_j)/(u_i + u_j) \le (u_i + u_j)/4$ if $u_i + u_j$ is even, with equality if $u_i = u_j$ and $(u_i u_j)/(u_i + u_j) \le ((u_i + u_j)/4) - (1/(u_i + u_j))$ if $u_i + u_j$ is odd, with equality if $|u_i - u_j| = 1$, and the result follows.

If $u_0 = u_2 = 0$ or $u_1 = u_3 = 0$, M is singular and taking its generalized inverse we find $Q = u_1(n - u_1)/(2n)$, $Q = u_2(n - u_2)/(2n)$, respectively. Hence $Q^* = n/8$ if n is even and $Q^* = (n/8) - 1/(8n)$ for n odd. ∎

Hence by taking the sequences AA, AB in equal or almost equal numbers, the design is optimal for estimating the difference of direct effects.

32.3.2   Optimal designs for residual effects

Here X_1 is the $(np) \times 1$ vector $(\delta_A - \delta_B)$, thus $X_{10} = (0\ 1)'$, $X_{11} = (0\ -1)'$, $X_{12} = (0\ 1)'$, $X_{13} = (0\ -1)'$. Also the first column of $W_{20}, W_{21}, W_{22}, W_{23}$ is the vector $\pi_1 = (1\ 0)'$ and the second column, which corresponds to the vector τ_A, is, respectively, $(1\ 1)'$, $(0\ 1)'$, $(1\ 0)'$, $(0\ 0)'$; then from (32.6)–(32.8) we obtain $R = n$, $q' = (q_1, q_2) = (u_0 - u_1 + u_2 - u_3, u_1 + u_2)$, $M = (m_{ij})$, $i, j = 1, 2$, $m_{11} = n$, $m_{12} = m_{21} = -u_1 + u_2$, $m_{22} = u_1 + u_2$, and then from (32.5)

$$Q = 2(u_0 u_3(u_1 + u_2) + u_1 u_2(u_0 + u_3))/((u_0 + u_3)(u_1 + u_2) + 4u_1 u_2). \quad (32.10)$$

Note that when $u_1 = u_2 = 0$, then M is singular and its generalized inverse has the elements: $m_{11} = 1/n$, $m_{12} = m_{21} = m_{22} = 0$; then $Q = 2u_0 u_3/(u_0 + u_3)$.

Theorem 32.3.2 *The optimal design for estimating $(\delta_A - \delta_B)/2$ is:*
     n even: $u_0 = u_3 = n/2$, $u_1 = u_2 = 0$, *then* $var((\hat{\delta}_A - \hat{\delta}_B)/2) = \sigma^2 (Q^*)^{-1} = \sigma^2 (2/n)$.
     n odd: $|u_0 - u_3| = 1$, $u_0 + u_3 = n$, $u_1 = u_2 = 0$, $var((\hat{\delta}_A - \hat{\delta}_B)/2) = \sigma^2 (Q^*)^{-1} = \sigma^2 (2n)/(n^2 - 1))$.

PROOF. If $u_1 u_2 > 0$, then from (32.10), $Q < 2u_0 u_3/(u_0 + u_3)$. If $u_1 u_2 = 0$, then from (32.10), $Q = 2u_0 u_3/(u_0 + u_3)$. The maximum value Q^* of Q is attained when
     n even: $u_0 = u_3 = n/2$, then $Q* = n/2$.
     n odd: $u_0 + u_3 = n$, $|u_0 - u_3| = 1$; then $Q^* = (n^2 - 1)/(2n)$. ∎

From this theorem we conclude that the optimal design for estimating $(\delta_A - \delta_B)/2$ is to take the sequences AA, BB with equal or almost equal number of units. For estimating $(\delta_A - \delta_B)$, the optimal design is the same but with $var(\hat{\delta}_A - \hat{\delta}_B) = 4\ var((\hat{\delta}_A - \hat{\delta}_B)/2)$

32.3.3   Optimal designs for direct and residual effects

Theorem 32.3.3 *If, in the model (32.1), we are estimating $\{(\tau_A - \tau_B), (\delta_A - \delta_B)/2\}$, $Q = (q_{ij})$ is a 2×2 matrix and the D optimal design, maximizing the determinant $|Q|$ of Q, is:*

$$n = 0 \quad \mod 4, \ u_0 = u_1 = u_2 = u_3 = n/4, \ |Q^*| = max|Q| = n^2/16,$$
$$n = 1 \quad \mod 4, \ u_0 = (n+3)/4, u_1 = u_2 = u_3 = (n-1)/4,$$
$$|Q^*| = (n-1)^2(n+2)/(16n),$$
$$n = 2 \quad \mod 4, \ u_0 = u_1 = (n+2)/4, u_2 = u_3 = (n-2)/4,$$
$$|Q^*| = (n^2 - 4)/16,$$
$$n = 3 \quad \mod 4, \ u_0 = (n-3)/4, u_1 = u_2 = u_3 = (n+1)/4,$$
$$|Q^*| = (n+1)^2(n-2)/(16n).$$

Any permutation of u_0, u_1, u_2, u_3 gives also a D optimal design.

PROOF. Here $b_1 = \{(\tau_A - \tau_B), (\delta_A - \delta_B)/2\}$ and $\text{var}(\hat{b}_1) = \sigma^2 Q^{-1}$, where $Q = (q_{ij})$ is a 2×2 matrix. In this case $X_1 = (\tau_A, (\delta_A - \delta_B))$ is a $(2n) \times 2$ matrix and $W = \pi_1$ is a $(2n) \times 1$ vector. From (32.5)–(32.8) find $q_{11} = \{(u_1 + u_2)(u_0 + u_3) + 4u_1 u_2\}/(2n)$, $q_{12} = q_{21} = -(u_0 u_1 + u_2 u_3 + 2u_1 u_2)/(2n)$, $q_{22} = (u_0 + u_2)/(2n)$.

The D optimal design maximizes $|Q| = (q_{11} q_{22} - (q_{12})^2)$; then $|Q| = (u_0 u_1 u_2 + u_0 u_1 u_3 + u_0 u_2 u_3 + u_1 u_2 u_3)/(4n)$. The maximum is attained if u_0, u_1, u_2, u_3 are as near to each other as possible, hence we have the result. ∎

Because the D optimal design remains invariant under a linear transformation of the parameters, the D optimal design for estimating $\{(\tau_A - \tau_B), (\delta_A - \delta_B)\}$ is the same with the design given in the above theorem.

Note that in the D optimal design the number of units, allocated to each one of the sequences AA, AB, BA, BB, must be as near to each other as possible.

Theorem 32.3.4 *If, in the model (32.1), we are interested in estimating $\theta = (1\,1)b_1 = \{(\tau_A - \tau_B) + (\delta_A - \delta_B)/2\}$, the optimal design is:*

$n = 0 \mod 2$, $u_0 = u_1 = k, u_2 = u_3 = (n-2k)/2$ with $\text{var}\hat{\theta} = \sigma^2(8/n)$.

$n = 1 \mod 2$, $|u_0 - u_1| = 1$, $u_0 + u_1 = n$ or $|u_2 - u_3| = 1$, $u_2 + u_3 = n$ with $\text{var}\hat{\theta} = \sigma^2(8n)/(n^2 - 1))$.

PROOF. $\text{var}\hat{\theta} = \sigma^2 g$ where $g = (11)Q^{-1}(11)' = (q_{11} + q_{22} - 2q_{12})/|Q|$; that is, $g = 2(u_0 + u_1)(u_2 + u_3)/\{u_0 u_1(u_2 + u_3) + u_2 u_3(u_0 + u_1)\}$.

If $n = 0 \mod 2$, $g \geq 8/n$ with equality only if $u_0 = u_1 = k, u_2 = u_3 = (n - 2k)/2$, $k = 1, 2, \ldots, n/2$.

If $n = 1 \mod 2$, then $g \geq 8/(n - (1/n))$ with equality only if $|u_0 - u_1| = 1, u_0 + u_1 = n$ or $|u_2 - u_3| = 1, u_2 + u_3 = n$. ∎

In the above design use the pair of sequences AA, BA or AB, BB with the number of allocated units as near to each other as possible.

32.3.4   The model with interaction

The model, with treatment-period interaction, is:

$$Y_{ijk} = \mu + \tau_{ij} + \pi_j + \delta_{i,j-1} + (\tau\pi)_{\tau_{(ij)},j} + \gamma_i + e_{ijk} \qquad (32.11)$$

with $(\tau\pi)_{\tau_{(ij)},j} \in \{(\tau\pi)_{A1}, (\tau\pi)_{A2}, (\tau\pi)_{B1}, (\tau\pi)_{B2}\}$.

Take the transformation $(\tau\pi) = ((\tau\pi)_{A1} - (\tau\pi)_{A2} - (\tau\pi)_{B1} + (\tau\pi)_{B2})$, $(\tau\pi)_{A2}$, $(\tau\pi)_{B1}$, $(\tau\pi)_{B2}$; then the corresponding vectors in the design matrix will be, respectively, $(\tau\pi)_{A1}$, $((\tau\pi)_{A1} + (\tau\pi)_{A2})$, $((\tau\pi)_{A1} + (\tau\pi)_{B1})$, and $(-(\tau\pi)_{A1} + (\tau\pi)_{B2})$.

Theorem 32.3.5 *(i) In the model (32.9) the parameters* $(\tau_A - \tau_B)$, $(\delta_A - \delta_B)$, $(\tau\pi)_{A1}$, $(\tau\pi)_{A2}$, $(\tau\pi)_{B1}$, $(\tau\pi)_{B2}$ *are not estimable.*

(ii) The optimal design for estimating $((\tau_A - \tau_B) + (\tau\pi)_{A2} - (\tau\pi)_{B1})$ *is the same with the optimal design for estimating* $(\tau_A - \tau_B)$ *in the model (32.1) and with the same variance.*

(iii) The optimal design in (32.9) for estimating $((\delta_A - \delta_B)/2 - (\tau\pi)/2)$ *is the same with the optimal design for estimating* $(\delta_A - \delta_B)/2$ *in the model (32.1) and with the same variance.*

PROOF. (i) The column vectors $(\tau\pi)_{A1}$, $(\tau\pi)_{A2}$, $(\tau\pi)_{B1}$, $(\tau\pi)_{B2}$, add up to $\mu = 1_{2n}$, so the corresponding parameters $(\tau\pi)_{A1}$, $(\tau\pi)_{A2}$, $(\tau\pi)_{B1}$, $(\tau\pi)_{B2}$, are not estimable. Also to the parameters $(\tau_A - \tau_B)$, $(\delta_A - \delta_B)/2$, $(\tau\pi)_{A1}$, $(\tau\pi)_{B2}$ the corresponding vectors τ_A, $(\delta_A - \delta_B)$, $(\tau\pi)_{A1}$, $(\tau\pi)_{B2}$ add up to $2(\gamma_0 + \gamma_2)$, hence the parameters $(\tau_A - \tau_B)$, $(\delta_A - \delta_B)/2$, are also not estimable.

(ii), (iii) The vectors of the design matrix corresponding to the parameters $((\tau_A - \tau_B) + (\tau\pi)_{A2} - (\tau\pi)_{B1})$, $((\delta_A - \delta_B)/2 - (\tau\pi)/2))$ are τ_A and $(\delta_A - \delta_B)$. The matrices X_{1i}, W_{2i} used in (32.6)–(32.8) to calculate Q from (32.5), are the same as in Section 32.3.1, hence we have the result. We have used the following vector relations $\tau_A - \pi_1 - (\tau\pi)_{A2} + (\tau\pi)_{B1} = 0$ and $(\delta_A - \delta_B) - \pi_1 + 2(\tau\pi)_{A1} = \gamma_0 - \gamma_1 + \gamma_2 - \gamma_3$. ∎

Theorem 32.3.6 *In the model (32.9) the D optimal design for estimating the parameters* $((\tau_A - \tau_B) + (\tau\pi)_{A2} - (\tau\pi)_{B1}, ((\delta_A - \delta_B)/2 - (\tau\pi)/2))$ *is the same as the optimal design for estimating* $((\tau_A - \tau_B), (\delta_A - \delta_B)/2)$ *in the model (32.1).*

PROOF. The vectors of the design matrix corresponding to the parameters $((\tau_A - \tau_B) + (\tau\pi)_{A2} - (\tau\pi)_{B1}, ((\delta_A - \delta_B)/2 - (\tau\pi)/2))$ are τ_A, $(\delta_A - \delta_B)$ so the proof follows the same steps as in Theorem 32.3.3. ∎

Remark 32.3.1 (i) The model (32.9) with treatment-period interaction is equivalent to the model (32.1) without interaction where the parameters $((\tau_A -$

$\tau_B), (\delta_A - \delta_B)/2)$ have been replaced by the parameters $((\tau_A - \tau_B) + (\tau\pi)_{A2} - (\tau\pi)_{B1}, ((\delta_A - \delta_B)/2 - (\tau\pi)/2))$, which are estimable.

(ii) The D optimal design remains invariant under a nonsingular linear transformation of the parameters.

Acknowledgements

Part of this work was done while the first author was visiting professor at the University of Cyprus. For the second author the project is cofinanced within Op. Education by the ESF (European Social Fund) and National Resources.

References

1. Carriere, K. C. and Reinsel, G. C. (1992). Investigation of dual-balanced crossover designs for two treatments, *Biometrics*, **48**, 1157–1164.

2. Carriere, K. C. and Reinsel, G. C. (1993). Optimal two-period repeated measurement design with two or more treatments, *Biometrika*, **80**, 924–929.

3. Carriere, K. C. and Huang, R. (2000). Crossover designs for two-treatment clinical trials, *Journal of Statistical Planning and Inference*, **87**, 125–134.

4. Cheng, C. S. and Wu, C. F. (1980). Balanced repeated measurements designs, *Annals of Statistics*, **11**, 29–50. Correction (1983), **11**, 349.

5. Grizzle, J. E. (1965). The two period change-over design and its use in clinical trials, *Biometrics*, **21**, 1272–1283.

6. Hedayat, A. S. and Yang, M. (2003). Universal optimality of balanced uniform crossover designs, *Annals of Statistics*, **31**, 978–983.

7. Hedayat, A. S. and Yang, M. (2004). Universal optimality for selected crossover designs, *Journal of the American Statistical Association*, **99**, 461–466.

8. Hedayat, A. S. and Zhao, W. (1990). Optimal two period repeated measurements designs, *Annals of Statistics*, **18**, 1805–1816.

9. Jones, B. and Kenward, M. G. (2003). *Design and Analysis of Cross-Over Trials*, Chapman and Hall, London, New York.

10. Kunert, J. (1983). Optimal design and refinement of the linear model with applications to repeated measurements designs, *Annals of Statistics*, **11**, 247–257.

11. Kunert, J. (1984). Optimality of balanced uniform repeated measurements designs, *Annals of Statistics*, **12**, 1006–1017.

12. Kunert, J. and Stufken, J. (2002). Optimal crossover designs in a model with self and mixed carryover effects, *Journal of the American Statistical Association*, **97**, 898–906.

13. Kushner, H. B. (1997). Optimality and efficiency of the two treatment repeated measurement design, *Biometrika*, **84**, 455–468. Corrigendum: *Biometrika* (1999), **86**, 234.

14. Kushner, H. B. (1998). Optimal and efficient repeated measurement designs-for uncorrelated observations, *Journal American Statistical Association*, **93**, 1176–1187.

15. Laska, E. M. and Meisner, M. (1985). A variational approach to optimal two treatment crossover designs: Application to carryover effect models, *Journal American Statistical Association*, **80**, 704–710.

16. Mathews, J. N. S. (1987). Optimal crossover designs for the comparison of two treatments in the presence of carryover effects and autocorrelated errors, *Biometrica*, **74**, 311–320.

17. Mathews, J. N. S. (1990). Optimal dual-balanced two treatment crossover designs, *Sankhya, Series B*, **52**, 332–337.

18. Searle, S. R. (1971). *Linear Models*, John Wiley & Sons, New York.

19. Senn, S. (1993). *Cross-Over Trials in Clinical Research*, John Wiley & Sons, New York.

20. Stufken, J. (1996). Optimal crossover designs. Designs and analysis of experiments, In *Handbook of Statistics 13*, (Eds., S. Ghosh and C. R. Rao), North-Holland, Amsterdam.

PART VIII

MEASURES OF DIVERGENCE, MODEL SELECTION, AND SURVIVAL MODELS

33

Discrepancy-Based Model Selection Criteria Using Cross-Validation

Joseph E. Cavanaugh,[1] **Simon L. Davies,**[2] **and Andrew A. Neath**[3]

[1]*Department of Biostatistics, The University of Iowa, Iowa City, IA, USA*
[2]*Pfizer Global Research and Development, Pfizer, Inc., New York, NY, USA*
[3]*Department of Mathematics and Statistics, Southern Illinois University, Edwardsville, IL, USA*

Abstract: A model selection criterion is often formulated by constructing an approximately unbiased estimator of an expected discrepancy, a measure that gauges the separation between the true model and a fitted approximating model. The expected discrepancy reflects how well, on average, the fitted approximating model predicts "new" data generated under the true model. A related measure, the estimated discrepancy, reflects how well the fitted approximating model predicts the data at hand.

In general, a model selection criterion consists of a goodness-of-fit term and a penalty term. The natural estimator of the expected discrepancy, the estimated discrepancy, corresponds to the goodness-of-fit term of the criterion. However, the estimated discrepancy yields an overly optimistic assessment of how effectively the fitted model predicts new data. It therefore serves as a negatively biased estimator of the expected discrepancy. Correcting for this bias leads to the penalty term.

Cross-validation provides a technique for developing an estimator of an expected discrepancy which need not be adjusted for bias. The basic idea is to construct an empirical discrepancy that evaluates an approximating model by assessing how accurately each case-deleted fitted model predicts the deleted case.

The preceding approach is illustrated in the linear regression framework by formulating estimators of the expected discrepancy based on Kullback's *I*-divergence and the Gauss (error sum of squares) discrepancy. The traditional criteria that arise by augmenting the estimated discrepancy with a bias adjustment term are the Akaike information criterion and Mallows' conceptual predictive statistic. A simulation study is presented.

Keywords and Phrases: AIC, Mallows' C_p, PRESS

33.1   Introduction

A model selection criterion is often formulated by constructing an approximately unbiased estimator of an expected discrepancy, a measure that gauges the separation between the true model and a fitted approximating model. The natural estimator of the expected discrepancy, the estimated discrepancy, corresponds to the goodness-of-fit term of the selection criterion.

The expected discrepancy reflects how well, on average, the fitted approximating model predicts "new" data generated under the true model. On the other hand, the estimated discrepancy reflects how well the fitted approximating model predicts the data at hand. By evaluating the adequacy of the fitted model based on its ability to recover the data used in its own construction, the estimated discrepancy yields an overly optimistic assessment of how effectively the fitted model predicts new data. Thus, the estimated discrepancy serves as a negatively biased estimator of the expected discrepancy. Correcting for this bias leads to the penalty term of the selection criterion.

Cross-validation provides a technique for developing an estimator of an expected discrepancy which need not be adjusted for bias. The basic idea involves constructing an empirical discrepancy that evaluates an approximating model by assessing how accurately each case-deleted fitted model predicts the deleted case.

Cross-validation facilitates the development of model selection procedures based on predictive principles. In this work, we attempt to establish a more explicit connection between cross-validation and traditional discrepancy-based model selection criteria, such as the Akaike (1973) information criterion and Mallows' (1973) conceptual predictive statistic.

In Section 33.2, we outline the framework for discrepancy-based selection criteria. In Section 33.3, we discuss the bias-adjustment approach for developing a model selection criterion, and in Section 33.4, we present the cross-validatory approach. Section 33.5 features examples of discrepancy-based selection criteria developed using both approaches. The linear regression framework is considered. In Section 33.6, we present simulation results to evaluate the performance of the criteria. Our results show that the cross-validatory criteria compare favorably to their traditional counterparts, offering greater protection from overfitting in small-sample settings.

33.2 Framework for Discrepancy-Based Selection Criteria

Suppose we have an n-dimensional data vector $y = (y_1, \ldots, y_n)'$, where the y_is may be scalars or vectors and are assumed to be independent. A parametric model is postulated for y. Let θ denote the vector of model parameters.

Let $F(y)$ denote the joint distribution function for y under the generating or "true" model, and let $F_i(y_i)$ denote the marginal distribution for y_i under this model. Let $G(y, \theta)$ denote the joint distribution function for y under the candidate or approximating model.

A *discrepancy* is a measure of disparity between $F(y)$ and $G(y, \theta)$, say $\Delta(F, G)$, which satisfies

$$\Delta(F, G) \geq \Delta(F, F).$$

A discrepancy is not necessarily a formal metric, which would additionally require that $\Delta(F, F) = 0$, that $\Delta(F, G)$ is symmetric in $F(y)$ and $G(y, \theta)$, and that $\Delta(F, G)$ satisfies the triangle inequality. However, the measure $\Delta(F, G)$ serves the same basic role as a distance; that is, as the dissimilarity between $F(y)$ and $G(y, \theta)$ becomes more pronounced, the size of $\Delta(F, G)$ should increase accordingly.

We consider discrepancies of the following form:

$$\Delta(F, G) = \Delta(\theta) = \sum_{i=1}^{n} \mathrm{E}_{F_i} \left\{ \delta_i(y_i; \theta) \right\}.$$

In the preceding, $\delta_i(y_i; \theta)$ represents a function that gauges the accuracy with which the ith case y_i is predicted under the approximating model (parameterized by θ).

Let $\widehat{\theta}$ denote an estimator of θ. The *overall discrepancy* results from evaluating the discrepancy between $F(y)$ and $G(y, \theta)$ at $\theta = \widehat{\theta}$:

$$\Delta(\widehat{\theta}) = \sum_{i=1}^{n} \mathrm{E}_{F_i} \left\{ \delta_i(y_i, \theta) \right\} |_{\theta = \widehat{\theta}}.$$

The *expected (overall) discrepancy* results from averaging the overall discrepancy over the sampling distribution of $\widehat{\theta}$:

$$\mathrm{E}_F \left\{ \Delta(\widehat{\theta}) \right\} = \sum_{i=1}^{n} \mathrm{E}_F \left\{ \mathrm{E}_{F_i} \left\{ \delta_i(y_i, \theta) \right\} |_{\theta = \widehat{\theta}} \right\}.$$

The *estimated discrepancy* is given by

$$\widehat{\Delta}(\widehat{\theta}) = \sum_{i=1}^{n} \delta_i(y_i, \widehat{\theta}).$$

Model selection criteria are often constructed by obtaining a statistic that has an expectation which is equal to $E_F\left\{\Delta(\widehat{\theta})\right\}$ (at least approximately). In the next two sections, we explore the bias-adjustment and cross-validatory approaches to obtaining such statistics.

33.3   The Bias-Adjustment Approach to Developing a Criterion

The overall discrepancy $\Delta(\widehat{\theta})$ is not a statistic because its evaluation requires knowledge of the true distribution $F(y)$. The estimated discrepancy $\widehat{\Delta}(\widehat{\theta})$ is a statistic and can be used to estimate the expected discrepancy $E_F\left\{\Delta(\widehat{\theta})\right\}$. However, $\widehat{\Delta}(\widehat{\theta})$ serves as a biased estimator.

Consider writing $E_F\left\{\Delta(\widehat{\theta})\right\}$ as follows,

$$E_F\left\{\Delta(\widehat{\theta})\right\} = E_F\left\{\widehat{\Delta}(\widehat{\theta})\right\} + \left[E_F\left\{\Delta(\widehat{\theta}) - \widehat{\Delta}(\widehat{\theta})\right\}\right].$$

The bracketed quantity on the right is often referred to as the *expected optimism* in judging the fit of a model using the same data as those which were used to construct the fit. The expected optimism is positive, implying that $\widehat{\Delta}(\widehat{\theta})$ is a negatively biased estimator of $E_F\left\{\Delta(\widehat{\theta})\right\}$. In order to correct for the negative bias, we must evaluate or approximate the bias adjustment represented by the expected optimism.

There are numerous approaches for contending with the bias adjustment. These approaches include deriving an asymptotic approximation for the adjustment [e.g., Akaike (1973)], deriving an exact expression [e.g., Hurvich and Tsai (1989)], or obtaining an approximation using Monte Carlo simulation [e.g., Bengtsson and Cavanaugh (2006)].

We now introduce a general cross-validatory estimate of the expected discrepancy that need not be adjusted for bias. As a model selection criterion, such an estimate has several advantages over a bias-adjusted counterpart.

First, the form of a cross-validatory criterion facilitates a convenient interpretation of the statistic as a measure of predictive efficacy. Broadly speaking, such a criterion evaluates an approximating model by gauging how accurately each case-deleted fitted model predicts a "new" datum, represented by the deleted case. The criterion provides a composite measure of accuracy resulting from the systematic deletion and prediction of each case. In contrast, the form of a bias-adjusted criterion is more esoteric, consisting of an additive combination of a goodness-of-fit term and a penalty term. These terms work in opposition to balance the competing modeling objectives of conformity to the data and parsimony. However, the connection between achieving such a balance and predictive efficacy is not transparent.

Second, a cross-validatory criterion serves as an exactly unbiased estimator of a cross-validatory expected discrepancy that may be viewed as a natural analogue of the expected discrepancy $\mathrm{E}_F\left\{\Delta(\widehat{\theta})\right\}$. This unbiasedness holds without imposing conditions that may restrict the applicability of the resulting criterion, conditions which are routinely required for the justifications of bias corrections.

Third, the difference between the cross-validatory expected discrepancy and its traditional counterpart converges to zero. Thus, in large sample settings, the cross-validatory criterion estimates the traditional expected discrepancy with negligible bias.

The key assumption for establishing the asymptotic equivalence of the cross-validatory and traditional expected discrepancies is that the difference in expectation between the full-data estimator and any case-deleted estimator is $o(n^{-1})$. The proof is provided in the appendix. For settings where the method of estimation is maximum likelihood and the approximating model is correctly specified or overspecified, the asymptotic condition on the estimators is verified.

33.4 The Cross-Validatory Approach to Developing a Criterion

Let $y[i]$ denote the dataset y with the ith case y_i excluded. Let $\widehat{\theta}[i]$ denote an estimator of θ based on $y[i]$.

Recall that the overall discrepancy is defined as

$$\Delta(\widehat{\theta}) = \sum_{i=1}^{n} \mathrm{E}_{F_i}\left\{\delta_i(y_i, \theta)\right\}|_{\theta=\widehat{\theta}}. \tag{33.1}$$

Now consider the following variant of the overall discrepancy:

$$\Delta^*(\widehat{\theta}[1], \dots, \widehat{\theta}[n]) = \sum_{i=1}^{n} \mathrm{E}_{F_i}\left\{\delta_i(y_i, \theta)\right\}|_{\theta=\widehat{\theta}[i]}. \tag{33.2}$$

The expected (overall) discrepancy corresponding to (33.1) is given by

$$\mathrm{E}_F\left\{\Delta(\widehat{\theta})\right\} = \sum_{i=1}^{n} \mathrm{E}_F\left\{\mathrm{E}_{F_i}\left\{\delta_i(y_i, \theta)\right\}|_{\theta=\widehat{\theta}}\right\}; \tag{33.3}$$

the expected (overall) discrepancy corresponding to (33.2) is given by

$$\mathrm{E}_F\left\{\Delta^*(\widehat{\theta}[1], \dots, \widehat{\theta}[n])\right\} = \sum_{i=1}^{n} \mathrm{E}_F\left\{\mathrm{E}_{F_i}\left\{\delta_i(y_i, \theta)\right\}|_{\theta=\widehat{\theta}[i]}\right\}. \tag{33.4}$$

Under the assumption that the difference in expectation between the full-data estimator $\widehat{\theta}$ and any case-deleted estimator $\widehat{\theta}[i]$ is $o(n^{-1})$, it can be established that the difference between $\mathrm{E}_F\left\{\Delta(\widehat{\theta})\right\}$ and $\mathrm{E}_F\left\{\Delta^*(\widehat{\theta}[1],\dots,\widehat{\theta}[n])\right\}$ is $o(1)$. (The proof is outlined in the appendix.) Hence, an unbiased estimator of (33.4) is approximately unbiased for (33.3).

Now the estimated discrepancy

$$\widehat{\Delta}(\widehat{\theta}) = \sum_{i=1}^{n} \delta_i(y_i, \widehat{\theta})$$

is *negatively biased* for (33.3). However, the empirical discrepancy defined as

$$\widehat{\Delta}^*(\widehat{\theta}[1],\dots,\widehat{\theta}[n]) = \sum_{i=1}^{n} \delta_i(y_i, \widehat{\theta}[i]) \tag{33.5}$$

is *exactly unbiased* for (33.4). The justification of this fact is straightforward.

Due to the fact that $\mathrm{E}_F\left\{\Delta^*(\widehat{\theta}[1],\dots,\widehat{\theta}[n])\right\} \approx \mathrm{E}_F\left\{\Delta(\widehat{\theta})\right\}$, it follows that $\widehat{\Delta}^*(\widehat{\theta}[1],\dots,\widehat{\theta}[n])$ is *approximately unbiased* for $\mathrm{E}_F\left\{\widehat{\Delta}(\widehat{\theta})\right\}$. Thus, the empirical discrepancy $\widehat{\Delta}^*(\widehat{\theta}[1],\dots,\widehat{\theta}[n])$:

(a) Estimates $\mathrm{E}_F\left\{\Delta^*(\widehat{\theta}[1],\dots,\widehat{\theta}[n])\right\}$ without bias.

(b) Estimates $\mathrm{E}_F\left\{\Delta(\widehat{\theta})\right\}$ with negligible bias for large n.

33.5   Examples in the Linear Regression Setting

Consider a setting where a continuous response variable is to be modeled using a linear regression model.

Under the approximating model, assume the y_i are independent with mean $x_i'\beta$ and variance σ^2. Let $\theta = (\beta'\sigma^2)'$. Furthermore, let $g(y,\theta)$ denote the approximating density for y, and let $g_i(y_i,\theta)$ denote the approximating density for y_i.

Kullback's I-divergence and the Gauss (error sum of squares) discrepancy have applicability to many modeling frameworks, including linear regression. In the context of model selection, the I-divergence may be defined as

$$\Delta_{\mathrm{I}}(\theta) = \mathrm{E}_F\left\{-2\ln g(y,\theta)\right\} = \sum_{i=1}^{n} \mathrm{E}_{F_i}\left\{\delta_i^{\mathrm{I}}(y_i;\theta)\right\}, \tag{33.6}$$

where $\delta_i^{\mathrm{I}}(y_i; \theta) = -2 \ln g_i(y_i, \theta)$. [See Linhart and Zucchini (1986, p. 18) and Hurvich and Tsai (1989, p. 299).] For the linear regression framework, the Gauss discrepancy may be expressed as

$$\Delta_{\mathrm{G}}(\theta) = \mathrm{E}_F \left\{ \sum_{i=1}^n (y_i - x_i'\beta)^2 \right\} = \sum_{i=1}^n \mathrm{E}_{F_i} \left\{ \delta_i^{\mathrm{G}}(y_i; \theta) \right\}, \qquad (33.7)$$

where $\delta_i^{\mathrm{G}}(y_i; \theta) = (y_i - x_i'\beta)^2$. [See Linhart and Zucchini (1986, p. 118).]

Provided that the approximating model of interest is correctly specified or overspecified, the Akaike information criterion provides an asymptotically unbiased estimator of the expected discrepancy corresponding to (33.6). In the present setting, AIC is given by

$$\mathrm{AIC} = -2 \ln g(y, \widehat{\theta}) + 2(p+1),$$

where p denotes the number of regression parameters, and $\widehat{\theta}$ denotes the maximum likelihood estimator (MLE) of θ. Under the additional assumption that the errors are normally distributed, the "corrected" Akaike information criterion, AICc, provides an *exactly* unbiased estimator of the expected discrepancy [Hurvich and Tsai (1989)]. AICc is given by

$$\mathrm{AICc} = -2 \ln g(y, \widehat{\theta}) + \frac{2(p+1)n}{n-p-2}.$$

Provided that the largest approximating model in the candidate collection is correctly specified or overspecified, a simple variant of Mallows' conceptual predictive statistic (with identical selection properties) provides an exactly unbiased estimator of the expected discrepancy corresponding to (33.7). Mallows' statistic is given by

$$C_p = \frac{\mathrm{SSE}}{\mathrm{MSE}_L} + (2p - n),$$

where SSE denotes the error sum of squares. The aforementioned variant is given by $(C_p + n)\mathrm{MSE}_L$, where MSE_L denotes the error mean square for the largest approximating model.

The cross-validatory criterion (33.5) based on the *I*-divergence (33.6) is given by

$$\sum_{i=1}^n -2 \ln g_i(y_i, \widehat{\theta}[i]),$$

where $\widehat{\theta}[i]$ represents the case-deleted MLE of θ. Assuming normal errors, the preceding reduces to

$$\sum_{i=1}^n \ln \hat{\sigma}_{-i}^2 + \sum_{i=1}^n \frac{(y_i - \hat{y}_{i,-i})^2}{\hat{\sigma}_{-i}^2},$$

where $\hat{y}_{i,-i}$ denotes the fitted value for y_i based on the case-deleted dataset $y[i]$, and $\hat{\sigma}^2_{-i}$ denotes the case-deleted MLE for σ^2. Davies *et al.* (2005) refer to the preceding criterion as the *predictive divergence criterion*, PDC. [See also Stone (1977).]

The cross-validatory criterion (33.5) based on the Gauss discrepancy (33.7) is given by

$$\sum_{i=1}^{n}(y_i - \hat{y}_{i,-i})^2,$$

the well-known PRESS (predictive sum of squares) statistic [Allen (1974)].

The preceding development indicates that PDC and PRESS may be respectively viewed as the cross-validatory analogues of AIC and C_p. In simulation studies, such cross-validatory criteria compare favorably to their traditional counterparts. In settings where the generating model is among the collection of candidate models under consideration, the cross-validatory criteria tend to select the correctly specified model more frequently and to select overspecified models less frequently than their bias-adjusted analogues. In the next section, we present representative sets from the simulation studies we have conducted.

33.6 Linear Regression Simulations

Consider a setting where samples of size n are generated from a true linear regression model of the form $y_i = 1 + x_{i1} + x_{i2} + x_{i3} + x_{i4} + x_{i5} + x_{i6} + \epsilon_i$, where $\epsilon_i \sim iid\ N(0,4)$. For every sample, nested candidate models with an intercept and k regressor variables ($k = 1, \ldots, 12$) are fit to the data. (Note that $p = k + 1$.) Specifically, the first model fit to each sample is based on only the covariate x_{i1}, the second is based on the covariates x_{i1} and x_{i2}, and so on. The sixth fitted model ($k = 6$, $p = 7$) is correctly specified. Subsequent fitted models are overspecified, because they contain the regressor variables for the generating model (x_{i1} through x_{i6}) in addition to extraneous covariates ($x_{i7}, \ldots, x_{i,12}$). All regressor variables are generated as *iid* replicates from a uniform distribution over the interval $(0, 10)$.

Suppose our objective is to search the candidate collection for the fitted model which serves as the best approximation to the truth. The strength of the approximation is reflected via the expected discrepancy, either (33.3) or (33.4).

We present six simulation sets based on the preceding setting. In the first three sets, we examine the effectiveness of AIC, AICc, and PDC in selecting the correctly specified model. In the next three sets, we examine the effectiveness of C_p and PRESS in achieving the same objective. We group the criterion selections into three categories: underfit (UF), correctly specified (CS), and overfit (OF).

Table 33.1. Selection results for AIC, AICc, PDC

				Criterion	
Set	n	Selections	AIC	AICc	PDC
		UF	0	1	18
1	25	CS	418	913	929
		OF	582	86	53
		UF	0	0	0
2	50	CS	606	815	870
		OF	394	185	130
		UF	0	0	0
3	75	CS	685	789	833
		OF	315	211	167

The results of sets 1–3 are presented in Table 33.1. These sets feature sample sizes of $n = 25, 50,$ and 75, respectively. In each set, PDC obtains the most correct selections, followed by AICc. The performance of AIC is relatively poor. In general, AIC favors overspecified models in settings where the sample size is insufficient to ensure the adequacy of the criterion's bias correction.

For the results from set 3, Figure 33.1 features a plot of criterion averages versus k. The expected overall discrepancies (33.3) and (33.4) are also plotted. The plot illustrates the exact unbiasedness of PDC for (33.4) and AICc for (33.3), yet also indicates the negative bias of AIC for (33.3) resulting from the poor bias approximation. This negative bias creates the criterion's propensity to favor over parameterized models.

Figure 33.1 also reflects the similarity of the curves for the expected overall discrepancies (33.3) and (33.4). As the sample size increases, the difference between these curves becomes negligible. Thus, in large sample settings, the selections of PDC, AICc, and AIC should agree. However, in smaller sample settings, where the predictive accuracy of the selected model may be greatly diminished by the inclusion of unnecessary covariates, PDC and its target discrepancy favor more parsimonious models.

The results of sets 4–6 are presented in Table 33.2. These sets feature sample sizes of $n = 15, 20,$ and 25, respectively. In sets 4 and 5, PRESS obtains more correct selections than C_p. This is mainly due to the difference in the behaviors of the targeted discrepancies: in smaller sample settings, (33.4) penalizes more heavily than (33.3) to protect against the inflation in predictive variability that accompanies the incorporation of extraneous regressors. However, in this setting, the asymptotic equivalence of (33.3) and (33.4) takes effect for relatively small n: in the third set, where n is 25, the selection patterns are the same for the two criteria.

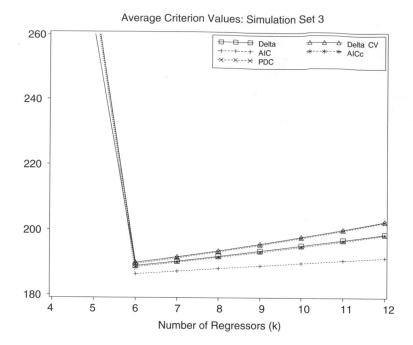

Figure 33.1. Expected discrepancies and criterion averages versus number of regressors (set 3).

Table 33.2. Selection results for C_p and PRESS

Set	n	Selections	Criterion	
			C_p	PRESS
		UF	22	19
4	15	CS	491	587
		OF	487	394
		UF	4	1
5	20	CS	634	671
		OF	362	328
		UF	0	0
6	25	CS	668	668
		OF	332	332

   The simulation results presented constitute a small yet representative sample from a larger simulation study. In general, our results show that cross-validatory criteria perform well relative to their traditional counterparts, offering greater protection from overfitting in smaller-sample settings, and exhibiting similar behavioral tendencies in larger-sample settings.

   In conclusion, cross-validatory model selection criteria provide an appealing alternative to traditional bias-adjusted selection criteria (such as AIC and C_p).

For many traditional expected discrepancies, a cross-validatory criterion may be easily formulated. Such a criterion is approximately unbiased for the traditional expected discrepancy, and exactly unbiased for an analogous expected discrepancy based on cross-validation. The preceding unbiasedness properties hold without requiring stringent conditions that may limit applicability. Moreover, the form of a cross-validatory criterion facilitates a convenient, intuitive interpretation of the statistic as a measure of predictive efficacy.

Acknowledgments

The authors wish to express their appreciation to an anonymous referee for valuable feedback which helped to improve the original version of this chapter.

Appendix

In what follows, we establish the asymptotic equivalence of (33.3) and (33.4); specifically

$$\mathrm{E}_F\{\Delta(\widehat{\theta})\} - \mathrm{E}_F\{\Delta^*(\widehat{\theta}[1], \ldots, \widehat{\theta}[n])\} = o(1). \tag{33.8}$$

We assume that the estimator $\widehat{\theta}$ converges weakly to some interior point θ_* of the parameter space Θ; that is, $\widehat{\theta} = \theta_* + o_p(1)$. Thus, we should also have $\widehat{\theta}[i] = \theta_* + o_p(1)$ for each $i = 1, \ldots, n$.

Let $\Delta_i(\theta) = \mathrm{E}_{F_i}\{\delta_i(y_i, \theta)\}$, so that

$$\Delta(\widehat{\theta}) = \sum_{i=1}^n \Delta_i(\widehat{\theta}), \qquad \Delta^*(\widehat{\theta}[1], \ldots, \widehat{\theta}[n]) = \sum_{i=1}^n \Delta_i(\widehat{\theta}[i]),$$

and

$$\Delta(\widehat{\theta}) - \Delta^*(\widehat{\theta}[1], \ldots, \widehat{\theta}[n]) = \sum_{i=1}^n \left[\Delta_i(\widehat{\theta}) - \Delta_i(\widehat{\theta}[i])\right]. \tag{33.9}$$

Our approach is to show that for each i,

$$\mathrm{E}_F\{\Delta_i(\widehat{\theta}) - \Delta_i(\widehat{\theta}[i])\} = o(n^{-1}). \tag{33.10}$$

Clearly, (33.10) in conjunction with (33.9) will establish (33.8).

We assume that $\Delta_i(\theta)$ has continuous first-order derivatives with respect to θ. Let $D_i(\theta) = \partial \Delta_i(\theta)/\partial \theta$. Using a first-order Taylor series expansion, we have

$$\Delta_i(\widehat{\theta}) = \Delta_i(\widehat{\theta}[i]) + D_i(\xi)'(\widehat{\theta} - \widehat{\theta}[i]), \tag{33.11}$$

where $\xi = \widehat{\theta}[i] + \lambda(\widehat{\theta} - \widehat{\theta}[i])$ for some $0 \leq \lambda \leq 1$. Thus, ξ converges to θ_*, and $D_i(\xi)$ converges to $D_i(\theta_*)$. From (33.11), we therefore have

$$\Delta_i(\widehat{\theta}) - \Delta_i(\widehat{\theta}[i]) = [D_i(\theta_*) + o_p(1)]'(\widehat{\theta} - \widehat{\theta}[i]). \tag{33.12}$$

Now assume that

$$\mathrm{E}_F\{(\widehat{\theta} - \widehat{\theta}[i])\} = o(n^{-1}). \qquad (33.13)$$

Because $D_i(\theta_*) = O(1)$, (33.13) together with (33.12) implies (33.10).

We now verify that (33.13) holds in a specific setting, namely one in which the method of estimation is maximum likelihood, and the approximating model is correctly specified or overspecified.

The latter assumption implies that the joint distribution function $F(y)$ under the generating model belongs to the same class as the joint distribution function $G(y, \theta)$ under the approximating model. We may therefore write $F(y)$ as $F(y, \theta_o)$, where θ_o is an interior point of Θ. Thus, θ_o defines the "true" parameter vector.

Let $L(\theta|y) = \prod_{i=1}^n g_i(y_i, \theta)$ denote the likelihood function for θ based on y. Assume that each of the likelihood contributions $g_i(y_i, \theta)$ is differentiable and suitably bounded: specifically, that for some function $h(\cdot)$ with $\int h(u)\, du < \infty$, we have

$$\left| \frac{\partial g_i(u, \theta)}{\partial \theta} \right| < h(u) \quad \text{for all } (u, \theta). \qquad (33.14)$$

For the overall likelihood $L(\theta|y)$, assume that $\ln L(\theta|y)$ has first- and second-order derivatives which are continuous and bounded over Θ. Let

$$V_n(\theta) = -\frac{1}{n} \ln L(\theta|y), \qquad V_n^{(1)}(\theta) = \frac{\partial V_n(\theta)}{\partial \theta}, \quad \text{and} \quad V_n^{(2)}(\theta) = \frac{\partial^2 V_n(\theta)}{\partial \theta \partial \theta'}.$$

Here, $\widehat{\theta} = \mathrm{argmin}_{\theta \in \Theta} V_n(\theta)$; that is, $\widehat{\theta}$ is the maximum likelihood estimator of θ.

Let $W_n(\theta) = \mathrm{E}_F\{V_n(\theta)\}$. Assume that as $n \to \infty$, $W_n(\theta)$ converges to a function $W(\theta)$ uniformly in θ over Θ, and that $W(\theta)$ has a unique global minimum at θ_o. Furthermore, suppose that $W(\theta)$ has first- and second-order derivatives which are continuous and bounded over Θ. Let $W^{(2)}(\theta) = (\partial^2 W(\theta))/(\partial\theta\partial\theta')$. Assume that $W^{(2)}(\theta)$ is positive definite in a neighborhood of θ_o.

Finally, assume that $V_n(\theta)$ converges to $W(\theta)$, that $V_n^{(2)}(\theta)$ converges to $W^{(2)}(\theta)$, and that the convergence is uniform in θ over Θ.

The preceding regularity conditions are typical of those used to ensure the consistency and the asymptotic normality of the maximum likelihood estimator of $\widehat{\theta}$. [See, for instance, Section 3 of Cavanaugh and Neath (1999).] In the setting at hand, the point of convergence θ_* for the estimator $\widehat{\theta}$ corresponds to the true parameter vector θ_o.

Expand $V_n^{(1)}(\widehat{\theta})$ about θ_o to obtain

$$\begin{aligned} 0 &= V_n^{(1)}(\widehat{\theta}) \\ &= V_n^{(1)}(\theta_o) + V_n^{(2)}(\widetilde{\theta})(\widehat{\theta} - \theta_o), \end{aligned}$$

where $\widetilde{\theta} = \theta_o + \gamma(\widehat{\theta} - \theta_o)$ for some $0 \leq \gamma \leq 1$. Then,

$$\widehat{\theta} = \theta_o - [V_n^{(2)}(\widetilde{\theta})]^{-1} V_n^{(1)}(\theta_o).$$

The preceding relation along with the assumed regularity conditions and the consistency of $\widehat{\theta}$ leads to

$$\widehat{\theta} = \theta_o - [W^{(2)}(\theta_o) + o_p(1)]^{-1}V_n^{(1)}(\theta_o).$$

Now without loss of generality, take $\widehat{\theta}[i] = \widehat{\theta}[1]$. Then we have

$$\widehat{\theta} - \widehat{\theta}[1] = -[W^{(2)}(\theta_o) + o_p(1)]^{-1}[V_n^{(1)}(\theta_o) - V_{n-1}^{(1)}(\theta_o)], \qquad (33.15)$$

where

$$V_n^{(1)}(\theta) = -\frac{1}{n}\sum_{i=1}^{n}\frac{\partial \ln g_i(y_i, \theta)}{\partial \theta} \quad \text{and} \quad V_{n-1}^{(1)}(\theta) = -\frac{1}{n-1}\sum_{i=2}^{n}\frac{\partial \ln g_i(y_i, \theta)}{\partial \theta}.$$

Note that

$$V_n^{(1)}(\theta_o) - V_{n-1}^{(1)}(\theta_o) = -\frac{1}{n}\frac{\partial \ln g_1(y_1, \theta_o)}{\partial \theta} - \frac{1}{n}V_{n-1}^{(1)}(\theta_o). \qquad (33.16)$$

Using (33.16) in conjunction with (33.15), we obtain

$$n(\widehat{\theta} - \widehat{\theta}[1]) = [W^{(2)}(\theta_o) + o_p(1)]^{-1}\left[\frac{\partial \ln g_1(y_1, \theta_o)}{\partial \theta} + V_{n-1}^{(1)}(\theta_o)\right]. \qquad (33.17)$$

Now the assumed regularity conditions along with the consistency of the maximum likelihood estimator allow us to conclude that the difference between $V_{n-1}^{(1)}(\theta_o)$ and $V_{n-1}^{(1)}(\widehat{\theta}[1]) = 0$ is $o_p(1)$, which implies that $V_{n-1}^{(1)}(\theta_o) = o_p(1)$. Moreover, one can argue that $E_F\{(\partial \ln g_1(y_1, \theta_o))/(\partial \theta)\} = 0$. This result is established by exchanging the order of differentiation and integration, which is permissible via the Lebesgue dominated convergence theorem under the imposed assumption (33.14). The preceding results along with (33.17) allow us to argue

$$E_F\{n(\widehat{\theta} - \widehat{\theta}[1])\} = o(1).$$

Thus, (33.13) is established.

References

1. Akaike, H. (1973). Information theory and an extension of the maximum likelihood principle, In *2nd International Symposium on Information Theory* (Eds., B. N. Petrov and F. Csáki), pp. 267–281, Akadémia Kiadó, Budapest.

2. Allen, D. M. (1974). The relationship between variable selection and data augmentation and a method for prediction, *Technometrics*, **16**, 125–127.

3. Bengtsson, T. and Cavanaugh, J. E. (2006). An improved Akaike information criterion for state–space model selection, *Computational Statistics and Data Analysis*, **50**, 2635–2654.

4. Cavanaugh, J. E. and Neath, A. A. (1999). Generalizing the derivation of the Schwarz information criterion, *Communications in Statistics—Theory and Methods*, **28**, 49–66.

5. Davies, S. L., Neath, A. A., and Cavanaugh J. E. (2005). Cross validation model selection criteria for linear regression based on the Kullback–Leibler discrepancy, *Statistical Methodology*, **2**, 249–266.

6. Hurvich, C. M. and Tsai, C. L. (1989). Regression and time series model selection in small samples, *Biometrika*, **76**, 297–307.

7. Linhart, H. and Zucchini, W. (1986). *Model Selection*, Wiley, New York.

8. Mallows, C. L. (1973). Some comments on C_p, *Technometrics*, **15**, 661–675.

9. Stone, M. (1977). An asymptotic equivalence of choice of model by cross-validation and Akaike's criterion, *Journal of the Royal Statistical Society, Series B*, **39**, 44–47.

34

Focused Information Criteria for the Linear Hazard Regression Model

Nils Lid Hjort

Department of Mathematics, University of Oslo, Oslo, Norway

Abstract: The linear hazard regression model developed by Aalen is becoming an increasingly popular alternative to the Cox multiplicative hazard regression model. There are no methods in the literature for selecting among different candidate models of this nonparametric type, however. In the present chapter a focused information criterion is developed for this task. The criterion works for each specified covariate vector, by estimating the mean squared error for each candidate model's estimate of the associated cumulative hazard rate; the finally selected model is the one with lowest estimated mean squared error. Averaged versions of the criterion are also developed.

Keywords and Phrases: Aalen's linear model, covariate selection, focused information criterion, hazard regression, model selection

34.1 Introduction: Which Covariates to Include?

We consider survival regression data of the usual form (T_i, δ_i, x_i) for individuals $i = 1, \ldots, n$, where x_i is a vector of say r covariates, among which one wishes to select those of highest relevance. Also, $T_i = \min\{T_i^0, C_i\}$ is the possibly censored life-length and $\delta_i = I\{T_i^0 < C_i\}$ the associated noncensoring indicator, in terms of underlying life-length T_i^0 and censoring time C_i for individual i.

Our framework is that of the linear hazard regression model introduced by Aalen (1980); see; for example, the extensive discussion in Andersen *et al.* (1993, Ch. 8) and Martinussen and Scheike (2006, Ch. 5), where the hazard rate for individual i may be represented as

$$h_i(u) = x_i^{\mathrm{t}} \alpha(u) = \sum_{j=1}^{r} x_{i,j} \alpha_j(u) \quad \text{for } i = 1, \ldots, n,$$

in terms of regressor functions $\alpha_1(u), \ldots, \alpha_r(u)$. These need to satisfy the requirement that the linear combination $x^t \alpha(u)$ stays nonnegative for all x supported by the distribution of covariate vectors. In other words, the associated cumulative hazard function

$$H(t \mid x) = \int_0^t x^t \alpha(u) \, du = x^t A(u) = \sum_{j=1}^r x_j A_j(t) \qquad (34.1)$$

is nondecreasing in t, for all x in the relevant covariate space; here we write $A_j(t) = \int_0^t \alpha_j(u) \, du$ for $j = 1, \ldots, r$.

Among questions discussed in this chapter is when we might do better with only a subset of the x covariates than with keeping them all. We focus specifically on the problem of estimating $H(t \mid x)$ of (34.1) well, for a specified individual carrying his given covariate information x. The full-model estimator

$$\widehat{H}(t \mid x) = \widehat{H}_{\text{full}}(t \mid x) = x^t \widehat{A}(t) = \sum_{j=1}^r x_j \widehat{A}_j(t) \qquad (34.2)$$

is one option, using the familiar Aalen estimators for $A_1, \ldots, A_r$ in the full model, keeping all covariates on board. Pushing some covariates out of the model leads to competing estimators of the type

$$\widetilde{H}_I(t \mid x) = \sum_{j \in I} x_j \widetilde{A}_{I,j}(t), \qquad (34.3)$$

where the index set I is a subset of $\{1, \ldots, r\}$, representing those covariates that are kept in the model, and where the $\widetilde{A}_{I,j}(t)$s for $j \in I$ are the Aalen estimators in the linear hazard rate model associated with the I covariates. Using $\widetilde{H}_I(t \mid x)$ instead of $\widehat{H}(t \mid x)$ will typically correspond to smaller variances but to modelling bias. Slightly more generally, bigger index sets I imply more variance but less modelling bias, and vice versa. Thus the task of selecting suitable covariates amounts to a statistical balancing game between sampling variability and bias.

In Section 34.2 we fix the framework and give proper definitions of full-model and submodel estimators. These are also expressed in terms of counting processes and at-risk processes. Links with martingale theory make it possible in Section 34.3 to accurately assess the bias and variance properties associated with a given candidate model. This is followed up in Section 34.4 by explicit methods for estimating bias and variance from the data. The focused information criterion (FIC) introduced in Section 34.5 acts by estimating the risk associated with each candidate model's estimator of the cumulative hazard function; the model we suggest being used in the end is the one with the lowest estimated risk. Weighted versions are also put forward. In an extended version of the present work the use of the methods for real data and in some simulation setups will be reported. This chapter ends with a list of concluding remarks in Section 34.7.

The brief introduction has so far taken model comparison as corresponding to accuracy of estimators of cumulative hazard rates $H(t \mid x)$. By a delta method argument this is also nearly equivalent to ranking models in terms of accuracy of estimates of survival probabilities $S(t \mid x) = \exp\{-H(t \mid x)\}$, where the estimates in question take the form

$$\widehat{S}_{\text{full}}(t \mid x) = \prod_{[0,t]}\{1 - x^{\text{t}}\,\widehat{A}(u)\} \quad \text{and} \quad \widetilde{S}_I(t \mid x) = \prod_{[0,t]}\Big\{1 - \sum_{j \in I} x_j\, \mathrm{d}\widetilde{A}_{I,j}(u)\Big\}.$$

[For details regarding notation for and properties of the product integral used on the right; see, for example, Andersen *et al.* (1993, Ch. II.6).] It is important to realise that a submodel I may work better than the full model, even if the submodel in question is not 'fully correct' as such; this is determined, among other aspects, by the sizes of the $\alpha_j(u)$ regressor functions that are left out of a model. This makes model selection different in spirit and operation than, for example, performing goodness-of-fit checks on all candidate models.

Aalen's linear hazard model is in many important respects different from Cox's proportional hazard model, also regarding the mathematical treatment of estimators and their properties; see Andersen *et al.* (1993, Ch. II.6). We note that focused information criteria and a general theory for model averaging estimators for the Cox model have been developed in Hjort and Claeskens (2006). Based on research in that and in the present chapter methods may be devised that can help select between 'the best Cox model' and 'the best Aalen model', in situations where that question is of relevance, but that theme is not pursued here.

34.2 Estimators in Submodels

This section properly defines the Aalen estimators $\widehat{A}$ and $\widetilde{A}_I$ involved in (34.2) and (34.3). It is convenient to define these in terms of the counting process and at-risk process

$$N_i(t) = I\{T_i \le t, \delta_i = 1\} \quad \text{and} \quad Y_i(u) = I\{T_i \ge u\}$$

for individuals $i = 1, \ldots, n$. We also need the martingales $M_i(t) = N_i(t) - \int_0^t Y_i(u)\,\mathrm{d}H_i(u)$, for which

$$\mathrm{d}N_i(u) = Y_i(u)x_i^{\text{t}}\,\mathrm{d}A(u) + \mathrm{d}M_i(u). \tag{34.4}$$

These are orthogonal and square integrable with variance processes

$$\langle M_i, M_i \rangle(t) = \int_0^t Y_i(u)h_i(u)\,\mathrm{d}u = \int_0^t Y_i(u)x_i^{\text{t}}\,\mathrm{d}A(u). \tag{34.5}$$

In other words, $M_i(t)^2 - \langle M_i, M_i \rangle(t)$ is another zero-mean martingale, implying in particular that the mean of (34.5) is equal to the variance of $M_i(t)$.

Now introduce the $r \times r$-size matrix function

$$G_n(u) = n^{-1} \sum_{i=1}^{n} Y_i(u) x_i x_i^{\mathrm{t}}. \tag{34.6}$$

The Aalen estimator $\widehat{A} = (\widehat{A}_1, \ldots, \widehat{A}_r)^{\mathrm{t}}$ in the full model corresponds to

$$\mathrm{d}\widehat{A}(u) = G_n(u)^{-1} n^{-1} \sum_{i=1}^{n} x_i \, \mathrm{d}N_i(u),$$

with integrated version

$$\widehat{A}(t) = \int_0^t G_n(u)^{-1} n^{-1} \sum_{i=1}^{n} x_i \, \mathrm{d}N_i(u) \quad \text{for } t \geq 0. \tag{34.7}$$

This also defines $\widehat{H}_{\mathrm{full}}(t \,|\, x)$ of (34.2). It is assumed here that at least r linearly independent covariate vectors x_i remain in the risk set at time t, making the inverse of G_n well defined for all $u \leq t$; this event has probability growing exponentially quickly to 1 as sample size increases, under mild conditions.

To properly define the competitor $\widetilde{H}_I(t \,|\, x)$ of (34.3), we use the notation $x_I = \pi_I x$ for the vector of those x_j components for which $j \in I$, for each given subset I of $\{1, \ldots, r\}$. In other words, π_I is the projection matrix of size $|I| \times r$, with $|I|$ the number of covariates included in I. For the given I, we partition the G_n function into blocks,

$$G_n(u) = \begin{pmatrix} G_{n,00}(u), & G_{n,01}(u) \\ G_{n,10}(u), & G_{n,11}(u) \end{pmatrix},$$

where

$$G_{n,00}(u) = \pi_I G_n(u) \pi_I^{\mathrm{t}} = n^{-1} \sum_{i=1}^{n} Y_i(u) x_{i,I} x_{i,I}^{\mathrm{t}}$$

is of size $|I| \times |I|$, and $G_{n,11}(u)$ is of size $q \times q$ with $q = r - |I|$, and so on. The Aalen estimator for the vector of A_j functions where $j \in I$ is

$$\widetilde{A}_I(t) = \int_0^t G_{n,00}(u)^{-1} n^{-1} \sum_{i=1}^{n} x_{i,I} \, \mathrm{d}N_i(u).$$

These are those at work in (34.3).

Using (34.4) we may write

$$n^{-1} \sum_{i=1}^{n} x_{i,I} \, \mathrm{d}N_i(u) = n^{-1} \sum_{i=1}^{n} Y_i(u) x_{i,I} x_i^{\mathrm{t}} \, \mathrm{d}A(u) + n^{-1} \sum_{i=1}^{n} x_{i,I} \, \mathrm{d}M_i(u),$$

which further leads to

$$
\begin{aligned}
\mathrm{d}\tilde{A}_I(u) = G_{n,00}(u)^{-1}\Big\{ & G_{n,00}(u)\,\mathrm{d}A_I(u) + G_{n,01}(u)\,\mathrm{d}A_{II}(u) \\
& + n^{-1}\sum_{i=1}^{n} x_{i,I}\,\mathrm{d}M_i(u) \Big\},
\end{aligned}
\tag{34.8}
$$

along with its integrated version. Here $II = I^c$ is the set of indexes not in I. This representation, basically in terms of a mean term plus martingale noise, is used in the next section to characterise means and variances of the (34.3) estimators. It again assumes that the G_n is invertible on $[0, t]$, an event having probability growing exponentially to 1 and therefore not disturbing the main analysis.

We remark that when the I model is used, then the Aalen estimator $\tilde{A}_I(t)$ does not directly estimate A_I, but rather the function $A_I(t) + \int_0^t G_{00}^{-1} G_{01}\,\mathrm{d}A_{II}$.

34.3 Bias, Variance, and Mean Squared Error Calculations

In this section we develop useful approximations for the mean squared error of each of the (34.3) estimators $\tilde{H}_I(t\,|\,x) = x_I^{\mathrm{t}}\tilde{A}_I(t)$. We assume that the censoring variables $C_1, \ldots, C_n$ are i.i.d. with some survival distribution $C(u) = \Pr\{C_i \geq u\}$, and that they are independent of the lifetimes T_i^0; the case of no censoring corresponds to $C(u) = 1$ for all u. It is furthermore convenient to postulate that $x_1, \ldots, x_n$ stem from some distribution in the space of covariate vectors. These assumptions imply, for example, that the G_n function of (34.6) converges with increasing sample size, say

$$
G_n(u) \to G(u) = \mathrm{E}_* Y(u) x x^{\mathrm{t}} = \mathrm{E}_* \exp\{-x^{\mathrm{t}} A(u)\} x x^{\mathrm{t}} C(u),
\tag{34.9}
$$

where E_* refers to expectation under the postulated covariate distribution. Also the mean function

$$
\bar{G}_n(u) = \mathrm{E}\,G_n(u) = n^{-1}\sum_{i=1}^{n} p_i(u) x_i x_i^{\mathrm{t}}
$$

converges to the same limit $G(u)$; here $p_i(u) = \mathrm{E}Y_i(u) = \exp\{-x_i^{\mathrm{t}} A(u)\}\,C(u)$. We finally assume that the $r \times r$-function $G(u)$ is invertible over the time observation window $u \in [0, \tau]$ of interest; this corresponds to $C(\tau)$ positive and to a nondegenerate covariate distribution. As in Section 34.2 there is a need to partition the $G(u)$ function into blocks $G_{00}(u), G_{01}(u)$, and so on; $G_{00}(u)$ has, for example, size $|I| \times |I|$. A similar remark applies to $\bar{G}_n(u)$.

Consider as in Section 34.1 a given individual with covariate information x. From representation (34.8),

$$
\begin{aligned}
x_I^{\mathrm t}\,\mathrm d\tilde A_I(u) &= x_I^{\mathrm t}\,\mathrm dA_I(u) + x_I^{\mathrm t}G_{n,00}(u)^{-1}G_{n,01}(u)\,\mathrm dA_{II}(u)\\
&\quad + n^{-1/2}x_I^{\mathrm t}G_{n,00}(u)^{-1}\,\mathrm dV_{n,I}(u)\\
&= x^{\mathrm t}\,\mathrm dA(u) + b_{I,n}(u)^{\mathrm t}\,\mathrm dA_{II}(u) + n^{-1/2}x_I^{\mathrm t}G_{n,00}(u)^{-1}\,\mathrm dV_{n,I}(u),
\end{aligned}
$$

in which V_n is the r-dimensional martingale process with increments

$$
\mathrm dV_n(u) = n^{-1/2}\sum_{i=1}^{n} x_i\,\mathrm dM_i(u), \tag{34.10}
$$

whereas $b_{I,n}$, defined by

$$
b_{I,n}(u) = G_{n,10}(u)G_{n,00}(u)^{-1}x_I - x_{II}, \tag{34.11}
$$

can be seen as a bias function (omitting at the moment x in the notation for this function). Its dimension is $q = r - |I|$. This leads to the representation

$$
\sqrt n\{x_I^{\mathrm t}\tilde A_I(t) - x^{\mathrm t}A(t)\} = \sqrt n\int_0^t b_{I,n}^{\mathrm t}\,\mathrm dA_{II} + x_I^{\mathrm t}\int_0^t G_{n,00}^{-1}\,\mathrm dV_{n,I}. \tag{34.12}
$$

The second term is a zero-mean martingale whereas the first term is a bias term, stemming from using model I that does not include all the components. We use (34.12) to develop good approximations to

$$
\mathrm{mse}_n(I) = \mathrm{mse}_n(I,t) = n\,\mathrm E\{\tilde H_I(t\,|\,x) - H(t\,|\,x)\}^2,
$$

the normalised mean squared error of the (34.3) estimator. We treat the covariate vectors $x_1,\dots,x_n$ as given; that is, our approximations are expressed directly in terms of these.

In view of the assumptions made in the beginning of this section, a first-order approximation to the mean of (34.12) is $\sqrt n\int_0^t \bar b_{I,n}^{\mathrm t}\,\mathrm dA_{II}$, because the second term has zero mean; here $\bar b_{I,n}(u) = \bar G_{n,10}(u)\bar G_{n,00}(u)^{-1}$. Also, $\int_0^t b_{I,n}^{\mathrm t}\,\mathrm dA_{II}$ and $\int_0^t \bar b_{I,n}^{\mathrm t}\,\mathrm dA_{II}$ are both close to the limit $\int_0^t b_I^{\mathrm t}\,\mathrm dA_{II}$, with high probability for large n, where $b_I(u) = G_{10}(u)G_{00}^{-1}x_I - x_{II}$.

To study the second term of (34.12), note that V_n of (34.10) is a zero-mean martingale with variance process $\langle V_n, V_n\rangle(t) = J_n(t)$, with $r \times r$-matrix increments

$$
\mathrm dJ_n(u) = n^{-1}\sum_{i=1}^{n} Y_i(u)x_i x_i^{\mathrm t}\, x_i^{\mathrm t}\,\mathrm dA(u).
$$

There is a well-defined limit function $J(u)$ with increments

$$
\mathrm dJ(u) = \mathrm E_* Y(u)xx^{\mathrm t}\,x^{\mathrm t}\,\mathrm dA(u) = \mathrm E_*\exp\{-x^{\mathrm t}A(u)\}xx^{\mathrm t}\,x^{\mathrm t}\,\mathrm dA(u)\,C(u)
$$

under the conditions stated above. Thus V_n converges in distribution to a Gaussian martingale V with increments $dV(u)$ having zero mean and variance matrix $dJ(u)$. It also follows that the second term of (34.12) converges in distribution,

$$x_I^{\mathrm{t}} \int_0^t G_{n,00}^{-1} \, dV_{n,I} \to_d x_I^{\mathrm{t}} \int_0^t G_{00}^{-1} \, dV_I,$$

which is normal with variance

$$\mathrm{var}(I, t) = x_I^{\mathrm{t}} \int_0^t G_{00}^{-1} \, dJ_{00} \, G_{00}^{-1} x_I.$$

The integral here is defined in the appropriate and natural Riemannian sense, and is also equivalent to a finite sum of ordinary integrals, found by writing out the quadratic form.

The first term of (34.12) is essentially nonrandom when compared with the second term. A more formal statement can be put forward in a framework of local asymptotic neighbourhoods, where $dA_{II}(u) = dD(u)/\sqrt{n}$, say; in this case,

$$\sqrt{n}\{\tilde{H}_I(t \mid x) - H(t \mid x)\} \to_d \int_0^t b(u)^{\mathrm{t}} \, dD(u) + \mathrm{N}(0, \mathrm{var}(I, t)).$$

Our main use of these considerations is the approximation to the normalised mean squared error;

$$\mathrm{mse}_n(I, t) \doteq \mathrm{sqb}(I, t) + \mathrm{var}(I, t), \tag{34.13}$$

where $\mathrm{var}(I, t)$ is defined above and

$$\mathrm{sqb}(I, t) = n\Big(\int_0^t \bar{b}_{I,n}^{\mathrm{t}} \, dA_{II}\Big)^2.$$

Remark There are often situations where it pays to exclude some covariates, even though their associated $\alpha_j(u)$ functions are nonzero. This is a consequence of the squared bias versus variance balancing game. For example, a submodel I is better than the full set, for the given covariate x, if $\mathrm{sqb}(I, t) + \mathrm{var}(I, t) \le 0 + \mathrm{var}(\mathrm{full}, t)$, which translates to

$$n\Big\{\int_0^t (G_{10}G_{00}^{-1} x_I - x_{II})^{\mathrm{t}} \, dA_{II}\Big\}^2 \le x^{\mathrm{t}} \int_0^t G^{-1} \, dJ \, G^{-1} x - x_I^{\mathrm{t}} \int_0^t G_{00}^{-1} \, dJ_{00} \, G_{00}^{-1} x_I.$$

This effectively describes a 'tolerance radius' around a given model, inside which the model is preferable to the full model, even when not perfectly valid. The inequality says that a certain linear combination of the $\alpha_j(u)$ functions for $j \notin I$ should not be too big, compared also to the sample size; for large n even small biases are costly, and the full model becomes preferable.

34.4   Estimating the Risks

We have seen that each candidate model I has an associated risk $\mathrm{mse}_n(I,t)$ of (34.13) when estimating the cumulative hazard function using $\widetilde{H}_I(t\,|\,x)$. Here we deal with the consequent task of estimating these risk quantities from data.

For the variance part we use

$$\widehat{\mathrm{var}}(I,t) = x_I^{\mathrm{t}} \int_0^t G_{n,00}^{-1}(u)\,\mathrm{d}\widehat{J}_{n,00}(u)\,G_{n,00}(u)^{-1}\,x_I,$$

wherein

$$\mathrm{d}\widehat{J}_n(u) = n^{-1}\sum_{i=1}^n Y_i(u)x_i x_i^{\mathrm{t}}\,x_i^{\mathrm{t}}\mathrm{d}\widehat{A}(u),$$

engaging the full-model Aalen estimator. The $|I|\times|I|$ block used for the variance estimation is $\pi_I\,\mathrm{d}\widehat{J}_n(u)\pi_I^{\mathrm{t}}$.

For the squared bias part, consider in general terms the quantity β^2, where $\beta = \int_0^t g^{\mathrm{t}}\,\mathrm{d}A_{II}$, for a specified q-dimensional function g; again, $q = r - |I|$. Considering $\widehat{\beta} = \int_0^t g^{\mathrm{t}}\,\mathrm{d}\widehat{A}_{II}$, employing the II part of the full-model Aalen estimator, we have

$$\mathrm{E}\,\widehat{\beta} \doteq \beta \quad\text{and}\quad \mathrm{Var}\,\widehat{\beta} \doteq n^{-1}\int_0^t g(u)^{\mathrm{t}}\,\mathrm{d}Q(u)\,g(u),$$

from results above, where we write

$$\mathrm{d}Q(u) = \{G(u)^{-1}\,\mathrm{d}J(u)\,G(u)^{-1}\}_{11}$$

for the lower right-hand $q \times q$ block of the matrix within brackets, the block associated with subset $II = I^c$. Thus $\mathrm{E}\,\widehat{\beta}^2 \doteq \beta^2 + n^{-1}\int_0^t g^{\mathrm{t}}\,\mathrm{d}Q\,g$, in its turn leading to the natural and nearly unbiased estimator

$$\left(\int_0^t g^{\mathrm{t}}\,\mathrm{d}\widehat{A}_{II}\right)^2 - n^{-1}\int_0^t g(u)^{\mathrm{t}}\,\mathrm{d}\widehat{Q}_n(u)\,g(u)$$

for β^2, where

$$\mathrm{d}\widehat{Q}_n(u) = \pi_{II}\{G_n(u)^{-1}\,\mathrm{d}\widehat{J}_n(u)\,G_n(u)^{-1}\}\pi_{II}^{\mathrm{t}}$$

is the empirical counterpart to $\mathrm{d}Q(u)$.

These considerations lead to the risk estimator

$$\widehat{R}(I,t) = \widehat{\mathrm{mse}}_n(I,t) = \max\{\widehat{\mathrm{sqb}}(I,t),0\} + x_I^{\mathrm{t}}\int_0^t G_{n,00}^{-1}\,\mathrm{d}\widehat{J}_{n,00}\,G_{n,00}^{-1}\,x_I,$$

where

$$\widehat{\mathrm{sqb}}(I,t) = n\left(\int_0^t b_{I,n}^{\mathrm{t}}\,\mathrm{d}\widehat{A}_{II}\right)^2 - \int_0^t b_{I,n}^{\mathrm{t}}\,\mathrm{d}\widehat{Q}_n\,b_{I,n}.$$

34.5   The FIC and the Weighted FIC

Here we show how risk estimation methods developed above lead to natural information criteria for model selection.

The first such is a *focused information criterion* that works for a given individual and a given time point at which we wish optimal precision for her survival probability estimate. For the given covariate x and time point t we calculate

$$\text{FIC} = \text{FIC}(I, x, t) = \max\{\widehat{\text{sqb}}(I, x, t), 0\} + \widehat{\text{var}}(I, x, t) \qquad (34.14)$$

for each candidate model I, where

$$\widehat{\text{sqb}}(I, x, t) = n\left(\int_0^t b_{I,n}^{\text{t}} \, d\widehat{A}_{II}\right)^2 - \int_0^t b_{I,n}^{\text{t}} \, d\widehat{Q}_n \, b_{I,n},$$

$$\widehat{\text{var}}(I, x, t) = x_I^{\text{t}} \int_0^t G_{n,00}^{-1} \, d\widehat{J}_{n,00} \, G_{n,00}^{-1} \, x_I.$$

We note that $b_{I,n}(u)$ of (34.11) depends on x and that the submatrices $G_{n,00}$ and so on of (34.9) depend on I. In the end one selects the model with smallest value of the FIC score number.

Note that FIC is sample-size dependent. In a situation with a given amount of nonzero bias $\int_0^t \bar{b}_I^{\text{t}} \, dA_{II}$, the $\widehat{\text{sqb}}$ component of FIC will essentially increase with n, whereas the variance component remains essentially constant. This goes to show that the best models will tolerate less and less bias as n increases, and for sufficiently large n only the full model (which has zero modelling bias) will survive FIC scrutiny.

There are various variations on the FIC above. For a given individual who has survived up to time t_1 it is the conditional survival probabilities

$$\Pr\{T^0 \geq t_2 \mid T^0 \geq t_1, x\} = \exp[-\{H(t_2 \mid x) - H(t_1 \mid x)\}]$$

that are of interest. The development and formulae above can be repeated mutatis mutandis with a given interval $[t_1, t_2]$ replacing $[0, t]$. This gives a machinery for selecting models that yield optimal estimation precision for conditional survival probabilities. It will also be useful in many applications to monitor FIC scores for important candidate models in terms of a 'gliding time window', say $[t - \delta, t + \delta]$; successful models should then have good FIC scores across time. We stress that it is not a paradox that one model might be particularly good at explaining the survival mechanisms involved for short life-lengths, whereas another model might be much better for understanding the survival of the longer life-lengths. Our FIC takes this on board, and makes an explicit model recommendation for each given time interval of interest.

Suppose now that a model is called for that works well in an average sense across a given set of (x, t) values, as opposed to a given (x, t). Consider in general terms

$$\mathcal{E}_n(I) = n \int \{\tilde{H}_I(t \,|\, x) - H(t \,|\, x)\}^2 \, \mathrm{d}w(t, x),$$

where $w(t, x)$ is a weight measure in the (x, t) space. This could, for example, take the form

$$\mathcal{E}_n(I) = (1/K) \sum_{j=1}^{K} n\{\tilde{H}_I(t \,|\, x_j) - H(t \,|\, x_j)\}^2, \qquad (34.15)$$

averaging across given covariate vectors $x_1, \ldots, x_K$. From (34.12), the random loss incurred using I is

$$\mathcal{E}_n(I) = \int \left\{ \sqrt{n} \int_0^t b_{I,n}(u, x)^{\mathrm{t}} \, \mathrm{d}A_{II}(u) + x_I^{\mathrm{t}} \int_0^t G_{n,00}(u)^{-1} \, \mathrm{d}V_{n,I}(u) \right\}^2 \mathrm{d}w(t, x),$$

writing now

$$b_{I,n}(u, x) = G_{n,10}(u) G_{n,00}(u)^{-1} x_I - x_{II}$$

with explicit mention of x in the notation.

Its associated risk, the expected loss, is by previous efforts closely approximated by the w-weighted risk

$$R_n(I) = \mathrm{E} \int \left[n \left\{ \int_0^t b_{I,n}(u, x)^{\mathrm{t}} \, \mathrm{d}A_{II}(u) \right\}^2 + x_I^{\mathrm{t}} \int_0^t G_{n,00}^{-1} \, \mathrm{d}J_{n,00} \, G_{n,00}^{-1} \, x_I \right] \mathrm{d}w(t, x).$$

We estimate the w-weighted squared bias and w-weighted variance contributions in turn. Define

$$\mathrm{w}\text{-}\widehat{\mathrm{sqb}}(I) = n \int \left\{ \int_0^t b_{I,n}(u, x)^{\mathrm{t}} \, \mathrm{d}\hat{A}_{II}(u) \right\}^2 \mathrm{d}w(t, x)$$
$$- \int \int_0^t b_{I,n}(u, x)^{\mathrm{t}} \, \mathrm{d}\hat{Q}_n(u) \, b_{I,n}(u, x) \, \mathrm{d}w(t, x),$$

which is an approximately unbiased estimator of the w-weighted squared bias term; and

$$\mathrm{w}\text{-}\widehat{\mathrm{var}}(I) = \int \widehat{\mathrm{var}}(I, x, t) \, \mathrm{d}w(t, x).$$

Our wFIC score, to be computed for each candidate model, is

$$\mathrm{wFIC}(I) = \max\{\mathrm{w}\text{-}\widehat{\mathrm{sqb}}(I), 0\} + \mathrm{w}\text{-}\widehat{\mathrm{var}}(I). \qquad (34.16)$$

Again, in the end the model achieving the lowest wFIC score is selected. This scheme in particular gives rise to an algorithm associated with the (34.15) loss, weighting evenly across a finite set of covariate vectors.

A special case worth recording is when t is fixed and w describes the covariate distribution. It is unknown, but may be approximated with the empirical distribution of covariates $x_1, \ldots, x_n$. This leads to wFIC(I) as in (34.16) with

$$
\text{w-}\widehat{\text{var}}(I) = n^{-1} \sum_{i=1}^{n} \widehat{\text{var}}(I, x_i, t)
$$

$$
= \text{Tr}\left\{ \left(\int_0^t G_{n,00}^{-1} \, d\widehat{J}_{n,00} \, G_{n,00}^{-1} \right) \left(n^{-1} \sum_{i=1}^{n} x_{i,I} x_{i,I}^{\text{t}} \right) \right\},
$$

whereas w-$\widehat{\text{sqb}}(I)$ may be written

$$
\sum_{i=1}^{n} \{ x_{i,I}^{\text{t}} \widehat{B}_I(t) - x_{i,II}^{\text{t}} \widehat{A}_{II}(t) \}^2 - n^{-1} \sum_{i=1}^{n} \int_0^t b_{I,n}(u, x_i)^{\text{t}} \, d\widehat{Q}_n(u) \, b_{I,n}(u, x_i),
$$

where

$$
\widehat{B}_I(t) = \int_0^t G_{n,00}(u)^{-1} G_{n,01}(u) \, d\widehat{A}_{II}(u).
$$

Remark Note that the wFIC method as defined here is subtly but crucially different from simply w-weighting of the individual pointwise FIC scores, regarding how the truncation of the squared bias estimate is carried out. In (34.16), the truncation to achieve nonnegativity of the estimate takes place after the w-weighting, making it different from w-weighting the collection of truncated sqb(I, x, t) terms. See in this connection also Claeskens and Hjort (2007).

34.6 Exact Risk Calculations

In the previous sections we were able to (i) develop formulae for risk functions and (ii) construct estimators for these. This led to model selection methods that may be used in any given application. The present section has a different aim, namely that of providing classes of case studies where the risk function formulae can be computed explicitly, thereby establishing a fair testing ground for model selection and model averaging methods. For reasons of space we are content to derive certain formulae under certain conditions, for biases and variances; these may then be used to form concrete illustrations and test cases that for reasons of space cannot be reported on in the present chapter.

Assume that the components $x_1, \ldots, x_r$ of the covariate vector x are distributed independently of each other, with Laplace transforms $\text{E}_* \exp(-\theta_j x_j) = \exp\{-M_j(\theta_j)\}$, say. Then

$$
\text{E}_* \exp(-\theta^{\text{t}} x) = \exp\{-M_1(\theta_1) - \cdots - M_r(\theta_r)\},
$$

from which follows, taking second-order derivatives with respect to the θ components, that

$$\mathrm{E}_* \exp(-\theta^t x) x_j x_k = \exp\left\{-\sum_{l=1}^r M_l(\theta_l)\right\}\{-M_j''(\theta_j)\delta_{j,k} + M_j'(\theta_j)M_k'(\theta_k)\},$$

in terms of first- and second-order derivatives of the M_j functions. This implies that the $r \times r$ limit function G of (34.9) may be expressed as

$$G(u) = f(u)\{D(u) + z(u)z(u)^t\}C(u).$$

Here $f(u) = \exp\{-\sum_{l=1}^r M_l(A_l(u))\}$; $D(u)$ is the diagonal matrix with elements $D_j(u) = -M_j''(A_j(u))$; and $z(u)$ is the vector with elements $z_j(u) = M_j'(A_j(u))$. For a candidate set I of covariates to include, the blocks of $G(u)$ can be read off from

$$G(u) = f(u)C(u)\left\{\begin{pmatrix} D_0 & 0 \\ 0 & D_1 \end{pmatrix} + \begin{pmatrix} z_0 \\ z_1 \end{pmatrix}\begin{pmatrix} z_0 \\ z_1 \end{pmatrix}^t\right\},$$

where D_0 and D_1 have components $D_j(u)$ where, respectively, $j \in I$ and $j \notin I$, and similarly z_0 and z_1 have components $z_j(u)$ where $j \in I$ and $j \notin I$. In particular,

$$G_{00}(u) = f(u)C(u)(D_0 + z_0 z_0^t) \quad \text{and} \quad G_{01}(u) = f(u)C(u)z_0 z_1^t,$$

leading in turn, via the matrix inversion formula

$$(D_0 + z_0 z_0^t)^{-1} = D_0^{-1} - \frac{1}{1 + z_0^t D_0^{-1} z_0} D_0^{-1} z_0 z_0^t D_0^{-1},$$

to a formula for $G_{00}(u)^{-1}G_{01}(u)$ and then to

$$\begin{aligned}
b_I(u) &= G_{10}(u)G_{00}(u)^{-1}x_I - x_{II} \\
&= z_1 z_0^t\left(D_0^{-1} - \frac{1}{1 + z_0^t D_0^{-1} z_0} D_0^{-1} z_0 z_0^t D_0^{-1}\right)x_I - x_{II} \\
&= z_1 \frac{z_0^t D_0^{-1} x_I}{1 + z_0^t D_0^{-1} z_0} - x_{II}.
\end{aligned}$$

Assume for a concrete example that $x_j \sim \mathrm{gamma}(a_j, b_j)$ for $j = 1, \ldots, r$, for which the Laplace transforms are $\{b_j/(b_j+\theta_j)\}^{a_j}$ with $M_j(\theta_j) = a_j\log(1+\theta_j/b_j)$. Then

$$M_j'(\theta_j) = \frac{\xi_j}{1 + \theta_j/b_j} \quad \text{and} \quad M_j''(\theta_j) = -\frac{\xi_j/b_j}{(1 + \theta_j/b_j)^2},$$

with $\xi_j = \mathrm{E}_* x_j = a_j/b_j$. This yields a bias function $b_I(u)$ with components

$$b_{I,j}(u) = \frac{g_I(u)}{1 + \sum_{j \in I} b_j \xi_j} \frac{\xi_j}{1 + A_j(u)/b_j} - x_j \quad \text{for } j \in II = I^c,$$

where $g_I(u) = \sum_{j \in I} \{b_j + A_j(u)\} x_j$. It follows that the important bias component of (34.12) may be written

$$\sqrt{n} \int_0^t b_I^{\mathrm{t}} \, \mathrm{d}A_{II} = \sqrt{n} \Big\{ \int_0^t \frac{g_I(u)}{1 + \sum_{j \in I} b_j \xi_j} \sum_{j \in II} \frac{\xi_j \alpha_j(u)}{1 + A_j(u)/b_j} \, \mathrm{d}u - x_{II}^{\mathrm{t}} A_{II}(t) \Big\}.$$

These bias functions are easily computed and displayed, for given covariate distributions and given hazard regression functions.

To handle the variance part of (34.13) we need an explicit formula for $\mathrm{d}J(u)$ and then for

$$G_{00}^{-1} \, \mathrm{d}J_{00} \, G_{00}^{-1} \quad \text{and} \quad G(u)^{-1} \, \mathrm{d}J(u) \, G(u)^{-1}.$$

We start with

$$\mathrm{E}_* \exp(-s\theta^{\mathrm{t}} x) x_j x_k = \exp\Big\{ -\sum_{l=1}^r M_l(s\theta_l) \Big\} \{ -M_j''(s\theta_j)\delta_{j,k} + M_j'(s\theta_j)M_k'(s\theta_k) \},$$

and then take the derivative w.r.t. s, and set $s = 1$ in the resulting equations. This yields

$$\begin{aligned}
\mathrm{E}_* \exp\{-\theta^{\mathrm{t}} x) x_j x_k \, \theta^{\mathrm{t}} x = {} & f^*(\theta)[\{M_j'''(\theta_j)\theta_j - g^*(\theta)M_j''(\theta_j)\}\delta_{j,k} \\
& - M_j'(\theta_j)M_k''(\theta_k)\theta_k - M_j''(\theta_j)M_k'(\theta_k)\theta_j \\
& + g^*(\theta)M_j'(\theta_j)M_k'(\theta_k)],
\end{aligned}$$

where

$$f^*(\theta) = \exp\Big\{ -\sum_{l=1}^r M_l(\theta_l) \Big\} \quad \text{and} \quad g^*(\theta) = \sum_{l=1}^r M_l'(\theta_l)\theta_l.$$

Let now $A_j(t) = \alpha_j t$ for $j = 1, \ldots, r$; that is, the α_j regressor functions are taken constant. The above leads with some further work to a formula for

$$\mathrm{E}_* \exp\{-x^{\mathrm{t}} A(u)\} x x^{\mathrm{t}} \, x^{\mathrm{t}} \, \mathrm{d}A(u) = f(u)\{E(u) + F(u)\} \, \mathrm{d}u,$$

where the $E(u)$ and $F(u)$ matrix functions are described below; also, $f(u) = \exp\{-\sum_{l=1}^r M_l(A_l(u))\}$ is as for the bias calculations above. The $E(u)$ is diagonal with elements

$$E_j(u) = M_j'''(A_j(u))\alpha_j - g(u)M_j''(A_j(u)),$$

where $g(u) = \sum_{l=1}^r M_l'(A_l(u))\alpha_l$. Next, $F(u)$ has (j, k) element

$$\begin{aligned}
-M_j'(A_j(u))M_k''(A_k(u))\alpha_k {} & - M_j''(A_j(u))M_k'(A_k(u))\alpha_j \\
& + g(u)M_j'(A_j(u))M_k'(A_k(u)).
\end{aligned}$$

These results may be used to compute the variance terms

$$x_I^{\text{t}} \int_0^t G_{00}^{-1} \, \mathrm{d}J_{00} \, G_{00}^{-1} \, x_I$$

and thereby the mean squared errors for different candidate models. These formulae may in particular be used for the case mentioned earlier, with independent gamma(a_j, b_j) distribution for the x_j components, and for which $M_j'''(\theta_j) = 2(\xi_j/b_j^2)/(1 + \theta_j/b_j)^3$.

Various concrete illustrations may now be given, for the specific case of independent gamma distributed covariates, to exhibit and examine various aspects and issues involved in model selection and model averaging. These relate in various ways to modelling bias versus estimation variance. We may, for example, show that when $\alpha_j(u)$s are small in size, then it may be best not to include these in the selected model, depending also on the sizes of x_I and x_{II}. We would also be able to illustrate how the complexity of the best model increases with higher sample size, and how the qualitative results depend on the relative spread of the distributions of covariates.

34.7   Concluding Remarks

Here we offer some concluding comments, some pointing to natural extensions of the material and methods we have presented above.

1. In a planned extended version of this chapter space will be given to analysis of a real dataset and to instructive simulation setups.

2. We have throughout used 'vanilla weights' for the Aalen estimators $\widehat{A}$ of (34.7). With more sophisticated weighting the estimator

$$\widehat{A}(t, k) = \int_0^t \left\{ n^{-1} \sum_{i=1}^n Y_i(u) k_i(u) x_i x_i^{\text{t}} \right\}^{-1} n^{-1} \sum_{i=1}^n x_i k_i(u) \, \mathrm{d}N_i(u)$$

may perform slightly better; see Huffer and McKeague (1991). Also for such schemes a FIC and wFIC methodology may be developed, generalising methods given in the present chapter.

3. A local asymptotic framework may be put up for the Aalen model, similar in spirit to that employed in Hjort and Claeskens (2003) and Claeskens and Hjort (2003) for purely parametric models. Here one would use hazard rates

$$h_i(u) = \sum_{j=1}^p x_{i,j} \alpha_j(u) + \sum_{j=1}^q z_{i,j} \delta_j(u)/\sqrt{n},$$

with $x_{i,j}$s protected covariates considered important to include in all candidate models, and $z_{i,j}$s the potentially discardable ones. A precise asymptotic description may now be given of all limiting risk functions, in terms of the $\delta_1, \ldots, \delta_q$ functions.

4. A fair question to ask is the behaviour of the final estimator, say

$$H^*(t \mid x) = \widetilde{H}_{\widehat{I}}(t \mid x),$$

where $\widehat{I}$ is the data-dependent set of finally included covariates. This is a complicated question without any easy answer. Inside the local asymptotic framework of (3), methods of Hjort and Claeskens (2003) may be used to describe the limit distribution of $\sqrt{n}\{H^*(t \mid x) - H(t \mid x)\}$, in terms of a nonlinear mixture of biased normals. This also opens the door to general model average strategies, as opposed to limiting inference methods to those that rely on deciding on only one model.

5. We have developed machinery for answering the question, "Should covariate j be included in the nonparametric Aalen model, or not?". More ambitiously and more laboriously, one can give not only two but three potential outcomes for each covariate: it might be excluded; it might be included nonparametrically; or it might be included parametrically. The latter possibility refers for example, to the model where $\alpha_j(u)$ is constant; see McKeague and Sasieni (1994) for treatment of such models. Again a FIC and a wFIC apparatus may be developed, requiring, however, more mathematical vigour.

Acknowledgements

This chapter reports on work carried out in the stimulating environment of the Centre of Advanced Study at the Norwegian Academy of Science and Letters, where Ørnulf Borgan and Odd Aalen organised a research group on Statistical Analysis of Complex Event History Data. Conversations with Axel Gandy were particularly fruitful.

References

1. Aalen, O. O. (1980). A model for nonparametric regression analysis of counting processes, In *Mathematical Statistics and Probability Theory* (Eds., W. Klonecki, A. Kozek, and J. Rosinski). *Proceedings of the 6th International Conference*, Wisla, Poland, pp. 1–25.

2. Andersen, P. K., Borgan, Ø., Gill, R., and Keiding, N. (1993). *Statistical Models Based on Counting Processes*, Springer-Verlag, Heidelberg.

3. Claeskens, G. and Hjort, N. L. (2003). The focused information criterion [with discussion], *Journal of the American Statistical Association*, **98**, 900–916 and 938–945.

4. Claeskens, G. and Hjort, N. L. (2008). Minimising average risk in regression models, *Econometric Theory*, to appear.

5. Hjort, N. L. and Claeskens, G. (2003). Frequentist average estimators [with discussion], *Journal of the American Statistical Association*, **98**, 879–899 and 938–945.

6. Hjort, N. L. and Claeskens, G. (2006). Focused information criteria and model averaging for the Cox hazard regression model, *Journal of the American Statistical Association*, **101**, 1449–1464.

7. Huffer, F. and McKeague, I. W. (1991). Weighted least squares estimation for Aalen's additive risk model, *Journal of the American Statistical Association*, **86**, 114–129.

8. McKeague, I. W. and Sasieni, P. D. (1994). A partly parametric additive risk model, *Biometrika*, **81**, 501–514.

9. Martinussen, T. and Scheike, T. H. (2006). *Dynamic Regression Models for Survival Data*, Springer-Verlag, New York.

35

On Measures of Information and Divergence and Model Selection Criteria

Alex Karagrigoriou[1] **and Takis Papaioannou**[2]

[1]*Department of Mathematics and Statistics, University of Cyprus, Nicosia, Cyprus*
[2]*Department of Statistics and Insurance Science, University of Piraeus, Piraeus, Greece and Department of Mathematics, University of Ioannina, Ioannina, Greece*

Abstract: In this chapter we discuss measures of information and divergence and model selection criteria. Three classes of measures, Fisher-type, divergence-type, and entropy-type measures, are discussed and their properties are presented. Information through censoring and truncation is presented and model selection criteria are investigated including the Akaike information criterion (AIC) and the divergence information criterion (DIC).

Keywords and Phrases: Measures of information and divergence, acid-test, additivity property, weighted distribution, censoring and truncation, model selection, AIC, DIC

35.1 Introduction

Measures of information appear everywhere in probability and statistics. They also play a fundamental role in communication theory. They have had a long history since the papers of Fisher, Shannon, and Kullback. There are many measures each claiming to capture the concept of information or simply being measures of (directed) divergence or distance between two probability distributions. Also there exist many generalizations of these measures. One may mention here the papers of Lindley and Jaynes who introduced entropy-based Bayesian information and the maximum entropy principle for determining probability models, respectively.

Broadly speaking there are three classes of measures of information and divergence: Fisher-type, divergence-type, and entropy (discrete and differential)-type measures. Some of them have been developed axiomatically (see, e.g., Shannon's entropy and its generalizations), but most of them have been established operationally in the sense that they have been introduced on the basis of their properties.

There have been several phases in the history of information theory: Initially we have (i) the development of generalizations of measures of information and divergence [f-divergence, (h-f)-divergence, hypoentropy, etc.], (ii) the synthesis (collection) of properties they ought to satisfy, and (iii) attempts to unify them. All this work refers to populations and distributions. Later on we have the emergence of information or divergence statistics based on data or samples and their use in statistical inference primarily in minimum distance estimation and for the development of asymptotic tests of goodness-of-fit or model selection criteria. Lately we have had a resurgence of interest in measures of information and divergence which are used in many places, in several contexts, and in new sampling situations.

The measures of information and divergence enjoy several properties such as nonnegativity, maximal information, and sufficiency, among others and statisticians do not agree on all of them. There is a body of knowledge known as statistical information theory which has made many advances but not achieved wide acceptance and application. The approach is more operational rather than axiomatic as is the case with Shannon's entropy.

There are several review papers that discuss the above points. We mention the following: Kendall (1973), Csiszar (1977), Kapur (1984), Aczel (1986), Papaioannou (1985, 2001), and Soofi (1994, 2000).

The aim of this chapter is to present recent developments on measures of information and divergences and model selection criteria. In particular, in Section 35.2 we present a number of measures of information and divergence and in Section 35.3 we discuss the most important properties of these measures. In Section 35.4 we review information and divergence under censoring including measures associated with weighted distributions and truncated data. Finally in Section 35.5 we cover issues related to model selection by discussing the well-known AIC criterion [Akaike (1973)] and introducing the divergence information criterion (DIC).

35.2 Classes of Measures

As mentioned earlier there are three classes of measures of information and divergence: Fisher-type, divergence-type, and entropy-type measures. In what follows assume that $f(x, \theta)$ is a probability density function (pdf) corresponding to a random variable X and depending on a parameter θ. At other places X follows a distribution with pdf f_1 or f_2.

35.2.1 Fisher-type measures

The Fisher measure of information introduced in 1925 is given by

$$I_X^F(\theta) = \begin{cases} E\left[\frac{\partial}{\partial\theta}\ln f(X,\theta)\right]^2 = -E\left[\frac{\partial^2}{\partial\theta^2}\ln f(X,\theta)\right], & \theta \text{ univariate} \\ \left\|E\left[\frac{\partial}{\partial\theta_i}\ln f(X,\theta)\frac{\partial}{\partial\theta_j}\ln f(X,\theta)\right]\right\|, & \theta\ k-\text{variate} \end{cases},$$

where $\|A_{i,j}\|$ denotes a $k \times k$ semidefinite matrix with $A_{i,j}$ the (i,j) element of the matrix. The above is the classical or expected information whereas the observed Fisher information where $\hat\theta$ an estimate of θ, is given by

$$\hat{I}_X^F(\theta) = \begin{cases} -\frac{\partial^2\ln f(X,\hat\theta)}{\partial\theta^2}, & 1 \text{ observation} \\ -\frac{\partial^2\ln f(\hat\theta|x_1,\ldots,x_n)}{\partial\theta^2}, & n \text{ observations}. \end{cases}$$

Finally the Fisher information number is given by

$$I_X^F = E\left[\frac{\partial\ln f(X)}{\partial X}\right]^2$$

or equivalently by

$$J_X^F(\theta) = -E\left[\frac{\partial^2\ln f(X)}{\partial X^2}\right] = E\left[\frac{\partial\ln f(X)}{\partial X}\right]^2 - [f'(b) - f'(a)],$$

where a and b are the endpoints of the interval of support of X.

Vajda (1973) extended the above definition by raising the score function to a power a, $a \geq 1$ for the purpose of generalizing inference with loss function other than the squared one which leads to the variance and mean squared error criteria. The corresponding measure for a univariate parameter θ is given by

$$I_X^V(\theta) = E\left|\frac{\partial}{\partial\theta}\ln f(X,\theta)\right|^a, \qquad a \geq 1.$$

In the case of a vector-parameter θ, Ferentinos and Papaioannou (1981) proposed as a measure of information $I_X^{FP}(\theta)$ any eigenvalue or special functions of the eigenvalues of Fisher's information matrix, such as the trace or its determinant.

Finally Tukey (1965) and Chandrasekar and Balakrishnan (2002) discussed the following measure of information,

$$I_X^{TB}(\theta) = \begin{cases} \frac{(\partial\mu/\partial\theta)^2}{\sigma^2}, & X \text{ univariate} \sim f(x,\theta), \theta \text{ scalar} \\ (\partial\mu/\partial\theta)'\Sigma^{-1}(\partial\mu/\partial\theta), & X \text{ vector}, \end{cases}$$

where μ and σ^2 (matrix Σ for the vector case) are the mean and the variance of the random variable X.

35.2.2   Measures of divergence

A measure of divergence is used as a way to evaluate the distance (divergence) between any two populations or functions. Let f_1 and f_2 be two probability density functions which may depend on an unknown parameter of fixed finite dimension. The most well-known measure of (directed) divergence is the Kullback–Leibler divergence which is given by

$$I_X^{KL}(f_1, f_2) = \int f_1 \ln(f_1/f_2) d\mu$$

for a measure μ. If f_1 is the density of $X = (U, V)$ and f_2 is the product of the marginal densities of U and V, I_X^{KL} is the well-known mutual or relative information in coding theory.

The additive and nonadditive directed divergences of order a were introduced in the 1960s and the 1970s [Renyi (1961), Csisczar (1963), and Rathie and Kannappan (1972)]. The so-called order a information measure of Renyi (1961) is given by

$$I_X^R(f_1, f_2) = \frac{1}{a-1} \ln \int f_1^a f_2^{1-a} d\mu, \qquad a > 0, \quad a \neq 1.$$

It should be noted that for α tending to 1 the above measure becomes the Kullback–Leibler divergence. Another measure of divergence is the measure of Kagan (1963) which is given by

$$I_X^{Ka}(f_1, f_2) = \int (1 - f_1/f_2)^2 f_2 \, d\mu.$$

Csiszar's measure of information [Csiszar (1963)] is a general divergence-type measure, known also as φ-divergence based on a convex function φ. Csiszar's measure is defined by

$$I_X^C(f_1, f_2) = \int \varphi(f_1/f_2) f_2 \, d\mu,$$

where φ is a convex function in $[0, \infty)$ such that $0\varphi(0/0) = 0$, $\varphi(u) \underset{u \to 0}{\to} 0$ and $0\varphi(u/0) = u\varphi_\infty$ with $\varphi_\infty = \lim_{u \to \infty}[\varphi(u)/u]$.

Observe that Csiszar's measure reduces to Kullback–Liebler divergence if $\varphi(u) = u \ln u$. If $\varphi(u) = (1-u)^2$ or $\varphi(u) = sgn(a-1)u^a$, $a > 0$, $a \neq 1$ Csiszar's measure yields the Kagan (Pearson's X^2) and Renyi's divergence, respectively.

Another generalization of measures of divergence is the family of power divergences introduced by Cressie and Read (1984) which is given by

$$I_X^{CR}(f_1, f_2) = \frac{1}{\lambda(\lambda+1)} \int f_1(z) \left[\left(\frac{f_1(z)}{f_2(z)} \right)^\lambda - 1 \right] dz, \qquad \lambda \in \mathbb{R},$$

where for $\lambda = 0, -1$ is defined by continuity. Note that the Kullback–Leibler divergence is obtained for λ tending to 0.

One of the most recently proposed measures of divergence is the BHHJ power divergence between f_1 and f_2 [Basu *et al.* (1998)] which is denoted by BHHJ, indexed by a positive parameter a, and defined as

$$I_X^{BHHJ}(f_1, f_2)$$
$$= \int \left\{ f_2^{1+a}(z) - \left(1 + \frac{1}{a}\right) f_1(z) f_2^a(z) + \frac{1}{a} f_1^{1+a}(z) \right\} dz, \qquad a > 0.$$

Note that the above family which is also referred to as a family of power divergences is loosely related to the Cressie and Read power divergence. It should be also noted that the BHHJ measure reduces to the Kullback–Leibler divergence for α tending to 0 and to the standard L_2 distance between f_1 and f_2 for $\alpha = 1$.

The above measures can be defined also for discrete settings. Let $P = (p_1, p_2, \ldots, p_m)$ and $Q = (q_1, q_2, \ldots, q_m)$ be two discrete finite probability distributions. Then the discrete version of Csiszar's measure is given by $I_X^C(P, Q) = \sum_{i=1}^m q_i \varphi(p_i/q_i)$ and the Cressie and Read divergence is given by

$$I_X^{CR}(P, Q) = \frac{1}{\lambda(\lambda + 1)} \sum_{i=1}^m p_i \left[\left(\frac{p_i}{q_i}\right)^\lambda - 1 \right], \quad \lambda \in R,$$

where again for $\lambda = 0, -1$ is defined by continuity. The discrete version of the BHHJ measure can be defined in a similar fashion.

For a comprehensive discussion about statistical inference based on measures of divergence the reader is referred to Pardo (2006).

35.2.3   Entropy-type measures

Let $P = (p_1, p_2, \ldots, p_m)$ be a discrete finite probability distribution associated with a r.v. X. Shannon's entropy is defined by

$$H_X^S = - \sum p_i \ln p_i.$$

It was later generalized by Renyi (1961) as entropy of order a:

$$H_X^R = \frac{1}{1-a} \ln \sum p_i^a, \qquad a > 0, \quad a \neq 1.$$

A further generalization along the lines of Csiszar's measure based on a convex function φ, known as φ-entropy, was proposed by Burbea and Rao (1982) and is given by $H_X^\varphi = - \sum_{i=1}^k \varphi(p_i)$. Finally, it is worth mentioning the entropy measure of Havrda and Charvat (1967):

$$H_X^C = \frac{1 - \sum p_i^a}{a - 1}, \qquad a > 0, \quad a \neq 1$$

which for $a = 2$ becomes the Gini–Simpson index. Other entropy-type measures include the γ-entropy given by

$$H_X^\gamma = \frac{1 - \left(\sum p_i^{1/\gamma}\right)^\gamma}{1 - 2^{\gamma-1}}, \qquad \gamma > 0, \qquad \gamma \neq 1$$

and the paired entropy given by

$$H_X^P = -\sum p_i \ln p_i - \sum (1 - p_i)\ln(1 - p_i),$$

where pairing is in the sense of $(p_i, 1 - p_i)$ [see, e.g., Burbea and Rao (1982)].

35.3 Properties of Information Measures

The measures of divergence are not formal distance functions. Any bivariate function $I_X(\cdot, \cdot)$ that satisfies the nonnegativity property, namely $I_X(\cdot, \cdot) \geq 0$ with equality iff its two arguments are equal can possibly be used as a measure of information or divergence. The three types of measures of information and divergence share similar statistical properties. Several properties have been investigated some of which are of axiomatic character and others of operational. Here we briefly mention some of these properties. In what follows we use I_X for either $I_X(\theta_1, \ldots, \theta_k), k \geq 1$, the information about $(\theta_1, \ldots, \theta_k)$ based on the r.v. X or $I_X(f_1, f_2)$, the measure of divergence between f_1 and f_2.

One of the most distinctive properties is the additivity property. The weak additivity property is defined as

$$I_{X,Y} = I_X + I_Y, \quad \text{if } X \text{ is independent of } Y$$

and the strong additivity is defined by

$$I_{X,Y} = I_X + I_{Y|X},$$

where $I_{Y|X} = E(I_{Y|X=x})$ is the conditional information or divergence of $Y|X$. The subadditivity and superadditivity properties are defined through weak additivity when the equal sign is replaced with an inequality:

$$I_{X,Y} \leq I_X + I_Y \quad \text{(subadditivity)}$$

and

$$I_{X,Y} \geq I_X + I_Y \quad \text{(superadditivity)}.$$

Observe that super- and subadditivity are contradictory. Subadditivity is not satisfied for any known measure except Shannon's entropy [see, e.g., Papaioannou (1985)]. Superadditivity coupled with equality iff X and Y independent is satisfied by Fisher's information number (Fisher's shift-invariant information) and mutual information [see, e.g., Papaioannou and Ferentinos (2005) and Micheas and Zografos (2006)]. Superadditivity generates measures of dependence or correlation whereas subadditivity stems from the conditional inequality (entropy).

Three important inequality properties are the conditional inequality given by

$$I_{X|Y} \leq I_X,$$

the nuisance parameter property given by

$$I_X(\theta_1, \theta_2) \leq I_X(\theta_1),$$

where θ_1 is the parameter of interest and θ_2 is a nuisance parameter and the monotonicity property (maximal information property) is given by

$$I_{T(X)} \leq I_X$$

for any statistic $T(X)$. Note that if $T(X)$ is sufficient then the monotonicity property holds as equality which shows the invariance property of the measure under sufficient transformations.

Let α_1 and α_2 be positive numbers such that $\alpha_1 + \alpha_2 = 1$. Also let f_1 and f_2 be two probability density functions. The convexity property is defined as

$$I_X(\alpha_1 f_1 + \alpha_2 f_2) \leq \alpha_1 I_X(f_1) + \alpha_2 I_X(f_2).$$

The order-preserving property has been introduced by Shiva *et al.* (1973) and shows that the relation between the amount of information contained in a r.v X_1 and that contained in another r.v. X_2 remains intact irrespective of the measure of information used. In particular, if the superscripts 1 and 2 represent two different measures of information then

$$I_{X_1}^1 \leq I_{X_2}^1 \rightarrow I_{X_1}^2 \leq I_{X_2}^2.$$

The limiting property is defined by

$$f_n \rightarrow f \quad \text{iff} \quad I_X(f_n) \rightarrow I(f) \quad \text{or} \quad I_X(f_n, f) \rightarrow 0,$$

where f_n is a sequence of probability density functions, f is a limiting probability density function, and $I(f_n)$ and $I(f_n, f)$ are measures of information based on one or two pdfs, respectively.

We finally mention the Ali–Silvey property: If $f(x, \theta)$ (or simply f_θ) has the monotone likelihood ratio property in x then

$$\theta_1 < \theta_2 < \theta_3 \rightarrow I_X(f_{\theta_1}, f_{\theta_2}) < I_X(f_{\theta_1}, f_{\theta_3}).$$

Other important properties concern loss of information and sufficiency in experiments. For details see Ferentinos and Papaioannou (1981) and Papaioannou (1985).

35.4 Information Under Censoring and Truncation

Let X be the variable of interest and Y the censoring variable. We observe (Z, δ) where $Z = \min(X, Y)$ and $\delta = I_{[X \leq Y]}$ an indicator function. The full likelihood for (Z, δ) is

$$L(z, \delta) = [f(z, \theta)\bar{G}(z, \theta)]^\delta [g(z, \theta)\bar{F}(z, \theta)]^{1-\delta},$$

where f and g are the pdfs of X and Y, F and G are the cdfs of X and Y, $\bar{G} = 1 - G$, and $\bar{F} = 1 - F$. The Fisher information about θ contained in (Z, δ) is given by

$$I^F_{(Z,\delta)}(\theta) = E\left(\frac{\partial}{\partial\theta}\log L(Z, \delta)\right)^2 = \int\limits_{-\infty}^{+\infty}\left(\frac{\partial}{\partial\theta}\log f\bar{G}\right)^2 dz + \int\limits_{-\infty}^{+\infty}\left(\frac{\partial}{\partial\theta}\log g\bar{F}\right)^2 dz.$$

Consider now f_1 and f_2 two different pdfs for the random variable X. Then the Csiszar's φ-divergence between f_1 and f_2 based on (Z, δ) is defined as

$$I^C_{(Z,\delta)}(f_1, f_2) = \int\limits_{-\infty}^{+\infty} f_2\bar{G}\varphi\left(\frac{f_1}{f_2}\right) dz + \int\limits_{-\infty}^{+\infty} g\bar{F}_2\varphi\left(\frac{\bar{F}_1}{\bar{F}_2}\right) dz.$$

The basic properties of the above (under censoring) measures of information have been investigated by Tsairidis *et al.* (1996).

In random censoring two additional properties introduced by Hollander *et al.* (1987, 1990) and called the "acid test properties" are appropriate. They are the maximal information property given by

(i) E[Information(X)] $\geq$ E[Information(Z, δ)] for every X, Y

and the censoring property given by

(ii) E[Information(Z_1, δ_1)] $\geq$ E[Information(Z_2, δ_2)] for every X, where (Z_i, δ_i) is the censored variable associated with Y_i, and $Y_1 <_{st} Y_2$. The censoring property indicates that as censoring increases, namely when $Y_1 <_{st} Y_2$, information decreases. The acid test properties are satisfied for any classical measure of information when censoring is noninformative.

Sometimes, particularly in quality control, random censoring is coarser (i.e., qualitative), where when we randomly inspect the items we record the value of δ (i.e., whether the item has failed before and we do not record the exact lifetime) and the inspection (censoring) time Y. This type of censoring is called quantal random censoring [Nelson (1982)]. For quantal random censoring, the distribution of δ given $Y = y$ is Bernoulli with probability of success $p = F(y, \theta)$. The conditional Fisher information is

$$I^{C(qrc)}_{(\delta,Y)|Y=y}(\theta) = \frac{(F'(y,\theta))^2}{F(y,\theta)(1 - F(y,\theta))}$$

and Csiszar's conditional divergence between f_1 and f_2 is

$$I^{C(qrc)}_{(\delta,Y)|Y=y}(f_1, f_2) = F_2(y)\varphi\left(\frac{F_1(y)}{F_2(y)}\right) + \bar{F}_2(y)\varphi\left(\frac{\bar{F}_1(y)}{\bar{F}_2(y)}\right),$$

where $\bar{F}_i(\cdot) = 1 - F_i(\cdot)$, $i = 1$, 2. Unconditionally we have the following Fisher and Csiszar quantal random censoring informations based on (δ, Y).

$$I^F_{qrc}(\theta) \equiv I^{F(qrc)}_{(\delta,Y)}(\theta) = \int_0^\infty g(y) \frac{(F'(y,\theta))^2}{F(y,\theta)(1 - F(y,\theta))} dy$$

and

$$I^C_{qrc}(f_1, f_2) \equiv I^{C(qrc)}_{(\delta,Y)}(f_1, f_2) = \int_0^\infty \left\{ g(y)F_2(y)\varphi\left(\frac{F_1(y)}{F_2(y)}\right) + \bar{F}_2(y)\varphi\left(\frac{\bar{F}_1(y)}{\bar{F}_2(y)}\right) \right\} dy,$$

respectively. The following results have been established [Tsairidis *et al.* (2001)],

$$I^F_{qrc}(\theta) \leq I^F_{(Z,\delta)}(\theta) \quad \text{and} \quad I^C_{qrc}(f_1, f_2) \leq I^C_{(Z,\delta)}(f_1, f_2),$$

that is, quantal random censoring, although less expensive, is less informative than complete random censoring.

Comparison of various statistics in terms of their information content has not received much attention or use in the statistical literature and practice. Below we report some recent results in the areas of weighted distributions, order statistics, and truncated data [see, e.g., Papaioannou *et al.* (2006)]. A weighted distribution is a distribution which has a density in its pdf; that is, if $f(x, \theta)$ is a density, we use a density proportional to $w(x)f(x, \theta)$ to make inferences about θ. Weighted distributions are used to model ascertainment bias. Iyengar *et al.* (1999) studied conditions under which the Fisher information about θ

obtained from a weighted distribution, is greater than the same information obtained from the original density $f(x,\theta)$, where $f(x,\theta)$ belongs to the exponential family of distributions. This is clearly a result on information. Thus, there are cases where the Fisher information about θ contained in an order statistic, is greater than the same information contained in a single observation. This follows from the fact that the distribution of an order statistic is a weighted distribution. It turns out that for the normal distribution with σ^2 known, $I^F_{X_{(k)}}(\theta) \geq I^F_X(\theta)$, where $X_{(k)}$ is the kth order statistic of a random sample $X_1, X_2, \ldots, X_k$ from $N(\theta, \sigma^2)$. This result is in agreement with our intuition, because the order statistic essentially involves the whole sample.

Several studies have shown that the tails of an ordered sample from a symmetric distribution contain more Fisher information about the scale parameter than the middle portion. Zheng and Gastwirth (2000, 2002) examined the Fisher information about the scale parameter in two symmetric fractions of order statistics data from four symmetric distributions. They showed that for the Laplace, logistic, and normal distributions, the extreme tails usually contain most of the Fisher information about the scale parameter, whereas the middle portion is less informative. For the Cauchy distribution the most informative two symmetric fractions are centered at the 25th and 75th percentiles.

Similar results as in the previous paragraph exist when we deal with truncated data, and in particular samples from truncated exponential distributions. Bayarri *et al.* (1989) give conditions under which for the Fisher information $I^F_X \geq I^F_Y$ or $I^F_X \leq I^F_Y$, where X follows an arbitrary exponential distribution of the form

$$f(x,\theta) = a(x)\exp(b(\theta)u(x)/c(\theta), \qquad \theta \in \Theta$$

and Y follows the truncated distribution

$$g(y,\theta) = \left\{ \begin{array}{ll} f(y,\theta)/s(\theta), & \text{for } y \in S \\ 0, & \text{otherwise.} \end{array} \right.$$

The set S, a subset of the sample space of X, is the truncation or selection set with $s(\theta) = P_\theta(X \in S) = \int_S f(x,\theta)dx$. A selection sample from the right tail of the normal distribution contains less Fisher information about the mean than an unrestricted random sample when the variance is known, but more information about the variance than an unrestricted random sample when the mean is known.

Other interesting informativity applications appear with the *residual lifetime* of a stationary renewal process or with truncated distributions. For details see Iyengar *et al.* (1999).

35.5   Model Selection Criteria

The measures of divergence are used as indices of similarity or dissimilarity between populations. They are also used either to measure mutual information concerning two variables or to construct model selection criteria. A model selection criterion can be considered as an approximately unbiased estimator of an expected "overall divergence," a nonnegative quantity that measures the "distance" between the true unknown model and a fitted approximating model. If the value of the criterion is small then the approximated model is good. The Kullback–Leibler measure was the one used by Akaike (1973) to develop the Akaike information criterion (AIC). Here we apply the same methodology used for AIC to the BHHJ divergence in order to develop the divergence information criterion (DIC).

Consider a random sample $X_1, \ldots, X_n$ from the distribution g (the true model) and a candidate model f_θ from a parametric family of models $\{f_\theta\}$, indexed by an unknown parameter $\theta \in \Theta$. To construct the new criterion for goodness-of-fit we consider the quantity:

$$W_\theta = \int \left\{ f_\theta^{1+a}(z) - \left(1 + a^{-1}\right) g(z) f_\theta^a(z) \right\} dz, \qquad a > 0 \qquad (35.1)$$

which is the same as the BHHJ divergence without the last term that remains constant irrespective of the model f_θ used. Observe that (35.1) can also be written as

$$W_\theta = E_{f_\theta} \left(f_\theta^a(Z) \right) - \left(1 + a^{-1}\right) E_g \left(f_\theta^a(Z) \right), \qquad a > 0. \qquad (35.2)$$

35.5.1   The expected overall discrepancy

The target theoretical quantity that needs to be estimated is given by

$$EW_{\hat\theta} = E\left(W_\theta \left| \theta = \hat\theta \right. \right), \qquad (35.3)$$

where $\hat\theta$ is any consistent and asymptotically normal estimator of θ. This quantity can be viewed as the average distance between g and f_θ up to a constant and is known as *the expected overall discrepancy between g and f_θ*.

Observe that the expected overall discrepancy can be easily evaluated. More specifically, the derivatives of (35.2) in the case where g belongs to the family $\{f_\theta\}$ are given by [see Mattheou and Karagrigoriou (2006)]:

$$(a) \qquad \frac{\partial W_\theta}{\partial \theta} = (a+1) \left[\int u_\theta(z) f_\theta^{1+a}(z) \, dz - E_g \left(u_\theta(z) f_\theta^a(z) \right) \right] = 0,$$

(b) $\dfrac{\partial^2 W_\theta}{\partial \theta^2} = (a+1)\left\{(a+1)\displaystyle\int [u_\theta(z)]^2 f_\theta^{1+a}(z)\,dz - \int i_\theta f_\theta^{1+a}dz\right.$

$\left. + E_g\left(i_\theta(z) f_\theta^a(z)\right) - E_g\left(a[u_\theta(z)]^2 f_\theta^a(z)\right)\right\} = (a+1)J\,,$

where $u_\theta = \partial/(\partial\theta)\,(\log(f_\theta))$, $i_\theta = -\partial^2/(\partial\theta^2)\,(\log(f_\theta))$ and $J = \int [u_\theta(z)]^2$ $f_\theta^{1+a}(z)\,dz$.

Using a Taylor expansion of W_θ around the true point θ_0 and for a p-dimensional *row-vector* parameter θ, we can show that (35.3) at $\theta = \hat{\theta}$ takes the form

$$EW_{\hat{\theta}} = W_{\theta_0} + \frac{(a+1)}{2}E\left[\left(\hat{\theta}-\theta_0\right)J\left(\hat{\theta}-\theta_0\right)'\right]. \qquad (35.4)$$

Observe that in the p-dimensional case i_θ and $[u_\theta(z)]^2$ represent $p \times p$ matrices.

35.5.2   Estimation of the expected overall discrepancy

In this section we construct an unbiased estimator of the expected overall discrepancy (35.4). First though we deal with the estimation of the unknown density g. An estimate of (35.2) w.r.t. g is given by replacing $E_g\left(f_\theta^a(Z)\right)$ by its sample analogue

$$Q_\theta = \int f_\theta^{1+a}(z)\,dz - \left(1+\frac{1}{a}\right)\frac{1}{n}\sum_{i=1}^{n} f_\theta^a(X_i) \qquad (35.5)$$

with derivatives given by

(a) $\dfrac{\partial Q_\theta}{\partial \theta} = (a+1)\left[\displaystyle\int u_\theta(z) f_\theta^{1+a}(z)\,dz - \frac{1}{n}\sum_{i=1}^{n} u_\theta(X_i) f_\theta^a(X_i)\right], \quad a>0,$

(b) $\dfrac{\partial^2 Q_\theta}{\partial \theta^2} = (a+1)\left\{(a+1)\displaystyle\int [u_\theta(z)]^2 f_\theta^{1+a}(z)\,dz - \int i_\theta f_\theta^{1+a}(z)\,dz\right.$

$\left. + \frac{1}{n}\sum_{i=1}^{n} i_\theta(z) f_\theta^a(z) - \frac{1}{n}\sum_{i=1}^{n} a[u_\theta(z)]^2 f_\theta^a(z)\right\}.$

It is easy to see that by the weak law of large numbers, as $n \to \infty$, we have:

$$\left[\frac{\partial Q_\theta}{\partial \theta}\right]_{\theta_0} \xrightarrow{P} \left[\frac{\partial W_\theta}{\partial \theta}\right]_{\theta_0} \quad \text{and} \quad \left[\frac{\partial^2 Q_\theta}{\partial \theta^2}\right]_{\theta_0} \xrightarrow{P} \left[\frac{\partial^2 W_\theta}{\partial \theta^2}\right]_{\theta_0}. \qquad (35.6)$$

The consistency of $\hat{\theta}$, expressions (35.5) and (35.6), and a Taylor expansion of Q_θ around the point $\hat{\theta}$ can be used to evaluate the expectation of the estimator Q_θ evaluated at the true point θ_0:

$$EQ_{\theta_0} \equiv E\left(Q_\theta \,|\, \theta = \theta_0\right) = EQ_{\hat{\theta}} + \frac{a+1}{2}E\left[\left(\hat{\theta}-\theta_0\right)J\left(\hat{\theta}-\theta_0\right)'\right] \equiv W_{\theta_0}.$$

As a result (35.4) takes the form: $EW_{\hat{\theta}} = E\left\{ Q_{\hat{\theta}} + (a+1) \left[\left(\hat{\theta} - \theta_0 \right) J \left(\hat{\theta} - \theta_0 \right)' \right] \right\}$.

It can be shown that under normality,

$$ J = (2\pi)^{-\frac{a}{2}} \left(\frac{1+a}{1+2a} \right)^{1+\frac{p}{2}} \Sigma^{-\frac{\alpha}{2}} \left[\mathrm{Var} \left(\hat{\theta} \right) \right]^{-1}, $$

where Σ is the asymptotic variance matrix of $\hat{\theta}$. Taking also into consideration that $\left(\hat{\theta} - \theta \right) \Sigma^{-\frac{\alpha}{2}} \left[\mathrm{Var} \left(\hat{\theta} \right) \right]^{-1} \left(\hat{\theta} - \theta \right)'$ has approximately a $\mathcal{X}_p^2$ distribution, the divergence information criterion defined as the asymptotically unbiased estimator of $EW_{\hat{\theta}}$ is given by

$$ DIC = Q_{\hat{\theta}} + (a+1) \left(2\pi \right)^{-\frac{a}{2}} \left(\frac{1+a}{1+2a} \right)^{1+\frac{p}{2}} p. $$

Note that the family of candidate models is indexed by the single parameter a. The value of a dictates to what extent the estimating methods become more robust than the maximum likelihood methods. One should be aware of the fact that the larger the value of a the bigger the efficiency loss. As a result one should be interested in small values of $a \geq 0$, say between zero and one.

The proposed DIC criterion could be used in applications where outliers or contaminated observations are involved. The prior knowledge of contamination may be useful in identifying an appropriate value of a. Preliminary simulations with a 10% contamination proportion show that DIC has a tendency of underestimation in contrast with AIC which overestimates the true model.

35.6   Discussion

In this chapter we attempted an overview of measures of information and divergence. We discussed several types of measures and several of the most important properties of these measures. We also dealt with measures under censoring and truncation as well as weighted distributions and order statistics. Finally we presented results related to the use of the measures of divergence in model selection criteria and presented a new divergence information criterion.

The measures of information and divergence have attracted the interest of the scientific community recently primarily due to their use in several contexts such as in communication theory and sampling situations. As a result, statisticians need to refocus on these measures and explore further their theoretical characteristics as well as their practical implications which constitute the main contributions in the field.

Acknowledgements

The authors would like to thank the referee for his comments which improved the presentation of the chapter. The second author would like to thank Professors Ferentinos and Zografos and Dr. Tsairidis for their longtime research collaboration which led to the development of the ideas mentioned in the first part of the chapter. Part of this work was done while the second author was visiting the University of Cyprus.

References

1. Aczel, J. (1986). Characterizing information measures: Approaching the end of an era, In *Uncertainty in Knowledge-Based Systems*, LNCS (Eds., B. Bouchon and R. R. Yager), pp. 359–384, Spinger-Verlag, New York.

2. Akaike, H. (1973). Information theory and an extension of the maximum likelihood principle, In *Proceedings of the 2nd International Symposium on Information Theory* (Eds., B. N. Petrov and F. Csaki), Akademiai Kaido, Budapest.

3. Basu, A., Harris, I. R., Hjort, N. L., and Jones, M. C. (1998). Robust and efficient estimation by minimising a density power divergence, *Biometrika*, **85**, 549–559.

4. Bayarri, M. J., DeGroot, M. H., and Goel, P. K. (1989). Truncation, information and the coefficient of variation, In *Contributions to Probability and Statistics. Essays in Honor of Ingram Olkin* (Eds., L. Gleser, M. Perlman, S. J. Press, and A. Sampson), pp. 412–428, Springer-Verlag, New York,

5. Burbea, J. and Rao, C. R. (1982). On the convexity of some divergence measures based on entropy functions, *IEEE Transactions on Information Theory*, **28**, 489–495.

6. Chandrasekar, B. and Balakrishnan, N. (2002). On a multiparameter version of Tukey's linear sensitivity measure and its properties, *Annals of the Institute of Statistical Mathematics*, **54**, 796–805.

7. Cressie, N. and Read, T. R. C. (1984). Multinomial goodness-of-fit tests, *Journal of the Royal Statistical Society*, **5**, 440–454.

8. Csiszar, I. (1963). Eine informationstheoretische ungleichung und ihre anwendung auf den beweis der ergodizitat von markoffischen ketten. *Magyar Tud. Akad. Mat. Kutato Int. Kozl.*, **8**, 85–108.

9. Csiszar, I. (1977). Information measures: A critical review, In *Transactions of the 7th Prague Conference*, pp. 73–86, Academia Prague.

10. Ferentinos, K. and Papaioannou, T. (1981). New parametric measures of information, *Information and Control*, **51**, 193–208.

11. Havrda, J. and Charvat, F. (1967). Quantification method of classification processes: Concept of structural a-entropy, *Kybernetika*, **3**, 30–35.

12. Hollander, M., Proschan, F., and Sconing, J. (1987). Measuring information in right-censored models, *Naval Research Logistics*, **34**, 669–681.

13. Hollander, M., Proschan, F., and Sconing, J. (1990). Information, censoring and dependence, In *Institute of Mathematical Statistics, Lecture Notes Monograph Series, Topics in Statistical Dependence*, **16**, 257–268.

14. Iyengar, S., Kvam, P., and Singh, H. (1999). Fisher information in weighted distributions, *The Canadian Journal of Statistics*, **27**, 833–841.

15. Kagan, A. M. (1963). On the theory of Fisher's amount of information (in Russian), *Doklady Academii Nauk SSSR*, **151**, 277–278.

16. Kapur, J. N. (1984). A comparative assessment of various measures of divergence, *Advances in Management Studies*, **3**, 1–16.

17. Kendall, M. G. (1973). Entropy, probability and information, *International Statistical Review*, **11**, 59–68.

18. Mattheou, K. and Karagrigoriou, A. (2006). A discrepancy based model selection criterion, In *Proceedings of the 18th Conference of the Greek Statistical Society*, pp. 485–494.

19. Micheas, A. C. and Zografos, K. (2006). Measuring stochastic dependence using ϕ-divergence, *Journal of Multivariate Analysis*, **97**, 765–784.

20. Nelson, W. (1982). *Applied Life Data Analysis*, John Wiley & Sons, New York.

21. Papaioannou, T. (1985). Measures of information, In *Encyclopedia of Statistical Sciences* (Eds., S. Kotz and N. L. Johnson), **5**, pp. 391–397, John Wiley & Sons, New York.

22. Papaioannou, T. (2001). On distances and measures of information: a case of diversity, In *Probability and Statistical Models with Applications*, (Eds., C. A. Charalambides, M. V. Koutras, and N. Balakrishnan), pp. 503–515, Chapman & Hall, London.

23. Papaioannou, T. and Ferentinos, K. (2005). On two forms of Fisher's measure of information, *Communications in Statistics—Theory and Methods*, **34**, 1461–1470.

24. Papaioannou, T., Ferentinos, K., and Tsairidis, Ch. (2007). Some information theoretic ideas useful in statistical inference. *Methodology and Computing in Applied Probability*, **9**(2), 307–323.

25. Pardo, L. (2006). *Statistical Inference Based on Divergence Measures*, Chapman & Hall, London.

26. Rathie, P. N. and Kannappan, P. (1972). A directed-divergence function of type β, *Information and Control*, **20**, 38–45.

27. Renyi, A. (1961). On measures of entropy and information, In *Proceedings of the 4th Berkeley Symposium on Mathematics, Statistics and Probability*, **1**, pp. 547–561, University of California Press, California.

28. Shiva, S., Ahmed, N., and Georganas, N. (1973). Order preserving measures of information, *Journal of Applied Probability*, **10**, 666–670.

29. Soofi, E. S. (1994). Capturing the intangible concept of information, *Journal of the American Statistical Society*, **89**, 1243–1254.

30. Soofi, E. S. (2000). Principal information theoretic approaches, *Journal of the American Statistical Society*, **95**, 1349–1353.

31. Tsairidis, Ch., Ferentinos, K., and Papaioannou, T. (1996). Information and random censoring, *Information Sciences*, **92**, 159–174.

32. Tsairidis, Ch., Zografos, K., Ferentinos, K., and Papaioannou, T. (2001). Information in quantal response data and random censoring. *Annals of the Institute of Statistical Mathematics*, **53**, 528–542.

33. Tukey, J. W. (1965). Which part of the sample contains the information? *Proceedings of the National Academy of Sciences, USA*, **53**, 127–134.

34. Vajda, I. (1973). X^2-divergence and generalized Fisher's information, *Transactions of the 6th Prague Conference*, Academia Prague, 873–886.

35. Zheng, G. and Gastwirth, J. L. (2000). Where is the Fisher information in an ordered sample? *Statistica Sinica*, **10**, 1267–1280.

36. Zheng, G. and Gastwirth, J. L. (2002). Do tails of symmetric distributions contain more Fisher information about the scale parameter? *Sankhya, Series B*, **64**, 289–300.

36

Entropy and Divergence Measures for Mixed Variables

Konstantinos Zografos

Department of Mathematics, University of Ioannina, Ioannina, Greece

Abstract: The roles of entropies and divergences in statistics and related fields are well known as indices of the diversity or variability and as pseudo-distances between statistical populations. The definition of these measures is extended in the case of mixed continuous and categorical variables, a case which is common in practice in the fields of medicine, behavioural sciences, and so on. The role of these indices in testing statistical hypothesis and as descriptive measures in the location model is clarified.

Keywords and Phrases: Location model, mixed variables, entropy, divergence

36.1 Introduction

Many times in practice the statistician is faced with mixed, continuous, and categorical variables. In medicine, for instance, variables such as sex, profession, smoking, and drinking are categorical whereas variables such as age, weight, height, and time per week for gymnastics are continuous. In this and similar situations, the vector random variables include both continuous and categorical components. There are several options to treat mixed data. If, for example, the qualitative variables can be subjected to some scoring system, then all variables can be treated as quantitative. In a similar manner, all the variables can be treated as qualitative if the quantitative variables might be categorized by grouping. Another approach is to analyze separately the continuous and the categorical parts of the data and then to combine the results. But all of the above procedures involve, according to Krzanowski (1983), some element of subjectivity. If, for example, we treat the continuous variables as categorical by grouping them, then this procedure results in a loss of information due to the grouping of observations. If we treat the continuous and the categorical variables separately and combine the results of the individual analyses then we will ignore possible associations and dependencies between the continuous and the categorical variables which may cause a false final decision. These reasons motivated several authors to adopt or generalize the location model, introduced by Olkin and Tate (1961) [cf. also Schafer (1997)], to study this type of mixed data. The location model helps to handle the joint distribution of mixed continuous and categorical variables and it has been used to formulate statistical tests, as well as discrimination and classification rules. Representative work in testing statistical hypothesis with mixed data are the papers by Afifi and Elashoff (1969), Bar-Hen and Daudin (1995), Morales *et al.* (1998), de Leon and Carrière (2000), Nakanishi (2003), and de Leon (2007). Allocation rules on this model were investigated, among others, by Krzanowski (1975), Vlachonikolis (1985), Balakrishnan *et al.* (1986), Cuadras (1989), Nakanishi (1996), Daudin and Bar-Hen (1999), and Boumaza (2004).

On the other hand, information-theoretic procedures are well known in statistics and related fields, and entropy and divergence measures provide useful tools in developing, for instance, statistical tests and allocation rules. We mention the review papers by Soofi (2000), Papaioannou (2001), and the recent book by Pardo (2006) for a discussion about several measures of information which appeared in the literature of the subject, the axiomatic characterization of the said measures, and statistical applications that are based on entropy and divergence measures. The use of entropies and divergences in the case of mixed variables is the subject of the papers by Krzanowski (1983), and recently by Bar-Hen and Daudin (1995), Morales *et al.* (1998), and Nakanishi (1996, 2003). To handle the joint distribution of mixed continuous and categorical variables, Krzanowski (1983) has considered the location model as it is introduced by Olkin and Tate (1961), whereas Bar-Hen and Daudin (1995) considered a generalization of the location model.

In Section 36.2, some preliminary concepts are presented with respect to the location model. This model is applied in Section 36.3 in order to derive measures of entropy and divergence in the mixed variables case. Sampling properties of the measures are investigated in the last section, 36.4, and applications for testing statistical hypothesis are also outlined.

36.2   The Model

The location model has been introduced by Olkin and Tate (1961) and has since been used in several disciplines in statistics and related fields. In order to present this model consider q continuous random variables $X_1, \ldots, X_q$ and d categorical random variables $Y_1, \ldots, Y_d$, where each Y_i is observed at k_i,

$i = 1, \ldots, d$, possible states y_{ij}, $i = 1, \ldots, d$ and $j = 1, \ldots, k_i$. Following Krzanowski (1983) and Bar-Hen and Daudin (1995), the d qualitative random variables define a multinomial vector Z with c possible states $z_1, \ldots, z_c$, where each of the $c = k_1 \times k_2 \times \cdots \times k_d$ states is associated with a combination of the values y_{ij}, $i = 1, \ldots, d$ and $j = 1, \ldots, k_i$ of the qualitative variables. Denote by p_m the probability of observing the state z_m, $m = 1, \ldots, c$,

$$p_m = \Pr(Z = z_m), \qquad m = 1, \ldots, c, \quad \text{with } \sum_{m=1}^{c} p_m = 1.$$

Conditionally on $Z = z_m$, $m = 1, \ldots, c$, the q continuous random variables $X = (X_1, \ldots, X_q)^T$ are described by a parametric density denoted by $f_{\xi_m}(x)$; that is,

$$f_{\xi_m}(x) = f(x | Z = z_m),$$

for $m = 1, \ldots, c$. In this context, the joint density, if it exists, with parameter θ of the random variables $X = (X_1, \ldots, X_q)^T$ and Z is

$$
\begin{aligned}
f_\theta(x, z) &= \sum_{m=1}^{c} f(x | Z = z_m) \Pr(Z = z_m) I_{z_m}(z) \\
&= \sum_{m=1}^{c} f_{\xi_m}(x) p_m I_{z_m}(z),
\end{aligned}
\tag{36.1}
$$

with $z \in \{z_1, \ldots, z_c\}$, and

$$I_{z_m}(z) = \begin{cases} 1, & \text{if } z = z_m \\ 0, & \text{otherwise} \end{cases}, \quad \text{for } m = 1, \ldots, c.$$

The conditional density $f_{\xi_m}(x) = f(x | Z = z_m)$, $m = 1, \ldots, c$, can be any parametric family of probability distributions. The classic location model, defined by Olkin and Tate (1961), considers that conditionally on $Z = z_m$, $m = 1, \ldots, c$, the q continuous random variables $X = (X_1, \ldots, X_q)^T$ jointly follow the multivariate normal distribution with location and scale parameters, respectively, μ_m and Σ_m, with Σ_m a positive definite matrix of order q, for $m = 1, \ldots, c$. If we denote by $f_{\xi_m}(x)$ this conditional density, then

$$f_{\xi_m}(x) = f(x | Z = z_m) = (2\pi)^{-\frac{q}{2}} |\Sigma_m|^{-\frac{1}{2}} \exp\left\{ -\frac{1}{2}(x - \mu_m)^T \Sigma_m^{-1}(x - \mu_m) \right\},$$

$$\tag{36.2}$$

where ξ_m is the $(q(q + 3)/2)$-dimensional parameter $\xi_m = (\mu_m, \Sigma_m)$. Bar-Hen and Daudin (1995) generalized the classic location model by considering $f_{\xi_m}(x) = f(x | Z = z_m)$ to be any parametric family of probability distributions and not necessarily the multivariate normal model (36.2). Hence, the joint density $f_\theta(x, z)$, given by (36.1), generalizes the well-known classic location model.

36.3   Entropy and Divergence in the Location Model

In this section the φ-entropy and the ϕ-divergence are defined and studied in
the generalized location model which has been defined previously by (36.1). The
φ-entropy is a general measure introduced by Burbea and Rao (1982), among
others. In the discrete case, φ-entropy has appeared previously in information-
theoretic literature. In fact, it is the relative entropy introduced independently
by Perez (1967) and Ben-Bassat (1978).

36.3.1 φ-entropy in the location model

Let μ_1 be the countable measure on $\mathcal{Z} = \{z_1, \ldots, z_c\}$ and μ_2 be the Lebesgue
measure on R^q. Denote by $\mu = \mu_1 \otimes \mu_2$ the product measure on $\mathcal{Z} \times R^q$. Then,
for a continuous concave function φ, $\varphi : (0, \infty) \to R$, the φ-entropy, if it exists,
of the joint density $f_\theta(x, z)$, given by (36.1), is defined by

$$H_\varphi(f_\theta) = \int \varphi(f_\theta(x, z)) d\mu, \qquad (36.3)$$

and it can be considered as a descriptive measure of the variability or diversity
of the mixed variables and hence of their joint distribution. If we apply (36.1),
then the φ-entropy is reduced to

$$H_\varphi(f_\theta) = \sum_{m=1}^{c} \int \varphi(p_m f_{\xi_m}(x)) d\mu_2. \qquad (36.4)$$

If $\varphi(x) = -x \ln x$, $x > 0$, then (36.3) leads to the well-known Shannon entropy
which is immediately obtained by (36.4) and it is given by

$$H_{Sh}(f_\theta) = - \sum_{m=1}^{c} p_m \ln p_m - \sum_{m=1}^{c} p_m \int f_{\xi_m}(x) \ln f_{\xi_m}(x) d\mu_2. \qquad (36.5)$$

Taking into account that $-\sum_{m=1}^{c} p_m \ln p_m$ is the Shannon entropy
$H_{Sh}(P)$ of the discrete probability distribution $P = (p_1, \ldots, p_c)$ and
$-\int f_{\xi_m}(x) \ln f_{\xi_m}(x) d\mu_2$ is the Shannon entropy $H_{Sh}(f_{\xi_m})$ of the parametric
density f_{ξ_m}, we conclude from (36.5) that the Shannon entropy $H_{Sh}(f_\theta)$ in the
location model (36.1), is analysed as

$$H_{Sh}(f_\theta) = H_{Sh}(P) + \sum_{m=1}^{c} p_m H_{Sh}(f_{\xi_m}). \qquad (36.6)$$

Equation (36.6) means that Shannon entropy in the location model is partitioned into two parts: the first is the Shannon entropy due to the qualitative

part of the data and the other is the convex combination of the Shannon entropies of the quantitive variables at the c states of the location model.

A more general entropy measure is Rényi's entropy of order λ which includes as a special case the Shannon entropy. Rényi's entropy and other important measures of entropy are not derived by a direct application of the φ-entropy (36.3). For this reason Pardo (2006, p. 21) has proposed the (h, φ)-entropy which is defined by

$$H_{h,\varphi}(f_\theta) = h\left(\int \varphi(f_\theta(x, z))d\mu\right), \tag{36.7}$$

where either $\varphi : (0, \infty) \to R$ is concave and $h : R \to R$, is differentiable and increasing or $\varphi : (0, \infty) \to R$ is convex and $h : R \to R$, is differentiable and decreasing. Rényi's entropy is obtained from (36.7) for $\varphi(x) = x^\lambda$, $x > 0$, and $h(x) = (1/(1 - \lambda))\log x$, for $\lambda > 0, \lambda \neq 1$; that is, Rényi's entropy is given by

$$H_R(f_\theta) = \frac{1}{1 - \lambda} \ln \int (f_\theta(x, z))^\lambda d\mu. \tag{36.8}$$

Shannon entropy $H_{Sh}(f_\theta) = -\int f_\theta(x, z) \ln f_\theta(x, z)d\mu$, is obtained from (36.8) for $\lambda \uparrow 1$. Other important entropy measures in the location model can be obtained from (36.7) for particular choices of the functions h and φ and appear in Table 1.1 of Pardo (2006, p. 20).

Example 36.3.1 As an example consider the Shannon entropy in the classic location model where conditionally on the state $Z = z_m$, $m = 1, \ldots, c$, the q continuous random variables $X = (X_1, \ldots, X_q)^T$ jointly follow the multivariate normal distribution (36.2) with location and scale parameters, respectively, μ_m and Σ_m, for $m = 1, \ldots, c$. In this case the mixed Shannon entropy (36.6) is analysed as follows,

$$H_{Sh}(f_\theta) = -\sum_{m=1}^c p_m \ln p_m + \sum_{m=1}^c p_m \left(\frac{p}{2} + \frac{p}{2} \ln(2\pi) + \frac{1}{2} \ln|\Sigma_m|\right).$$

It does not depend on the mean vectors μ_m, $m = 1, \ldots, c$, of the multivariate normal distributions which describe the continuous random variables $X_1, \ldots, X_q$ at the states $Z = z_m$, $m = 1, \ldots, c$. In the homoscedastic normal case, $\Sigma_1 = \Sigma_2 = \cdots = \Sigma_c = \Sigma$, the Shannon entropy is simplified

$$H_{Sh}(f_\theta) = -\sum_{m=1}^c p_m \ln p_m + \frac{p}{2} + \frac{p}{2} \ln(2\pi) + \frac{1}{2} \ln|\Sigma|.$$

Similar examples can be derived for the case where the conditional densities $f_{\xi_m}(x)$, $m = 1, \ldots, c$, are members of the elliptic family of multivariate distributions. Explicit expressions of $H_{Sh}(f_{\xi_m})$ for members of the elliptic family are available in Zografos (1999) and Zografos and Nadarajah (2005).

36.3.2 ϕ-divergence in the location model

In order to define measures of divergence in the location model, suppose that the continuous and the categorical variables $X_1, \ldots, X_q$ and $Y_1, \ldots, Y_d$ are observed on the members of two populations π_1 and π_2. Each of the populations is described by the generalized location model (36.1) with joint density

$$
\begin{aligned}
f_{\theta_i}(x, z) &= \sum_{m=1}^{c} f_i(x|Z = z_m) p_{im} I_{z_m}(z) \\
&= \sum_{m=1}^{c} f_{\xi_{im}}(x) p_{im} I_{z_m}(z),
\end{aligned}
\tag{36.9}
$$

respectively, where p_{im} denotes the probability of observing the state z_m in the population π_i, and $f_{\xi_{im}}$ the joint density of $X_1, \ldots, X_q$ at the state z_m of the population π_i, $i = 1, 2$ and $m = 1, \ldots, c$.

The ϕ-divergence of f_{θ_1} and f_{θ_2} is defined by

$$
D_\phi(f_{\theta_1}, f_{\theta_2}) = \int f_{\theta_2}(x, z) \phi\left(\frac{f_{\theta_1}(x, z)}{f_{\theta_2}(x, z)}\right) d\mu,
\tag{36.10}
$$

where ϕ is a real convex function defined on $(0, \infty)$, which, moreover, satisfies appropriate conditions that ensure the existence of the above integral [cf. Pardo (2006, p. 5)]. An application of (36.9) leads to the equivalent expression

$$
D_\phi(f_{\theta_1}, f_{\theta_2}) = \sum_{m=1}^{c} p_{2m} \int f_{\xi_{2m}}(x) \phi\left(\frac{p_{1m} f_{\xi_{1m}}(x)}{p_{2m} f_{\xi_{2m}}(x)}\right) d\mu_2.
\tag{36.11}
$$

Special choices of the convex function ϕ lead to the Kullback–Leibler directed divergence, the Cressie and Read's power divergence, and the distances considered by Krzanowski (1983), as well. D_ϕ is a measure of the distance between populations π_1 and π_2 in the sense that $D_\phi(f_{\theta_1}, f_{\theta_2})$ attains its minimum value $\phi(1)$ if and only if $f_{\theta_1}(x, z) = f_{\theta_2}(x, z)$.

For $\phi(x) = x \ln x$, (36.11) is reduced to the Kullback–Leibler divergence in the mixed variables case, which is given by

$$
D_{KL}(f_{\theta_1}, f_{\theta_2}) = \sum_{m=1}^{c} p_{1m} \ln \frac{p_{1m}}{p_{2m}} + \sum_{m=1}^{c} p_{1m} \int f_{\xi_{1m}}(x) \ln \frac{f_{\xi_{1m}}(x)}{f_{\xi_{2m}}(x)} d\mu_2.
\tag{36.12}
$$

Taking into account that $D_{KL}(P_1, P_2) = \sum_{m=1}^{c} p_{1m} \ln(p_{1m}/p_{2m})$ is the Kullback–Leibler divergence of the discrete probability distributions $P_i = (p_{i1}, \ldots, p_{ic})$, $i = 1, 2$, and $D_{KL}(f_{\xi_{1m}}, f_{\xi_{2m}}) = \int f_{\xi_{1m}}(x) \ln[f_{\xi_{1m}}(x)/f_{\xi_{2m}}(x)] d\mu_2$ is the Kullback–Leibler divergence of the distributions $f_{\xi_{1m}}$ and $f_{\xi_{2m}}$, the above equation is equivalently stated

$$
D_{KL}(f_{\theta_1}, f_{\theta_2}) = D_{KL}(P_1, P_2) + \sum_{m=1}^{c} p_{1m} D_{KL}(f_{\xi_{1m}}, f_{\xi_{2m}}),
$$

and therefore the Kullback–Leibler divergence in the mixed variables case shares common property with the Shannon entropy, as formulated by (36.6).

In a similar manner, for $\phi(x) = [x^{\lambda+1} - x - \lambda(x-1)]/[\lambda(\lambda+1)]$, $\lambda \neq 0, -1$, (36.11) is reduced to the Cressie and Read (1984) power divergence family in the mixed variables case. This generalized divergence is formulated as follows,

$$D_{CR}(f_{\theta_1}, f_{\theta_2}) = \frac{1}{\lambda(\lambda+1)} \left\{ \sum_{m=1}^{c} \frac{p_{1m}^{\lambda+1}}{p_{2m}^{\lambda}} \int \frac{f_{\xi_{1m}}^{\lambda+1}(x)}{f_{\xi_{2m}}^{\lambda}(x)} d\mu_2 - 1 \right\}. \tag{36.13}$$

An interesting divergence measure which is not included in the ϕ-divergence is the density power divergence which has been recently introduced by Basu *et al.* (1998) for developing a robust estimation procedure. This divergence between f_{θ_1} and f_{θ_2} is defined by

$$D_a(f_{\theta_1}, f_{\theta_2}) = \int \left\{ f_{\theta_2}^{1+a}(x, z) - \left(1 + \frac{1}{a}\right) f_{\theta_1}(x, z) f_{\theta_2}^{a}(x, z) + \frac{1}{a} f_{\theta_1}^{1+a}(x, z) \right\} d\mu,$$

or

$$\begin{aligned} D_a(f_{\theta_1}, f_{\theta_2}) &= \sum_{m=1}^{c} \int \left\{ p_{2m}^{1+a} f_{\xi_{2m}}^{1+a}(x) - \left(1 + \frac{1}{a}\right) p_{1m} p_{2m}^{a} f_{\xi_{1m}}(x) f_{\xi_{2m}}^{a}(x) \right. \\ &\quad \left. + \frac{1}{a} p_{1m}^{1+a} f_{\xi_{1m}}^{1+a}(x) \right\} d\mu_2, \end{aligned}$$

in view of the generalized location models (36.9). For $a \to 0$, $D_a(f_{\theta_1}, f_{\theta_2})$ leads to the Kullback–Leibler divergence $D_{KL}(f_{\theta_1}, f_{\theta_2})$.

Example 36.3.2 Suppose that conditionally on the state $Z = z_m$, $m = 1, \ldots, c$, the q continuous random variables $X = (X_1, \ldots, X_q)^T$ jointly follow the multivariate normal distribution (36.2) with location and scale parameters, respectively, μ_{im} and Σ_{im}, for $m = 1, \ldots, c$, in the ith population π_i, $i = 1, 2$. This means that the joint densities $f_{\xi_{1m}}$ and $f_{\xi_{2m}}$ are the densities of the $N_q(\mu_{1m}, \Sigma_{1m})$ and $N_q(\mu_{2m}, \Sigma_{2m})$ distributions, respectively. In this case, based on results of Pardo (2006, p. 45–47), it can be shown that the mixed Kullback–Leibler divergence is obtained from (36.12) for

$$\begin{aligned} \int f_{\xi_{1m}}(x) \ln \frac{f_{\xi_{1m}}(x)}{f_{\xi_{2m}}(x)} d\mu_2 &= \frac{1}{2}(\mu_{1m} - \mu_{2m})^T \Sigma_{2m}^{-1}(\mu_{1m} - \mu_{2m}) \\ &\quad + \frac{1}{2} tr\left(\Sigma_{2m}^{-1}\Sigma_{1m} - I\right) + \frac{1}{2}\ln \frac{|\Sigma_{2m}|}{|\Sigma_{1m}|}, \end{aligned} \tag{36.14}$$

whereas the Cressie–Read power divergence is obtained from (36.13), for

$$\int f_{\xi_{1m}}^{\lambda+1}(x) f_{\xi_{2m}}^{-\lambda}(x) d\mu_2 = \frac{|(\lambda+1)\Sigma_{2m} - \lambda\Sigma_{1m}|^{-1/2}}{|\Sigma_{1m}|^{\lambda/2} |\Sigma_{2m}|^{-(\lambda+1)/2}}$$

$$\times \exp\left\{ \frac{\lambda(\lambda+1)}{2} v_m^T [(\lambda+1)\Sigma_{2m} - \lambda\Sigma_{1m}]^{-1} v_m \right\},$$

where $v_m = \mu_{1m} - \mu_{2m}$, $m = 1, \dots, c$.

36.4 Sampling Properties

In practice, training samples are available from the population described by $f_\theta(x, z)$ or the populations π_i, which are described by $f_{\theta_i}(x, z)$, $i = 1, 2$. Based on these samples, we are interested in the study of the sampling behaviour of $H_\varphi(f_\theta)$, or to test the hypothesis of homogeneity of the two populations or to construct minimum distance rules for the allocation of a new observation as coming from one of the populations considered. In these cases an estimator of $H_\varphi(f_\theta)$ or $D_\phi(f_{\theta_1}, f_{\theta_2})$ can be used as a test statistic for testing homogeneity or it can be used as the main tool in order to define a minimum distance allocation rule. An estimator of $H_\varphi(f_\theta)$ or $D_\phi(f_{\theta_1}, f_{\theta_2})$ can be obtained, on the basis of a random sample of size n from $f_\theta(x, z)$, or on the basis of two independent random samples of sizes n_i, from the populations $f_{\theta_i}(x, z)$, $i = 1, 2$. Let $\widehat{\theta}$ denote the maximum likelihood estimator (m.l.e.) of θ and $\widehat{\theta}_i$ denote the m.l.e. of θ_i, $i = 1, 2$. Then, the sample estimators $H_\varphi(f_{\widehat{\theta}})$ and $D_\phi(f_{\widehat{\theta}_1}, f_{\widehat{\theta}_2})$ of H_φ and D_ϕ are obtained from (36.3) and (36.10), if we replace the unknown parameters by their m.l.e., in the formulas for $H_\varphi(f_\theta)$ and $D_\phi(f_{\theta_1}, f_{\theta_2})$. The said estimators are the φ-entropy of $f_{\widehat{\theta}}$ and the ϕ-divergence of $f_{\widehat{\theta}_1}$ and $f_{\widehat{\theta}_2}$, defined, respectively, by

$$\widehat{H}_\varphi = H_\varphi(f_{\widehat{\theta}}) = \int \varphi(f_{\widehat{\theta}}(x, z)) d\mu, \tag{36.15}$$

and

$$\widehat{D}_\phi = D_\phi(f_{\widehat{\theta}_1}, f_{\widehat{\theta}_2}) = \int f_{\widehat{\theta}_2}(x, z) \phi\left(\frac{f_{\widehat{\theta}_1}(x, z)}{f_{\widehat{\theta}_2}(x, z)} \right) d\mu. \tag{36.16}$$

In the next sections we derive the asymptotic distributions of the statistics $H_\varphi(f_{\widehat{\theta}})$ and $D_\phi(f_{\widehat{\theta}_1}, f_{\widehat{\theta}_2})$.

36.4.1 Asymptotic distribution of $H_\varphi(f_{\widehat{\theta}})$

Assume that the probability vector $P = (p_1, \dots, p_c)$ depends on a τ-dimensional parameter η; that is, $P = P(\eta)$, with $\eta \in R^\tau$. Suppose also that the joint parametric density $f_{\xi_m}(x)$ of $X = (X_1, \ldots, X_q)^T$ at the state $Z = z_m$, $m = 1, \ldots, c$, depends on the κ-dimensional parameter $\xi_m \in R^\kappa$, $m = 1, \ldots, c$. Under this notation the generalized location model is formulated as

$$f_\theta(x, z) = \sum_{m=1}^c f_{\xi_m}(x)p_m(\eta)I_{z_m}(z),$$

and it depends on the $(\tau + \kappa c)$-dimensional parameter

$$\theta = (\eta^T, \xi_1^T, \ldots, \xi_c^T)^T = (\theta_1, \theta_2, \ldots, \theta_{\tau+\kappa c})^T.$$

In order to estimate $H_\varphi(f_\theta)$, consider a random sample of size n from the mixed population $f_\theta(x, z)$. Denote by

$$\widehat{\theta} = (\widehat{\eta}^T, \widehat{\xi}_1^T, \ldots, \widehat{\xi}_c^T)^T = (\widehat{\theta}_1, \widehat{\theta}_2, \ldots, \widehat{\theta}_{\tau+\kappa c})^T,$$

the m.l.e. of the parameter θ, and the sample estimator of $H_\varphi(f_\theta)$ is now defined by (36.15). The asymptotic distribution of $H_\varphi(f_{\widehat{\theta}})$ is stated in the next proposition. The proof is obtained by following partly the lines of the proof of Theorem 2.1 in Pardo (2006, p. 60) and it is outlined in the sequel.

Proposition 36.4.1 *Under the classical regularity conditions of the asymptotic statistics [cf. for instance, Pardo (2006, p. 58–60)],*

$$\sqrt{n}\left(\widehat{H}_\varphi - H_\varphi\right) \xrightarrow[n\to\infty]{\mathcal{L}} N\left(0, \sigma_\varphi^2(\theta)\right),$$

where

$$
\begin{aligned}
\sigma_\varphi^2(\theta) &= T^T I_F(\theta)^{-1} T \\
&= T_0^T I_F(\eta)^{-1} T_0 + \sum_{m=1}^c \frac{1}{p_m(\eta)} T_m^T I_F(\xi_m)^{-1} T_m,
\end{aligned}
$$

with T being the $(\tau + \kappa c)$-dimensional vector with elements $t_i = \frac{\partial}{\partial\theta_i}H_\varphi(f_\theta) = \int \varphi'(f_\theta(x, z))\frac{\partial}{\partial\theta_i}f_\theta(x, z)d\mu$, $i = 1, \ldots, \tau + \kappa c$, T_0 the τ-dimensional vector with elements

$$T_{0i} = \sum_{m=1}^c \left(\frac{\partial}{\partial\eta_i}p_m(\eta)\right)\int \varphi'\left(p_m(\eta)f_{\xi_m}(x)\right)f_{\xi_m}(x)d\mu_2, \qquad 1 \le i \le \tau,$$

and T_m a κ-dimensional vector with elements

$$T_{mi} = p_m(\eta)\int \varphi'\left(p_m(\eta)f_{\xi_m}(x)\right)\frac{\partial}{\partial\xi_{mi}}f_{\xi_m}(x)d\mu_2,$$

for $i = 1, \ldots, \kappa$ and $m = 1, \ldots, c$. $I_F(\eta)$ is used to denote the Fisher information matrix of the discrete probability distribution $P(\eta) = (p_1(\eta), \ldots, p_c(\eta))$ and $I_F(\xi_m)$ is the Fisher information matrix of the parametric family $f_{\xi_m}(x)$, $m = 1, \ldots, c$.

PROOF. The first-order Taylor expansion of $\widehat{H}_\varphi$, considered as a function of $\widehat{\theta}$, around θ gives

$$\widehat{H}_\varphi - H_\varphi = \sum_{i=1}^{\tau+\kappa c} t_i(\widehat{\theta}_i - \theta_i) + o(||\widehat{\theta} - \theta||).$$

Simple algebra leads to $t_i = T_{0i}$, $1 \le i \le \tau$ and $t_i = T_{mj}$, for $i = \tau+(m-1)\kappa+j$, $m = 1, \ldots, c$ and $j = 1, \ldots, \kappa$. Hence, the $(\tau + \kappa c)$-dimensional vector T can be equivalently written as $T = (T_0^T, T_1^T, \ldots, T_c^T)^T$ where the vectors T_0 and T_m, $m = 1, \ldots, c$, have been defined in the proposition. Hence

$$\widehat{H}_\varphi - H_\varphi = T^T(\widehat{\theta} - \theta) + o(||\widehat{\theta} - \theta||). \tag{36.17}$$

Taking into account that $\widehat{\theta}$ is the m.l.e. of θ,

$$\sqrt{n}(\widehat{\theta} - \theta) \xrightarrow[n\to\infty]{\mathcal{L}} N\left(0, I_F(\theta)^{-1}\right), \tag{36.18}$$

and, based on Pardo (2006, p. 61), $\sqrt{n}o(||\widehat{\theta} - \theta||) = o_P(1)$. After some algebraic manipulations it can be shown that the Fisher information matrix $I_F(\theta)$ of the parametric family $f_\theta(x, z)$ is the block diagonal matrix,

$$I_F(\theta) = diag\left(I_F(\eta), p_1(\eta)I_F(\xi_1), \ldots, p_c(\eta)I_F(\xi_c)\right),$$

which completes the proof of the proposition, in view of (36.17) and (36.18). ■

Remark 36.4.1 (a) If we consider Shannon entropy $H_{Sh}(f_\theta)$, then the proposition is valid with

$$T_{0i} = \sum_{m=1}^{c} H_{Sh}(f_{\xi_m})\frac{\partial}{\partial \eta_i}p_m(\eta) - \sum_{m=1}^{c}\left(\frac{\partial}{\partial \eta_i}p_m(\eta)\right)\ln p_m(\eta),$$

for $1 \le i \le \tau$ and $H_{Sh}(f_{\xi_m}) = -\int f_{\xi_m}(x)\ln f_{\xi_m}(x)d\mu_2$. Moreover,

$$T_{mi} = -p_m(\eta)\int \left(\frac{\partial}{\partial \xi_{mi}}f_{\xi_m}(x)\right)\ln f_{\xi_m}(x)d\mu_2, \quad i = 1, \ldots, \kappa, \quad m = 1, \ldots, c.$$

(b) Following the steps of the proof of Corollary 2.1 in Pardo (2006, p. 61) the asymptotic distribution of the (h, φ)-entropy, defined by (36.7), is

$$\frac{\sqrt{n}\left(\widehat{H}_{h,\varphi} - H_{h,\varphi}\right)}{h'\left(\int \varphi(f_\theta(x, z))d\mu\right)} \xrightarrow[n\to\infty]{\mathcal{L}} N\left(0, \sigma_\varphi^2(\theta)\right),$$

where $\sigma_\varphi^2(\theta)$ is given in Proposition 36.4.1.

(c) Proposition 36.4.1 can be used in various settings in order to construct confidence intervals and to test various statistical hypotheses in the location model, expressed by means of the φ-entropy H_φ. In this context, all the testing procedures of Section 2.3 of Pardo (2006) can be presented by means of the generalized location model. In this direction, presented in the sequel is a test for the equality of entropies of r independent mixed populations. It is well known that Shannon entropy and other general entropic indices may be regarded as descriptive quantities such as the median, mode, and variance [cf., among others, Guerrero-Cusumano (1996) and Song (2001)]. Hence a test for the equality of entropies can be considered as a test procedure for testing the equality of descriptive measures of two or more populations which are discriminated by means of a set of continuous and categorical variables.

In this case we are interested in testing the hypothesis,

$$H_0 : H_\varphi(f_{\theta_1}) = H_\varphi(f_{\theta_2}) = \cdots = H_\varphi(f_{\theta_r}),$$

against the alternative

$$H_a : \text{There are } i, j \in \{1, \ldots, r\},\ i \neq j,\ \text{such that } H_\varphi(f_{\theta_i}) \neq H_\varphi(f_{\theta_j}).$$

For testing the above hypotheses we can use the test statistic

$$\sum_{i=1}^{r} \frac{n_i (H_\varphi(f_{\widehat{\theta}_i}) - \overline{D})^2}{\sigma_\varphi^2(\widehat{\theta}_i)},$$

with a chi-square null distribution with $r - 1$ degrees of freedom, and

$$\overline{D} = \left(\sum_{i=1}^{r} \frac{n_i}{\sigma_\varphi^2(\widehat{\theta}_i)} \right)^{-1} \sum_{i=1}^{r} \frac{n_i H_\varphi(f_{\widehat{\theta}_i})}{\sigma_\varphi^2(\widehat{\theta}_i)}.$$

36.4.2 Asymptotic distribution of $D_\phi(f_{\widehat{\theta}_1}, f_{\widehat{\theta}_2})$

Assume as above that under the population π_i, $i = 1, 2$, the probability vector $P_i = (p_{i1}, \ldots, p_{ic})$ depends on a τ-dimensional parameter η_i; that is, $P_i = P_i(\eta_i) = (p_1(\eta_i), \ldots, p_c(\eta_i))$, with $\eta_i \in R^\tau$ and $p_{im} = p_m(\eta_i)$, $i = 1, 2$, $m = 1, \ldots, c$. Suppose also that the joint parametric density $f_{\xi_{im}}(x)$ of $X = (X_1, \ldots, X_q)^T$ at the state $Z = z_m$, $m = 1, \ldots, c$, depends on the κ-dimensional parameter $\xi_{im} \in R^\kappa$, $m = 1, \ldots, c$ and $i = 1, 2$. Following ideas in Bar-Hen and Daudin (1995), we can distinguish between two kinds of parameters in the model: those which depend on the populations and noisy parameters which are independent from the populations. To see this let's consider the next example.

Example 36.4.1 Suppose that conditionally on the state $Z = z_m$, $m = 1, \ldots, c$, the q continuous random variables $X = (X_1, \ldots, X_q)^T$ jointly follow the multivariate normal distribution (36.2) with location parameters μ_{im},

$m = 1, \ldots, c$, and common scale matrix Σ, in the ith population π_i, $i = 1, 2$. This means that the joint densities $f_{\xi_{1m}}$ and $f_{\xi_{2m}}$ are the densities of the $N_q(\mu_{1m}, \Sigma)$ and $N_q(\mu_{2m}, \Sigma)$ distributions, respectively. In this case taking into account (36.12) and (36.14),

$$
\begin{aligned}
D_{KL}(f_{\theta_1}, f_{\theta_2}) \\
= \sum_{m=1}^{c} p_m(\eta_1) \ln \frac{p_m(\eta_1)}{p_m(\eta_2)} + \frac{1}{2} \sum_{m=1}^{c} p_m(\eta_1)(\mu_{1m} - \mu_{2m})^T \Sigma^{-1}(\mu_{1m} - \mu_{2m}).
\end{aligned}
$$

In this framework, suppose that the mean is modeled with an analysis of variance model, $\mu_{im} = \mu + \alpha_i + \beta_m$, $i = 1, 2$, $m = 1, \ldots, c$, where α is the population effect and β is the categorical state effect. In this case we observe that β is not included in the expression of the divergence $D_{KL}(f_{\theta_1}, f_{\theta_2})$ because $\mu_{1m} - \mu_{2m} = \alpha_1 - \alpha_2$. Therefore β_m, $m = 1, \ldots, c$, can be considered as a noisy parameter.

Motivated by the above example, suppose that the τ-dimensional parameter η_i includes a noisy and a structural part; that is, $\eta_i = ((\eta_i^0)^T, (\eta_i^1)^T)^T = (\eta_{i1}, \ldots \eta_{ia}, \eta_{i(a+1)}, \ldots, \eta_{i(a+r)})^T$, where $\eta_i^0 = (\eta_{i1}, \ldots \eta_{ia})^T$ are the noisy parameters and $\eta_i^1 = (\eta_{i(a+1)}, \ldots, \eta_{i(a+r)})^T$ are the structural parameters. Moreover, we assume that the noisy parameters coincide, $\eta_{1j} = \eta_{2j}$, $j = 1, \ldots, a$, in the two populations π_1 and π_2. In a similar manner we suppose that the parameters ξ_{im}, $i = 1, 2$, $m = 1, \ldots, c$, include a noisy and a structural part, $\xi_{im} = ((\xi_{im}^0)^T, (\xi_{im}^1)^T)^T = (\xi_{im1}, \ldots \xi_{im\ell}, \xi_{im(\ell+1)}, \ldots, \xi_{im(\ell+s)})^T$ and $\xi_{1mj} = \xi_{2mj}$, $j = 1, \ldots, \ell$, are noisy parameters that coincide in the two populations. Under this notation, the generalized location model

$$
f_{\theta_i}(x, z) = \sum_{m=1}^{c} f_{\xi_{im}}(x) p_m(\eta_i) I_{z_m}(z),
$$

in the ith population, $i = 1, 2$, depends on the $[(a + r) + (\ell + s)c]$-dimensional parameter $\theta_i = \left((\eta_i^0)^T, (\eta_i^1)^T, (\xi_{i1}^0)^T, (\xi_{i1}^1)^T, \ldots, (\xi_{ic}^0)^T, (\xi_{ic}^1)^T\right)^T$, $i = 1, 2$. Hence populations π_1 and π_2 depend on the parameters $\theta_1^T = (\theta_{11}, \ldots, \theta_{1k}, \theta_{1(k+1)}, \ldots, \theta_{1M})$ and $\theta_2^T = (\theta_{21}, \ldots, \theta_{2k}, \theta_{2(k+1)}, \ldots, \theta_{2M})$, respectively, with $M = [(a+r) + (\ell + s)c]$, $k = a + \ell c$ and $\theta_{1j} = \theta_{2j}$, $j = 1, \ldots, k$, are noisy parameters.

In order to estimate $D_\phi(f_{\theta_1}, f_{\theta_2})$, consider two random samples of sizes n_1 and n_2 from the mixed populations $f_{\theta_1}(x, z)$ and $f_{\theta_2}(x, z)$, respectively. Denote by $\widehat{\theta}_i = (\widehat{\theta}_{i1}, \ldots, \widehat{\theta}_{ik}, \widehat{\theta}_{i(k+1)}, \ldots, \widehat{\theta}_{iM})^T$ the m.l.e. of the parameter θ_i, $i = 1, 2$, and the sample estimator of $D_\phi(f_{\theta_1}, f_{\theta_2})$ is now defined by (36.16). The asymptotic distribution of $D_\phi(f_{\widehat{\theta}_1}, f_{\widehat{\theta}_2})$ is stated in the next proposition. The proof is obtained by an application of Theorem 3.1 of Morales et al. (1998) and it is therefore omitted.

Proposition 36.4.2 *Assume that the classical regularity conditions of the asymptotic statistics are satisfied. Under the hypothesis of homogeneity of the populations π_1 and π_2, that is, under the null hypothesis $H_0 : \theta_1 = \theta_2$, we have for $n_1, n_2 \to \infty$, that*

$$\frac{2n_1 n_2}{n_1 + n_2} \frac{D_\phi(f_{\widehat{\theta}_1}, f_{\widehat{\theta}_2}) - \phi(1)}{\phi''(1)} \xrightarrow[n_1, n_2 \to \infty]{\mathcal{L}} \chi^2_{r+sc},$$

provided that $\phi''(1) \neq 0$.

Similar asymptotic results have been obtained previously by Bar-Hen and Daudin (1995) and Nakanishi (2003), considering Jeffreys' divergence which is defined [cf. Kullback (1959, p. 6)] by $J(f_{\theta_1}, f_{\theta_2}) = D_{KL}(f_{\theta_1}, f_{\theta_2}) + D_{KL}(f_{\theta_2}, f_{\theta_1})$.

Proposition 36.4.2 can be used in several disciplines and contexts in order to state and test various statistical hypotheses which are formulated on the basis of the parameters of the location model. We present, in the examples which follow, two applications of the above proposition. For more details we refer to the paper by Morales *et al.* (1998).

Example 36.4.2 Consider the case $s = 0$. This is the case where the parameters ξ_{im} coincide for $i = 1, 2$ and $m = 1, \ldots, c$, and therefore the populations π_1 and π_2 are discriminated on the basis of their probabilities of observing the state $Z = z_m$, $m = 1, \ldots, c$. In this case the estimated ϕ-divergence is reduced to

$$\widehat{D}_\phi = \sum_{m=1}^{c} p_m(\widehat{\eta}_2) \phi\left(\frac{p_m(\widehat{\eta}_1)}{p_m(\widehat{\eta}_2)}\right),$$

and under the null hypothesis $H_0 : \eta_1 = \eta_2$,

$$\frac{2n_1 n_2}{n_1 + n_2} \frac{\widehat{D}_\phi - \phi(1)}{\phi''(1)} \xrightarrow[n_1, n_2 \to \infty]{\mathcal{L}} \chi^2_r,$$

where r is the number of the structural parameters.

Example 36.4.3 Suppose now that $r = 0$; that is, $p_m(\eta_1) = p_m(\eta_2)$, or $p_{1m} = p_{2m}$, $m = 1, \ldots, c$. In this case the null hypothesis $H_0 : \theta_1 = \theta_2$ is equivalent to the hypothesis $H_0 : \xi_{1m} = \xi_{2m}$, $m = 1, \ldots, c$ and

$$\widehat{D}_\phi = \sum_{m=1}^{c} \widehat{p}_{2m} \int f_{\widehat{\xi}_{2m}}(x) \phi\left(\frac{f_{\widehat{\xi}_{1m}}(x)}{f_{\widehat{\xi}_{2m}}(x)}\right) d\mu_2.$$

The asymptotic distribution of $\widehat{D}_\phi$ is χ^2_{sc}, according to the Proposition 36.4.2.

In the particular case where $X|Z = z_m$ follows a multivariate normal distribution $N_q(\mu, \Sigma_{im})$ under the ith population π_i, $i = 1, 2$ and $m = 1, \ldots, c$, then the null hypothesis $H_0 : \theta_1 = \theta_2$ is equivalent to the hypothesis of homogeneity of the dispersion matrices $H_0 : \Sigma_{1m} = \Sigma_{2m}$, $m = 1, \ldots, c$, and under this hypothesis,

$$\frac{2n_1 n_2}{n_1 + n_2} \frac{\widehat{D}_\phi - \phi(1)}{\phi''(1)} \xrightarrow[n_1, n_2 \to \infty]{\mathcal{L}} \chi^2_{c[q(q+1)/2]}.$$

36.5 Conclusions

The previous asymptotic results are based on the assumption that the sample sizes n_1 and n_2 from the populations π_1 and π_2 are large relative to the possible states c of the location model. In the opposite case some of the frequencies will be small or zero and the corresponding parameter estimates will be poor or unobtainable. Iterative estimation procedures have been proposed by Krzanowski (1975) in order to overcome this problem. Moreover, Nakanishi (2003) performed a simulation study in order to get an idea about the sample size which is necessary to test some hypotheses. According to this study more than $10 \times q$ observations are necessary in each of the c-cells, where q is the number of the continuous variables. This idea is very rough, but it is perhaps a precept for applications.

Acknowledgements

A part of this chapter was done while the author was visiting the department of mathematics and statistics of the University of Cyprus the spring semester of 2006.

References

1. Afifi, A. A. and Elashoff, R. M. (1969). Multivariate two sample tests with dichotomous and continuous variables. I. The location model, *Annals of Mathematical Statistics*, **40**, 290–298.

2. Balakrishnan, N., Kocherlakota, S., and Kocherlakota, K. (1986). On the errors of misclassification based on dichotomous and normal variables, *Annals of the Institute of Statistical Mathematics*, **38**, 529–538.

3. Bar-Hen, A. and Daudin, J. J. (1995). Generalization of the Mahalanobis distance in the mixed case, *Journal of Multivariate Analysis*, **53**, 332–342.

4. Basu, A., Harris, I. R., Hjort, N. L., and Jones, M. C. (1998). Robust and efficient estimation by minimising a density power divergence, *Biometrika*, **85**, 549–559.

5. Ben-Bassat, M. (1978). ƒ-entropies, probability of error, and feature selection, *Information and Control*, **39**, 227–242.

6. Boumaza, R. (2004). Discriminant analysis with independently repeated multivariate measurements: An L^2 approach, *Computational Statistics and Data Analysis*, **47**, 823–843.

7. Burbea, J. and Rao, C. R. (1982). On the convexity of some divergence measures based on entropy functions, *IEEE Transactions on Information Theory*, **28**, 489–495.

8. Cressie, N. and Read, T. R. C. (1984). Multinomial goodness-of-fit tests, *Journal of the Royal Statistical Society, Series B*, **46**, 440–464.

9. Cuadras, C. M. (1989). Distance analysis in discrimination and classification using both continuous and categorical variables, In *Recent Developments in Statistical Data Analysis and Inference*. (Ed., Y. Dodge), pp. 459–473, North-Holland, Amsterdam.

10. Daudin, J. J. and Bar-Hen, A. (1999). Selection in discriminant analysis with continuous and discrete variables, *Computational Statistics and Data Analysis*, **32**, 161–175.

11. de Leon, A. R. (2007). One-sample likelihood ratio tests for mixed data, *Communications in Statistics—Theory and Methods*, **36**, 129–141.

12. de Leon, A. R. and Carriere, K. C. (2000). On the one sample location hypothesis for mixed bivariate data, *Communications in Statistics—Theory and Methods*, **29**, 2573–2561.

13. Guerrero-Cusumano, J. (1996). A measure of total variability for the multivariate t distribution with applications to finance. *Information Sciences*, **92**, 47–63.

14. Krzanowski, W. J. (1975). Discrimination and classification using both binary and continuous variables. *Journal of the American Statistical Association*, **70**, 782–790.

15. Krzanowski, W. J. (1983). Distance between populations using mixed continuous and categorical variables, *Biometrika*, **70**, 235–243.

16. Kullback, S. (1959). *Information Theory and Statistics*, John Wiley & Sons, New York.

17. Morales, D., Pardo, L., and Zografos, K. (1998). Informational distances and related statistics in mixed continuous and categorical variables, *Journal of Statistical Planning and Inference*, **75**, 47–63.

18. Nakanishi, H. (1996). Distance between populations in a mixture of categorical and continuous variables. *J. Japan Statist. Soc.*, **26**, 221–230.

19. Nakanishi, H. (2003). Tests of hypotheses for the distance between populations on the mixture of categorical and continuous variables, *Journal of the Japanese Society of Computational Statistics*, **16**, 53–62.

20. Olkin, I. and Tate, R. F. (1961). Multivariate correlation models with mixed discrete and continuous variable, *Annals of Mathematical Statistics*, **32**, 448–465.

21. Papaioannou, T. (2001). On distances and measures of information: A case of diversity, In *Probability and Statistical Models with Applications* (Eds., C. A. Charalambides, M. V. Koutras, and N. Balakrishnan), pp. 503-515, Chapman & Hall, New York.

22. Pardo, L. (2006). *Statistical Inference Based on Divergence Measures*, Chapman & Hall, New York.

23. Perez, A. (1967). Risk estimates in terms of generalized f-entropies, In *Proceedings of the Colloquium on Information Theory*, Vol. II, János Bolyai Mathematical Society, Budapest, pp. 299–315.

24. Schafer, J. L. (1997). *Analysis of Incomplete Multivariate Data*, Chapman & Hall, New York.

25. Song, K-S. (2001). Rényi information, loglikelihood and an intrinsic distribution measure, *Journal of Statistical Planning and Inference*, **93**, 51–69.

26. Soofi, E. S. (2000). Principal information theoretic approaches, *Journal of the American Statistical Association*, **95**, 1349–1353.

27. Vlachonikolis, I. G. (1985). On the asymptotic distribution of the location linear discriminant function, *Journal of the Royal Statistical Association, Series B*, **47**, 498–509.

28. Zografos, K. (1999). On maximum entropy characterization of Pearson's type II and VII multivariate distributions, *Journal of Multivariate Analysis*, **71**, 67–75.

29. Zografos, K. and Nadarajah, S. (2005). Expressions for Rényi and Shannon entropies for multivariate distributions, *Statistics & Probability Letters*, **71**, 71–84.

PART IX
New Statistical Challenges

Clinical Trials and the Genomic Evolution: Some Statistical Perspectives

Pranab Kumar Sen

Department of Biostatistics, University of North Carolina at Chapel Hill, NC, USA

Abstract: During the past four decades, clinical trials, having their genesis in biometric and epidemiologic studies, have been going through an evolutionary transition from simple biometric type to (randomized) multiphase placebo-controlled trials to active controlled equivalence trials to adaption of dynamic treatment regimens, all generally relating to symptomatic diagnostics. In this scenario, a newcomer is bioinformatics with its battery of thousands of genes, interacting with the disease/disorder complexities as well as with environmental stressors of diverse types. Although the impact of genomics is not yet totally clear, statistical challenges are mounting, and there is a dire need for development of novel and largely nonstandard methodology to cope with the basic statistical modeling and inference tasks. Some of these perspectives are appraised here with due consideration of their impact on modern clinical trials.

Keywords and Phrases: ACET, CSI, cost-benefit, FDR, interim analysis, meta analysis, PCS, PCT, RST

37.1 Introduction

In a little over a period of three decades, clinical trials (CT) have mushroomed in a variety of human health studies, with a variety of objectives, having a variety of interdisciplinary perspectives, and diverse implementational motives. CT are designed by human beings, mostly for human beings, incorporating mostly human subjects, and supposedly for human benefit. Yet in this human venture there are some inhuman features that warrant critical appraisal. Using human subjects in scientific (and mostly exploratory) studies may generally trigger *medical ethics, cost-benefit perspectives,* and a variety of other concerns. In order to control some of these disturbing concerns, often, subhuman primates are advocated as precursors or surrogates of human beings with usually different dose levels as well as periods of exposure, albeit there remains a basic query: How to extrapolate stochastics from mice to man? Can the basic principles of animal studies or *dosimetry* be validated in clinical trials designated for human being?

There is a basic qualm on the main objective of a clinical trial: *symptomatic effects* versus true disease–disorder detection and cure. Drug developers, pharmaceutical groups, and regulatory agencies focus on treatments to relieve symptoms which may not totally or adequately match treatment objectives. Bioethics and public advocates have voiced concern on clinical trials in third-world countries, the affordability of usual *high-cost drugs* being a major issue in this cost-benefit context. WHO and public health authorities all over the world are trying to identify effective and affordable regimens for many developing countries. These medical ethics, economic resources, and operational restraints often mar the routine use of standard statistical tools for drawing valid conclusions from CT.

The last but not the least important factor with profound impact on CT is the ongoing genomics evolution where the search for disease genes and gene–environment interaction has posed challenging statistical as well as computational tasks for coping with the basic need for development of valid and effective statistical tools for modeling and drawing conclusions from such complex trials. There is a shift of emphasis from symptomatic endpoints to genetic undercurrents, mostly in an oligogenic setup, for which standard statistical tools are of limited utility. In this study, the complexity of modern CT and the genomics undercurrents are highlighted with due special emphasis on statistical perspectives.

37.2   Biometry to Clinical Trial Methodology

There are some basic differences between dosimetry or animal studies and CT. The former can be conducted in a fairly controlled laboratory setup, validating the use of standard statistical inference tools. However, in a CT, human beings cannot be put under such controlled laboratory setups, and as such, the enormous disparity in physical characteristics and many other epidemiologic endpoints call for highly nonstandard statistical modeling and analysis. That is why *placebo-controlled trials* (PCT) are used extensively in development of new pharmaceuticals. In the early phase of development of CT, such PCTs were mostly advocated and underlying constraints were validated, at least to a certain extent. However, there are allegations that PCT are invariably unethical when known effective therapy is available for the condition being treated or studied, regardless of the condition or the consequences of deferring treatments. The 1997 Helsinki Declaration by the World Medical Association (WMA) has clearly laid down the basic ethical principles for clinical trials: In any medical study, every patient, including those of a control group, if any, should be assured of the best proven diagnostic and therapeutic methods. Most often, in a PCT, this ethics is violated by the very composition of the placebo group. Based on this declaration, patients asked to participate in a PCT must be informed of the existence of any effective therapy, must be able to explore the consequences of deferring such therapy with the investigator, and must provide fully informed consent. To eliminate some of these drawbacks, *active controlled equivalence trials* (ACET) have therefore been advocated for comparing an existing treatment with a targeted one. They may show whether a new therapy is superior (or inferior) to an existing one, but may not possess other characteristics of PCTs [Temple and Ellenberg (2000) and Sen (2001)]. Basically, in ACET, statistical reasoning has to be adapted with due respect to most of these complexities.

In many chronic disease and carcinogenic studies, the same treatment may not be followed through the entire period following the detection of the disease or disorder. For example, in breast cancer studies, initially after the disease has been detected for a patient, a particular treatment may be allotted. If over a specified period of time, say a month, the drugresponse is not within an expected limit, the treatment regimen is changed or a different dose may be used to suit the protocol better. In an extreme case, no treatment is allotted due to the prevailing health condition which may not allow the patient to be subjected to such high-potency drugs with identified side effects. This scenario has led to the development of the so-called *randomized clinical trials for dynamic regimens*. Dynamic treatment regimens are adjusted to the need and prevailing conditions (progress) of a patient but are governed by the principles of medical ethics, cost-benefit (i.e., affordability and efficacy), and other clinical constraints and adaptable optimality considerations. This is not a cross-over design but more in line with outcome-dependent longitudinal (or follow-up) data models. Clearly, much of the simplicity of randomized clinical trials may be lost in this complex constrained environment and as a result, statistical modeling as well as analysis could be generally much more complex.

No matter if it is a PCT or an ACET, or even a randomized clinical trial with dynamic treatment regimens, there are numerous underlying constraints calling for novel *constrained statistical inference* (CSI) tools [Silvapulle and Sen (2004)] for statistical analysis. There is another feature common to both PCT and ACETs. In CT, it is typically a longitudinal data model, so it may be desirable in such a follow-up study to have *interim analysis* to monitor the accumulating clinical evidence in the light of statistical perspectives. Although this feature has led to the evolution of *time-sequential* statistical methodology, there remains much to update this novel branch of CSI (constrained statistical inference) in light of the underlying constraints and complications. It is usually desirable to look into the accumulating datasets at regular time intervals, and statistically deciding whether an *early termination* of the trial can be made in favor of the new therapy (if that is to be advocated in the drug market) so that patients can be switched to a better health perspective. Thus, usually, a *repeated significance testing* (RST) scheme, often in a restrained setup, underlies statistical modeling and analysis of clinical trials. In conventional *group sequential tests* (GST) usually one assumes independent and homogeneous increments for the associated stochastic processes. This is generally not the case in interim analysis related RST. *Progressively censoring schemes* (PCS) were introduced by Chatterjee and Sen (1973) to formulate the general methodology of *time-sequential* procedures; suitable martingale characterizations underlie most of these developments [Sen (1981, 1999a, 2001)]. Faced with a need to update this approach in a more general framework to suit the ACET, let us consider the following statistical scenario.

37.3   Interim Analysis and Statistical Tests

Consider a typical constrained statistical interim analysis scheme relating to a comparative CT where an existing therapy and a new one are to be compared with respect to their therapeutic efficacy, side effects as well as cost-benefit perspectives. Although a trial may be planned for a predetermined duration of time, the above considerations usually advocate a monitoring of the trial, either on a continual time basis or more conveniently at regular time intervals when no drastic effect is anticipated within a small time interval. The interim analysis relates to monitoring of the accumulating evidence at time points

$$t_1 < \cdots < t_K \text{ for some specified } K, \tag{37.1}$$

spanning a preplanned period of study $T = (0, t_K)$. If, at an early (or intermediate) time point t_k, there appears to be a significant difference (in favor of the new drug), then the trial is to be terminated at that point. The null hypothesis (H_0) relates to no difference over the entire period T and the alternative (H_1) to the new being better than the existing. We frame the null hypothesis H_{0r} that up to the time point t_r there is no difference between the two therapies, and let H_{1r} be the alternative that for the first time, at time point t_r, there is a difference in favor of the new drug, for $r = 1, \ldots, K$. Then, restricted to the time domain T, we may note that there is a nested nature of these hypotheses. The null hypothesis H_0 is accepted only when all the H_{0r} are accepted, whereas the alternative hypothesis H_1 is accepted when at least one of the K exclusive hypotheses $H_{1r}, 1 \le r \le K$ is accepted. Hence we write

$$H_0 = \bigcap_{r=1}^{K} H_{0r}, \qquad H_1 = \bigcup_{r=1}^{K} H_{1r}. \qquad (37.2)$$

Note that the tenacity of the null hypothesis up to an intermediate point t_r may not preclude a significant difference at a later time, whereas a significant difference at any time point precludes a no-difference scenario over the entire span of the study. That is why the acceptance of the null hypothesis is deferred to the end of the trial although rejection may occur earlier. Furthermore, based on the accumulating data set up to the time point t_r, we construct a suitable test statistic $\mathcal{L}_r$ for testing H_{0r} versus H_{1r}, $r = 1, \ldots, K$. This is essentially a RST problem in a constrained environment, and the nature of the null and alternative hypotheses immediately calls for the [Roy (1953)] UIP (*union intersection principle*). There are, however, some notable differences between the clinical trial and usual multiple hypothesis testing problems. The UIP has a finite intersection/union mode that makes it more cumbersome to incorporate appropriately. Furthermore, accumulating datasets have a nested structure that may preclude independence and homogeneity of increments. Because of clinical and ethical undercurrents, first we appraise the potential constraints.

Restraint 1: The component hypotheses are nested. For each $r(= 1, \ldots, K)$, H_{1r} is a one-sided alternative.

Restraint 2: For different $r(= 1, \ldots, K)$, the different test statistics $\mathcal{L}_r$ are not independent, and the pattern of their dependence may not follow a Markov chain.

Restraint 3: Early termination of the trial is associated with the acceptance of H_{1r}, for some $r < K$. It might be also due to significant adverse side effects of the treatment, irrespective of the accumulating statistical evidence.

Restraint 4: Explanatory variables provide useful statistical information, and hence, need to be included as far as possible, albeit increasing model complexity and CSI protocols.

Restraint 5: Conventional (log-)linear regression models may not be appropriate. Some of the explanatory variables (viz., smoking, physical exercise, diabetic, etc.) may be binary, or at best, categorical. Even if they were quantitative, often for data recording, they are reported as categorical.

Restraint 6: Informative censoring: Censoring due to noncompliance (e.g., dropout or failure due to other causes) may not be independent of the placebo-treatment setup.

Restraint 7: Surrogate endpoint: Often, the primary endpoint may be costly from data collection perspectives, and some closely related or associated (by symptoms, e.g.) variables, termed surrogate endpoints are used as substitutes. The statistical model for the surrogate endpoint could be quite different from the primary one. Furthermore, multiple endpoints may also crop up in such studies. Standard parametric multivariate CSI tools may not be properly usable.

Restraint 8: Assessment of statistical quality of accumulating data with due respect to the underlying clinical and statistical restraints could be a major task.

Restraint 9: Parametric models may not suit the purpose. Nonparametrics and semiparametrics may perform better. However, the underlying restraints in semiparametrics may generally need critical appraisal. Nonparametrics may fare better but may require larger sample sizes to be of good quality and efficacy.

Restraint 10: Data mining: The advent of genomics is increasingly advocating for a large number of endpoints and explanatory variables, and knowledge discovery and data mining (KDDM) tools are being advocated more and more. This does not, however, diminish the primary concern: to what extent is statistical inference not compromised or invalidated by data mining?

Suppose now that taking into account most of these restraints, albeit in approximate forms, it is possible to observe the partial dataset $\mathcal{D}_t$ up to the time point t, so that $\mathcal{D}_t$ is nondecreasing (accumulating) in $t \in T$. Let $\mathcal{F}_t$ be the history process up to the time point t, so that $\mathcal{F}_t$ is nondecreasing in $t \in T$. Furthermore, suppose that if all the (n) observations were available (i.e., the dataset includes all responses and all explanatory variables), then for testing H_0 against a restricted alternative H_1, we would have a desirable test statistic which we denote by $\mathcal{L}_n$. In a parametric setup, $\mathcal{L}_n$ could be a version of the likelihood ratio statistic or some of its variants such as the partial likelihood (score), penalized likelihood score, and so on. In semiparametrics, pseudo-likelihood, quasi-, or profile likelihood statistics might be usable. In nonparametrics, rank statistics have more appeal. At this stage, it might be better to force a distinction between PCT and ACET with respect to underlying statistical models. In PCT, the placebo or control group having no drugs or treatments may often qualify for the Cox (1972) *proportional hazards model* (PHM) and as such, semiparametrics, based on the PHM structure may have a natural appeal. On the other hand, in ACET, in the presence of existing drugs, the control group structure may be largely compromised, and as a result, a PHM needs to be justified in the specific context under study. The advantage of the PHM lies in more efficient inference for the finite-dimensional regression parameters at the cost of reduced efficiency for the baseline (unknown) survival function. Thus, if the objective is to infer on the baseline hazard function, a PHM-based analysis may be misleading unless the PHM structure can be at least approximately justified. Thus, depending on the objectives of a trial, the choice of nonparametric versus semiparametric models has to be decided, there being no clear-cut option, in general. Available sample size has a basic role to play in this context too.

With a suitable choice of a model and relating statistical perspectives, we may set without any loss of generality $E(\mathcal{L}_n | H_0) = 0$. Let us then define

$$\mathcal{L}_n(t) = E_{H_0}\{\mathcal{L}_n \mid \mathcal{F}_t\}, \qquad t \geq 0. \tag{37.3}$$

Then, under fairly general regularity assumptions, under H_0,

$$\{\mathcal{L}_n(t), \mathcal{F}_t; t \geq 0\} \quad \text{is a zero mean martingale (array)}, \tag{37.4}$$

although this martingale characterization may not generally hold when the null hypothesis is not true. Typically, we may construct the partial sequence (array) of projected statistics at every successive failure point, resulting in a discrete time parameter process, or more generally, we can construct a continuous time parameter process by usual linear segmenting between successive failure points. Even so, under such reconstructions, $\mathcal{L}_n(t)$ may not have independent and stationary increments, even under the null hypothesis. Our task is to set a time sequential or RST procedure based on the reduced and discretized time-parameter process $\{\mathcal{L}_n(t_j), \ j \leq K\}$. Thus, we are confronted with suitable CSI procedures amenable to RST or interim analysis. Intuitively, we could conceive of an array of cut-off points: $\{C_{nr}, r = 1, \ldots, K\}$, such that if $\mathcal{L}_n(t_1) \geq C_{n1}$, we stop the trial along with the rejection of H_0; if not, we go to the next time period t_2 and then if $\mathcal{L}_n(t_2) \geq C_{n2}$, we stop at that time along with the rejection of the null hypothesis. Otherwise we proceed to the next time period. In this way, the process continues, and if for the first time, for some $k \leq K$, $\mathcal{L}_n(t_k) \geq C_{nk}$, we reject the null hypothesis at that point and stop the trial. Thus, we proceed to accept the null hypothesis only when $\mathcal{L}_n(t_j) < c_{nj}, \forall j \leq K$ after continuing the trial to its target time t_K.

The basic problem is to control the type I error rate (i.e., the probability of rejecting the null hypothesis when it is actually true) without sacrificing much power in such an interim analysis scheme. This, in turn, requires a skilful choice of the cut-off points $C_{nr}, r \leq K$, which generally depend not only on the $t_k, k \leq K$ but also on the accumulated statistical information at these points, and the latter is generally unknown or, at least, not properly estimable at the start of the trial. In this respect, we appraise the role of UIP along with other competitors. Group sequential tests, formulated mostly in the late 1970s, make explicit use of normal distribution and equal increment assumptions which may not be generally true in such a time-sequential setup. Even so, they needed extensive computation of the cut-off points. For some of these details, we refer to Sen (1999a). Led by the basic weak convergence results for progressively censored linear rank statistics [Chatterjee and Sen (1973)] some of these computational complexities have been eliminated considerably.

Typically, by virtue of the martingale property, there exists a (random) time-parameter transformation (induced by the partial information) by which the process $\{\mathcal{L}_n(t), t \in T\}$ can be written as $\mathbf{W}_{n,T} = \{W_{n,T}(u), u \in [0,1]\}$ such that under the null hypothesis, $\mathbf{W}_{n,T}$ converges weakly to a Brownian motion on $[0,1]$. By the same transformation, the usual calendar time points $t_r, r = 1, \ldots, K$ are converted into (random) information time points $u_1 < \cdots < u_K$. Thus, we reduce the problem to a multivariate one-sided alternative hypothesis testing the CSI problem for which the UIT sketched in detail in Silvapulle and Sen (2004, Chapters 3–5) works out well. Basically, we have to construct the $W_{n,T}(u_r), r \geq 1$, and find a suitable cut-off point τ_{α^*} and a significance level α^* such that for a chosen α,

$$P\{W_{n,T}(u_r)/\sqrt{u_r} < \tau_{\alpha^*}, \forall r \, |H_0\} \leq \alpha. \tag{37.5}$$

Because a Brownian motion process $W(t), t \in [0,1]$ has irregular behavior with respect to the square root boundary as $t \to 0$, technically, we need that u_1 is away from 0. If the u_r are scattered over $(0,1]$ and K is large, a more convenient way of computing the cut-off points would be to appeal to the boundary-crossing probability of standard Brownian motion over one-sided square root boundaries; DeLong (1981) has provided detailed tables for these. This approximation is quite good when K is larger than 10, as is often the case of clinical trials with long-range follow-up time. Here also, the tabulated critical values correspond to some small truncation at 0 [i.e., over the range $[\epsilon, 1]$, for some positive ϵ (small)]. This weak invariance principle also avoids the need to specify the exact information times needed for the GST. There is an allied RST procedure considered by Chatterjee and Sen (1973) [and DeMets and Lan (1983)] where the weak convergence to Brownian motion has been incorporated in the utilization of (one-sided) linear boundaries (and a more general spending function approach). If a square root boundary is chosen then for the DeMets–Lan spending function approach too, their formula works out only when a truncation point $\epsilon > 0$ is fixed in advance, and the critical level depends on this point: the smaller the value of is ϵ, the larger will be the critical value. In many studies, the flat boundary considered in Chatterjee and Sen (1973) works out well. For rank-based procedures, often, for not so large samples, under suitable hypotheses of invariance, permutation tools provide scope for good approximations. The spirit of UIP is inherent in such interim analysis too.

There is a basic difference in this setup with the classical (group) sequential procedure. In the latter case, when the null hypothesis is not true, we may have a drifted Wiener process with a linear drift, so that well-known results on boundary crossing of a Wiener process with linear boundaries can be used to confer on power properties. In the present case, even for contiguous or local alternatives, we do not have a linear drift function, and as a result, most of these results are not directly applicable. Furthermore, the nature of alternative hypotheses may depend on the difference pattern, if any, of the two survival functions (viz., early difference but no significant difference at a later point versus accumulated curvilinear difference over time), so that nothing in general can be said about power optimality even in an asymptotic setup. Fortunately, the weak invariance principle, discussed above, has opened the doors for extensive simulation work for studies of performance characteristics of different boundaries under different alternatives. Some of these findings also apply for ACET's with minor modifications.

In the above setup, if we consider more complex designs, such as randomized clinical trials with dynamic treatment regimens, the test statistic $\mathcal{L}_n$ will generally be more complex, and as a result, although the definition in (37.3) remains intact and the martingale property in (37.4) may still be true, the $\mathcal{L}_n(t)$ may not be attracted to a Gaussian process (in distribution and under null hypothesis). For example, in a CSI setup, the terminal statistic $\mathcal{L}_n$ may have the so-called chi-square bar distribution, and as a result, the projected $\mathcal{L}_n(t)$ may not be (asymptotically) normal even under suitable null hypothesis. Thus, much of the present research interest centers around such CSI problems in complex clinical trials so as to effectively institute interim analysis in a valid statistical manner. Multiplicity of treatment regimens and CSI environments with all other restraints of clinical trials indeed constitutes a challenging statistical task. Furthermore, there could be a totally different interpretation of early termination of the trial under such dynamic regimens. It could be due to the fact that none of the treatment regimens may suit a patient who may therefore need special treatment violating the general principles that govern randomized clinical trials. Moreover, if prolongation of life, even under compromised health conditions, is the main objective of a treatment protocol then treatment preference could be on different grounds, and a comparative clinical trial methodology would be of limited utility. Thus, cancer clinical trials have been modeled and analyzed in a somewhat different manner, and there is still ample room for development of further statistical methodology. Some of these points are further elaborated in the next section.

37.4   Genomics Impact

With the advent of genomics and bioinformatics, in general, clinical trials are also encountering some challenging tasks. Instead of the conventional symptomatic effect approach, there is a new emphasis on pharmacogenomics dealing with the drug responses and the detection of disease genes along with the gene-environment interaction. Recalling that there may be thousands of genes which in a polygenic mode may not have individually significant impact but a large number of them in synergy may have significant (joint) impact, clinical trials are charged with not only finding the genes associated (causally or statistically) with a specific (group of) disease(s) but also their pharmacokinetics and pharmacodynamics with specific drug development. Instead of clinical trials with human subjects it calls for additional refinements: microarray and proteomics studies in clinical trials setup at the molecular level with tissues or cells. For example, in the IBD (inflammatory bowel disease), in a microarray setup, gene expression levels (for a large number of genes) for people not afflicted with the disorder may be compared with similar microarrays for afflicted groups at various level of afflictions, resulting in a very high-dimensional MANOVA model with low sample size (as such microarray studies are excessively expensive). Although this subject matter is beyond the scope of the present study, at least it could be emphasized that because of the enormous cost in conducting such trials, multicenter trials are needed for pooling relatively smaller information from the individual centers and also multiple endpoints typically arise in such composite studies. Typically, we encounter a matrix of statistics, individually from the centers and within each center, for the multiple endpoints. Although these centers may be treated as independent, the intracenter responses for the different endpoints are not. Confined to within-center perspectives, typically, we have a vector-valued stochastic process, and as before, we have a constrained environment (probably in greater complexity due to large dimensions). Therefore, even if we are able to construct a martingale array (in a multidimensional setup), formulating CSI procedures in a proper manner could be a formidable task. Bessel process approximations for multidimensional stochastic processes in clinical trials have been studied in the literature [viz., Sen (1981, Chapter 11)].

There is a challenging task of incorporating such distributional approximations in the formulation of statistical inference procedures for restrained environments. The prospects for multivariate CSI analysis, displayed in detail in Silvapulle and Sen (2004) need to be appraised further. In such genomics-oriented clinical trials, interim analysis rests on a totally different base, and the main concern is the proper accommodation of high-dimensional low sample size scenarios. Even in the conventional case of multivariate normal distributions when the dimension p is large and the sample size n is smaller than p, usual multivariate analysis of variance tests are not usable, and a dimension reduction may throw away some statistical information and thereby reduce the precision of statistical conclusions. It is our belief that UIP, because of its flexibility and amenity to more complex models, would be a trump card in this context too. For some related work, we may refer to Sen (2006) where other pertinent references are cited.

We conclude with some pertinent remarks on the role of UIP in meta-analysis, as is currently adapted in multicenter clinical trials and genomic studies. Multicenter clinical trials, although generally conducted under not-so-homogeneous environments (e.g., different geographical or demographic strata, age/culture differences), have a common objective of drawing statistical conclusions that pertain to a broader population. Consider in this vein, $C(\geq 2)$ centers, each one conducting a clinical trial with the common goal of comparing a new treatment with an existing one or a control or placebo. Because such centers pertain to patients with possibly different cultural and racial demographic profiles, diet and physical exercise habits, and so on, and they may have somewhat different clinical norms too, the intracenter test statistics $\mathcal{L}_c$, $c = 1, \ldots, C$, used for CSI/RST, although they could be statistically independent, might not be homogeneous enough to pull directly. This feature may thus create some impasses in combining these statistics values directly into a pooled one to enhance the statistical information. Meta-analysis, based on observed significance levels (OSL) or p-values, is commonly advocated in this context. Recall that under the null hypothesis (which again can be interpreted be the intersection of all the center null hypotheses), the p-values have the common uniform $(0, 1)$ distribution, providing more flexibility to adopt UIP in meta-analysis. Under restricted alternatives, these OSL values are left-tilted (when appropriate UIT are used) in the sense that the probability density is positively skewed over $(0, 1)$ with high density at the lower tail and low at the upper. Let us denote the p-values by

$$P_c = P\{\mathcal{L}_c \geq \text{the observed value} \,|H_0\}, c = 1, \ldots, C. \tag{37.6}$$

The well-known Fisher's test is based on the statistic

$$F_n = \sum_{c=1}^{C}\{-2 \log P_c\}, \tag{37.7}$$

which, under the null hypothesis, has the central chi-square distribution with $2C$ degrees of freedom. This test has some desirable asymptotic properties. There are many other tests based on the OSL values. The well-known step-down procedure [Roy (1958)] has also been adapted in this vein [cf. Subbaiah and Mudholkar (1980) and Sen (1983)], and they have been amended for CSI and RST as well [cf. Sen (1988)]. One technical drawback observed in this context is the insensitivity (to small to moderate departures from the null hypothesis) of such tests (including the Fisher's) when C is large, resulting in nonrobust and, to a certain extent, inefficient procedures. Thus, alternative approaches based on the OSL values have been explored more recently in the literature.

In the evolving field of bioinformatics and genomics, generally, we encounter an excessively high-dimensional dataset with inadequate sample size to induce the applicability of standard CSI or even conventional statistical inference tools.

On top of that, in genomics, the OSL values to be combined (corresponding to different genes) may not be independent, creating another layer of difficulty with conventional meta-analysis. This led to the development of multiple hypothesis testing in large dependent data models based on OSL values. This field is going through an evolution, and much remains to be accomplished. It is possible to use Bonferroni-type inequalities wherein for each gene a test statistic is formulated separately and its *p*-value computed. If we are to judge these *p*-values simultaneously for all the K genes, we need to fix the individual level of significance as $\alpha^* = \alpha/K$. Thus, if K is large, α^* will be so small that virtually it would be powerless for detecting any significant ones. One way to minimize this conservative property is to consider the information contained in the ordered *p*-values with cut-off points dependent on the orders. In this spectrum, the Simes (1986) theorem occupies a focal point. Simes (1986) was probably unaware of the classical Ballot theorem in stochastic processes [Karlin (1969)], which is the same result in terms of the empirical distribution, and hence, we refer to this as the Ballot–Simes theorem. Let there be K null hypotheses (not necessarily independent) H_{0k}, $k = 1, \ldots, K$ with respective alternatives (which possibly could be restricted or constrained as in clinical trials or microarray studies) H_{1k}, $k = 1, \ldots, K$. We thus come across the same UIP scheme by letting H_0 be the intersection of all the component null hypotheses, and H_1 be the union of the component alternatives. Let $P_k, k = 1, \ldots, K$ be the OSL values associated with the hypotheses testing H_{0k} versus H_{1k}, for $k = 1, \ldots, K$. We denote the ordered values of these OSL values by $P_{K:1}, \ldots, P_{K:K}$. If the individual tests have continuous null distributions then the ties among the P_k (and hence, among their ordered values) can be neglected, in probability. Assuming independence of the P_k, the Simes theorem states that

$$P\{P_{K:k} > k\alpha/K, \forall k = 1, \ldots, K | H_0\} = 1 - \alpha. \tag{37.8}$$

It is a nice illustration of how the UIP is linked to the extraction of extra statistical information through ordered OSL values, albeit the strong assumption of independence of the *p*-values (under H_0) needs to be critically appraised in any specific application.

It did not take long time for applied mathematical statisticians to make good use of the Simes–Ballot theorem in CSI and multiple hypothesis testing problems. The above results pertain to tests for an overall null hypothesis in the UIP setup. Among others, Hochberg (1988) considered a variant of the above result:

$$P\{P_{K:j} \geq \alpha/(K - j + 1), \forall j = 1, \ldots, K | H_0\} = 1 - \alpha, \tag{37.9}$$

and incorporated this result in a multiple testing framework. Benjamini and Hochberg (1995) introduced the concept of false discovery rate (FDR) in the context of multiple hypothesis testing, and illustrated the role of the

Ballot–Simes theorem in that context. The past ten years have witnessed a phenomenal growth of research literature in this subfield with applications to genomics and bioinformatics. The basic restraint in this respect is the assumption of independence of the P_j, $j = 1, \ldots, K$, and in bioinformatics, this is hardly the case. Sarkar (1998) and Sarkar and Chang (1997) incorporated the MTP_2 (multivariate total positivity of order 2) property to relax the assumption of independence to a certain extent. Sarkar (2000, 2002, 2004) has added much more to this development with special emphasis on controlling FDR in some dependent cases. The literature is too large to cite adequately, but our primary emphasis here is to stress how UIP underlies some of these developments and to focus on further potential work.

Combining OSL values, in whatever manner, may generally involve some loss of information when the individual tests are sufficiently structured to have coherence that should be preserved in the meta-analysis. We have seen earlier how guided by the UIP, progressive censoring in clinical trials provided more efficient and interpretable testing procedures. The classical Cochran–Mantel–Haenszel (CMH) procedure is a very notable example of this line of attack. In a comparatively more general multiparameter CSI setting, Sen (1999b) has emphasized the use of the CMH procedure in conjunction with the OSL values to induce greater flexibility. The field is far from being saturated with applicable research methodology. The basic assumption of independence or specific type of dependence is just a part of the limitations. A more burning question is the curse of dimensionality in CSI problems. Typically, there K is large and the sample size n is small (i.e., $K >> n$). In the context of clinical trials in genomics setups, Sen (2007) has appraised this problem with due emphasis on the UIP. Conventional test statistics (such as the classical LRT) have awkward distributional problems so that usual OSL values are hard to compute and implement in the contemplated CSI problems. Based on the Roy (1953) UIP but on some nonconventional statistics, it is shown that albeit there is some loss of statistical information due to the curse of dimensionality, there are suitable tests that can be implemented relatively easily in high-dimension low sample size environments. In CSI for clinical trials in the presence of genomics undercurrents, there is tremendous scope for further developments of statistical methodology along this line.

References

1. Benjamini, Y. and Hochberg, Y. (1995). Controlling the false discovery rate: A practical and powerful approach to multiple testing, *Journal of the Royal Statistical Society, Series B*, **57**, 289–300.

2. Chatterjee, S. K. and Sen, P. K. (1973). Nonparametric testing under progressive censoring, *Calcutta Statistical Association Bulletin*, **22**, 13–50.

3. Cox, D. R. (1972). Regression models and life tables (with discussion), *Journal of the Royal Statistical Society, Series B*, **34**, 187–220.

4. DeLong, D. M. (1981). Crossing probabilities for a square root boundary by a Bessel process, *Communications in Statitics—Theory and Methods*, **10**, 2197–2213.

5. DeMets, D. L. and Lan, K. K. G. (1983). Discrete sequential boundaries for clinical trials, *Biometrika*, **70**, 659–663.

6. Hochberg, Y. (1988). A sharper Bonferroni procedure for multiple tests of significance, *Biometrika*, **75**, 800–802.

7. Karlin, S. (1969). *A First Course in Stochastic Processes*, Academic Press, New York.

8. Roy, J. (1958). Step-down procedures in multivariate analysis, *Annals of Mathematical Statistics*, **29**, 1177–1188.

9. Roy, S. N. (1953). On a heuristic method of test construction and its use in multivariate analysis, *Annals of Mathematical Statistics*, **24**, 220–238.

10. Sarkar, S. K. (1998). Some probability inequalities for ordered MTP_2 random variables: A proof of the Simes conjecture, *Annals of Statistics*, **26**, 494–504.

11. Sarkar, S. K. (2000). A note on the monotonicity of the critical values of a step-up test, *Journal of Statistical Planning and Inference*, **87**, 241–249.

12. Sarkar, S. K. (2002). Some results on false discovery rate in multiple testing procedures, *Annals of Statistics*, **30**, 239–257.

13. Sarkar, S. K. (2004). FDR-controlling stepwise procedures and their false negative rates, *Journal of Statistical Planning and Inference*, **125**, 119–137.

14. Sarkar, S. K. and Chang, C.-K. (1997). The Simes method for multiple hypothesis testing with positively dependent test statistics, *Journal of the American Statistical Association*, **92**, 1601–1608.

15. Sen, P. K. (1981). *Sequential Nonparametrics: Invariance Principles and Statistical Inference*, John Wiley & Sons, New York.

16. Sen, P. K. (1983). A Fisherian detour of the step-down procedure, In *Contributions to Statistics: Essays in Honour of Norman L. Johnson*, pp. 367–377, North Holland, Amsterdam.

17. Sen, P. K. (1988). Combination of statistical tests for multivariate hypotheses against restricted alternatives, In *Advances in Multivariate Statistical Analysis* (Eds., S. Dasgupta and J. K. Ghosh), pp. 377–402, Indian Statistical Institute, Calcutta.

18. Sen, P. K. (1999a). Multiple comparisons in interim analysis, *Journal of Statistical Planning and Inference*, **82**, 5–23.

19. Sen, P. K. (1999b). Some remarks on the Stein-type multiple tests of significance, *Journal of Statistical Planning and Inference*, **82**, 139–145.

20. Sen, P. K. (2001). Survival analysis: Parametrics to semiparametrics to pharmacogenomics, *Brazilian Journal of Probability and Statistics*, **15**, 201–220.

21. Sen, P. K. (2006). Robust statistical inference for high-dimension low sample size problems with applications to genomics, *Austrian Journal of Statistics*, **35**, 197–214.

22. Sen, P. K. (2007). Union-intersection principle and constrained statistical inference, *Journal of Statistical Planning and Inference*, **137**(11), 3741–3752.

23. Silvapulle, M. J. and Sen, P. K. (2004). *Constrained Statistical Inference: Inequality, Order and Shape Restrictions*, John Wiley & Sons, New York.

24. Simes, R. J. (1986). An improved Bonferroni procedure for multiple tests of significance, *Biometrika*, **73**, 751–754.

25. Subbaiah, P. and Mudholkar, G. S. (1980). Testing significance of a mean vector – a possible alternative to Hotelling T^2, *Annals of the Institute of Statistical Mathematics*, **32**, 43–52.

26. Temple, R. and Ellenberg, S. S. (2000). Placebo-controlled trials and active-controlled trials in the evaluation of new treatments, I: Ethical and scientific issues. *Ann. Inter. Med. 133*, 455–463.

27. Tsai, M.-T. and Sen, P. K. (2005). Asymptotically optimal tests for parametric functions against ordered functional alternatives, *Journal of Multivariate Analysis*, **95**, 37–49.

Index

Aalen's linear model 487
Accelerated failure time models 3
Accelerated lifetime model 225
Accrual stopping 447
ACET 537
Acid-test 503
Additivity property 503
Aging distributions 69
AIC 473, 503
AIDS 275
Air quality 349
Annoyances 349
Asymptotic normality 405
Average run length 199

Bayesian decision theory 447
Bessel process 109
Biodemography 275
Bootstrap and resampling 171

Censoring 3
Censoring and truncation 503
Change detection 199
Chi-squared test 295
Clinical trials 333
Cluster data 55
Clusters 3
Complete sufficient statistic 435
Concentration inequality 187
Conditional moment generating
        function 319
Confidence bands 171
Confidence interval 405
Consistency 405
Continuous time 55
Correlated survival data 3
Cost-benefit 537
Covariate selection 487
Cross-effect 3
CSI 537

Deconvolution 419
Degradation 69
Degradation failure time 83
Degradation models 95
Demand 153
DIC 503
Diffusion process 385
Direct effects 461
Discrete time 3
Divergence 519

Empirical estimator 419
Entropy 519
Epidemiology 275
Errors in variables 23
Exact inference 319
Exponential distribution 319
Exponential family of
        distributions 199
Extended Cox models 3
Extreme values 259

Failure rate 69, 137
FDR 537
Focused information criterion 487
Frailty 43, 307
Functional 435

Generalized birth and death
        processes 95
Goodness-of-fit test 295, 385
Graphical diagnostics 43

Hazard rate 55, 127
Hazard regression 487
Health care planning 369
Heteroscedasticity 33
Hierarchical modeling 369
Hitting time moments 405
HIV infection rate 275
Hybrid censoring 319

Hypotheses testing 385

Incomplete follow-up 275
Incomplete repair 127
Information integration 369
Inhomogeneity problems 3
Integral functional 405
Interim analysis 537
Interval censoring 295, 307
Inverse problem 275
Item response theory 333

Kernel density estimators 171

L_2-type test 225
Lexis diagram 213
Life-testing 319
Lifetime data 43
Linear autoregression 419
Location model 519
Logistic model 3
Loss function 447
Lower confidence bound 319

Mallows' C_p 473
Markov chain 419
Markov reward model 153
Maximum likelihood 137
Maximum likelihood and moment
        type estimators 241
Maximum likelihood estimator 319
Mean remaining lifetime 69
Measures of information and
        divergence 503
Meta analysis 537
Mixed models 333
Mixed variables 519
Model selection 487, 503
Modified chi-squared tests 241
Multiple crossings 33
Multi-state system 153
Multivariate normal distribution 199

Nelson-Aalen estimator 83
Nested plan 199
Nonlinear mixed regression 83
Nonlinear models 23
Nonparametric estimation 307, 405
Nonparametric functional estimation 171

Nonparametric inference 213
Nonparametric regression estimation 225
Nonparametric statistics 187
Nonproportional hazards 33
Nonrandomized decision rule 447
Nuisance parameter 447

Optimal maintenance 127
Optimal nested plan 199

Parametric regression 225
Partial observation 419
PCS 537
PCT 537
Pearson's chi-squared test 241
Perception quality of life 349
Performability 405
Periodic skipping 419
Poisson mixture 137
Poisson process 127, 385
PRESS 473
Progressive censoring 319
Projection matrix 461
Proportional hazards 23, 33, 43
Psychometrical models 349

Quality control 369
Quality of life 333
Quasi-stationary state
        probabilities 95

Random skipping 419
Rasch models 333
Regenerative process 109
Regression tests 259
Reliability 405
Reliability and survival analysis 241
Reliability measure 153
Renewal process 127
Resampling 225
Rescaled observations 187
Residual effects 461
Right censoring 55
Right-censored data 213
RST 537

Selection-bias 213
Self-exciting process 385
Semi-Markov process 405

Shared frailty 43
Simulation 225
Skeleton estimates 187
Software debugging 137
Software error 137
Stochastic process 435
Stopping boundary 447
Structure and power of modified
          chi-squared tests 241
Survival analysis 295, 369
Survival data 3, 55
Survival in wild 275

Time-varying effect 33
Transportation metric 187

Traumatic failure time 83
Treatment-period interaction 461
Triangular test 333
Truncated gamma density 319
Truncation 3
Type I Pareto distribution 259
Type II Pareto distribution 259

Utility theory 369

Virtual age 69, 127

Weighted distribution 503
Weighting or biasing function 213
Wiener process 109

Printed in the United States of America